TUBERCULOSIS

LUNG BIOLOGY IN HEALTH AND DISEASE

Executive Editor

Claude Lenfant
Director, National Heart, Lung and Blood Institute
National Institutes of Health
Bethesda, Maryland

ADDITIONAL VOLUMES IN PREPARATION

The opinions expressed in these volumes do not necessarily represent the views of the National Institutes of Health.

TUBERCULOSIS

A COMPREHENSIVE INTERNATIONAL APPROACH

Edited by

Lee B. Reichman

University of Medicine and Dentistry of New Jersey—
New Jersey Medical School and University Hospital
and New Jersey Medical School National Tuberculosis Center
Newark, New Jersey

Earl S. Hershfield

University of Manitoba
Faculty of Medicine
Winnipeg, Manitoba, Canada

Marcel Dekker, Inc.   **New York • Basel • Hong Kong**

Library of Congress Cataloging-in-Publication Data

Tuberculosis : a comprehensive international approach / edited by Lee B.
Reichman, Earl S. Hershfield.
     p.   cm. -- (Lung biology in health and disease ; v. 66)
    Includes bibliographical references and index.
    ISBN 0-8247-8852-4 (alk. paper)
    1. Tuberculosis.   I. Reichman, Lee B.   II. Hershfield,
Earl S.   III. Series
    [DNLM: 1. Tuberculosis.   W1 LU62 v. 66 1993 / aWF 200 T8805
1993]
    RC311.T826 1993
    616.9'95--dc20
    DNLM/DLC
    for Library of Congress   93-20307
                                              CIP

The publisher offers discounts on this book when ordered in bulk quantities.
For more information, write to Special Sales/Professional Marketing at the
address below.

This book is printed on acid-free paper.

Marcel Dekker, Inc.
270 Madison Avenue, New York, New York 10016

Current printing (last digit):
10 9 8 7 6 5 4 3 2

PRINTED IN THE UNITED STATES OF AMERICA

To the memory of Dr. Julia M. Jones,
who was my inspiration in devoting my scientific career to tuberculosis
and public health.

—L. B. R.

To the memory of my father, Dr. C. Sheppy Hershfield (1904–1989),
whose concepts of social justice for all had a profound influence on my life.

—E. S. H.

Introduction

As the editors of this volume, Lee B. Reichman and Earl S. Hershfield, say in their preface: "tuberculosis is an ancient disease. . . . it has been both feared and respected . . . (and) glamorized. . . ."

It is, however, to René Théophile Hyacinthe Laënnec that the first scholarly description of the "Phthisie Pulmonaire" must be attributed (*De l'auscultation médiate*, 1818). Since then, much has been written about what is now called tuberculosis by all. But the romantics had another name for this disease: consumption! In 1853, Samuel Sheldon Fitch published *Six Discourses on the Functions of the Lungs; and Causes, Prevention and Cure of Pulmonary Consumption, Asthma and Diseases of the Heart; on the Laws of Life; and on the Mode of Preserving Male and Female Health to an Hundred Years.*

Fitch was a Philadelphia physician who was highly respected in his community and beyond it. In fact, one of his colleagues praised the fact that "his ideas are not crude and confused, as those of quack lecturers invariably are," and a judge in Baltimore commented: "The Doctor has effected many extraordinary cures in this section of the country . . . after all other means had totally failed."

This volume, simply titled *Tuberculosis: A Comprehensive International Approach*, is a prescription to preserve male and female health to a great age.

In the years following World War II, there was great expectation that phthisis, or consumption, or tuberculosis would disappear, at least in the so-called Western countries. Indeed, stringent public health measures and the development of new drugs led to a considerable reduction in the incidence and prevalence of the disease in these countries. But, little did we know!

The ease with which long distances between countries could be covered, the deepening of existing—and the development of new—social and economic problems throughout the world, even in countries that thought themselves forever protected, led to a severe resurgence of tuberculosis. At the same time, its treatment became much more difficult. Today, the world is faced with a vast and grave problem if we want to preserve "male and female health. . . ." Certainly, research is and will be an important tool, but it will take much more than that: most notably, a will to address this problem.

This book is a comprehensive description of the problem facing us all, but it is also a blueprint for what needs to be done. Many distinguished researchers, clinicians, and public health officials have contributed to it. Nearly all the continents and many countries are represented. Further, no such book has been published for a very long time.

The readers who are familiar with the series of monographs Lung Biology in Health and Disease will soon recognize that no previous volume has addressed all the aspects of a problem as this one does. I am extremely grateful to Drs. Reichman and Hershfield for their willingness to undertake this project and for the remarkable quality of their effort. They and their authors have undoubtedly made a great contribution to solving a worldwide problem.

Claude Lenfant, M.D.
Bethesda, Maryland

Preface

Tuberculosis is an ancient disease. In the past it has been both feared and respected. Despite being glamorized in literature, drama, opera, its effects have led to death, disfigurement, and disability. It has wiped out young people in the prime of their lives; it has devastated families.

The history of tuberculosis parallels the socioeconomic ills of humankind. Endemic in many populations, it rose to epidemic proportions with the advent of overcrowding, undernutrition, lack of fresh water, and poor sewage disposal. When susceptible populations were exposed for the first time, the epidemic flourished. In the long fight against this disease, treatments often evolved from fear and ignorance. Individuals with tuberculosis were isolated, treated with various potions, and subjected to a variety of surgical interventions. The advent of the mass radiograph for early diagnosis and the development of potent antituberculous medications and highly effective treatment regimens raised the hope that eradication of this disease was possible.

However, the inability of governments to develop appropriate national tuberculosis control programs has hindered the fight against this disease. The lack of patient adherence to prescribed regimens has led to the development of relapses, often with drug-resistant organisms. Finally, the appearance on the world scene of widespread human immunodeficiency virus infection has increased tuberculosis rates worldwide, in both developing and developed countries.

It is against this background that we offer *Tuberculosis: A Comprehensive International Approach*. This book represents a complete consideration of this disease from the historical, theoretical, practical, and operational points of view. Hopefully the various chapters will provide the reader with valuable information so that appropriate treatment regimens and control programs can be developed to ensure that those infected fully benefit from the most recent advances.

We are proud to include contributions from many of the world's leading authorities on tuberculosis. Their combined knowledge forms the basis of the current principles and practices embodied in this volume. We are especially honored that the List of Contributors includes many of our mentors and teachers as well as our colleagues. We would like to thank the contributors and their secretarial staffs for their assistance in meeting our deadline. Ms. Jean Norwood and Ms. Janet Haywood were invaluable in organizing and coordinating the work. Our Production Editor, Elaine Grohman, was of great assistance in helping us put the work together and carry it to production. To Dr. Claude Lenfant, Executive Editor of the Lung Biology in Health and Disease series, we wish to express our heartfelt thanks for his most cheerful counsel and encouragement.

We acknowledge the support and patience of our wives, Rose Reichman and Betty Anne Hershfield, and our children, Daniel and Deborah Gar Reichman, and Jeffrey, David, and Bryan Hershfield.

Lee B. Reichman
Earl S. Hershfield

Contributors

L. Fred Ayvazian, M.D. Professor of Medicine, University of Medicine and Dentistry of New Jersey–New Jersey Medical School, Newark, and Chief, Pulmonary Section, Department of Veterans Affairs Medical Center, East Orange, New Jersey

John B. Bass, Jr., M.D. Professor of Medicine, Vice-Chairman, Department of Internal Medicine, and Director, Division of Pulmonary and Critical Care Medicine, University of South Alabama College of Medicine, Mobile, Alabama

M. Miles Braun, M.D., M.P.H.* National Research Service Award Fellow and Master of Public Health Student, Department of Epidemiology, The Johns Hopkins University School of Hygiene and Public Health, Baltimore, Maryland

Joseph L. Breault, M.D., M.P.H.T.M. Department of Family Medicine, Ochsner Clinic, New Orleans, Louisiana

Eric Brenner, M.D. Consulting Medical Epidemiologist, EPI Resources, Columbia, South Carolina

---

Present affiliation: Senior Clinical Investigator, Epidemiology and Biostatistics Program, National Cancer Institute, National Institutes of Health, Bethesda, Maryland.

Philip W. Brickner, M.D. Chairman, Department of Community Medicine, St. Vincent's Hospital and Medical Center of New York, New York, New York

Jaap F. Broekmans, M.D., M.P.H. Director, Royal Netherlands Tuberculosis Association, The Hague, The Netherlands

George M. Cauthen, Sc.D. Epidemiologist, Division of Tuberculosis Elimination, National Center for Prevention Services, Centers for Disease Control and Prevention, Atlanta, Georgia

Pierre Chaulet, M.D. Professor, Department of Tuberculosis and Lung Disease, Hôpital de Beni Messous, Centre Hospitalier Universitaire d'Alger-Ouest, Algiers, Algeria

H. J. Chum, M.D. Tuberculosis and Leprosy Unit, National Tuberculosis and Leprosy Programme, Ministry of Health, Dar-es-Salaam, Tanzania

George W. Comstock, M.D., Dr.P.H. Alumni Centennial Professor of Epidemiology, The Johns Hopkins School of Hygiene and Public Health, Baltimore, Maryland

Thomas M. Daniel, M.D. Professor of Medicine and International Health, Department of Medicine, and Director, Center for International Health, Case Western Reserve University School of Medicine, and University Hospitals of Cleveland, Cleveland, Ohio

Paul T. Davidson, M.D. Director of Tuberculosis Control, County of Los Angeles, Department of Health Services, Public Health Programs, and Clinical Professor of Medicine, University of Southern California School of Medicine, Los Angeles, California

Jerrold J. Ellner, M.D. Professor of Pathology and Medicine, Case Western Reserve University School of Medicine, and Chief, Division of Infectious Diseases, Department of Medicine, University Hospitals of Cleveland, Cleveland, Ohio

Donald A. Enarson, M.D. Professor, Department of Medicine, University of Alberta, Edmonton, Alberta, Canada, and Director of Scientific Activities, International Union Against Tuberculosis and Lung Disease, Paris, France

Sue C. Etkind, R.N., M.S. Director, Division of Tuberculosis Control, Massachusetts Department of Public Health, Boston, Massachusetts

Charles P. Felton, M.D. Clinical Professor of Medicine, Columbia University College of Physicians and Surgeons, and Chief, Pulmonary Division, Department of Medicine, Harlem Hospital Center, New York, New York

Jean G. Ford, M.D. Instructor of Clinical Medicine, Columbia University College of Physicians and Surgeons, and Division of Pulmonary Medicine, Harlem Hospital Center, New York, New York

Pattisapu R. J. Gangadharam, Ph.D. Professor of Medicine, Microbiology, and Pathology and Director of Mycobacteriology Research, University of Illinois College of Medicine at Chicago, Chicago, Illinois

Lawrence J. Geiter, M.P.H. Chief, Clinical Research Branch, Division of Tuberculosis Elimination, Centers for Disease Control and Prevention, Atlanta, Georgia

Jeffrey Glassroth, M.D. Marquardt Professor of Medicine, Northwestern University Medical School, Chicago, Illinois

M. Gninafon, M.D. Director, National Centre of Pneumophthisiology, Cotonou, Benin

Robert C. Good, Ph.D. National Center for Infectious Diseases, Centers for Disease Control and Prevention, Atlanta, Georgia

Jacques H. Grosset, M.D. Professor of Bacteriology and Virology, Faculté de Médecine Pitíe-Salpêtrière, Paris, France

Earl S. Hershfield, M.D., F.R.C.P.C. Professor, Departments of Medicine and Community Health Sciences, University of Manitoba, Faculty of Medicine, Winnipeg, Manitoba, Canada

Philip C. Hopewell, M.D. Professor of Medicine, University of California at San Francisco, and Chief, Division of Pulmonary and Critical Care Medicine, San Francisco General Hospital, San Francisco, California

Michael E. Jones, M.D. Medical Epidemiologist, Section of Epidemiology, Division of Public Health, State of Alaska, Anchorage, Alaska

Arata Kochi, M.D., M.P.H. Programme Manager, Tuberculosis Programme, World Health Organization, Geneva, Switzerland

Jure Manfreda, M.D. Associate Professor of Medicine, University of Manitoba, Faculty of Medicine, Winnipeg, Manitoba, Canada

John M. McAdam, M.D. Attending Physician, Department of Community Medicine, St. Vincent's Hospital and Medical Center of New York, New York, New York

Reynard J. McDonald, M.D. Associate Professor of Clinical Medicine and Director, Division of Geriatric Medicine, University of Medicine and Dentistry of New Jersey–New Jersey Medical School, Newark, New Jersey

John P. Middaugh, M.D. Chief, Section of Epidemiology, Division of Public Health, State of Alaska, Anchorage, Alaska

Edward A. Nardell, M.D. Assistant Professor of Medicine, Harvard Medical School; The Cambridge Hospital, Cambridge, and Tuberculosis Control Officer, Massachusetts Department of Public Health, Boston, Massachusetts

Daniel S. Nyangulu, M.B., Ch.B., M.P.H. Tuberculosis Programme Coordinator and Acting Chief Community Health Officer, Ministry of Health, Lilongwe, Malawi

Richard J. O'Brien, M.D. Chief, Research and Development Unit, Tuberculosis Programme, World Health Organization, Geneva, Switzerland

Frances R. Ogasawara, C.H.E.S. Formerly Associate Managing Director, American Lung Association, New York, New York

Pamela Hutchins Orr, M.D., F.R.C.P.C. Assistant Professor, Department of Medicine, Medical Microbiology, and Community Health Sciences, University of Manitoba, Faculty of Medicine, Winnipeg, Manitoba, Canada

Carol Pozsik, R.N. Director, Tuberculosis Control Division, South Carolina Department of Health and Environmental Control, Columbia, South Carolina

Lee B. Reichman, M.D., M.P.H. Professor, Departments of Medicine and Preventive Medicine and Community Health, University of Medicine and Dentistry of New Jersey–New Jersey Medical School and University Hospital, and Director, New Jersey Medical School National Tuberculosis Center, Newark, New Jersey

Hans L. Rieder, M.D. Deputy Chief, Division of Epidemiology and Infectious Diseases, Federal Office of Public Health, Liebefeld-Berne, Switzerland

Richard L. Riley, M.D. Petersham, Massachusetts; Professor Emeritus of Medicine and Environmental Health Sciences, The Johns Hopkins University, Baltimore, Maryland

Annik Rouillon, M.D., M.P.H. Formerly Executive Director, International Union Against Tuberculosis and Lung Disease, Paris, France

M. Angélica Salomão, M.D. National Director of Health, Ministry of Health, Maputo, Republic of Mozambique

John A. Sbarbaro, M.D., M.P.H. Professor of Medicine and Preventive Medicine and Vice Chairman of Clinical Affairs, University of Colorado Health Sciences Center, Denver, Colorado

Lawrence L. Scharer, M.D. Director, Pulmonary Division, Department of Medicine (Roosevelt Site), St. Luke's–Roosevelt Hospital Center, New York, New York

Dixie E. Snider, Jr., M.D., M.P.H. Assistant Director for Science, National Center for Prevention Services, Centers for Disease Control and Prevention, Atlanta, Georgia

Jeffrey R. Starke, M.D. Assistant Professor, Department of Pediatrics, Baylor College of Medicine, Houston, Texas

Karel Styblo, M.D. Director, Tuberculosis Surveillance Research Unit, International Union Against Tuberculosis and Lung Disease, Paris, France

H. G. ten Dam Scientist, Tuberculosis Unit, Division of Communicable Diseases, World Health Organization, Geneva, Switzerland

Noureddine Zidouni, M.D. Clinique de Pneumo-Phtisiologie, Hôpital de Beni Messous, Centre Hospitalier Universitaire d'Alger-Ouest, Algiers, Algeria

Contents

PART FIVE: THE FUTURE

1

History of Tuberculosis

L. FRED AYVAZIAN

University of Medicine and Dentistry of New Jersey–New Jersey Medical School
Newark, New Jersey

Department of Veterans Affairs Medical Center
East Orange, New Jersey

I. Introduction

Paleopathologists identify skeletal deformities characteristic of tuberculosis in fossils of paleolithic and neolithic fauna; some believe the disease afflicted animals that inhabited the earth before the advent of mankind. In documented history, records from the Hindu literature of 2000 B.C. described a "slow wasting fever" in elephants, and the civilization of the ancient Nile Valley reported phthisis among its domesticated cattle. Phthisis, the most destructive of cattle diseases, became so rampant among the animals of Europe that from the Middle Ages through the 18th century it led to periods of human famine (Steele and Ranney, 1958; Francis, 1958; Myers and Steele, 1969). Pathogens of great antiquity, the human, bovine, and avian strains of the tubercle bacillus are thought to have derived from a common stock, and it is not known when speciation occurred.

Evidence of human tuberculosis, most convincingly as spinal gibbus, has been unearthed in petrified bones that date to 8000 B.C., as well as in the hunchbacks depicted in statuettes and figurines of ancient artworks. Graphic instances of Pott's disease are seen in the mummified reliquiae from pre-Dynastic

Egypt and pre-Columbian Peru; a study of a remarkably preserved Incan child of A.D. 700 demonstrated microscopic acid-fast bacilli in smears taken from a psoas abscess. There is evidence that a large sanatorium for treating victims of phthisis existed in Egypt about 1000 B.C. (Dubos and Dubos, 1952; Dubos, 1982). An affliction of mankind from the dawn of civilization, tuberculosis is accurately described ("lung fever," with emaciation, cough, and the expectoration of blood) in the earliest writings and classical texts of Chinese, Greek, and Roman physicians. Neither the Old nor the New Testament, however, contains references to tuberculosis, possibly because these writings dealt predominantly with pastoral, nonurban peoples (Dubos, 1968).

The oldest code of laws in the world—formulated by the Babylonian monarch Hammurabi between 1948 and 1905 B.C. and engraved onto a stone pillar now in the Louvre—makes reference to a chronic affliction that was very probably tuberculosis (Keers, 1978). Hippocrates (460–370 B.C.) traditionally is credited with the first authentic accounts of clinical phthisis (Major, 1932), a term at first limited to conditions with wasting, but subsequently connoting pulmonary disease. A unified pathological entity, however, was not recognized (the Greeks performed no autopsies), although Hippocrates noted the tubercles (phymata) in the tissues of cattle, sheep, and swine.

Aristotle (384–322 B.C.) described scrofula in hogs and believed phthisis to be contagious, but the alternative theory of heredity as the main causative factor had strong popular support. Galen (A.D. 131–201), who also lacked a base in pathology, characterized clinical phthisis (tabes, marasmus, phthoe) as a bleeding ulceration of the lungs, possibly resulting from trauma or from vitiated body humors aspirated from upper airways. Galen favored a contagious etiology over the hereditary concept and he advised against intimate contact with consumptives. For centuries, medical thinking did not deviate far from the dogma of Galen (Garrison, 1913).

The school of medicine in Alexandria, founded in 332 B.C., practiced human dissection but—using healthy prisoners, who were dissected alive—contributed little to the study of morbid anatomy. Over a millennium later, in the late 1400s, the birth of modern anatomy and the almost simultaneous invention of the printing press began to define the pathology of disease and to disseminate this new teaching through the emerging technologies of publication. Vesalius (1514–1574), the great Renaissance anatomist, corrected Galen's errors, while other anatomists established the principles of human dissection and began to correlate symptoms with postmortem findings. Cavities (vomicae) were reported in consumptive lungs and "miners' phthisis" was described. In *De Contageone*, Fracatorius (1483–1553) postulated contagion from exhaled particles from diseased lungs, and he first applied the term "fomites" to infected clothing and utensils; many regard Fracatorius as the founder of modern epidemiology (Keers, 1978; Guthrie, 1945).

II. The 17th and 18th Centuries

The 17th and 18th centuries saw major advances in both the pathological and clinical diagnosis of phthisis. Sylvius (1617–1655) stressed the importance of the anatomical tubercle in lung and extrathoracic tissues, introducing a new concept into medical thought, and he linked phthisis and scrofula. Willis (1621–1675) described miliary and chronic fibroid (noncavitary) postmortem findings. Benjamin Marten (1704–1782), a physician lost to history, left behind *A New Theory of Consumptions More Especially of a Phthisis or Consumption of the Lungs*, a book then ignored and still obscure but vindicated 150 years after its writing, which described clinical tuberculosis (night sweats and all), disputed the theories of "malignant humors," and offered the alternative of contagious transmission by "minute living Creatures" that are "inimical to our Natures" and "capable of subsisting in our Juices and Vessels." Marten warned that consumption may be caught by a "sound Person" by the breath emitted from diseased lungs, possibly not through "slender conversation" but by "habitual lying in the same Bed with a consumptive Patient, constantly eating and drinking with him" (Keers, 1978).

The early 1800s also saw advances in physical diagnosis of lung diseases, specifically Auenbrugger's discovery of the method of percussion and Laënnec's invention of the stethoscope. Remembering his innkeeper-father's practice of tapping on casks to estimate the level of wine, Auenbrugger, who had a good musical ear, applied the technique to the examination of the thorax, and he spent years correlating percussion note with postmortem findings. Laënnec, a physician of many accomplishments and contributions despite lifelong debility, first attempted direct auscultation of breath and voice sounds with the awkward placement of the examiner's ear directly to the patient's chest wall. Inspired by children listening to sounds of scratching transmitted along a length of wood, Laënnec refined this game into the technique for mediate auscultation, using first a quire of paper rolled into a tube and then the 1-ft cylinder of wood that became the forerunner of the flexible biaural instrument now the symbol of the modern physician (Major, 1932). The nomenclature and vocabulary that Laënnec created for auscultation remain in use today. Chronically ill with depression and tuberculosis, Laënnec nevertheless wrote profusely, published a pulmonary textbook (over 100 pages devoted to phthisis, at a time when a quarter of all deaths in Paris were attributed to the disease), and promoted a unification concept for tuberculosis. The generic designation "tuberculosis" was suggested by Schönlein in 1839 for all manifestations of phthisis, recognizing the tubercle as the fundamental anatomical lesion (Major, 1932).

In continental Europe and Victorian England, the sum of these scientific accomplishments failed to imbalance romantic notions of consumption as a numinous visitation, a spiritualizing and purifying disease exemplified in literature and opera by the courtesan, the lunger, the poitrinaire of Dumas, Dickens, Stevenson, Alcott, Thoreau, Puccini, and the Goncourt brothers. Thousands pilgrimaged to monarchs to receive "touch therapy" for scrofula, popular with Clovis the Frank in the fifth century and still going strong in 1712 when Samuel Johnson sought the hand of Queen Anne. A taste for the sickly was reflected in the wan heroines portrayed in the pre-Raphaelite paintings of Rosetti and Morris, and languid pallor became such a desirable feminine attribute that the popular use of rouge was abandoned and replaced by whitening powder (Dubos, 1982). Consumption was referred to as the muse of literature, the planet Earth as the grave-paved star. Shakespeare acknowledged the "healing benediction" of the royal touch in *Macbeth*, gave Beatrice a consumptive lover in *Much Ado About Nothing*, and in *The Tempest* he characterized pleuritic chest pain ("Side stitches, that shall pen thy breath up").

In support of the Frascatorius theory of contagion, Italy and Spain briefly in the 18th century legislated prophylactic measures against and introduced compulsory notification of phthisis. Far more widespread was the largely unquestioning view that the disease was transmissible only by an obscure hereditary defect, and it was little feared, with isolation never imposed as strictly as for leprosy. In some cultures, affliction decreased eligibility for marriage and for certain occupations; it implied poverty and stigmatized families, often being denied and kept from death records; others associated consumption with genius and otherworldly attributes. Therapies included dietetic measures, hygienic regimens, and bizarre practices. Horseback riding and sea voyages were seen to have intrinsic value as well as a bonus benefit from motion sickness. Remedies utilized bloodletting, blistering, purging, starving, vomiting, cupping, the application of leeches and counterirritants, and vogues in medication that included human fat (obtained from executioners), despite the work of Pierre Louis (1787–1872)—of the Paris school of clinical pathology—who used medical statistics to show the futility of such "heroic" measures (Teller, 1988). Centuries of such nonscientific chaos ended with the bacteriological era launched by Koch in 1882 and the discovery of diagnostic radiology by Roentgen in 1896.

An infective transmission of phthisis is implicit in the thinking behind some ancient practices and in the writings of Aristotle, Galen, and others, but not until Villeman did the concept advance beyond hunch to the realm of scientific method. Using animals, Villeman (1827–1892) demonstrated that tuberculosis is a specific infection due to an inoculable agent. Although other laboratories repeated the experiments and verified the results, many hesitated to apply animal studies to humans. The Académie de Médicine rebuffed Villeman's work, and in the United States, Austin Flint and W. H. Welch, in the fifth edition of *The Principles and Practice of Medicine*, published in 1881 just months before the announcement of Koch's discovery, discounted the doctrine of contagion of phthisis, favoring instead hereditary disposition, unfavorable climate, sedentary indoor life, defective ventilation, deficiency of light, and depressing emotions. "Never," observed Dubos, "did a textbook statement become so soon and so completely outmoded" (Dubos, 1950). Several late-century experimenters—Pasteur, Lister, Metchnikoff, Hansen, Ehrlich—pioneered importantly in the burgeoning field of bacteriology, but not with the prompt professional and popular impact of Koch's announcement in 1882. The ensuing scientific revolution finally discredited the environmentalist school of "miasmic" theorists and left the contagionists in control of the public health movement.

III. The Work of Robert Koch

Robert Koch (1843–1910), a German physician not entirely satisfied with hometown practice, on his 28th birthday received from his wife a Hartnach microscope, a gift synergistic with his appetite for gadgetry and inquisitiveness. Installing a small laboratory in a corner of his consultation room, he turned his attention to the study of microbes in relation to infectious diseases. The microbe responsible for anthrax (earlier described by a veterinary surgeon named Pollender) was isolated by Koch, who then, innovating the hanging-drop technique, was able to watch the development of bacilli from forms later designated as spores, to grow the bacilli in culture, and to transmit the disease to healthy animals. Koch rapidly won recognition and acclaim with a series of scientific accomplishments, the most historic being the demonstration on March 29, 1882 to the Berlin Physiologic Society that he had identified the tubercle bacillus and convicted it of causing consumption by fulfilling his self-imposed postulates for proof of a cause-effect relationship between germ and disease. (This formulation, originally suggested by Henle in 1840, henceforth became designated as "Koch's postulates.")

Appointed to the Imperial Health Office, Koch recruited such pupils as Gaffky and Löffler and went on to such further bacteriological discoveries as the bacilli for typhoid, glanders, and diphtheria. Continuing his interest in tuberculosis, Koch demonstrated in guinea pigs differing reactions following secondary and primary infection (the Koch phenomenon), and he produced a glycerine extract of dead tubercle bacilli initially called "lymph" and later "tuberculin." Apparently under political pressure, the composition of this extract was at first kept secret, although it was promoted as an effective therapeutic weapon. This aroused worldwide excitement and caused massive migrations of the phthisic to Berlin in search of the cure. Then widely regarded as an embarrassment to his career, tuberculin in time proved to be therapeutically useless but of enormous value diagnostically, and Koch the scientist was recognized with a Nobel Prize in 1905 (Teller, 1988; Sakula, 1979, 1982; Grange and Bishop, 1982).

Koch's work also had an impact on attitudes toward tuberculosis, approaches to therapy, and the sanatorium movement.

There is evidence back to antiquity that at various times consumptives collected at specific sites, but often more for segregation and disposal than for therapy or for hygienic concerns. An early change to a humanitarian approach is represented by the Brompton Hospital for Consumption and Diseases of the Chest, founded in 1841 "as an asylum for consumptive patients and as a means for furthering knowledge of the disease." Formalized and structured sanatoria took consumption out of the darkened and hermetic bedroom and relocated it at sites imagined to have therapeutic attributes, often at mountain altitudes aromatic with pine and spruce, but also at seashores or at spas with mineral waters. The earliest documented example of open-air seaside therapy is the Royal Bathing Infirmary for Scrofula established at Margate, England in 1791 by a fashionable Quaker physician named Lettsom, who observed that fishermen did not suffer from scrofula. Also freely using many other practices then in vogue, he is remembered chiefly for his rhyme:

When any sick to me apply,
I physics, bleeds and sweats 'em.
If after that they choose to die
Why Verily!
                                                    I lettsom.

Brehman, linking an alleged immunity to phthisis among high-altitude dwellers with his conviction that the cure was aided by an active heart pumping a vigorous supply of blood to the lungs, in 1859 established in the Silesian Mountains the first modern institution exclusively for tuberculosis, imposing a number of dietary and hygienic regulations that included daily exercise. This came to serve as a prototype sanatorium, although others—Dettweiler's in the Taurus Mountains (1876), Walther's at 1500 feet in the Black Forest—architecturally and by regimen promoted rest in fresh air, particularly until fever subsided and weight was regained. In the years following 1882, especially as it became clear that Koch's tuberculin had no place in therapeutics, the sanatorium movement spread beyond central Europe to Britain, abandoning altitude for coastal and riverside locations (Pratt, 1944; Dubos and Dubos, 1952; Grigg, 1958; Keers, 1978; Caldwell, 1988; Sigerist, 1961).

IV. The American Experience

In America, both the sanatorium movement and hygienic campaigns borrowed extensively from European experience. Victorian England instituted measures to cope with filth and misery, but little progress in public health was seen in the

United States prior to the Civil War and the cholera epidemic of 1857. The public's greatest medical fears were yellow fever, cholera, and typhoid, all with far more explosive symptoms and rapid mortality than had tuberculosis. The Channing Home, a small endowed facility in Boston, opened in 1857 as a refuge for tuberculous women, providing mainly terminal nursing care. In 1875, Joseph Gleitsmann from Bavaria established the Mountain Sanatorium for Pulmonary Disease in Ashville, North Carolina, but failed to attract wide attention. Credit for popularizing the sanatorium concept in America is traditionally given to Edward Livingston Trudeau, whose personal affliction was diagnosed by Edward Janeway in 1872 and who turned his tuberculosis into a movement he helped pioneer. After a year of progressive debility, Trudeau journeyed to a primitive area of New York's Adirondack mountains for a last hunting trip. Following a remarkable improvement, Trudeau drew from his personal and anecdotal experience to publish a depiction of the Adirondacks as a health resort for consumptives; this led directly to the growth of the village of Saranac Lake specifically and the environs in general as a center for those seeking cure. In 1884, Trudeau built a simple shack ("Little Red") furnished with two cots, two chairs, a washstand, a wood stove, and a kerosene lamp for a total cost of $100 (Meade, 1972), and in February 1885 he admitted as his first patients two tuberculous sisters (with pulmonary and Pott's disease). Trudeau was quick to accept the sanatorium concepts of Brehman and Dettweiler (favoring rest over activity) and to adopt the methods of Koch (even persevering with "tuberculin therapy" long after it was discredited). He established a laboratory and attempted largely self-taught research (some contemporaries characterized Trudeau as more *bricoleur* than scientist) but showed a major talent for eliciting contributions from the wealthy and for promoting his Adirondack Cottage Sanatorium as a fashionable charity. Renamed in 1915 at his death, the Trudeau Sanatorium established routines that became the prototype for many subsequent facilities in America (with staffing, often, with Trudeau-trained personnel).

Under such disciplinarians as Lawrason Brown, the "cure" developed from a simple hospitalization into a doctrinal commitment to health, a regimentalized community whose cultic rituals extended even to elaborate instructions for wrapping up in blankets on the open-air porch. The highest or "complete" category of disciplined inactivity did not permit the arms behind the head, reading, or listening to the radio. All patients, at every level of rest, were required to observe the universal daily rest period, and the town itself was so geared into sanatorium routine that station WNBZ in Saranac Lake went off the air between 2:00 and 4:00 P.M. Emotionally segregating, many sanatoria additionally achieved physical isolation by their nature as outlying communities with private post offices, railroad stations, power generators, and icehouses. Filled to the last bed, popular sanatoria overflowed their patients (or new arrivals on waiting lists) into neighboring boarding houses and luxury hotels (Gallo, 1985) or such subspecialized units as "Infantoria" and "Preventoria" (designed to isolate newborns and children from infected parents). Decades of preoccupation with fresh air and mountain altitudes as primary therapeutic elements eventually lost emphasis to bed rest alone, allowing accommodation for masses of poor consumptives for treatment at local urban institutions: "Home Hospitals," day camps, tent cities, shack colonies, even moored ferry boats (Major, 1932; Meade, 1972; Bignall, 1982; Taylor, 1986; Caldwell, 1988).

Habits from the sanatorium "cure" often endured for life. Henry Sewall, the 1930 Trudeau medalist, who in 1889 examined his own sputum and realized his "hostship of that acid-fact bacillus," traveled to Saranac Lake, and briefly served under Trudeau as the sanatorium's first resident physician as well as laboratory worker and patient taking the "cure," spent most of a subsequent distinguished academic career in Denver. After his death at the age of 81 in 1936, his obituary reported: "A few minutes before Dr. Henry Sewall, world-famous physician and physiologist, died Wednesday at his home here, he reached for tablet and pencil at the bedside. With faltering fingers he wrote down the time and his temperature and noted that his skin was moist. Then he died" (Webb, 1946).

The first major American contribution to the modern history of tuberculosis was the so-called "Tuberculosis Movement." From its inception in the late 19th century to its maturity in 1917, the Movement scrutinized the complex interactions between science and medicine, public health, social concerns, and economic conditions and began to shape modern policies for disease control. Widespread attitudes of fatalism and despair began to yield under evidence that the disease was both preventable and curable. The works of Pasteur, Villeman, and others correlated consumption with population density and poverty, giving focus to public health campaigns. The use of Koch's tuberculin not for therapy but as a diagnostic tool redefined the detection of human bacillary infection and served also to reveal that disease in cattle, a dangerous pool for contagion to humans, was far more widespread than previously suspected. The gigantic human costs of tuberculosis included devastating degrees of family wreckage, destitute parents forced to send their children to work, and institutions filled with children orphaned by this specific disease. Harvey Cushing, in his biography of Sir William Osler, tells that of the Johns Hopkins Medical School class of 1899, 5 of 19 developed consumption, one fatally (Francis, 1947, 1958; Steele and Ranney, 1958; Amberson, 1966; Wright et al., 1990). Zealous crusaders campaigned for kissing on the forehead instead of the lips, opening windows, abolition of the common drinking cup, and the use of spittoons. "Straphangers" in subways and buses protested against the absorbent and "unsafe" overhead straps of leather for the use of standees, and the straps were replaced by loops of metal (*New York Times*, June 23, 1982). Tuberculosis, out of the closet, had become a popular concern.

In the early 1900s a number of pioneer American bacteriologists (William H. Welch, Hermann M. Biggs) traveled to Germany and returned to apply their new studies to public health. In 1892, Biggs became the head of the Division of Pathology, Bacteriology, and Disinfection of the New York City Department of Health, and he made it the first such department in the world that used routine bacteriology in the diagnosis of disease. Biggs carefully planned and brilliantly led a comprehensive program for tuberculosis control that became a model for officials throughout the United States and Europe. His recommendations included education of the public, precautionary measures against the spread of infection, separation and isolation of tuberculous patients, the assignment of inspectors to visit and disinfect the apartments of consumptives, sputum examination for disease detection, and the reporting of all cases of tuberculosis. In 1897, Cincinnati converted a smallpox hospital into the first municipal tuberculosis hospital in the nation (Burke, 1938; Keers, 1978; Caldwell, 1988).

This need for new public health measures inspired the first organization created to cope with a single disease. Lawrence F. Flick, who felt that the health of the people was a governmental responsibility, agitated for a comprehensive program to combat tuberculosis and in 1892 spearheaded the organization of the Pennsylvania Society for the Prevention of Tuberculosis.

Ohio and New York soon followed. These early crusades recognized the limiting aspects to professional domination and followed Flick's principles of cooperation between physicians and laypersons, volunteer groups and public agencies, actively welcoming the efforts of spouses, women, anyone with missionary enthusiasm. Many small and, often, rival organizations, municipal and state, coalesced into larger and more powerful units that ultimately became a historic national organization (today's American Lung Association and American Thoracic Society) with a constitutional committee that included Flick, Osler, Biggs, Trudeau, and Welch. The 1904 inauguration at Atlantic City selected Edward Livingston Trudeau as president and, abandoning morbid warnings, adopted the upbeat attitude that mankind need no longer be the passive victim of tuberculosis and that the careful consumptive need not be dangerous. A major theme was the drain by tuberculosis of the nation's vitality; major hygienic campaigns addressed such issues as infant mortality and prison reform. Health hints and slogans were printed on the backs of streetcar transfers, on posters and pamphlets distributed to hotel rooms and church bulletins, schools, store windows, and community centers, always with the symbol of the double-barred cross. The movement spread rapidly and the last of the state associations (South Carolina) was organized in 1917 (Dubos and Dubos, 1952; Grigg, 1958; Wilson, 1979; Teller, 1988).

Emily Bissell, a dedicated lifelong volunteer with many outstanding achievements, in 1907 borrowed from Denmark the fund-raising strategy of Christmas stamps with the hope of raising $300 for an insolvent Delaware sanatorium, and she collected the astonishing sum of $3000. Under Red Cross sponsorship, stamp sales became nationwide in 1908 and in 1911 was converted into the annual Christmas Seal Campaign of the National Tuberculosis Association (as the society was then known), using the double-barred cross, fashioned after the Cross of Lorraine, as its emblem. The success of the seals with the general public transformed the movement into a cause that millions joined, and it provided a major financial subsidy for the national society and its units (*American Lung Association Bulletin*, 1979; Ayvazian, 1980).

The earliest American tuberculosis associations sponsored mainly educational, diagnostic, and treatment programs and left the primacy of scientific investigation to European centers. When World War I disrupted the flow of research information to the United States, the National Association for the Study and Prevention of Tuberculosis set up a Committee on Research. In March 1917, it launched publication of the *American Review of Tuberculosis* and in 1921 began to distribute research grants (Teller, 1988).

Attention to the specific needs of blacks with tuberculosis, however, was slow to develop. Sanatoria, back to Trudeau's, did not welcome blacks, or they practiced segregation at the few allowing admission. Attempts at organizing black societies and sanatoria (often along church lines) were few and transient, due mainly to poverty. The efforts of whites for blacks often seemed motivated by the menace of a pool of contagion—their cooks and laundresses—left unattended, a public health concern of self-interest and not a matter of charity. (Early in the century, the annual mortality from tuberculosis for the nation's nine million blacks was over three times the white rate; indeed, so advanced was the disease when first diagnosed that professional workers had the impression that tuberculosis differed in blacks and that they did not get it in lesser forms.)

Not until the 1930s did the enormous problem of tuberculosis among blacks become a major concern of the movement, and the dual goals of cure and detention led to the creation of two distinct types of hospital facilities, some available only for terminal cases. Reasoning that blacks would be more likely to use the services of black physicians and visiting nurses, advanced training programs for such professionals were offered, but the major forces for black social projects lagged until the Depression and the New Deal (housing reform, food to the needy, welfare payments to tuberculous breadwinners) and the disease provisions of the 1935 Social Security Act. In the 1950s these separate efforts gradually acquired unity of purpose and increasingly shifted the protection of public health from local to state and to federal responsibility. In 1964, the Civil Rights Act gave hospital desegregation legal sanction, but in many cases sanatoria had phased out before integration was achieved (Payne, 1949; Dubos and Dubos, 1952; Torchia, 1975).

Many prechemotherapy patients showed favorable in-sanatorium response, but follow-up studies revealed such sobering long-range results as death in over 60% of discharged patients within 6 years (17% of the ''cured,'' 51% of the ''arrested,'' and 72% of the ''improved''). ''Cured'' physicians and nurses often remained as sanatorium staff, many intermittently requiring periods of retreatment. Some sanatoria adopted the policy of admitting only potentially ''curable'' patients and excluding the hopeless. In the 1930s, such discouraged apathy gradually gave way to innovative methods of collapse therapy: pneumothorax, pneumoperitoneum, phrenic nerve crush, and thoracoplasty.

That collapsing the lung might assist the healing of a tuberculous cavity was first suggested in 1771 in the writings of Edmond Claud Bourru, librarian to the Faculté de Médecine in Paris (Burke, 1938). In the early 1800s, sporadic reports described symptomatic improvement in tuberculosis patients after pleural effusions and spontaneous pneumothorax, and James Carson in Liverpool demonstrated that induced collapse of one lung did not interfere with a rabbit's activities (Keers, 1978). Eventually, in 1888, Carlo Forlanini of the medical school in Pavia, Italy induced the first artificial pneumothorax, using a simple home-constructed pumping mechanism to inject nitrogen intrapleurally, and over the next 18 years he published reports of 25 treated cases (Sakula, 1983). J. B. Murphy of the Cook County Infirmary in Chicago independently noted that Civil War chest injuries that resulted in lung collapse rarely caused ''unpleasant symptoms''; he published descriptions of pneumothorax induced with a trochar (1898) and pioneered in using roentgenography as a therapeutic guide. In 1908 Christian Saugman introduced the two-bottle-and-manometer pneumothorax apparatus for bedside use. Amberson lucidly reviewed his use of therapeutic pneumothorax at the Loomis Sanatorium in New York's Catskill Mountains between 1911 and 1925 (Amberson and Peters, 1925). During the next 25 years, the technique became the most widely used and important sanatorium adjunct to bed rest. Effective collapse of the lung was sometimes prevented by stringy pleural adhesions that kept cavities open, prompting Jacobeus to invent the thoracoscope (1912) for the closed method of cutting these adhesions with cautery (intrapleural pneumonolysis) and achieving sufficient lung collapse for cavity closure. By the end of World War II, the alternate techniques of pneumoperitoneum, phrenic nerve crush, and thoracoplasty also became commonly selected collapse procedures.

In 1933, Banyai accidentally injected air into the peritoneal cavity during a pneumothorax refill and noted improvement in the pulmonary lesions; others also reported healing of tuberculous cavities while pneumoperitoneum was being tried for abdominal tuberculosis. These observations, as well as the improvement in tuberculosis observed during pregnancy, led to the widespread employment of pneumoperitoneum as a therapeutic measure that was less hazardous than pneumothorax, always fully reversible, and augmented in the degree of lung collapse by the supine posture of bed rest. Although used since 1911 (Sturz) for the treatment of lower-lobe cavities, phrenic-nerve interruption or crush, at the supraclavicular level, to achieve diaphragmatic paralysis became coupled with pneumoperitoneum for substantially greater diaphragmatic rise and unilateral compression, but with the cost of possibly irreversible functional loss, respiratory impairment, and mediastinal "flutter." Extrapleural pnuemothorax and plombage—creating a space between costal periosteum and parietal pleura and inserting a "plomb" of paraffin, oil, bone fragments, or lucite spheres—also came into use but generated new complications and were not long in vogue.

V. Surgical Procedures and Vaccination

The story of surgery in the treatment of tuberculosis is excellently reviewed in a collection of articles commemorating the centenary of Koch's discovery (Gaensler, 1982). Thoracoplasty—rib resection to diminish the volume of the thoracic cavity—was first performed for empyema (Schede, 1890) and over the next two decades extended from the removal of sectional segments to the entire lengths of ribs 2–9 (for more effective pulmonary compression). Mechanical complications resulting from deribbed hemithorax ultimately led to the practice of preserving periosteum in order to restore some skeletal stability following new bone formation. During the 10 years before chemotherapy for tuberculosis, the technically refined procedure of thoracoplasty was 80% successful in closing cavities and eliminating tubercle bacilli from sputum, with well-preserved pulmonary function and low operative mortality. The original German literature on permanent collapse therapy and the subsequent refinement of thoracoplasty is reviewed in a textbook by John Alexander (Alexander, 1925). Alexander, a pioneer thoracic surgeon, wrote the textbook while being treated for vertebral tuberculosis at Trudeau Sanatorium, working supine in a plaster cast and Bradford frame and an inverted rack of his own design to accommodate a book above him and an angled typewriter so that he could read and write in his enforced immobility (Meyer, 1991).

Prior to specific chemotherapy, surgery into tuberculous lung was complicated by tissue infection, spread of disease, fistula formation, or empyema, and it was reserved for situations where collapse procedures had failed or could not be offered at all. Shortly after streptomycin became available intrathoracic forms of chest surgery (lobectomy, segmentectomy, decortication, extrapleural pneumonectomy) enjoyed a revival and remained in vogue until long-term studies certified complete sterilization of tuberculous lesions under chemotherapy alone. The career of the multistaged and deforming procedure of thoracoplasty, however, virtually ended.

Attempts to vaccinate against tuberculosis antedate the advent of antimicrobial drugs. In the early 1900s, Calmette and Guérin were able to attenuate a strain of *Mycobacterium bovis* (BCG) after 231 passages through media containing glycerine and ox bile and to show that this BCG strain was unable to produce progressive lesions in experimental animals. First used in Paris in 1921, BCG vaccination, particularly for children at high risk, gained popularity across Europe. After trials with oral and subcutaneous administration, an intradermal injection technique appeared to cause no significant untoward reactions. The benefit from the vaccine, however, was disputed by such authorities as Petroff in the United States. The 1930 disaster in Lubeck, Germany, in which 67 children died after vaccination, generated decades of distrust, although the incident was shown to result not from authentic BCG but from the accidental use of virulent tubercle bacilli stored in the same refrigerator. By 1945, however, this method for preventing tuberculosis again was back in use. Further experience appeared to show that the vaccine conferred good protection against tuberculosis, although present strains of vaccine are reported to vary in protection in a range from 0 to 80%. Explanations offered for this disparity include quality of vaccine, partial protection from previous nontuberculous mycobacterial infection, route of vaccine administration, and regulation of dosage. Clinicians commonly agreed, however, on BCG's efficacy with children (childhood tuberculosis was found to reappear in European countries in which vaccine use was suspended), and it is widely recommended that BCG be administered as early in life as possible. Evidence also suggests that the more serious forms of tuberculosis (miliary, meningitis) are prevented by BCG vaccination. It is regarded as one of the safest of live vaccines now in use (except with immunosuppressed individuals, who may develop local or disseminated bovine tuberculosis), but its efficacy for adults is still in dispute. A number of investigators are actively pursuing approaches toward vaccine improvement or redesign, including attempts to fortify BCG to overexpress the protective antigens of *M. tuberculosis* (Luelmo, 1982; Caldwell, 1988; MMWR, 1988, 1991; Stover et al., 1991).

VI. Antibiotic Therapy

The history of phthisis is as ancient as humanity itself, but its scientific milestones are recent and few. Villemin's demonstration and Koch's certification that tuberculosis is an infection transmittable by inoculum ranks high, together with the use of Roentgen's rays for diagnosis and the chemotherapeutic revolution ushered in by streptomycin. The many former treatments of consumption ranged from the harmlessly useless to the harmfully grotesque and without scientific legitimacy. Koch's "tuberculin cure" was defensible by the logic of the day but is now judged a negative episode in his career. Amberson's trial with gold in 1931 represents an early example of the modern randomized study (the putative benefit carried over to the use of gold in rheumatoid arthritis, then thought akin to phthisis). In the later 1930s, improvement was reported in both experimental and clinical tuberculosis with some sulfonamide and complex sulfone compounds, but with considerable hematological toxicity. In the 1940s, streptomycin—the first antibiotic effective against Gram-negative bacteria and the tubercle bacillus—rewrote tuberculosis history (Amberson et al., 1931; Dubos and Dubos, 1952; Keers, 1978; Teller, 1988.)

Accepting the Nobel Prize in Medicine in 1952, Selman Waksman quoted from Ecclesiasticus: "The Lord hath created medicines out of the earth and he that is wise will not abhor them." Waksman's interest in the microbiology of the soil began during his undergraduate years (1911–1916) at Rutgers College of Agriculture. Noting that bacteria pathogenic to animals and humans eventually find their way to the soil, from which they promptly disappear, he postulated the existence of soil-inhibiting microbes antagonistic to human pathogens. In 1941, Waksman, now a soil microbiologist, coined the word "antibiotic" to designate antibacterial substances derived from actinomycetes and fungi. Streptomycin, a product of *Streptomyces griseus* (originally isolated in 1916 as *Actinomycete griseus* and rediscovered and renamed in 1943), was tabulated in a 1944 report according to in vitro antibiotic activity against 22 listed bacteria, one of which was the tubercle bacillus. Taking this hint of antituberculous antibiotic activity into his research laboratory, William Feldman at the Mayo Clinic showed that under treatment with streptomycin the spleens of guinea pigs experimentally infected with virulent human tubercle bacilli were rendered morphologically negative and noninfectious, a circumstance never before observed in the animal model. Also in 1944, Pfuetze (collaborating with Feldman and Hinshaw) was the first to treat human tuberculosis with streptomycin, dramatically "curing" a 21-year-old woman "in the last stages," despite the administration of five courses, each of only 10–18 days' duration, over a 15-month period, without a companion drug. (Ten years later the woman was well, married, with three children.) Clinical results from large-scale controlled trials—conducted by the American Trudeau Society (now the American Thoracic Society) and the Veterans Administration—were presented in 1946, establishing the unprecedented value of streptomycin as an antituberculosis agent but revealing two serious problems: the toxicity of streptomycin (chiefly damage to the eighth cranial nerve) and the emergence of drug-resistant bacilli in most of the patients treated. In the course of these studies, Feldman developed tuberculosis and became the patient of Hinshaw, his colleague, and also one of the first humans to receive combined antituberculosis drug therapy [the sulfone Promin, streptomycin, and *para*-aminosalicylic acid (PAS)], with complete recovery (Comroe, 1978; D'Esopo, 1982; Sakula, 1988).

Working from Bernheim's report that both benzoic and salicylic acids stimulated oxygen uptake in tubercle bacilli, Jorgen Lehmann in Sweden searched for competitive inhibitors of these acids and eventually demonstrated that PAS exerted in vitro bacteriostatic activity against *M. tuberculosis*; by 1946 he confirmed favorable results in treating tuberculosis both in experimental animals and in humans. Confronting the problem of the emergence of bacterial drug resistance with streptomycin monotherapy, combined streptomycin-PAS trials were undertaken in both Britain and the United States. By 1950, the unequivocal success of combined drug chemotherapy of tuberculosis was clearly established.

The complex nature and high cost of modern chemotherapeutic research proved to be insurmountable for the modestly funded individual worker and shifted to the research teams of giant pharmaceutical companies. The discovery of the next major antituberculosis agent was apparently simultaneous by three groups, working in the United States at Hoffmann–La Roche and at the Squibb Institute for Medical Research and in Germany at the Farbenfabriken Bayer. So hopeful was the preliminary laboratory antituberculous activity of isonicotinic acid hydrazide (INH) that an immediate clinical trial seemed justified. This, conducted by Robitzek and Selikoff at Staten Island's Sea View Hospital in New York in 1951 and 1952, showed marked and rapid improvement in 44 consecutive patients with "acute progressive caseopneumonic tuberculosis." Premature and unauthorized publicity, describing sensationalized "miracle" results, confused early clinical reports, but INH soon proved to be potent, cheap, orally effective, well accepted, and of low toxicity. Again, bacillary resistance limited the use of the drug singly, indicating the continued need for multidrug regimens in tuberculosis. The remarkable enhancement of any regimen by the addition of INH initiated a reappraisal of centuries-old concepts of tuberculosis healing; properly chosen drug combinations administered for sufficient duration proved to be the sole requirement for the complete cure of uncomplicated disease, pulmonary or extrapulmonary. The traditional therapeutic options of prolonged hospitalization, bed rest, collapse measures, surgery, and rehabilitation one by one lost their priorities. Outpatient supervision of chemotherapy, however, soon demonstrated the primal importance of patient cooperation (Raleigh, 1982; D'Esopo, 1982; Caldwell, 1988).

During the 1950s a number of new antituberculosis drugs—the injectables viomycin, capreomycin, and amikacin and the orals pyrazinamide, thioacetazone, ethionamide, and cycloserine—became available for clinical use, all with significant toxicities and side effects. Developed by Lederle Laboratories in the 1960s, ethambutol proved to be an excellent oral medication with low toxicity and few side effects, and it soon replaced PAS (24 pills a day, often sickening the patient) as the companion for INH. The next major advance after INH was rifampin.

In 1957, a number of Gram-negative organisms were isolated from a soil sample collected at a pine arboretum near St. Raphael on the Côte d'Azur, and these organisms were found to exert activity against *M. tuberculosis*. First numbered ME/83, then called *Streptomyces mediterranei*, and later reclassified as *Nocardia mediterranea*, the strain yielded an antibiotic extract laboratory-nicknamed ''Rififi''(an argot word meaning a struggle among gangsters), the title of a French movie then popular in Europe. Ultimately named rifampin or rifampicin, the antibiotic went into clinical trial in 1967 and, administered orally, proved to be rapidly absorbed, produced a high serum level, and exerted marked antituberculous bactericidal effect. As with INH, the discovery of rifampin was heralded as opening a new area in tuberculosis chemotherapy. In combinations with INH, rifampin sterilized more rapidly than any other matching of drugs, the one unfortunate aspect being the high cost of rifampin. By the 1970s, this pair of drugs became established as the best multidrug regimen for tuberculosis. The addition of pyrazinamide to INH and rifampin made a short-term (4–6 month) regimen a successful option, which in part atoned for the high cost of the new drug (Sensi, 1982, 1983).

The single exception to multidrug antituberculosis chemotherapy is the INH ''chemoprophylaxis'' program, which actually amounts to the prevention of overt disease by the single-drug treatment of subclinical (''latent'') tuberculosis. The concept evolved from (1) the availability of a safe, inexpensive oral drug bactericidal for tubercle bacilli, (2) the ability of INH to prevent death, disease, and even tuberculin reactivity in guinea pigs challenged with virulent tubercle bacilli, and (3) the early observation that single-drug INH chemotherapy could prevent complications, particularly meningitis, in children with miliary or primary tuberculosis. The program was tested in large cooperative studies, first with children by the U.S. Public Health Service in 1955 and subsequently in adults throughout the world. Despite compelling evidence to its support, the INH chemoprophylaxis program coped with controversy from outset and has never been maximally implemented as a public health policy.

Phthisiologists have a long history of community, with societies, a specific literature, an international union, cooperative studies that generated a therapeutic renaissance for tuberculosis and defined new patterns for all fields clinical investigation. Successful antituberculosis chemotherapy initially couraged safer thoracic surgery but ultimately served to eliminate not only cisional procedures but all collapse measures as well. Optimistic prediction foresaw the global eradication of tuberculosis within a few decades. Through 1950s and 1960s, tuberculosis sanatoria were phased out and phthisiotherapy was bequeathed to the ''mainstream'' of medicine with little effort to integrate established expertise into the national health structure. Unfortunately, the mainstream was not prepared for this inheritance as an outright gift and has been slow to develop enthusiasm for the care and treatment of tuberculosis. The redesignation of tuberculosis resulted also in a self-defeating loss of centers of excellence to provide research and teaching facilities. The emergence of human immunodeficiency virus (HIV) infection and the problem of patient noncompliance with drug therapy have also played into the persistence of tuberculosis as a major public health problem, and eradication remains an unfulfilled vision.

The World Health Organization estimates that a third of the global population is infected with the tubercle bacillus: 95% of the developing world, 5% of industrialized countries. Tuberculosis is the number 1 cause of disability and death, with close to three million fatalities each year. Epidemic since early urbanization, the disease is thought now to occur in waves that affect different communities at different times. In the populations of Western Europe and white North America, the epidemic achieved its peak as the 18th century moved into the 19th. Epidemiologists judge that tuberculosis mortality in England and Wales began to decline in the 1850s, antedating official control programs, and that by the 1930s it had halved. The black population of sub-Saharan Africa was affected in the early 1900s and may now be at midepidemic. Each recent wave appears to peak rapidly and then to begin a slow decline. Early in the epidemic, tuberculosis strikes heavily at young adults, while in later stages of the declining wave, it gradually becomes a disease of older persons. The reason for the natural decline is unknown and seems essentially unaided by human efforts. Traditional medical interpretations, possibly self-congratulatory, include such interventive measures as isolation of cases and BCG vaccination, but the role and importance of curative medicine is widely disputed. Humanitarian and biological interpretations point to public health measures, social reform, an increase in resistance in a population, or a progressive reduction in the dose of tubercle bacilli acquired at primary infection (Dubos and Dubos, 1952; Teller, 1988).

The potential for modern chemotherapeutic tuberculosis control was dramatically depicted among the Eskimo population of the Yukon and Kuskokwim Delta. In 1950, the rates of infection (25% per year) and disease were the highest ever reported in medical literature; by 1970, the incidence of new infection was so low it could not be measured with accuracy. This was attributed to the effectiveness of the case-finding and treatment program of the state and federal and public health authorities together with a highly cooperative population (Comstock, 1986; Grzybowski, 1991).

On a larger scale, the introduction of chemotherapy caused a fall in mortality from tuberculosis and a slower fall in morbidity. Also, since the introduction of chemotherapy, the rate of natural tuberculosis decline in many developed countries has accelerated from 1–2% to 8–10% a year. Poor chemotherapy, prolonging life without cure, leaves more sources of infection in the community, achieving a humanitarian purpose but not a public health goal.

Primary resistance to antituberculosis drugs, common in developing countries, is a consequence of poor treatment often unsupervised by trained personnel. When drug resistance, primary or secondary, extends beyond INH and includes rifampin, it confounds both standard antituberculosis combined-drug regimens and INH chemoprophylaxis for contact cases. Multidrug-resistant tuberculosis, tuberculosis among the HIV infected, the noncompliant patient who discontinues treatment as symptoms improve, the search for new drugs suitable for shorter courses of chemotherapy, and strategies toward the goal of eradication of tuberculosis early in the 21st century are all concerns of subsequent chapters in this volume.

References

Alexander, J. (1925). *The Surgery of Pulmonary Tuberculosis*. Lea & Febiger, Philadelphia.

Amberson, J. B. (1966). A retrospect of tuberculosis: 1865–1965. *Am. Rev. Respir. Dis.* **93**:343–351.

Amberson, J. B., and Peters, A. (1925). Pulmonary tuberculosis: its treatment by induced pneumothorax. In *Thoracic Surgery*. Vol. II. Edited by H. Lilienthal. WB Saunders, Philadelphia, pp. 320–442.

Amberson, J. B., McMahon, B. T. and Pinner, M. (1931). A clinical trial of sanocrysin in pulmonary tuberculosis. *Am. Rev. Tuberc.* **24**:401–435.

American Lung Association Bulletin: Seventy-Fifth Anniversary (1979). Editorial: "Well, Emily, see what you can do." **65** (4):2.

Ayvazian, L. F. (1980). The fifty-five Trudeau medalists (1926–1980): a seventy-fifth anniversary review. *Am. Rev. Respir. Dis.* **121**:753–775.

Bignall, J. R. (1982). A century of treating tuberculosis. *Tubercle* **63**:19–22.

Burke, R. M. (1938). *A Historical Chronology of Tuberculosis*. Charles C Thomas, Springfield, IL.

Caldwell, J. (1988). *The Last Crusade: The War on Consumption, 1862–1954*. Atheneum, New York.

Comroe, J. H. (1978). Pay dirt: the story of streptomycin. *Am. Rev. Respir. Dis.*, 117: Part I: From Waksman to Waksman, pp. 773–781; Part II: Feldman and Hinshaw, Lehmann, pp. 957–968.

Comstock, G. W. (1986). Tuberculosis—a bridge to chronic disease epidemiology. *Am. J. Epidemiol.* **124**:1–16.

D'Esopo, N. D. (1982). Clinical trials in pulmonary tuberculosis. *Am. Rev. Respir. Dis.* **125**(Part 2):85–93.

Dubos, R. (1950). *Louis Pasteur, Free Lance of Science*. Little Brown, Boston.

Dubos, R. (1968). *Man, Medicine and Environment*. Pall Mall Press, London.

Dubos, R. (1982). The romance of death. *Am. Lung Assoc. Bull.* **68**(2):5–6.

Dubos, R., and Dubos, J. (1952). *The White Plague*. Little Brown, Boston.

Francis, J. (1947). *Bovine Tuberculosis*. Staples Press, London.

Francis, J. (1958). *Tuberculosis in Animals and Man*. Cassell, London.

Gaensler, E. A. (1982). The surgery for pulmonary tuberculosis. *Am. Rev. Respir. Dis.* **125**(Part 2):73–84.

Gallo, P. (1985). *Cure Cottages of Saranac Lake*. Historic Saranac Lake, Saranac Lake, NY.

Garrison, F. H. (1913). *An Introduction to the History of Medicine*. WB Saunders, Philadelphia.

Grange, J., and Bishop, P. (1982). "Uber Tuberkulose," a tribute to Robert Koch's discovery of the tubercle bacillus, 1882. *Tubercle* **62**:3–17.

Grigg, E. R. N. (1958). The arcana of tuberculosis. *Am. Rev. Tuberc. Pulm. Dis.* **78**:151–172, 426–453, 583–595.

Grzybowski, S. (1991). Tuberculosis in the Third World. *Thorax* **46**:689–691.

Guthrie, D. (1945). *A History of Medicine*. Thomas Nelson, London.

Keers, R. Y. (1978). *Pulmonary Tuberculosis, a Journey down the Centuries*. Bailliere Tindall, London.

Luelmo, F. (1982). BCG vaccination. *Am. Rev. Respir. Dis.* **125**(Part 2): 70–72.

Major, R. H. (1932). *Classic Descriptions of Disease*. Charles C Thomas, Springfield, IL.

Meade, G. M. (1972). Edward Livingston Trudeau, M.D. *Tubercle* **53**:229–250.

Meyer, J. A. (1991). Tuberculosis, the Adirondacks, and coming of age for thoracic surgery. *Ann. Thorac. Surg.* **52**:881–885.

MMWR (1988). Use of BCG vaccines in the control of tuberculosis. **37**(43):663–675.

MMWR (1991). Nosocomial transmission of multidrug-resistant tuberculosis among HIV-infected persons. **40**(34):590.

Myers, J. A., and Steele, J. H. (1969). *Bovine Tuberculosis: Control in Man and Animals*. Warren H. Green, St. Louis.

Payne, H. M. (1949). The problem of tuberculosis control among American Negroes. *Am. Rev. Tuberc.* **60**:332–342.

Pratt, J. H. (1944). The evolution of rest treatment of pulmonary tuberculosis. *Am. Rev. Tuberc.* **50**:185–201.

Raleigh, J. (1982). Chemotherapy rings the bell. *Am. Lung Assoc. Bull.* (special anniversary issue) **68**(2):14.

Sakula, A. (1979). Robert Koch (1843–1910): founder of the science of bacteriology and discoverer of the tubercle bacillus. *Br. J. Dis. Chest* **73**:389–294.

Sakula, A. (1982). Robert Koch: Centenery of the Discovery of the Tubercle Bacillus, 1882. *Thorax* **37**:246–251.

Sakula, A. (1983). Carlo Forlanini, inventor of artificial pneumothorax for treatment of pulmonary tuberculosis. *Thorax* **38**:326–332.

Sakula, A. (1988). Selman Waksman (1888–1973), discoverer of streptomycin: a centensry review. *Br. J. Dis. Chest* **82**:23–31.

Schede, M. (1890). Die Behandlung der Empyeme. *Verhandl Cong Innere Med.* *(Wiesbaden)*, 41.

Sensi, P. (1982). Rifampin. In *Chronicles of Drug Discovery*. Vol. I. Edited by J. S. Bindra and D. Lednicer. Wiley, New York.

Sensi, P. (1983). History of development of rifampin. *Rev. Infect. Dis.* **5**(suppl 3):S402–S406.

Sigerist, H. E. (1961). *A History of Medicine*. Vol. II. Oxford University Press, New York, p. 131.

Steele, J. H., and Ranney, A. F. (1958). Animal tuberculosis. *Am. Rev. Tuberc. Pulm. Dis.* **77**:908–922.

Stover, C. K., de la Cruz, V. F., Fuerst, T. R., Burlein, J. E., Benson, L. A., Bennett, L. T., Bansal, G. P., Young, J. F., Lee, M. H., Hatfull, G. F., Snapper, S. B., Barletta, R. G., Jacobs, W. R., and Bloom, B. R. (1991). New use of BCG for recombinant vaccines. *Nature* 351:456–460.

Taylor, R. (1986). *Saranac, America's Magic Mountain*. Houghton Mifflin, Boston.

Teller, M. E. (1988). *The Tuberculosis Movement*. Greenwood Press, New York.

Torchia, M. M. (1975). The tuberculosis movement and the race question, 1890–1950. *Bull. Hist. Med.* **49**(2):152–168.

Webb, G. B. (1946). *Henry Sewall, Physiologist and Physician*. The Johns Hopkins Press, Baltimore, p. 160.

Wilson, J. L. (1979). History of the American Thoracic Society. *Am. Rev. Respir. Dis.* **119**: Part I: pp. 177–184, Part II: pp. 327–335, Part III: pp 521–530.

Wright, K. W., Monroe, J., and Beck, F. (1990). A history of the Ray Brook State Tuberculosis Hospital. *NY State J. Med.* **90**:406–413.

Part One

BASIC ASPECTS

2

Epidemiology of Tuberculosis

GEORGE W. COMSTOCK

The Johns Hopkins School of Hygiene
and Public Health
Baltimore, Maryland

GEORGE M. CAUTHEN

National Center for Prevention Services
Centers for Disease Control
and Prevention
Atlanta, Georgia

I. Introduction

Tuberculosis is still a leading contender for the dubious distinction of being the most important plague of mankind. The World Health Organization recently estimated that 1700 million people have been infected with *Mycobacterium tuberculosis*, and that each year, 8 million develop tuberculosis in a recognizable form and 2.9 million die from it (Kochi, 1991). Accentuating the impact of tuberculosis on the world's well-being is its concentration among young adults throughout most of the developing world and its airborne spread from person to person, especially to household members. As noted in Chapter 1, tuberculosis has been exacting a toll for many centuries. Of particular interest from an epidemiological point of view is the reported frequency of skeletal lesions suggestive of tuberculosis among pre-Columbian populations of North American (Buikstra and Cook, 1981). While such lesions were occasionally noted in skeletons of the Late Woodland peoples (A.D. 800–1050), their successors, the Mississippians, had a much higher frequency of tuberculosis-like bony lesions, associated with their coming together in larger and relatively permanent settlements.

That tuberculosis and crowding go together is now so generally accepted that the reason(s) for the association is rarely considered. Is it solely because crowding increases the risk of becoming infected if infectious cases are present? Is it because there is something associated with crowding that makes it more likely that an infected person will develop tuberculous disease? Is it some combination of these sets of risks? Answers to these questions comprise the "etiological epidemiology" of tuberculosis.

This chapter will first address etiological epidemiology by reviewing what is known about risk factors for becoming infected with tubercle bacilli, then risk factors for developing disease given that infection has occurred, and finally risk factors for relapse following apparent cure or spontaneous healing of the disease. This approach is consistent with the oft-stated goals of tuberculosis control: (1) prevent the uninfected from becoming infected; (2) prevent the infected from developing tuberculous disease; and (3) prevent relapse, disability, and death among those who have tuberculosis.

"Administrative epidemiology" will then be reviewed. This aspect of epidemiology deals with the occurrence of tuberculosis based on routine reporting or special surveys. These data are vital for tuberculosis control workers and other persons interested in health policy who must know the distribution of cases by time, place, and personal characteristics regardless of what caused these distributions.

II. Etiological Epidemiology

A. Risk of Becoming Infected with Tubercle Bacilli

Causes of Tuberculous Infection

Three related organisms—*M. tuberculosis*, *M. africanum*, and *M. bovis*—are the necessary causes of tuberculosis. *M. tuberculosis* is by far the most common. *M. africanum* is rarely found outside of northwestern Africa, and disease due to *M. bovis* is limited in developed countries by widespread pasteurization of milk and in the developing world by the low consumption of milk along with the practice of boiling much that is consumed.

The probability of having been infected with one of the three tubercle bacilli is assessed by the size of induration caused by the tuberculin test.

Risk of Infection by Time and Place

The best estimate of the decrease in the risk of becoming infected for residents of the United States comes from the extensive and carefully standardized tuberculin testing of Navy recruits (Lowell et al., 1969; Rust and Thomas, 1975). Among white males aged 17–21 years, the proportion of positive reactors fell from 6.6% in 1949–1951 to 3.1% in 1967–1968. Subsequent testing on a routine basis showed the prevalence of positive reactors among all recruits to be 1.2% in 1986 (Cross and Hyams, 1990). While the mean age of recruits had probably

Table 1 Prevalence and Average Annual Incidence of Positive Reactors to 5 Tuberculin Units of PPD-S Among U.S. Navy Recruits, Lifetime Residents of One County, Aged 17–21 Years, 1958–1965, for the States and Metropolitan Areas with the Highest and Lowest Values

	Positive reactors(%)[a]	Average annual incidence(%)[b]
Conterminous United States	3.8	0.22
Kentucky	7.8	0.45
North Dakota	1.3	0.07
Metropolitan Baltimore	9.2	0.54
Metropolitan Minneapolis–St. Paul	2.2	0.12

[a]Induration of 10+ mm to 5 Tuberculin Units of PPD-S.
[b]Average over period of 1940–1965, assuming the average age of recruits to be 18 years.
Source: Edwards et al., 1969.

changed little since 1950, the 1986 study population included sizable proportions of nonwhites, who in the earlier study had much higher proportions of infected persons than the white recruits. In addition, the positive reactors throughout this period undoubtedly included some who were infected with nontuberculous mycobacteria and not with *M. tuberculosis*. Correcting for this mixture of infections led to an estimate that only 1.4% of the white male recruits tested in 1968 had been infected with *M. tuberculosis* (Rust and Thomas, 1975).

Results of skin-testing U.S. Navy recruits in the period 1958–1965 have been reported in considerable detail (Edwards et al., 1969).Although the prevalence of infection has changed since that time, the relative rankings by area of lifetime residence and other characteristics must be similar today. The prevalence of tuberculin reactors among these white male recruits aged 17–21 years and the average annual incidence of acquiring new infections during their lifetime is shown in Table 1 for all 48 conterminous states as well as for the states and metropolitan areas with the highest and lowest prevalence of tuberculin reactors in 1958–1965.

The likelihood of having been infected among household contacts of infectious cases of tuberculosis has also declined with time, at least in the United States (Comstock, 1975). In Williamson County, Tennessee, in the period 1931–1955, 67% of household contacts aged 5–9 years were positive tuberculin reactors. In a large study of contacts in 1958, this proportion was 48%. In 1986, less than 30% of close contacts of all ages were positive tuberculin reactors (Rieder et al., 1989).

It is believed that the risk of becoming infected has been falling throughout most of the world, most rapidly in industrialized nations and least in sub-Saharan Africa and the Indian subcontinent, where the annual rate of decline is estimated to be less than 3% per year (Kochi, 1991). Reasonably good estimates can be obtained in countries where there are enough children and young adults who have not been vaccinated with BCG to allow the risk to be estimated (Styblo, 1976, 1991). For example, in the Netherlands the risk of becoming infected was 0.5% per year in 1950 and only 0.02% in 1971. In contrast, several African countries had an estimated risk of becoming infected of 3.0% per year in 1950, with only a slight decrease during the next 20 years. Similar findings were reported from a rural area of South India (Tuberculosis Prevention Trial, Madras, 1980). Among children 1–4 years of age at the initial examination, the average annual risk of infection during the next 4 years was estimated to be 2.8%, with some evidence of a decrease during the 4-year period.

The most dramatic decrease in the risk of infection was documented among the Inuit residents of the Yukon and Kuskokwim River deltas in Alaska (Kaplan et al., 1972). In 1949–1951, 34% of children under the age of 3 years were infected with tubercle bacilli, equivalent to an average annual risk of becoming infected of approximately 25% per year. An intensive program of case finding and treatment, supplemented by isoniazid preventive therapy, was instituted. By 1963–1964, only 0.2% were infected, and in 1969–1970, there were no reactors among 534 tested children.

Personal Risk Factors for Acquiring Infections

Degree of Contact and Intensity of Exposure

Because tuberculosis is a communicable disease primarily spread by the airborne route, it is not surprising that the risk of an uninfected person becoming infected is strongly associated with the probability of coming in contact with someone with infectious tuberculosis, the closeness or intimacy of that contact, its duration, and the degree of infectiousness of the case. Crowding increases both the likelihood of coming into contact with a case and the closeness of the contact. The Navy recruit testing program illustrates the risk associated with urban or rural residence for white males aged 17–21 years (Lowell et al., 1969). Lifetime residents of metropolitan areas had a prevalence of positive tuberculin reactors of 4.2%; lifetime residents of farms, 2.8%; and lifetime residents of other nonmetropolitan areas, an intermediate 3.6%.

The associations of infection risk with closeness of contact, with factors related to race, and with the degree of infectiousness of the source case are shown in Table 2 (Grzybowski et al., 1975). In the Canadian provinces of British Columbia and Saskatchewan, Indian contacts were more likely to have been infected than whites, probably because Indian households were more crowded. For both Indians and whites, infection risk was greater if the contact was intimate (household associates or sweethearts) than if it was casual (other friends, fellow employees). If sputum of the source case contained so many tubercle bacilli that

Table 2 Age-Adjusted[a] Percentages of Positive Tuberculin Reactors Among White and Indian Children Aged 0–14 Years in British Columbia and Saskatchewan, by Sputum Status of Source Case, 1966–1971

Sputum status of source case	Race and closeness of tuberculosis contact			
	Indian children		White children	
	Intimate	Casual	Intimate	Casual
Positive smear	44.7	37.4	34.7	10.1
Positive culture only	27.7	15.6	8.9	2.4
Negative culture	25.7	18.7	7.2	3.3

[a]Adjusted to age distribution of total study population aged 0–14 years.
Source: Grzybowski et al., 1975.

they were demonstrable by microscopic examination of a stained sputum smear, the risk of infecting a contact was also greatly increased. In this population, there was only equivocal evidence that patients with positive sputum cultures were more infectious than those with negative cultures. In other populations, the infectiousness of patients with positive sputum cultures was appreciably greater than those with negative cultures (Loudon and Spohn, 1969).

Other characteristics of the source case are related to the prevalence of positive tuberculin reactions among children who are household contacts (Grzybowski et al., 1975). Extent of pulmonary involvement was strongly associated with infectivity: 62% of contacts of cases with far-advanced disease were reactors, compared to only 16% reactors among contacts to minimal cases. Also related to the risk of infection was cough frequency, which decreased appreciably during the first week of chemotherapy. Similar findings were noted in a study in Mysore State, India (Raj Narain et al., 1966).

Duration of Exposure

Duration of exposure is important in comparing the infectiousness of tuberculosis with other communicable diseases. Although an occasional tuberculous patient can be as infectious as a child with measles (Riley et al., 1962), in most instances the proportion of exposed contacts who become infected with tubercle bacilli is much lower than the risk of infection from patients with other acute communicable diseases. When the duration of exposure is taken into account, the average tuberculosis patient has a low degree of infectiousness per unit of time.

Foreign Residence

There is little evidence that a period of foreign residence is associated with an important risk of infection for persons born in the United States. Navy recruits who had lived abroad at a time when tuberculosis was common even in many developed countries were only slightly more likely to be tuberculin reactors than lifetime residents of this country (Lowell et al., 1969). At least some of the difference must have resulted from BCG vaccinations received in the foreign country. The fact that the excess risk was so low is probably attributable to the lifestyle of most expatriate Americans, most of whose exposures must have occurred in public places and have been very short in duration.

Age

There is some evidence that the risk of acquiring infections increases with age during the period from infancy to early adult life (Sutherland and Fayers, 1975), probably because of increasingly numerous contacts with other persons. Although tuberculin sensitivity, once acquired as a result of infection with tubercle bacilli, persists for many years, the prevalence of positive tuberculin reactions tends to level off around 50–60 years of age. In some populations, there is even a decreased prevalence in older ages, possibly because the infecting bacilli in some persons had died out at an early age.

Sex and Race

In nearly all populations around the world, males are more likely to have been infected than females, again probably reflecting their opportunity for more and varied contacts in most societies. This was clearly illustrated in a large tuberculin testing program among New York City school employees (Reichman and O'Day, 1978; Comstock and O'Brien, 1991). The prevalence of positive reactors was also higher among nonwhites that whites and among residents of poor areas than among employees living in well-to-do areas. Indeed, in the latter, the prevalence of positive reactors was equally low among whites and nonwhites.

Chemotherapy of Source Case

Effective chemotherapy of the source case appears to reduce infectiousness rapidly, perhaps even more rapidly than is indicated by results of sputum examinations (Loudon and Spohn, 1969; Kamat et al., 1966; Riley and Moodie, 1974; Riley et al., 1962). Although isoniazid-resistant organisms have reduced virulence for guinea pigs, there is no indication that drug resistance per se has any effect on infectiousness for humans (Snider et al., 1985). However, when source cases with drug-resistant organisms had a history of prior and probably ineffective treatment, their contacts were at increased risk of being infected. It is likely that this increased risk resulted from the longer duration of exposure that is associated with multiple episodes of treatment.

Institutionalization

Both voluntary and involuntary confinement in two types of institutions has also been shown to be associated with an increased risk of becoming infected with tubercle bacilli. In a continuing survey of nursing homes in Arkansas, it was found that the risk of becoming a positive tuberculin reactor was 3.5% per year even if there had been no recognized tuberculosis cases in the home within the previous 3 years (Stead et al., 1985). Periodic tuberculin testing in an elderly population in poor health can be misleading in individuals because of the relatively high degree of instability of the tuberculin reaction in such persons (Perez-Stable et al., 1988). Using the two-step procedure at the time of initial testing will identify many of the conversions due to "boosting" (anamnestic reaction) which might otherwise be subsequently classified as new infections (Perez-Stable et al., 1988; Barry et al., 1987).

The problem of identifying new tuberculosis infections in correctional institutions is not so difficult because boosted reactions are relatively infrequent in this age group (Thompson et al., 1979). Repeated tuberculin testing in a large state prison with 7–18 tuberculosis cases per year showed a conversion rate from a negative to a positive tuberculin test of 9% per year (Stead, 1978). Since that time, tuberculosis has been recognized as a serious threat because of gross overcrowding in correctional institutions and the ease of air-borne spread of infection (Centers for Disease Control, 1989b).

A growing problem concerns tuberculosis transmission in shelters for the homeless. The presence of an untreated infectious case of tuberculosis in these often crowded, poorly ventilated buildings confers a considerable risk of infection for the other clients and the shelter personnel (Nolan et al., 1991).

Intrinsic Susceptibility

A review of the foregoing shows that the determinants of becoming infected are extrinsic to the exposed person, or, in other words, environmental. However, there is evidence that there may also be an intrinsic risk factor. When exposed similarly in nursing homes and prisons, blacks were more likely to become positive tuberculin reactors than whites (Stead et al., 1990). While the reason(s) for this difference is unknown, the existence of differences between groups in the risk of becoming infected when exposed makes it likely that there are also differences between individuals that have not yet been detected.

B. Risk of Developing Tuberculosis Following Infection

Relatively few studies have been able to investigate the factors that influence whether or not an infected person will develop tuberculosis. Although most of them were done 25 or more years ago, the relative risks are still likely to be relevant.

Time and Place

The change in risk of disease occurring after infection is not known with respect to calendar time. There are, however, some data showing that the risk of disease is highest shortly after receipt of infection and that it declines thereafter. Findings from a controlled trial of isoniazid prophylaxis among contacts of active tuberculosis cases and a trial among mental hospital patients can be combined to yield a reasonable estimate (Ferebee, 1970). In these two trials, 1472 persons allocated to the placebo regimen converted from a negative to a positive tuberculin reaction at some time within the first study year. Fifty-four percent of the new cases that developed during a 7-year period occurred during that first year, the year in which they became reactors. Twenty-nine percent developed during the next 3 years, and 17% during the last 3 years. In South India, the risk of developing tuberculosis was 2.6% within the first year after infection and only 0.5% during the next 3 years (Krishna Murthy et al., 1976).

Incidence of tuberculosis among tuberculin reactors varies by place, probably related to intensity of exposure. Among 265,488 tuberculin reactors with negative chest radiographs who participated in a mass campaign in 1950–1952 in Denmark (exclusive of Copenhagen), the average annual incidence over the next 12 years was 29 per 100,000 (Horwitz et al., 1969). At the other extreme was the Inuit population in the Yukon-Kuskokwim delta of Alaska, where the average annual incidence rate from 1957 to 1964 was over 500 per 100,000 persons with initially negative chest radiographs, virtually all of whom were tuberculin reactors (Comstock et al., 1967). In Denmark in the 1960s, rural tuberculin reactors 15–44 years of age had a risk of subsequently developing tuberculosis that was only 60% of the risk for their urban counterparts (Horwitz et al., 1969).

Personal Characteristics

Age

Among tuberculosis contacts in British Columbia and Saskatchewan, Canada, who had positive tuberculin reactions, the frequency of active tuberculosis discovered during a 6-month period following diagnosis of the index case varied markedly with the age of the contact (Grzybowski et al., 1975). The inverse association with age held true for total active cases as well as those whose diagnosis was confirmed by sputum examination. A similar pattern by age was observed in South India (Krishna Murthy et al., 1976). The higher risk among younger contacts may have resulted in part from the fact that a higher proportion of infections among young people are likely to have been recent.

The incidence of tuberculosis among tuberculin reactors by age was investigated as a by-product of a controlled trial of BCG vaccination in Puerto Rico (Comstock et al., 1974b). Among 82,269 tuberculin reactors aged 1–18 years who were followed for 18–20 years, 1400 cases of tuberculosis were identified. As shown in Figure 1, there were two peaks of incidence. One occurred among children in the 1- to 4-year age group, probably reflecting the fact that

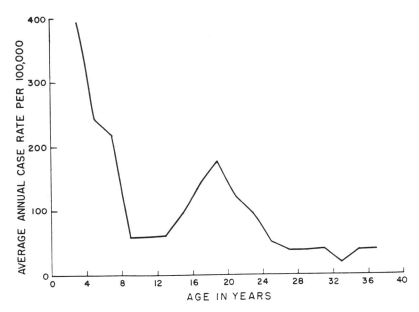

Figure 1 Incidence of tuberculosis among Puerto Rican children who were reactors to tuberculin, by age when tuberculosis was first diagnosed. (Reprinted with permission from Comstock et al., 1974b.)

these infections must have been recent. The second peak occurred during late adolescence and early adult life and was experienced by all birth cohorts as they passed through this period of life. A similar peak was noted among British adolescents though at a slightly lower age (Sutherland, 1966). The cause of increased incidence at this age, even for persons infected in early childhood, is unknown. The risk among older adults is not well established, but all evidence points to the persistence of at least a low risk of developing tuberculosis during the lifetime of infected persons. For this reason, life expectancy becomes a major determinant of the lifetime risk of developing tuberculosis among tuberculin reactors.

Sex

In both a low-prevalence area, Denmark, and a high-prevalence area, Alaska, male and female reactors showed a peak of incidence around 25–34 years of age, with female rates being higher during this period and slightly lower than male reactor rates at older ages (Horwitz et al., 1969; Comstock et al., 1967). In striking contrast was the experience of strong tuberculin reactors identified in the controlled trial of BCG vaccination in South India (Tuberculosis Prevention

Table 3 Age-Adjusted[a] Prevalence of Active Tuberculosis Among *Infected* Tuberculosis Contacts in British Columbia and Saskatchewan by Race, Type of Contact, and Sputum Status of Source Case 1966–1971

Sputum status of source case	Prevalence (%)			
	Indian contacts		White contacts	
	Intimate	Casual	Intimate	Casual
Positive smear	14.4	10.0	14.0	8.2
Positive culture only	5.1	3.9	5.0	6.2
Negative culture	3.0	0	2.3	0

[a]Adjusted to age distribution of total study population.
Source: Grzybowski et al., 1975.

Trial, Madras, 1980). During the first $7\frac{1}{2}$ years of follow-up observation, the average annual age-adjusted new case rate among persons over the age of 15 years was 160 per 100,000 for male reactors and only 54 for females. This discrepancy was present at all ages but was most marked after the age of 35 years.

Race

Race per se appears to have little influence on the risk of disease once infection has occurred. Case rates were not significantly different among black and white reactors in Georgia and Alabama (Comstock and Palmer, 1966) or among Navy recruits (Comstock et al., 1974a). As can be seen in Table 3, Indian and white reactors in Canada also had similar rates when age, intimacy of contact, and infectiousness of source case had been controlled (Grzybowski et al., 1975).

Dosage of Infection

The findings shown in Table 3 also bear on the relationship of dosage of infection to the risk of developing tuberculosis (Grzybowski et al., 1975). All the subjects in this study were tuberculin reactors and can be considered to have been infected. Because the risk of disease was greatest among those exposed to the most infectious cases and among those with the closest contact, the conclusion seems inescapable that persons infected with larger numbers of tubercle bacilli are at greater risk than those infected with smaller numbers of organisms.

A study in Mysore State, India also showed that among contacts who were strongly positive tuberculin reactors, development of pulmonary disease was most likely among those with the most intense exposure, i.e., the contacts most likely to have received larger doses of infections (Raj Narain et al., 1973).

Size of Tuberculin Reaction

It has been known for several decades that infections with nontuberculous mycobacteria often cause tuberculin sensitivity but rarely result in disease, and also that cross-reactions caused by these organisms are usually smaller than those caused by *M. tuberculosis* (Palmer et al., 1959). Consequently, it is not surprising that where nontuberculous mycobacterial infections are present, small tuberculin reactions are less likely to be caused by infections with tubercle bacilli and hence are less likely to be associated with a risk of subsequent disease than larger reactions. The importance of this risk was illustrated by a study of Puerto Rican children (Comstock et al., 1974a). Children with reactions measuring 16 mm or more in diameter to 1 Tuberculin Unit of a purified tuberculin had a subsequent risk of tuberculous disease more than five times greater than children with reactions of 6–10 mm following a test with 10 Tuberculin Units of a purified tuberculin. The prognostic importance of this widely available risk factor has only recently been recognized in recommended standards for tuberculosis control (American Thoracic Society, 1990).

Immunosuppression

The fact that the great majority of persons do not develop tuberculosis after they have been infected indicates the ability of the normal immune system to hold the infecting organisms in abeyance or even in some instances to eradicate them. Treatment with immunosuppressive agents can upset this balance, as can infections with the human immunodeficiency virus (HIV). Tuberculosis is reported to be rampant in populations who have dual infections with both the tubercle bacillus and the human immunodeficiency virus. An illustration of the magnitude of this risk is afforded by a longitudinal study among intravenous drug users in New York City (Selwyn et al., 1989). No cases of tuberculosis were observed among 298 reactors who were HIV-negative, compared to eight among 215 HIV-positive persons. Seven of the tuberculosis cases occurred among 36 who were known to have been positive tuberculin reactors and who had not received isoniazid chemoprophylaxis, a case rate of nearly 20,000 per 100,000.

The well-documented, temporary loss of tuberculin sensitivity following measles has been equated with immunosuppression, and hence increased susceptibility to activation of a latent tuberculosis infection. However, a careful review of the pertinent literature failed to substantiate the widespread belief that measles predisposes tuberculin reactors to the development of tuberculous disease (Flick, 1976).

Relative Weight

Among the few benefits of being overweight is its association with protection against tuberculosis. Among white male recruits with positive tuberculin reactions and negative chest radiographs on entry to the Navy, those who were 10%

or more underweight were 3.4 times more likely to develop tuberculosis than those who were 10% or more overweight (Edwards et al., 1971).

Socioeconomic Status

There is almost no evidence on the relationship of social and economic factors to the development of tuberculous disease among tuberculin reactors. In Muscogee County, Georgia, the incidence of tuberculosis among reactors during the period 1950–1962 showed no association with the quality of their housing as recorded in a private census in 1946 (Comstock and Palmer, 1966). This held true for both whites and blacks. There are no data on reactors living under conditions of extreme deprivation, although anecdotal evidence indicates a high risk.

C. Risk of Reactivation of Disease

The third risk to be considered in etiological epidemiology is relapse, namely the risk of developing active disease following spontaneous or therapeutically associated "cure." Relatively little is known about these risks except for those related to chemotherapy.

Inadequate Chemotherapy

Chemotherapy has made an almost miraculous improvement in the prognosis for persons who develop tuberculosis. Conscientious adherence to an appropriate regimen comes close to guaranteeing a lasting cure (American Thoracic Society, 1986; Fox, 1968). It is not surprising, therefore, that poor compliance with therapy is a major risk factor not only for treatment failure, but also for relapse after apparent cure (Stead and Jurgens, 1973; Nakielna et al., 1975; Kopanoff et al., 1988). Presence of drug-resistant tubercle bacilli is also an important risk factor for relapse. In 12 controlled trials of short-course chemotherapy, patients with bacilli resistant to streptomycin or isoniazid were much more likely to relapse than patients with bacilli sensitive to these drugs (Mitchison and Nunn, 1986).

Time

The risk of relapse by calendar time has clearly been influenced by the markedly reduced risk following the introduction of chemotherapy. In Denmark, after the introduction of isoniazid into the therapeutic regimen, the relapse rate fell from nearly 13% to 6% (Horwitz, 1969).

The risk of relapse by time following completion of therapy has also been influenced by the introduction of chemotherapy. Prior to its introduction, relapse was most likely to occur shortly after treatment stopped (Comstock, 1962; Edwards et al., 1972); after chemotherapy was introduced, relapses were less likely during the year or two following adequate treatment (Pamra et al., 1976; Chan-Yeung et al., 1971).

Age, Sex, and Race

Relapse rates by age do not show a consistent pattern. In untreated persons whose disease was judged to be inactive or fibrotic at the time of diagnosis, reactivation was less likely with increasing age (Comstock, 1962; Springett, 1972). Among persons whose disease became inactive after treatment, relapse rates went up with age in Denmark (Horwitz, 1969) and showed no significant trend with age in India (Pamra et al., 1976). There was a tendency for relapse rates to be somewhat higher in males than females (Horwitz, 1969; Pamra et al., 1976; Springett, 1972) though not in all populations (Nakielna et al., 1975). Reactivation rates were more common among Canadian Indians than other Canadians (Nakielna et al., 1975) and in the state of Georgia, more common among blacks than whites (Comstock, 1962).

Socioeconomic Status

Among blacks in Georgia, degree of skin pigmentation was not related to the risk of relapse, suggesting that socioeconomic factors might be more important than race per se (Comstock, 1962). Another indication that social or economic factors might play a role came from a geographic comparison of relapse rates in Denmark (Horwitz, 1969). Relapse rates among residents of Copenhagen were higher than among persons living in the more rural areas of Denmark.

Extent of Disease

In Georgia and in Europe, reactivation in untreated persons was much more likely among persons with extensive fibrotic disease than among those with only minimal lesions (Comstock, 1962; International Union Against Tuberculosis Committee on Prophylaxis, 1982). A similar finding was reported among previously treated patients in Wisconsin and South Africa (Stead and Jurgens, 1973; Cowie et al., 1989).

III. Administrative Epidemiology

Information on tuberculosis morbidity and mortality is voluminous compared to that which is available for etiological epidemiology. Even so, most of it is based on official reports and can be related only to time, place, race, sex, and age. Hard data on other risk factors are sparse. The available information on many aspects of administrative epidemiology is included in other chapters.

A. Time and Place

The reported incidence of tuberculosis in the United States had been declining at an average rate of 6% each year for several decades until 1985 (Centers for

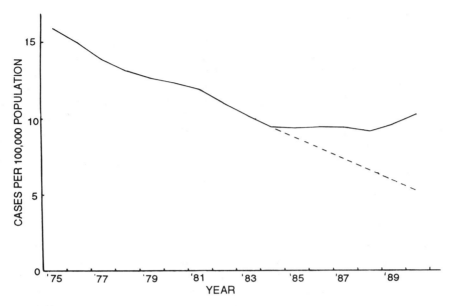

Figure 2 Reported cases of tuberculosis per 100,000 by year, United States, 1975–1990, with estimated number of cases if rate of decline from 1975 to 1985 had continued. (Adapted from Robinson and Comstock, 1992.)

Disease Control, 1990b, 1991). Since that time, the case rate has risen from 9.3 per 100,000 in 1985 to 10.3 in 1990. As shown in Figure 2, a continuation of the previous downward trend would have brought the case rate in 1990 to half of that which was actually reported. Much of the excess in observed cases over those expected can be attributed to the high incidence of tuberculosis among persons dually infected with tubercle bacilli and the human immunodeficiency virus (HIV). This is particularly noticeable in the New York City metropolitan area and in Florida. However, the decline in tuberculosis case rates in small cities and rural areas also came to a halt in 1985 (Robinson and Comstock, 1992). It is likely that the considerable reduction in tuberculosis control efforts during the past decade has also contributed to the resurgence of tuberculosis (Brudney and Dobkin, 1991).

Tuberculosis is more common in large cities than in rural areas (Centers for Disease Control, 1991; Medical Research Council Tuberculosis and Chest Diseases Unit, 1986). In the United States in 1975 and 1989, the rates were highest in cities with populations greater than 500,000, intermediate in smaller cities, and lowest in rural areas and towns with populations less than 100,000. The rate of decrease for that 14-year period was only 21% in the largest cities compared to 47% in the least densely populated areas (Centers for Disease Control, 1977, 1991). Even so, half the cases came from the rural areas and small towns in 1989.

A number of other developed countries have experienced a slowing in the rate of decline of their tuberculosis case rates, and Japan has had a reversal (Kochi, 1991). Although firm data are hard to obtain for most underdeveloped nations, it appears that in general there has been a slow downward trend. A major exception is sub-Saharan Africa where the high frequency of persons infected with both HIV and *M. tuberculosis* has resulted in a dramatic increase in tuberculosis (Kochi, 1991).

Influx of immigrants from areas where the prevalence of tuberculosis is high can also affect temporal trends in some areas. In British Columbia, Canada, tuberculosis case rates decreased from 1970 to 1985 except for the city of Vancouver (Enarson et al., 1989). On investigation, it was found that the failure of the rates to decline in Vancouver was due to selective immigration into the poorer areas of the city of a group of high-risk, socially disadvantaged immigrants.

Not all the considerable geographical differences can be explained by stage of economic development, immigration, or prevalence of HIV infections. Case rates within the original European Community varied from 7.4 to 31.9 per 100,000 in 1983; among six members of the Eastern Bloc, the range was 20.3 to 72.8 (Tala, 1987). The Netherlands and four of the Scandinavian countries had the lowest rates. Rates in England and Wales ranged from 3.1 in Anglia to 37.0 per 100,000 in some boroughs of London in 1983 (Medical Research Council Tuberculosis and Chest Diseases Unit, 1986), while among the 50 United States the case rate in 1988–1989 ranged from 0.8 in Wyoming to 17.3 in New York (Centers for Disease Control, 1991). Unfortunately, interpretation of geographical variations is more difficult than generally recognized. Within the United States in 1989, the percentage of pulmonary cases not bacteriologically confirmed varied from 0.8 to 32.1 percent among states with 20 or more reported cases (Centers for Disease Control, 1991). Considerable variations between nations in both the extent and nature of cases of pulmonary tuberculosis have also been recorded (Horwitz and Comstock, 1973).

B. Age, Race, and Sex

In the United States, case rates are low in infancy and decrease slightly during childhood (Centers for Disease Control, 1991). After adolescence, they show a generally steady increase with age (Fig. 3). White rates are lower than nonwhite rates; female rates are lower than male rates. In underdeveloped countries, the highest reported rates are likely to be among young adults (Raj Narain et al., 1973; Styblo, 1991). In India, females have higher rates than males in young adult life, while in Tanzania, male rates are higher throughout adult life.

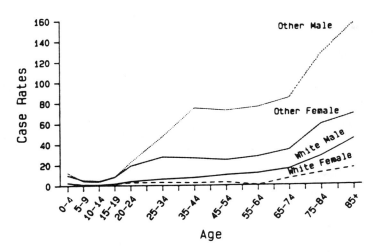

Note: Case rate per 100,000 population.

Figure 3 Tuberculosis case rates, United States, 1989, by race, sex, and age. (Reprinted from Centers for Disease Control, 1991.)

The age-adjusted trends in tuberculosis rates in the United States are shown in Figure 4 by race and sex for the years 1977–1989 (Centers for Disease Control, 1991; National Center for Health Statistics, 1985). For all four race-sex groups, there is a general downward trend through 1984. During this period, the average percentage decline each year was almost identical for the four groups. After 1984, the rates level off, and even increase somewhat for nonwhite males and females in 1989.

C. Socioeconomic Status

The association of tuberculosis with poor socioeconomic status has long been noted (Lowell et al., 1969; Osler and McCrae, 1926) and perhaps is even stronger today. Decades ago, homeless men in New York City's skid row were found to have high rates of tuberculosis (Chaves et al., 1961); a similar excess was noted among unmarried men living in central Copenhagen (Horwitz, 1971). The situation has been aggravated recently by the increase in homeless persons and the continued high frequency of tuberculosis among them (VonVille et al., 1991). Further aggravation comes from the tendency of poor immigrants to crowd into large cities (Enarson et al., 1989; Froggatt, 1985). Their tuberculosis risk reflects the prevalence of the disease in their native countries; the risk decreases with their duration of stay in their adopted homes (Enarson et al., 1990; Sutherland et al., 1984; Centers for Disease Control, 1987; Nolan and Elarth, 1988).

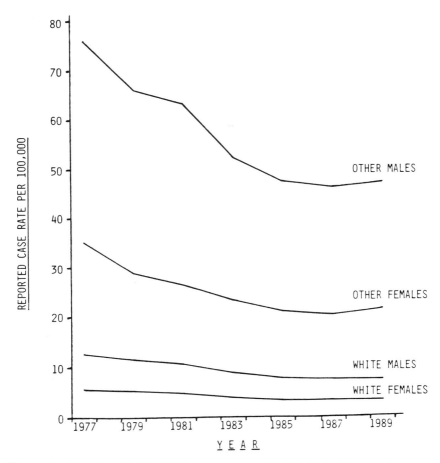

Figure 4 Age-adjusted tuberculosis case rates per 100,000, United States, 1977–1989, by race and sex. (Data from National Center for Health Statistics, 1985, and Centers for Disease Control, 1986, 1991.)

D. Institutional Living

Poverty being associated with crime, it is not surprising that tuberculosis is often a problem among inmates of correctional institutions. Various surveys have estimated the frequency of tuberculosis to be increasing among such populations and to be three to six times higher than expected from rates in the general population (Centers of Disease Control, 1989b).

Tuberculosis among persons living and working in nursing homes and other facilities providing long-term medical care has only recently been recognized as a problem (Stead et al., 1985). A survey of 29 states suggested that the case rate for patients was approximately 50% higher and the rate among employees was three times higher than expected from the rates in similar age-sex groups in the general population (Centers for Disease Control, 1990a).

E. Special Medical Situations

A variety of medical conditions are associated with tuberculosis. Although these risk factors are presumably limited to persons already infected with *M. tuberculosis*, studies to substantiate this presumption are few and rarely definitive. By far the most important is immunosuppression, particularly that resulting from infection with the human immunodeficiency virus (Centers for Disease Control, 1989a; Braun et al., 1991). Other causes of immunosuppression that are also accompanied by an increased tuberculosis risk are treatment with immunosuppressive drugs including prolonged adrenocorticosteroid therapy, some hematological and reticuloendothelial diseases such as leukemia and lymphoma, and end-stage renal disease (American Thoracic Society, 1986).

Silicosis has long been linked with tuberculosis, so much so that silicotuberculosis is an accepted disease entity. Although the causal nature of this association is largely based on uncontrolled reports (Snider, 1978), silica dust has been shown to have an adverse effect on tuberculosis in animals (Rich, 1944).

Diabetes, too, has been accepted as a risk factor for tuberculosis for a long time (Pinner, 1945). Two studies in the 1950s indicated that the prevalence among diabetics was approximately four times that in a comparable general population, and that the risk was greatest among those with severe diabetes (Boucot et al., 1952; Oscarsson and Silwer, 1958).

Alcoholism and drug addiction are also associated with tuberculosis, although it is not clear whether these diseases increase susceptibility to tuberculosis, or whether conditions conducive to substance abuse are similar to those leading to tuberculosis. In any case, alcoholism was well known to physicians in tuberculosis sanatoria, since 10–30% of patients were reported to be alcoholics (Lowell et al., 1969). Current surveys also show the high prevalence of tuberculosis among alcoholics and drug addicts (Friedman et al., 1987).

F. Genetic Susceptibility

In the 19th century, it was commonly believed that tuberculosis was a hereditary disease (Dubos and Dubos, 1952). In the early part of the present century, Karl Pearson and Raymond Pearl each attempted to disentangle the hereditary and environmental factors that led to the familial concentration of tuberculosis (Pinner, 1945), investigations that were continued in the Williamson County Tuberculosis Study by Ruth Puffer (Puffer, 1944). Subsequent studies of monozygotic and dizygotic twins indicated that some degree of susceptibility was inherited (Comstock, 1978).

Because of these indications of genetic susceptibility, investigators have looked for associations of tuberculosis with various genetic markers. Among Inuits in Alaska, tuberculosis was more prevalent among persons with blood groups B and AB than among those with blood groups O or A (Overfield and Klauber, 1980). Although various human leukocyte antigen types have also been suspected of playing a role in tuberculosis susceptibility, no consistent associations have been found (Hwang et al., 1985; Hawkins et al., 1988).

G. Nontuberculous Mycobacterial Infections

In a series of experiments unlikely to be rivaled in size and sophistication, Palmer and associates showed that infections with a variety of mycobacteria increased the resistance of guinea pigs against tuberculosis (Palmer and Long, 1966). Evidence of protection was also found among British adolescents, who reacted only to a strong dose of tuberculin, and U.S. Navy recruits, who reacted to antigens prepared from *M. avium-intracellulare* or *M. scofulaceum* but not to the intermediate dose of PPD-tuberculin (Hart and Sutherland, 1977; Edwards et al., 1973). These findings were not confirmed in a large study in Puerto Rico (Comstock et al., 1974a) although it is possible that the nonreactors to the strong dose of tuberculin were like some of Palmer's guinea pigs who failed to react even after two injections of nontuberculous mycobacteria but still showed evidence of some protection. Although the question is unsettled, there is a strong possibility that human infections with nontuberculous mycobacteria do confer some protection against tuberculosis.

H. Psychosocial Stress

Although medical scientists are often hesitant to study the possible effects of mind on the body, there have been persistent hints in the tuberculosis literature that psychological, social, and economic stresses have an adverse effect on tuberculosis (Downes and Price, 1942; Hendricks, 1949; Holmes, 1956). Stress is a common thread running throughout the risk factors of poverty, marital disruption, institutionalization, and substance abuse. A study that controls for many other risk factors involved Navy recruits (Comstock et al., 1974c). White, black, and Filipino men who were tuberculin reactors on entry to the Navy had very similar housing, diet, and income during the first 4 years of their enlistment. Case rates among white and black reactors decreased during this period; case rates among Filipinos increased, possibly because of stresses associated with separation from families and with being a small minority with few social supports.

IV. Conclusion

Although this review of risk factors seems lengthy, it should be noted that much of the information rests on only a few studies and that many of them were performed 30–40 years ago. A particular concern is the current risk of disease following tuberculous infection in a variety of populations. Even small and individually nondefinitive studies of this and other risks would be helpful if they all pointed to the same conclusion. Increased knowledge of current risks of infection and subsequent disease could help greatly in efforts to bring tuberculosis back under control and, in developed countries, could even lead to its elimination in the near future.

References

American Thoracic Society (1986). Treatment of tuberculosis and tuberculosis infection in adults and children. *Am. Rev. Respir. Dis*. **134**:355–363.

American Thoracic Society (1990). Diagnostic standards and classification of tuberculosis. *Am. Rev. Respir. Dis*. **142**:725–735.

Barry, M. A., Regan, A. M., Kunches, L. M., Harris, M. E., Bunce, S. A., and Craven, D. E. (1987). Two-stage tuberculin testing with control antigens in patients residing in two chronic disease hospitals. *J. Am. Geriatr. Soc*. **35**:147–153.

Boucot, K. R., Dillon, E. S., Cooper, D. A., Meier, P., and Richardson, R. (1952). Tuberculosis among diabetics. The Philadelphia survey. *Am. Rev. Respir. Dis*. **65**(No. 1, Part 2):1–50.

Braun, M. M., Badi, N., Ryder, R. W., Baende, E., Mukadi, Y., Nsuami, M., Matela, B., Willame, J-C., Kaboto, M., and Heyward, W. (1991). A retrospective cohort study of the risk of tuberculosis among women of childbearing age with HIV infection in Zaire. *Am. Rev. Respir. Dis*. **143**:501–504.

Brudney, K., and Dobkin, J. (1991). Resurgent tuberculosis in New York City. Human immunodeficiency virus, homelessness, and the decline of tuberculosis control programs. *Am. Rev. Respir. Dis*. **144**:745–749.

Buikstra, J. E., and Cook, D. C. (1981). Pre-Columbian tuberculosis in West-Central Illinois: prehistoric disease in biocultural perspective. In *Prehistoric Tuberculosis in the Americas*. Edited by J. E. Buikstra. Northwestern University Archeological Program, Evanston, IL, pp. 115–139.

Centers for Disease Control (1977). Tuberculosis in the United States, 1975. HEW Publication No. (CDC) 77-8322. Public Health Service, Atlanta, GA.

Centers for Disease Control (1986). 1981–1984 tuberculosis in the United States. HHS Publication No. (CDC) 86-8322. Public Health Service, Atlanta, GA.

Centers for Disease Control (1987). Tuberculosis among Asians/Pacific Islanders—United States, 1985. *MMWR* **36**:331–334.

Centers for Disease Control (1989a). Tuberculosis and human immunodeficiency virus infection: recommendations of the Advisory Committee for Elimination of Tuberculosis (ACET). *MMWR* **38**:236–250.

Centers for Disease Control (1989b). Prevention and control of tuberculosis in correctional institutions: recommendations of the Advisory Committee for Elimination of Tuberculosis. *MMWR* **38**:313–325.

Centers for Disease Control (1990a). Prevention and control of tuberculosis in facilities providing long-term care to the elderly: recommendations of the Advisory Committee for Elimination of Tuberculosis. *MMWR* **39**(RR-10):7–20.

Centers for Disease Control (1990b). Summary of notifiable diseases, United States, 1990. *MMWR* **39**(53):56–57.

Centers for Disease Control (1991). Tuberculosis statistics in the United States, 1989. HHS Publication No. (CDC) 91-8322. Public Health Service, Atlanta, GA.

Chan-Yeung, M., Galbraith, J. D., Schulson, N., Brown, A., and Grzybowski, S. (1971). Reactivation of inactive tuberculosis in Northern Canada. *Am. Rev. Respir. Dis.* **104**:861–865.

Chaves, A. D., Robins, A. B., and Abeles, H. (1961). Tuberculosis case finding among homeless men in New York City. *Am. Rev. Respir. Dis.* **84**:900–901.

Comstock, G. W. (1962). Untreated inactive pulmonary tuberculosis: risk of reactivation. *Public Health Rep.* **77**:461–470.

Comstock, G. W. (1975). Frost revisited: the modern epidemiology of tuberculosis. *Am. J. Epidemiol.* **101**:363–382.

Comstock, G. W. (1978). Tuberculosis in twins: a re-analysis of the Prophit Survey. *Am. Rev. Respir. Dis.* **117**:621–624.

Comstock, G. W., and O'Brien, R. J. (1991). Tuberculosis. In *Bacterial Infections of Humans. Epidemiology and Control*, 2nd ed. Edited by A. S. Evans and P. S. Brachman, Plenum Press, New York, pp. 745–771.

Comstock, G. W., and Palmer, C. E. (1966). Long-term results of BCG vaccination in the southern United States. *Am. Rev. Respir. Dis.* **93**:171–183.

Comstock, G. W., Ferebee, S. H., and Hammes, L. M. (1967). A controlled trial of community-wide isoniazid prophylaxis in Alaska. *Am. Rev. Respir. Dis.* **95**:935–943.

Comstock, G. W., Livesay, V. T., and Woolpert, S. F. (1974a). Evaluation of BCG vaccination among Puerto Rican children. *Am. J. Public Health* **64**:283–291.

Comstock, G. W., Livesay, V. T., and Woolpert, S. F. (1974b). The prognosis of a positive tuberculin reaction in childhood and adolescence. *Am. J. Epidemiol.* **99**:131–138.

Comstock, G. W., Edwards, L. B., and Livesay, V. T. (1974c). Tuberculosis morbidity in the U.S. Navy: its distribution and decline. *Am. Rev. Respir. Dis.* **110**:572–580.

Cowie, R. L., Langton, M. E., and Becklake, M. R. (1989). Pulmonary tuberculosis in South African gold miners. *Am. Rev. Respir. Dis.* **139**:1086–1089.

Cross, E. R., and Hyams, K. C. (1990). Tuberculin skin testing in US Navy and Marine Corps personnel and recruits, 1980–86. *Am. J. Public Health* **80**:435–438.

Downes, J., and Price, C. R. (1942). The importance of family problems in the control of tuberculosis. *Milbank Mem. Fund Q.* **20**:7–22.

Dubos, R., and Dubos, J. (1952). *The White Plague. Tuberculosis, Man and Society.* Little, Brown, Boston.

Edwards, L. B., Acquaviva, F. A., Livesay, V. T., Cross, F. W., and Palmer, C. E. (1969). An atlas of sensitivity to tuberculin, PPD-B, and histoplasmin in the United States. *Am. Rev. Respir. Dis.* **99**(No. 4, Part 2):1–132.

Edwards, L. G., Livesay, V. T., Acquaviva, F. A., and Palmer, C. E. (1971). Height, weight, tuberculous infection, and tuberculous disease. *Arch. Environ. Health* **22**:106–112.

Edwards, L. B., Doster, B., Livesay, V. T., and Ferebee, S. H. (1972). Tuberculosis risk in persons with "fibrotic" lesions. *Bull. Int. Un. Tuberc.* **47**:151–156.

Edwards, L. B., Acquaviva, F. A., and Livesay, V. T. (1973). Identification of tuberculous infected. Dual tests and density of reaction. *Am. Rev. Respir. Dis.* **108**:1334–1339.

Enarson, D. A., Wang, J-S., and Dirks, J. M. (1989). The incidence of active tuberculosis in a large urban area. *Am. J. Epidemiol.* **129**:1268–1276.

Enarson, D. A., Wang, J. S., and Grzybowski, S. (1990). Case-finding in the elimination phase of tuberculosis: tuberculosis in displaced people. *Bull. IUATLD* **65**(2–3):71–72.

Ferebee, S. H. (1970). Controlled chemoprophylaxis trials in tuberculosis. A general review. *Adv. Tuberc. Res.* **17**:28–106.

Flick, J. A. (1976). Does measles really predispose to tuberculosis? *Am. Rev. Respir. Dis.* **114**:257–265.

Fox, W. (1968). The John Barnwell Lecture. Changing concepts in the chemotherapy of pulmonary tuberculosis. *Am. Rev. Respir. Dis.* **97**:767–790.

Friedman, L. N., Sullivan, G. M., Bevilaqua, R. P., and Loscos, R. (1987). Tuberculosis screening in alcoholics and drug addicts. *Am. Rev. Respir. Dis.* **136**:1188–1192.

Froggatt, K. (1985). Tuberculosis: spatial and demographic incidence in Bradford, 1980–82. *J. Epidemiol. Commun. Health* **39**:20–26.

Grzybowski, S., Barnett, G. D., and Styblo. K. (1975). Contacts of cases of active pulmonary tuberculosis. *Bull. Int. Un. Tuberc.* **50**:90–106.

Hart, P. D'A., and Sutherland, I. (1977). BCG and vole bacillus vaccines in the prevention of tuberculosis in adolescence and early adult life. *Br. Med. J.* **2**:293–295.

Hawkins, B. R., Higgins, D. A., Chan, S. L., Lowrie, D. B., Mitchison, D. A., and Girling, D. J. (1988). HLA typing in the Hong Kong Chest Service/British Medical Research Council study of factors associated with the breakdown to active tuberculosis of inactive pulmonary lesions. *Am. Rev. Respir. Dis.* **138**:1616–1621.

Hendricks, C. M. (1949). Psychosomatic aspects of tuberculosis. In *The Fundamentals of Pulmonary Tuberculosis and Its Complications*. Edited by E. W. Hayes. Charles C Thomas, Springfield, IL.

Holmes, T. H. (1956). Multidiscipline studies of tuberculosis. In *Personality, Stress and Tuberculosis*. Edited by P. J. Sparer. International Universities Press, New York.

Horwitz, O. (1969). Public health aspects of relapsing tuberculosis. *Am. Rev. Respir. Dis.* **99**:183–193.

Horwitz, O. (1971). Tuberculosis risk and marital status. *Am. Rev. Respir. Dis.* **104**:22–31.

Horwitz, O., and Comstock, G. W. (1973). What is a case of tuberculosis? The tuberculosis case spectrum in eight countries evaluated from 1235 case histories and roentgenograms. *Int. J. Epidemiol.*, **2**:145–152.

Horwitz, O., Wilbek, E., and Erickson, P. A. (1969). Epidemiological basis of tuberculosis eradication. 10. Longitudinal studies on the risk of tuberculosis in the general population of a low prevalence area. *Bull. WHO* **41**:95–113.

Hwang, C-H., Khan, S., Ende, N., Mangura, B. T., Reichman, L. B., and Chou, J. (1985). The HLA-A, -B, and -DR phenotypes and tuberculosis. *Am. Rev. Respir. Dis.* **132**:382–385.

International Union Against Tuberculosis Committee on Prophylaxis. (1982). Efficacy of various durations of isoniazid preventive therapy for tuberculosis: five years of follow-up in the IUAT trial. *Bull. WHO* **60**:555–564.

Kamat, S. R., Dawson, J. J. Y., Devadatta, S., Fox, W., Janardhanam, B., Radhakrishna, S., Ramakrishnan, C. V., Somasundaram, P. R., Stott, H., and Velu, S. (1966). A controlled study of the influence of segregation of tuberculous patients for one year on the attack rate of tuberculosis in a 5-year period in close family contacts in south India. *Bull. WHO* **34**:517–532.

Kaplan, G. J., Fraser, R. I., and Comstock, G. W. (1972). Tuberculosis in Alaska, 1970. The continued decline of the tuberculosis epidemic. *Am. Rev. Respir. Dis.* **105**:920–926.

Kochi, A. (1991). The global tuberculosis situation and the new control strategy of the World Health Organization. *Tubercle* **72**:1–6.

Kopanoff, D. E., Snider, D. E., Jr., and Johnson, M. (1988). Recurrent tuberculosis: why do patients develop disease again? *Am. J. Public Health* **78**:30–33.

Krishna Murthy, V. V., Nair, S. S., Gothi, G. D., and Chakraborty, A. K. (1976). Incidence of tuberculosis among newly infected population and in relation to the duration of infected status. *Indian J. Tuberc.* **33**:3–7.

Loudon, R. G., and Spohn, S. K. (1969). Cough frequency and infectivity in patients with pulmonary tuberculosis. *Am. Rev. Respir. Dis.* **99**:109–111.

Lowell, A. M., Edwards, L. B., and Palmer, C. E. (1969). *Tuberculosis*. Harvard University Press, Cambridge, MA, pp. 129–166.

Medical Research Council Tuberculosis and Chest Diseases Unit (1986). The geographical distribution of tuberculosis notifications in a national survey of England and Wales in 1983. *Tubercle* **67**:163–178.

Mitchison, D. A., and Nunn, A. J. (1986). Influence of initial drug resistance on the response to short-course chemotherapy of pulmonary tuberculosis. *Am. Rev. Respir. Dis.* **133**:423–430.

Nakielna, E. M., Cragg, R., and Grzybowski, S. (1975). Lifelong follow-up of inactive tuberculosis: its value and limitations. *Am. Rev. Respir. Dis.* **112**:765–772.

National Center for Health Statistics: *Vital Statistics of the United States, 1980*. (1985). *Volume II, Mortality, Part A*. DHHS Publication No. (PHS) 85-1101. Public Health Service, U.S. Government Printing Office, Washington, D.C.

Nolan, C. M., and Elarth, A. M. (1988). Tuberculosis in a cohort of southeast Asian refugees. *Am. Rev. Respir. Dis.* **137**:805–809.

Nolan, C. M., Elarth, A. M., Barr, H., Mahdi Saeed, A., and Risser, D. R. (1991). An outbreak of tuberculosis in a shelter for homeless men. *Am. Rev. Respir. Dis.* **143**:257–261.

Oscarsson, P. N., and Silwer, H. (1958). II. Incidence of pulmonary tuberculosis among diabetics. Search among diabetics in the county of Kristianstad. *Acta Med. Scand.* **161**(Suppl 335):23–48.

Osler, W., and McCrae, T. (1926). *The Principles and Practice of Medicine*, 10th ed. D. Appleton, New York, p. 161.

Overfield, T., and Klauber, M. R. (1980). Prevalence of tuberculosis in Eskimos having blood group B gene. *Hum. Biol.* **52**:87–92.

Palmer, C. E., and Long, M. W. (1966). Effects of infection with atypical mycobacteria on BCG vaccination and tuberculosis. *Am. Rev. Respir. Dis.* **94**:553–568.

Palmer, C. E., Edwards, L. B., Hopwood, L., and Edwards, P. Q. (1959). Experimental and epidemiologic basis for the interpretation of tuberculin sensitivity. *J. Pediatr.* **55**:413–429.

Pamra, S. P., Prasad, G., and Mathur, G. P. (1976). Relapse in pulmonary tuberculosis. *Am. Rev. Respir. Dis.* **113**:67–72.

Perez-Stable, E. J., Flaherty, D., Schecter, G., Slutkin, G., and Hopewell, P. C. (1988). Conversion and reversion of tuberculin reactions in nursing home residents. *Am. Rev. Respir. Dis.* **137**:801–804.

Pinner, M. (1945). *Pulmonary Tuberculosis in the Adult. Its Fundamental Aspects.* Charles C Thomas, Springfield, IL, p. 190.

Puffer, R. R. (1944). *Familial Susceptibility to Tuberculosis.* Harvard University Press, Cambridge, MA.

Raj Narain, Nair, S. S., Ramanatha Rao, G. R., and Chandrasekhar, P. (1966). Distribution of tuberculous infection and disease among households in a rural community. *Bull. WHO* **34**:639–654.

Raj Narain, Naganna, K., and Murthy, S. S. (1973). Incidence of pulmonary tuberculosis. *Am. Rev. Respir. Dis.* **107**:992–1001.

Reichman, L. B., and O'Day, R. (1978). Tuberculous infection in a large urban population. *Am. Rev. Respir. Dis.* **117**:705–712.

Rich, A. R. (1944). *The Pathogenesis of Tuberculosis.* Charles C Thomas, Springfield, IL. pp. 636–637.

Rieder, H. L., Cauthen, G. M., Comstock, G. W., and Snider, D. E. Jr. (1989). Epidemiology of tuberculosis in the United States. *Epidemiol. Rev.* **11**:79–98.

Riley, R. L., and Moodie, A. S. (1974). Infectivity of patients with pulmonary tuberculosis in inner city homes. *Am. Rev. Respir. Dis.* **110**:810–812.

Riley, R. L., Mills, C. C., O'Grady, F., Sultan, L. U., Wittstadt, F., and Shivpuri, D. N. (1962). Infectiousness of air from a tuberculosis ward. Ultraviolet irradiation of infected air: comparative infectiousness of different patients. *Am. Rev. Respir. Dis.* **85**:511–525.

Robinson, D. B., and Comstock, G. W. (1992). Tuberculosis in a small semirural county. *Public Health Rep.* **107**:179–182.

Rust, P., and Thomas, J. (1975). A method for estimating the prevalence of tuberculosis infection. *Am. J. Epidemiol.* **101**:311–322.

Selwyn, P. A., Hartel, D., Lewis, V. A., Schoenbaum, E. E., Vermund, S. H., Klein, R. S., Walker, A. T., and Friedland, G. H. (1989). A prospective study of the risk of tuberculosis among intravenous drug users with human immunodeficiency virus infection. *N. Eng. J. Med.* **320**:545–550.

Snider, D. E., Jr. (1978). The relationship between tuberculosis and silicosis. *Am. Rev. Respir. Dis.* **118**:455–460.

Snider, D. E. Jr., Kelly, G. D., Cauthen, G. M., Thompson, N. J., and Kilburn, J. O. (1985). Infection and disease among contacts of tuberculosis cases with drug-resistant and drug-susceptible bacilli. *Am. Rev. Respir. Dis.* **132**:125–132.

Springett, V. H. (1972). Tuberculosis risk in persons with "fibrotic" lesions. *Bull. Int. Un. Tuberc.* **47**:157–159.

Stead, W. W. (1978). Undetected tuberculosis in prison. *JAMA* **240**:2544–2547.

Stead, W. W., Lofgren, J. P., Warren, E., and Thomas C. (1985). Tuberculosis as an endemic and nosocomial infection among the elderly in nursing homes. *N. Engl. J. Med.* **312**:1483–1487.

Stead, W. W., Senner, J. W., Reddick, W. T., and Lofgren, J. P. (1990). Racial differences in susceptibility to infection by *Mycobacterium tuberculosis*. *N. Engl. J. Med.* **322**:422–427.

Styblo, K. (1976). Surveillance of tuberculosis. *Int. J. Epidemiol.* **5**:63–68.

Styblo, K. (1991). The impact of HIV infection on the global epidemiology of tuberculosis. *Bull. IUATLD* **66**:27–32.

Sutherland, I. (1966). The evolution of clinical tuberculosis in adolescents (abstract). *Tubercle* **47**:308.

Sutherland, I., and Fayers, P. M. (1975). The association of the risk of tuberculous infection with age. TSRU Report No. 3. *Bull. Int. Un. Tuberc.* **51**:70–81.

Sutherland, I., Springett, V. H., and Nunn, A. J. (1984). Changes in tuberculosis notification rates in ethnic groups in England between 1971 and 1978–79. *Tubercle* **65**:83–91.

Tala, E. (1987). Registration of tuberculosis in Europe. *Bull. Int. Un. Tuberc. Lung Dis.* **62**(1–2):74–76.

Thompson, N. J., Glassroth, J. L., Snider, D. E., Jr., and Farer, L. S. (1979). The booster phenomenon in serial tuberculin testing. *Am. Rev. Respir. Dis.* **119**:587–597.

Tuberculosis Prevention Trial, Madras. (1980). Trial of BCG vaccines in South India for tuberculosis prevention. *Indian J. Med. Res.* **72**(Suppl):1–74.

VonVille, P., Holtzhauer, F., Long, T., Phurrough, A., Murphy, D., Mortensen, B. K., Horst, G., and Halpin, T. J. (1991). Tuberculosis among residents of shelters for the homeless—Ohio, 1990. *MMWR* **40**:869–877.

3

Bacteriology of Tuberculosis

JACQUES H. GROSSET

Faculté de Médecine Pitié-Salpêtrière
Paris, France

I. General Characteristics of the Tubercle Bacillus

Although tubercle bacilli include all members of the "tuberculosis complex," e.g., *Mycobacterium tuberculosis*, *M. bovis*, *M. africanum*, and *M. microti* or "vole bacillus," a rarely encountered organism closely related to *M. tuberculosis*, this latter species will be considered as type species of tubercle bacilli because of its clinical importance.

A. Physical and Chemical Characteristics

Optical Microscopy

M. tuberculosis is a thin rod, with round extremities, 2–5 µm long and 0.2–0.3 µm thick. Nonmotile, without capsule, spore, and true branching, it is difficult to stain with usual staining methods. But stained with the classic carbol fuchsin or Ziehl-Neelsen method, it resists decolorization with strong mineral acids and alcohol, hence the term "acid-alcohol fast," and appears at microscope examination as curved or straight small red or pink rods. Stained with a fluorochrome dye, it appears as fluorescent under blue light. In pathological specimens, it occurs as single rod or small packs or even cords.

In aging cultures or in clinical specimens from patients on chemotherapy, tubercle bacilli are frequently not solidly stained, an appearance probably related to loss of viability. Acid-alcohol fastness of *M. tuberculosis*, which is not constant at all stages in the growth cycle, may disappear when the organism is submitted to the action of isoniazid, a thioamide, or even high concentrations of penicillin.

Electron Microscopy

The cell wall of *M. tuberculosis*, like that of other mycobacteria, has a total thickness of about 20 nm and appears to consist of an inner, electron-dense layer surrounded by an outer, electron-transparent layer (Draper, 1982). No outer membrane covers the outer layer of the wall, as is the case with Gram-negative bacteria. Mycobacteria are therefore structurally related to the Gram-positive bacteria, which have no such outer membrane.

The inner membrane or plasma membrane, which limits the cytoplasm, has the classic triple-layered shape. The cytoplasm of mycobacteria contains an elongated fibrillar mass of DNA in the center of the cell, numerous ribosomes, polyphosphate granules, and lipid droplets or vacuoles.

Chemical Cell Wall Structure and Composition

The mycobacterial wall structure has many similarities with that of other bacteria. The basic or "backbone" structure is the peptidoglycan, a polymer of *N*-acetylglucosamine and *N*-acetylmuramic acid common to almost all bacteria. More specific are the lipopolysaccharide side chains that are branched on the muramic acids. The lipopolysaccharide is made of arabinogalactan, a polysaccharide present among bacteria of the genera *Mycobacterium*, *Corynebacterium*, and *Nocardia*, which is esterified at its distal end with mycolic acids (Fig. 1). These are fatty acids with about 70 carbon atoms, which are also present in *Corynebacteria* and *Nocardia* but with smaller molecular weights and constitute the major part of the outer layer of the cell wall. Arabinogalactan moiety, which is used as antigen in the Middebrook and Dubos serological test (Grange, 1984), is immunologically active but cross-reacts with antisera prepared against corynebacteria and nocardia as well as all mycobacterial species. Mycolic acids play a major role in acid fastness of mycobacteria (Barsdale and Kim, 1977).

In addition to the above components, *M. tuberculosis* is capable of synthesizing a wide variety of other complex molecules, associated with the outer layer of cell wall (Minnikin, 1982). Among them, sulfatides or sulfated acyl trehaloses might play a role in virulence because they prevented phagosome-lysosome fusion in cultured macrophages infected with *M. tuberculosis*. The "cord factor," a trehalose dimycolate, initially thought to be characteristic of

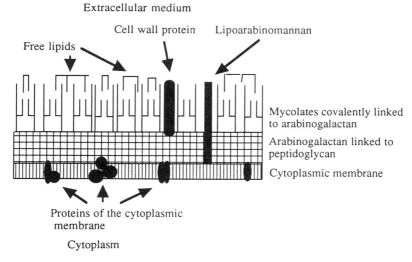

Figure 1 Scheme of mycobacterial cell wall.

virulent strains, has been demonstrated in all mycobacterial species. Mycosides are either phenol-phtiocerol glycosides or peptidoglycolipids. Among the former, mycosides A, related to the phenolic glycolipid of *M. leprae*, have been isolated from *M. kansasii*, mycosides B from *M. bovis*, and mycosides G from *M. marinum*. Mycobacterial peptidoglycolipids, termed C mycosides, have been isolated from *M. avium-intracellulare* and *scrofulaceum* strains (MAIS complex). They have been shown to have phage-binding properties and to be serologically active and type specific and are used in a seroagglutination technique for identification and classification. Finally, several waxes, especially phtiocerol dimycocerosates, and triacylglycerols or triglycerides have been isolated from *M. tuberculosis* strains. Their presence increases the overall impermeability of the mycobacterial cell wall.

Walls of *M. tuberculosis* also contain proteins and peptides, which have strong tuberculin-like activity. In addition, a protein acting as receptor for iron uptake has been isolated from *M. smegmatis* (Hall et al., 1987) and, more recently, a structural protein that has some similarities with the outer membrane protein F or OmpF of *E. coli*, and a L-glutamine polymer that might be a reservoir of carbon and nitrogen (Hirschfield et al., 1990).

Because of its thickness and high content in lipids, the cell wall of *M. tuberculosis* is much more impermeable to hydrophilic molecules than that of *E. coli* or even *P. aeruginosa* (Jarlier and Nikaido, 1990). The penetration of hydrophilic molecules, at least those of low size, such as glycerol or isoniazid, might rely on wall-associated proteins that would play the same role as porins in Gram-negative bacteria, whereas the penetration of hydrophobic molecules, such as rifampin or macrolides, might be ensured by dissolution into the cell wall lipids.

The high content of lipid in the cell wall is responsible not only for the extreme hydrophobicity of mycobacterial cells, but also for the resistance of mycobacteria to chemical injury, in other words to decontamination procedures using sulfuric acid, sodium hydroxide, and/or detergents. On the other hand, it explains why *M. tuberculosis* is as susceptible as other bacteria to heat, X- and UV rays, and alcohol. In addition, *M. tuberculosis* keeps its viability for weeks at +4°C and for years at −70°C.

Mycobacterial Antigens

Soon after the discovery of the tubercle bacillus, Robert Koch prepared a concentrated, sterile filtrate from heat-killed liquid culture (Koch, 1891a), which he named "old tuberculin" (OT). It soon became apparent that tuberculosis patients reacted to the injection of OT more rapidly and intensely than uninfected persons, and the intradermal skin test with OT became part of the diagnosis of tuberculosis infection. However, being a crude extract of tubercle bacillus, OT contained a number of antigens, and subsequent investigators tried to purify these antigens.

The first efforts led to the preparation of purified protein derivatives (PPDs) of OT. Although PPDs are widely used as antigens in immunology, epidemiology, and clinical medicine, they are complex mixtures and for that reason have been subjected to innumerable attempts at purification to increase their specificity. Among the major antigens of *M. tuberculosis* and *M. bovis* that have been described, polysaccharide antigens, especially arabinogalactan, arabinomannan, and D-glucan, are probably similar or identical for all mycobacterial species. Protein antigens, antigen 5, a protein of apparent cytoplasmic origin, and antigen 6, a major extract of culture filtrate, have no more specificity than PPD (Daniel, 1984). Peptidoglycolipids or C mycosides of MAIS complex are type-specific. Antibodies against them are currently used for the serological typing of MAIS-complex strains. Peptidoglycolipids of *M. tuberculosis* cannot be used as specific antigens.

In recent years, it has been possible to obtain recombinant proteins by cloning the genes of dominant antigens into *E. coli*. The dominant 65–kDa protein appeared to be a stress protein common to numerous procaryotic and eukaryotic cells but having a *M. tuberculosis*–specific epitope (Shinnick, 1987) of promising value for immunologic diagnosis.

B. Nutrition and Growth

M. tuberculosis has two main growth characteristics: it does not grow on ordinary culture media but only on enriched media containing an egg-potato base or a serum (albumin) base; it has a slow rate of growth, the generation time of the cells in best conditions of culture being 17–18 hr, and the first appearance of grossly visible colonies taking 2–4 weeks. However, *M. tuberculosis* does not require any particular growth factor or vitamin, even though various compounds potentiate its in vitro growth. This is the case for bovine serum albumin, egg yolk, and even catalase. The beneficial effect of these compounds is probably due to their absorption of toxic moieties that are present in any culture medium.

M. tuberculosis is a strict aerobe equipped with catalase, peroxydase, and superoxide-dismutase, whose growth rate is highly dependent on the oxygen tension. When it is high, as in the tuberculosis cavity of the lung, *M. tuberculosis* multiplies freely; when it is much lower, as in the caseous foci of the lung, *M. tuberculosis* multiplies slowly or not at all (Wayne, 1976). Carbon dioxide either as $NaHCO_3/Na_2CO_3$ in the medium or as CO_2 in the gas phase above the medium up to 8% considerably improves the growth of isolates from clinical specimens (Ratledge, 1982).

M. tuberculosis can oxidize an extremely wide range of compounds. The preferred carbon sources for growth of *M. tuberculosis* in the laboratory are, by order of preference, glycerol, pyruvate, or glucose. On the other hand, the growth of *M. bovis*, a species closely related to *M. tuberculosis*, is favored by pyruvate and inhibited by high concentrations of glycerol. Citrate used as ferric ammonium citrate is usually part of the culture medium and provides a source of iron for the organism.

Asparagine is usually the preferred source of nitrogen for growth of *M. tuberculosis*. However, glutamine, aspartic acid, glutamate, or even NH^+_4 salts can substitute for asparagine, and even alanine has been reported as being the best nitrogen source (Ratledge, 1982). Besides carbon and nitrogen sources, *M. tuberculosis* requires four major inorganic elements for growth, potassium (k), magnesium (Mg), sulfur (S), phosphorus (P), and trace elements such as iron, zinc, and probably manganese. All elements are present in usual semisynthetic culture media as well as in the human body.

C. Genetics of *M. tuberculosis*

The development of basic studies on the genetics of the genus *Mycobacterium* and especially of *M. tuberculosis* has long been hampered by the slow growth rate of the pathogenic mycobacteria, the difficulty of building systems for exchange of genetic material between mycobacterial strains, and also by the hazards in manipulating such a highly infectious organism as *M. tuberculosis*.

The Nucleic Acids of M. tuberculosis

M. tuberculosis has a genome weighing $3.01–3.13 \times 10^6$ kDa, while that of *E. coli* weighs 2.5×10^6 kDA and those of other culturable ("atypical") mycobacteria weigh between 3.92 and 5.5×10^6 kDa. Its content of guanine (G) plus cytosine (C), found to range from 66.1 to 71.4% of the total base content, is higher than that of other bacteria. By DNA-DNA hybridization among the genomes of mycobacterial species, it has been shown that *M. tuberculosis*, *M. bovis*, and *M. africanum* have strong DNA homology. Although *M. tuberculosis*, *M. bovis*, and *M. africanum* have clear-cut cultural, biochemical, and epidemiological characteristics, from a genetic point of view they should be considered as varieties of the same species more than as distinct species (Wayne, 1984).

Repeated species-specific DNA sequences have been identified in the chromosome of *M. tuberculosis* (Clark-Curtiss, 1990). Some of them have strong analogies with mobile genetic elements, known as insertion sequences (IS), that have the property of integrating at numerous sites of the bacterial chromosome. For example, the insertion sequence IS6110 is homologous to the *E. coli* insertion sequence IS3411 (Clark-Curtiss, 1990). The digestion of the *M. tuberculosis* chromosome with restriction endonucleases gives DNA fragments of different sizes, which can be separated by electrophoresis and revealed by staining. They appear as a succession of bands ranked according to the molecular weights of each restriction fragment. The banding patterns different from one DNA to another are referred to as restriction fragment-length polymorphisms (RFLP) or genomic fingerprints. As the distribution of insertion sequences, IS6110 for example, is variable from one strain to another among the *M. tuberculosis* species, the use of a specific DNA probe, for example IS6110 probe, to examine the DNA fragments obtained by RFLP simplifies the genomic fingerprinting and is, at present, the most elaborate technique to characterize individual strains of *M. tuberculosis* and conduct scientifically based epidemiological studies.

By the use of recombinant DNA technology, specific genes of *M. tuberculosis* have been identified and cloned. These include genes for stress or heat-shock proteins and genes for ribosomal RNA (rRNA). Interestingly, *M. tuberculosis*, like other slow-growing mycobacteria, has only a single copy of rRNA gene (Bercovier et al., 1986) while fast-growing mycobacteria have two copies and *E. coli* has seven copies. This might be related to the slow growth of *M. tuberculosis*. Although the majority of the identified genes are highly conserved (e.g., have many nucleotide sequences common to other mycobacterial species and unrelated species), some species-specific differences in sequence are found among mycobacteria, particularly in some variable regions of DNA or even rRNA. If isotopic or nonisotopic enzyme-labeled complementary DNA sequences of these variable regions are prepared, they can be used as probes because they would specifically hybridize with the corresponding so-called variable region. Since rRNA is present in approximately 10,000 copies per bacterial cell, a DNA probe having rRNA as target is in theory 10,000 times more sensitive than a DNA probe having DNA as target. This explains why nucleic acid probes complementary to rRNA have been developed commercially for the identification of *M. tuberculosis* complex, *M. avium*, *M. intracellulare*, and *M. gordonae* pure cultures (McFadden et al., 1990).

Unfortunately, DNA probes are not sensitive enough to directly detect *M. tuberculosis* in clinical specimens. However, the enzymatic amplification of DNA by the polymerase chain reaction (PCR) has revolutionized DNA probe technology (Saiki et al., 1985). Using PCR, one can increase the amount of specific DNA regions up to the limit of probe detection. The technique, relatively simple to perform and exquisitely sensitive, is highly promising although at present very costly.

As mycobacterial genetics is rapidly advancing, one might expect definite progress in diagnosis, in epidemiology, and hopefully in prevention and treatment of tuberculosis as of other infectious diseases (Stover et al., 1991).

Mutation, Drug Resistance

Like all bacterial genomes, the mycobacterial genome is subject to a wide range of mutations. Mutants affecting colony morphology and time for appearance, biochemical and virulence characteristics, and drug sensitivity are of major interest in view of their importance for the diagnosis, treatment, and epidemiological surveillance of tuberculosis. An example of the spontaneous mutations that have occurred is given by the different geographic varieties of *M. tuberculosis* complex. In Europe and the Americas, the organisms grow slowly in culture as well-developed (eugonic), rough colonies with a characteristic buff color. In Africa, they often grow much more slowly, as minute flat and rough colonies, with a matte color (*M. africanum*). In South-East Asia, they are small and smooth like *M. bovis* colonies but with characteristic *M. tuberculosis* buff color, while the colonies of *M. bovis* are not pigmented. However, if subpassaged on pyruvate-containing medium, the small (dysgonic) colonies of *M. bovis* often give rise to large, rough colonies having the same morphology as *M. tuberculosis* colonies. An historical example of such mutation is the bacillus Calmette Guérin (BCG), *M. bovis* in genetic origin and *M. tuberculosis* in colony morphology.

Mutation affecting sensitivity to antituberculous agents is of prime importance in view of their medical consequences. Mutants resistant to streptomycin, isoniazid, rifampin, pyrazinamide, and ethambutol have been selected in the test tube and during the course of chemotherapy in humans. At least three factors appear to be important for selecting drug-resistant mutants. The first is the proportion of resistant mutants in normally susceptible or "wild" strains of tubercle bacilli, which ranges from 1 per 10^5 to 1 per 10^8 (Canetti et al., 1963). The second is the size of the bacillary population from which drug-resistant mutants are intended to be selected. The larger the bacillary population, the higher the chance it contains resistant mutants. In practice, resistant mutants are easy to select among 10^8 cells—the usual bacillary content of lung cavity—of normally susceptible *M. tuberculosis*. The third factor is the antimicrobial quality of the drug used. The more bactericidal the drug, the easier the selection of mutants, of course on condition that the drug is used alone.

The genes responsible for drug resistance in tubercle bacilli have not yet been identified. But a classic feature of a mutant resistant to a given drug is to remain susceptible to other drugs. Clinicians take advantage of that feature in always treating patients with a combination of drugs, each of them being active against the mutants resistant to other drugs.

Mycobacteriophages and Phage Typing

The first isolation of a bacteriophage or phage that was capable of infecting and lysing mycobacteria (mycobacteriophage) was reported in 1947. However, phages capable of infecting *M. tuberculosis* were reported only in 1954 (Crawford and Bates, 1984). Some strains being susceptible to phage lysis and others resistant, the possibility of subdividing *M. tuberculosis* by phage typing was raised in 1966 (Crawford and Bates, 1984). At present, 12 mycobacterial typing phages, human (MTPH) are recommended (Rado et al., 1975) for typing *M. tuberculosis* strains. Unfortunately, only four phage types are officially recognized, Ao, Aox, B, and C. Type B is common in Europe and the Americas, and type A in Japan and Hong Kong. No relation exists between phage typing and drug resistance.

D. The Microbial Populations in the Lesions of Human Tuberculosis

M. tuberculosis is not a toxin producer. Its pathogenicity for humans is therefore linked to its capacity to survive and multiply inside the human body and to the immune reactions of the infected host. *M. tuberculosis* is spread almost exclusively by the airborne route. A few bacillary units are inhaled by a new host and are deposited on the alveolar surface, where they are ingested by the alveolar macrophages and begin to multiply inside them. Within a few weeks after infection, at least in the immunocompetent host, the infected host mounts a specific cell-mediated immune response in which activated T lymphocytes and macrophages play a major role. As a result, the host becomes tuberculin positive and the pulmonary tissue where the bacilli have multiplied undergoes a semisolid necrosis, termed caseous necrosis, in which the bacilli are freed up for macrophages.

The presence of toxic substances of tissue origin and the low oxygen tension in the foci of caseation are not favorable for bacillary multiplication, so the bacilli begin to diminish rapidly in number. In an immunodeficient host, for example in a case of HIV infection and especially in the late stage of AIDS, cell-mediated immunity is hampered, the tuberculin skin test remains negative, and caseous necrosis is lacking. In such cases, tubercle bacilli remain and continue to multiply inside macrophages.

In an immunocompetent host, if the semisolid caseous necrosis undergoes softening and liquefaction, the liquid material is drained via the bronchi and cavitation occurs in the area of destroyed lung. As a consequence, oxygen tension rises and conditions become favorable for intense bacillary multiplication. From the cavity, bacilli disseminate, are ingested by macrophages, which undergo caseation, and then new caseous foci result in the already infected patients as well as in newly infected contacts.

In the course of these events, the environment of *M. tuberculosis* changes to such an extent that three different microbial subpopulations can be identified in lesions of human tuberculosis. The first is a subpopulation of organisms that are actively multiplying at neutral pH, in the thin layer of liquefied caseous necrosis covering the interior of the cavity wall. Because of its active metabolic state, that subpopulation responds well to antituberculous drugs, but, because of its size, up to 1×10^9 organisms (Canetti, 1965), it contains drug-resistant mutants that can be selected by monotherapy.

The second is a subpopulation of organisms inside macrophages or inside areas of recent caseous necrosis at an acid pH. This subpopulation does not multiply as freely as that located on the surface of the cavity wall and is limited in number: less than 10^6 organisms. Because it is in an active metabolic state, it responds as well as the preceding subpopulation to antituberculous drugs on the condition that the drugs penetrate inside cells and/or are active at an acid pH. Because of its limited size, this subpopulation does not contain drug-resistant mutants.

The third is a subpopulation of organisms located in the semisolid caseous necrosis, a very unfavorable environment for metabolic activity. That subpopulation decreases spontaneously in number or, if the local conditions become momentarily favorable, multiplies intermittently. It does not contain drug-resistant mutants but, because of its inactive metabolic state, does not respond well to antituberculosis drugs and even tends to persist despite adequate therapy (Mitchison and Dickinson, 1978; Grosset, 1980).

II. Bacteriology for Diagnosis and Monitoring the Treatment of Tuberculosis

A diagnosis of tuberculosis may be suggested by clinical symptoms, radiological, and/or histological findings. However, the only definite diagnosis of tuberculosis depends on the recognition of the etiological agent in clinical specimens. Smear examination is a rapid but relatively unsensitive (at least 10^4 organisms per milliliter are required for microscopic examination to be positive) and unspecific (all mycobacterial species are acid fast) method for recognizing tubercle bacilli in a clinical specimen. Like other organisms, tubercle bacilli are best recognized by culture and identification. But unlike other organisms, tubercle bacilli require several weeks for growth and identification when routine procedures are applied. For this reason, new techniques have been or are being developed to reduce the time required for culture and identification. In addition, new tests based on immunology, biochemistry, and genetic engineering, aimed at avoiding the necessary step of culture and thus at giving a rapid diagnosis of tuberculosis, are currently under development. Although highly promising, these new procedures must be evaluated for accuracy, reproductibility, and cost-effectiveness before they can be used in routine diagnosis. However, because of their interest and importance, they will be examined separately from the conventional procedures, which are still highly relevant in countries with a high incidence of tuberculosis and even in the majority of other countries.

A. Biological Safety

Biological safety is of crucial importance in laboratories dealing with *M. tuberculosis* bacteriology because workers in the mycobacteriology laboratory are exposed to infectious aerosols that are generated by manipulations of tubercle bacilli. Therefore, all work involving specimens or cultures, such as making smears, decontaminating clinical specimens and inoculating them onto culture media, preparing pure suspensions of tubercle bacilli for drug susceptibility testing and inoculating them onto culture media, and performing biochemical tests, must be carried out safely. Manipulations must be made in a separate room under negative pressure and equipped with a biological safety cabinet, either a class I negative-pressure or a class II laminar-flow safety cabinet. Centrifugation should be done in sealed centrifuge cups to prevent aerosols in case of leakage. Workers should wear laboratory coats or gowns, mouth pipetting should be prohibited, and all persons leaving the laboratory should leave their laboratory coat and wash their hands with good soap.

B. Conventional Procedures in Mycobacteriology

Specimen Collection and Transport

A number of clinical specimens may be submitted to the laboratory for search for mycobacteria. The quality of the results depends in large part on the quality of their collection and transport, of their repetition, and sometimes of their conservation. For the diagnosis of tuberculosis, specimens must be collected before chemotherapy begins. The collection containers should be clean, and sterile if the specimen is taken from a closed space (spinal fluid, pleural effusion, abscess, etc.). They should be delivered to the laboratory as soon as possible. If delays in delivery or processing are anticipated, specimens should be kept at

+4°C to prevent the growth of contaminants and preserve the viability of mycobacteria. In case of transportation, the collection container must be sealed to prevent leakage and cushioned to prevent breakage according to regulations.

Sputum or Sputum-Containing Specimens

Three spontaneously produced specimens of sputum are usually collected in clean but not sterile containers. If a sputum sample cannot be produced, a satisfactory specimen can be obtained by nebulization, gastric lavage, laryngal swabs, bronchoscopy, bronchial brushing, and so forth (Kubica, 1984).

Extrapulmonary Specimens

Acid-fast bacilli are usually of limited number in clinical specimens from extrapulmonary disease. Therefore, those specimens (pleural, pericardial, spinal, synovial, and ascitic fluids, blood, bone marrow, surgical biopsy, etc.) from closed lesions normally free of organisms other than mycobacteria must be collected aseptically and transported to the laboratory in sterile containers. Thus they will not have to be submitted to digestion and decontamination procedures that may harm the viability of bacilli. Special emphasis should be given to the collection of blood for culture of mycobacteria in subjects with HIV infection. Ten-milliliter samples of blood may be collected using the "isolator" or lysis-centrifugation system, which permits the laboratory worker to safely lyse mononuclear cells and centrifuge blood in the same container before inoculating the sediment directly onto culture media.

Specimens expected to be contaminated, e.g., urine, may be collected in containers similar to those used for sputum specimens. Before collection of urine, the external genitalia should be washed and early-morning, midstream specimens collected on 3 consecutive days.

Microscopy

The examination of stained smear under the microscope is the first step in the search for acid-fast bacilli in the laboratory. Direct smear on a glass slide of necrotic or blood-tinged particles of the specimen, usually sputum, is done in most laboratories of the world. Often, especially when all specimens are processed for culture, a portion of the digested, decontaminated specimen is used for preparing a concentrated smear.

A wide variety of acid-fast staining procedures is available (Kubica, 1984). The most classic is the carbol fuchsin or Ziehl-Neelsen stain. After staining, the slide should be scanned under the oil immersion lens (100×) of an ordinary microscopy. Acid-fast bacilli appear as pink-red thin rods against a blue background when methylene blue is used as counterstain. In many laboratories, particularly those having a large number of smears to examine daily, fluorescent acid-fast staining methods are used because fluorochrome-stained smears are easier and more rapid to scan. Auramine O is used as primary fluorochrome dye. After decolorization with acid-alcohol preparation, the slide is counter-stained with either potassium permangate or acridine orange or thiazine red and read with a fluorescent microscope under a low magnification lens (25 or 40×) without immersion oil (Kubica, 1984). Acid-fast bacilli appear as green fluorescent thin rods.

Whatever the staining method used, the number of acid-fast bacilli (AFB) observed in smears should be reported in a quantitative way (Kubica, 1984). This is of prime importance for assessing the gravity of the disease at the time of diagnosis and monitoring patient response to therapy.

Culture

Digestion and Decontamination

Most clinical specimens, except those collected from closed aseptic lesions, are contaminated with more rapidly growing organisms and should be decontaminated to eliminate these organisms before culture is attempted. One decontaminates specimens by mixing them with chemical compounds (acid, alkali, quaternary ammonium) that kill contaminant organisms more rapidly than tubercle bacilli. As tubercle bacilli are frequently included in organic debris, for example mucus globules in the sputum, specimens must, first, be digested or liquefied with detergents or enzymes. In practice, both digestion and decontamination are processed simultaneously by using either a single compound with both capacities, for example sodium hydroxide, or a mixture of two compounds, for example N-acetyl-L-cysteine and sodium hydroxide, sodium dodecyl-sufate (sodium lauryl sulfate) and sodium hydroxide, benzalkonium chloride and trisodium phosphate (Kubica, 1984). At the end of the procedure, decontaminated specimens are generally centrifuged, the supernate decanted, and the sediment neutralized with a diluted acid solution. All procedures must be critically timed to minimize the killing of tubercle bacilli by the decontaminating agent.

Quality control should ensure that the specimens are being decontaminated adequately without killing excessive numbers of mycobacteria. A simple procedure is to control the percentage of contaminated cultures. Above 5% indicates the digestion-contamination procedure is insufficient; below 2% indicates the procedure is too strong and kills too many mycobacteria.

Some procedures, using slow-acting compounds, such as Pancreatin-Desogen or cetylpiridinium chloride–sodium chloride, can be used for the digestion-decontamination of specimens that have to be transported for several days before culture.

Culture Medium

Numerous culture media are available, but the most commonly used are egg media, modified Löwenstein-Jensen and Ogawa, and agar media, Middlebrook 7H10, 7H11, and 7H12 (Kubica, 1984). For all types of media the pros and the cons may be listed. Egg media are more laborious to prepare but are less expensive than agar media, and the morphology of colonies is more typical. They do not require additional CO_2-enriched atmosphere to initiate primary growth of mycobacteria and may be placed in screw-capped tubes. Conversely, agar media are easier to prepare, permit a more rapid detection of growth but require CO_2-enriched atmosphere to initiate primary growth of mycobacteria and therefore should be placed in plates (Petri dishes). For these reasons, egg media are more commonly used in countries where tuberculosis is still highly prevalent. On the other hand, agar media that are better standardized than egg media are often required in scientific research. Selective drug-containing media have also been proposed (Mitchison et al., 1972) to control contamination on primary isolation. Although useful in some circumstances, these media are not used in routine practice.

From two to six tubes or plates of plain culture medium should be inoculated with 0.1–0.5 ml of the decontaminated or the aseptically processed specimen. In countries where *M. bovis* and/or *M. africanum* may be suspected, one or two tubes or plates of pyruvate-containing medium may be inoculated in supplement, because sodium pyruvate enhances growth of both organisms. The number of tubes to be inoculated depends on many factors among which the space available in the incubator and the clinical importance of the specimen (for example, CSF) are prominent. All inoculated media should be incubated at 35°–37°C.

Regardless of the kind of medium used, the media should be examined within a few days after inoculation. This permits early recognition of rapidly growing mycobacteria and of contaminated cultures. For the latter, new clinical specimens should be obtained, submitted to digestion-decontamination, and cultured. Incubation should continue for at least 6 weeks, at best 3 months, with weekly examination of cultures of evidence of growth. Culture is reported as positive as soon as colonies of characteristic morphology and constituted of acid-fast bacilli, are recognized. The report of culture should contain the amount of growth (number of colonies) recorded in a semiquantitative way: for example, no colonies; exact number if less than 50; 50–100; 100–200; or more than 200 colonies in case of confluent growth.

Identification of Tubercle Bacilli

The careful observation of pigment production and colonial morphology facilitates the differential identification of the isolated mycobacteria. Typical colonies of *M. tuberculosis* are rough and headed-up or eugonic and develop in 3–4 weeks with a characteristic buff color. At isolation, colonies of *M. bovis* do not develop before 1 month of culture, are smooth, tiny or dysgonic, and white. However, colonies of *M. bovis* BCG have growth and morphology characteristics similar to those of *M. tuberculosis*. Colonies of *M. africanum* may appear still later,

Table 1 Identification of Tubercle Bacilli

Mycobacteria	Colonies		Niacin production	Nitrate reduction	Catalase at 68°C	Growth on TCH
	Morphology	Pigmentation				
M. tuberculosis	R	e	buff	+	+	−	+
M. bovis	S	d	white	−	−	−	−
M. bovis BCG	R	e	buff	−	−	−	−
M. africanum	R	d	buff	−to+	−to+	−	−to+
"Atypicals"	S to R	d to e	different	−	−to+	+	+

R = rough; S = smooth; e = eugonic; d = dysgonic; + = positive; − = negative; TCH = thiophen-2-carboxylic hydrazid (2 mg/liter).

are rough, flat, with a buff color. Colonies of "atypical" mycobacteria may produce pigment after exposure to light (photochromogens, such as *M. kansasii* and *M. marinum*) or even when grown in the dark (scotochromogens, such as *M. gordonae*). Other species of atypical mycobacteria (rapid growers and nonphotochromogens) have nonpigmented colonies and may be easily confused with colonies of *M. tuberculosis*. For this reason, three standard biochemical tests should be used for the confirmed identification of the tubercle bacilli, namely niacin production, nitrate reduction, and search for heat-labile catalase activity. Another test used to separate *M. tuberculosis* and *M. bovis* is growth in medium containing 2 mg/liter of thiophen-2-carboxylic acid hydrazid (TCH) (Bönicke, 1958). As shown in Table 1, *M. tuberculosis*, the organism responsible for human tuberculosis, produces niacin, reduces nitrates, and grows on TCH, whereas atypical mycobacteria, often opportunistic organisms, produce a heat-stable catalase. Differentiation between the varieties of tubercle bacilli relies on colony morphology and pigmentation, niacin production, and nitrate reduction, as well as growth on TCH-containing medium. Elaborate species differentiation of "atypical" mycobacteria is accomplished with a series of tests, including growth at different temperatures; pigment production including determination of photochromogenicity and scotochromogenicity; biochemical tests; and drug susceptibility (Kubica, 1984). Because numerous mycobacterial species other than *M. tuberculosis* are frequently recovered from human sources in the clinical laboratory (Table 2), the importance of species differentiation should not be underestimated.

Drug Susceptibility

Indications

Drug sensitivity testing is the logical complement of *M. tuberculosis* isolation. However, newly diagnosed, previously untreated patients are usually started on therapy well before pretreatment drug susceptibility results are known. Thus sys-

Table 2 Mycobacterial Species Isolated[a] in the Clinical Laboratory of Pitié-Salpêtrière Hospital, Paris in 1979 and 1989

Mycobacteria	Species	Positive cultures in 1979		Positive cultures in 1989	
		No.	%	No.	%
Tubercle bacilli	*M. tuberculosis*	637	67	380 (88)	45 (29.5)
	M. bovis	0	—	3 (0)	0.3
	M. bovis BCG	0	—	2 (1)	0.2 (0.3)
	M. africanum	12	1.3	8 (0)	0.9
Potentially	*M. kansasii*	12	1.3	16 (10)	1.9 (3.3)
pathogenic	*M. marinum*	0	—	0	—
"atypical"	*M. szulgaï*	0	—	50 (18)	5.9 (6)
mycobacteria	*M. xenopi*	2	0.2	0	—
	M. scrofulaceum	0	—	0	—
	M. avium-intracellulare	5	0.5	133 (111)	158 (372)
	M. ulcerans	1	0.1	0	—
	M. fortuitum	19	2	35 (3)	4.1 (1)
	M. chelonae	19	2	12 (2)	1.4 (0.6)
Usually a	*M. gordonae*	166	17	179 (62)	21.2 (20)
nonpathogenic	*M. flavescens*	55	5.8	6 (2)	0.7 (0.6)
"atypical"	*M. terrae complex*	3	0.3	15 (1)	1.8 (0.3)
mycobacteria	*M. vaccae-aurum complex*	19	2	0	—
	M. gastri	0	0	2	0.2
Total		950	100	841 (298)	100 (100)

[a]With sodium dodecylsulfate method as digestion-decontamination procedure and Loewenstein-Jensen as culture medium.
(   ), clinical specimens from HIV-positive persons.

tematic drug sensitivity tests cannot be considered a prerequisite or even a need, particularly in countries where a standard regimen is recommended by national programs. However, systematic drug sensitivity testing may be fully justified in other circumstances and for surveying primary drug resistance in the community (WHO, 1991). The patients for whom drug susceptibility tests are indicated may be ranked in the following order of priority:

1. Chronic cases: patients who remain smear- and/or culture-positive after completing a retreatment regimen under supervision.

2. Smear-positive failure cases: patients who remain smear- and/or culture-positive 5 months or more after the start of chemotherapy *or*

patients who interrupted the treatment after 1–5 months of chemotherapy and are subsequently found to be smear- and/or culture-
positive.

3. Relapse cases: patients declared cured in the past who again have ac-
    tive smear- and/or culture-positive tuberculosis.

4. New cases: patients who have never taken tuberculosis drugs for more
    than 1 month.

For patients (1) and (2), a drug sensitivity test is the only means to determine the drugs to be prescribed; for patients (3), a drug sensitivity test permits one to determine whether relapse may be due to resistant organisms; for
patients (4), a drug sensitivity test permits one to detect primary drug resistance
and to conduct surveys of primary drug resistance.

Procedures to Be Used

The proportion method, which is the generally accepted method for determining
resistance to tubercle bacilli, is based on macroscopic growth of the organisms
on a solid either egg- or agar-based medium containing a uniform, specified
concentration of drug, called "critical" concentration. Every culture of *M. tuberculosis* contains a mixture of drug-susceptible and drug-resistant organisms,
the proportion of the latter being about 10^{-6} in wild strains of *M. tuberculosis*.
The critical concentration (Table 3) is the one that inhibits the growth of susceptible organisms without affecting the growth of the drug-resistant mutants
that are present. Comparison between the growth of *M. tuberculosis* on drug-
free medium and that on medium containing the critical concentration of the
drug permits one to evaluate the proportion of drug-resistant mutants and hence
to determine the susceptibility or the resistance of the tested strain to the drug.

Table 3 Critical Concentration of Drugs for Susceptibility Testing
Using 7H10, 7H11, or Löwenstein-Jensen (LJ) Media

Drugs	Drug concentration (mg/liter)		
	7H10	7H11	LJ
Isoniazid	0.2	0.2	0.2
Rifampin	1	1	40
Pyrazinamide	25	?	200
Ethambutol	5	7.5	2
Streptomycin	2	2	4
PAS	2	8	0.5

Source: From Canetti et al. (1963) and Hawkins et al. (1991).

Table 4 Dilutions of Decontaminated Specimens for Inoculation in Direct Drug Susceptibility Testing

No. of AFB per immersion field	Suspensions to be inoculed
Less than 1	Undiluted and 10^{-2}
1–9	10^{-1} and 10^{-3}
10 and more	10^{-2} and 10^{-4}

Source: From Hawkins et al. (1991).

Drug-susceptibility tests are routinely performed on either Löwenstein-Jensen, 7H10, or 7H11 medium. The medium may be inoculated directly (direct test) with the decontaminated smear-positive specimen or with a suspension prepared from a pure culture (indirect test). In the direct test, the inoculum size is adjusted on the basis of the expected number of viable organisms in the decontaminated specimen, as indicated in Table 4. In the indirect test, a homogeneous suspension of the primary culture growth is diluted to 10^{-3} and 10^{-5} mg wet weight per milliliter. In both cases, the two dilutions must be inoculated, under the volume of 0.1 or 0.2 ml, onto drug-containing (at the critical concentration) and drug-free media to provide a valid interpretation by the proportion method (Canetti et al., 1963). Susceptibility or resistance is determined by the proportion of colonies that grow on media prepared with and without the drug. If that proportion is higher than the "critical" proportion, usually 1% (Table 5), the strain is considered to be resistant; if it is lower, then the strain is considered to be susceptible. In practical terms, if the growth on a drug-containing medium

Table 5 Criteria of Drug Resistance: Critical Proportions of Colonies on Critical Drug Concentrations in Löwenstein-Jensen Medium

Drug	Critical drug concentrations (mg/liter)	Critical proportion of colonies
Isoniazid	0.2	1%
Rifampin	40	1%
Pyrazinamide	200	10%
Ethambutol	2	1%
Streptomycin	4	1%
PAS	0.5	1%

inoculated with the 10^{-3} dilution is greater than the growth on drug-free medium inoculated with the 10^{-5} dilution, then the strain is considered to be resistant.

When performed carefully in a laboratory with enough expertise, drug susceptibility tests give accurate and reliable results, except for pyrazinamide. Pyrazinamide, a drug active only at an acid pH, should be incorporated in a medium with pH 5.5. At this pH, only 1–10% of the inoculated *M. tuberculosis* grow on control, drug-free, medium. Thus it is important to determine whether the acidity by itself is responsible for the poor or absence of growth on pyrazinamide-containing medium, e.g., for the apparent susceptibility of the strain to pyrazinamide. On the other hand, if the pH is too high, pyrazinamide is inactive, and the strain will grow on pyrazinamide-containing medium and be considered resistant to pyrazinamide. To ensure that the acid medium is really at the requested pH, in addition to pyrazinamide-containing medium at pH 5.5, the strain should be inoculated onto control tubes at normal pH (6.6) and at acid pH (5.5). The growth on controls at pH 5.5 should be 1–10% of the growth on controls at pH 6.6. If not, the test should be repeated with newly prepared media. This explains why pyrazinamide susceptibility tests are not routinely performed.

Other Methods. Besides the proportion methods, two methods have been widely used to determine drug susceptibility of tubercle bacilli by indirect test: the absolute concentration method and the resistance ratio method (Canetti et al., 1963). In the absolute concentration method, results are expressed in terms of the lowest concentration of drug that inhibits growth of a carefully controlled inoculum. Because it is difficult to standardize the inoculum, the method is not recommended. In the resistance ratio method, which follows the same general procedure as the absolute concentration method, parallel sets of drug test media are inoculated with the standard H37Rv strain and the patient strain. Resistance is then expressed as the ratio of the minimal inhibitory concentration (MIC) for the patient strain to the MIC for the H37Rv strain. A resistance ratio superior or equal to 4 is indicative of drug resistance. This method has been employed in British Medical Research Council chemotherapy trials.

C. New Procedures in Mycobacteriology

Rapid Detection of Growth

A rapid radiometric respirometry method has been developed to detect mycobacterial growth. Known as the BACTEC TB system (Becton Dickinson Diagnostic Instrument Systems, Towson, MD), it is based on the measurements of $^{14}CO_2$ produced by the growth of tubercle bacilli in a liquid medium containing carbon 14-labeled palmitic acid as the only carbon source. As an increase in the $^{14}CO_2$ amount is more rapidly detected than colonies on a solid medium, the average detection time of in vitro growth of *M. tuberculosis* was 8 days with the BACTEC TB system versus 18 days with conventional media in a multicenter study of acid-fast smear-positive specimens (Roberts et al., 1991). In another study using acid-fast smear negative specimens, the average detection time was 14 days with the BACTEC TB system versus 26 days with conventional media (Morgan et al., 1983).

In practice, 0.5-ml aliquots of the decontaminated specimen are added to vials of 4 ml Middlebrook 7H12 broth containing an antibiotic mixture consisting of polymyxin B, amphotericin B, nalidixic acid, trimethoprim, and Azlocillin (Good and Mastro, 1989). It is recommended that simultaneous inoculation of conventional media be performed in addition to the Bactec media because some strains of *M. tuberculosis* grow on one primary isolation medium and not on the other. As soon as a significant amount of $^{14}CO_2$ is produced, it is necessary to perform an acid-fast smear from the culture vial and to subculture to recover the mycobacteria.

The BACTEC TB has three other advantages. First, a radiometric blood culture system (BACTEC 13A) may be used to recover mycobacteria from blood. Second, culture of *M. tuberculosis* can be identified with the BACTEC TB system by testing resistance to para-nitro-alpha-acetylamino-β-hydroxypropiophénone (NAP). Growth of the three varieties of tubercle bacilli (*M. tuberculosis*, *M. bovis*, and *M. africanum*), or *M. tuberculosis* complex, is not affected by NAP that inhibits the growth of all other *Mycobacterium* species ("atypicals"). The NAP test is complete within 5 days. Third, the BACTEC TB system may also be used for antimicrobial susceptibility testing and is as reliable as conventional methods for testing susceptibility of *M. tuberculosis* to isoniazid, rifampin, ethambutol, and streptomycin, and possibly pyrazinamide in the near future (Hawkins et al., 1991). The basic principle of the test using the BACTEC TB system is similar to that of the proportion method. Two inocula, one of which is 100-fold diluted, are used so that the proportion of resistant mutants may be extrapolated from the amounts of $^{14}CO_2$ produced.

New Identification Tests

In addition to the NAP test, two new tests may be used to identify rapidly (within 2 hr) the mycobacteria isolated in pure culture, namely mycolic acid pattern and genetic homology. Another test, genomic fingerprinting, is useful to characterize *M. tuberculosis* strains and to trace their distribution in the community.

Mycolic Acid Pattern

Mycobacteria contain large amounts of lipids, particularly mycolic acids. From species to species, the type and the amount of mycolic acids vary in such a way that by high-performance liquid chromatography (HPLC), thin-layer chromatography, or, better, gas-liquid chromatography (GLC) species-specific patterns of the mycolic acids may be determined. The method requires 10^7 to 10^8 mycobacterial cells, is reproducible, and is in use in a few specialized laboratories.

Determination of Genetic Homology (Genetic Probes)

DNA probes that hybridize specifically with corresponding mycobacterial DNA or RNA have been developed. The first were ^{125}I-labeled single-stranded DNA probes complementary to the ribosomal RNA (rRNA) of the target organisms, *M. tuberculosis* complex, *M. avium*, and *M. intracellulare*. At present, nonisotopic nucleic acid probes have been developed and are commercially available (GenProbe, San Diego, CA). These probes use a chemiluminescent acridinium ester-labeled single-stranded DNA sequence complementary also to the rRNA of the target mycobacteria. The acridinium ester label associated with the hybrids is detected using a luminometer. The probes are specific and sensitive for the identification of *M. tuberculosis* complex, *M. avium*, *M. intracellulare*, *M. avium* complex, and *M. gordonae* obtained in pure culture. They can be applied to mycobacterial cells recovered from colonies obtained on solid media as well as from culture in BACTEC broth, but they are not sensitive enough to be applied to the search of *M. tuberculosis* in clinical specimens. The cost and ease of the method make it useful and valuable for clinical laboratories.

Genomic Fingerprinting (RFLP) for Epidemiological Surveys

Organisms that belong to the *M. tuberculosis* species have, like other organisms, nucleotide sequences of their chromosome that vary from strain to strain but not within a given strain. The variability can be seen when chromosomal DNA is purified and cleaned into pieces of different lengths with restriction endonucleases (enzymes that cut DNA at specific sites). After separation on an agarose gel, the DNA pieces or fragments of several different strains distribute in a polymorphic banding pattern characteristic of each strain. This method of genomic analysis is known as restriction fragment length polymorphism (RFLP). If two patients are infected with the same strain, the banding pattern of their DNA is similar; if they are infected with different strains, the banding pattern is different (Clark-Curtiss, 1990).

By choosing probes that specifically hybridize within the highly variable nucleotide sequences, for example the IS6110 probe, the differences between strains are accentuated and the interpretation of the banding pattern simplified (Thierry et al., 1990). At present, RFLP is the only precise and reliable tool for strain typing, thus for tracing strains in the community.

New Methods for Rapid Diagnosis of Tuberculosis

Recent progress in biochemistry, immunology, and molecular genetics of mycobacteria are leading the way for rapid diagnosis of tuberculosis. Though the already developed or in-development methods for rapid diagnosis are technically highly promising, none of them is, at the present time, available for routine use in the clinical laboratory.

Detection of Tuberculostearic Acid

Tuberculostearic acid is a fatty acid produced by almost all bacterial species belonging to *Mycobacterium, Nocardia*, and *Actinomyces* genera. Thus, its detection in clinical specimens is not specific but only suggestive of tuberculosis, no more but no less than the detection of acid-fast bacilli is suggestive of *M. tuberculosis*. As a consequence, the detection of small amount of tuberculostearic acid in cerobrospinal fluid by using gas chromatography-mass spectrometry with selected ion monitoring is highly indicative of tuberculous meningitis (Brooks et al., 1987; French et al., 1987; Larsson et al., 1987). The procedure, which requires only 8 hr, is much more sensitive than smear examination and almost as sensitive as conventional culture.

Immunodiagnosis of Tuberculosis

The tuberculin skin test is well established for immunodiagnosis of tuberculosis infection since the description by Robert Koch of the exaggerated reaction that appeared when tubercle bacilli were inoculated in the skin of previously infected guinea pigs. However, it is also well established (Chaparas, 1984) that much of the skin sensitivity to tuberculin in humans throughout the world is due to infection with mycobacteria other than *M. tuberculosis*, because of the common antigens shared by mycobacterial species. What holds true for skin test diagnosis of tuberculosis infection holds true also for the serodiagnosis of tuberculosis.

The first serodiagnostic test was performed in 1898 by Arloing and Courmont (Arloing and Courmont, 1904), who reported that tubercle bacilli could be agglutinated by the serum of tuberculosis patients. However, there was no agglutination with about 10% of the patient sera and agglutination with about 10% of the control sera. Since that time, many attempts have been made to overcome these deficiencies by using more and more sophisticated procedures, such as immunoelectrophoresis, hemagglutination tests, fluorescent antibody tests, radioimmunoassay, and enzyme-linked immunosorbent assay (ELISA), and more and more well-characterized antigens, but without much success (Chaparas, 1984; Roberts et al., 1991). It is wise to admit that as long as specific antigen(s) or epitope(s) of *M. tuberculosis complex* are not available to the clinical laboratory, there is no hope for serodiagnosis of tuberculosis, because of lack of specificity. But specificity alone is not sufficient. Sensitivity also is required for a valuable serodiagnostic test. Unfortunately, both are not yet associated (Chan et al., 1990; Charpin et al., 1990).

Nucleic Acid Amplification

For the hybridization of the nucleic acid probes with the complementary sequence of the target *M. tuberculosis* to be detectable, the tested sample should contain more than 10^6 mycobacterial cells. As this amount is not attained in clinical specimens, nucleic acid probes cannot be used, at present, for the direct detection of mycobacteria in clinical specimens.

An elegant means to overcome the lack of sensitivity of direct detection by probes in clinical specimens is to submit, first, the few mycobacteria present in clinical specimens to nucleic acid amplification using polymerase chain reaction (PCR) and then to reveal the amplified mycobacterial DNA by specific nucleic acid probes. The method has already been applied to the diagnosis of other bacterial and viral diseases (Tenover, 1991). Because the present DNA may be amplified one million times, as few as 10–100 *M. tuberculosis* cells may be detected in a clinical specimen. The total procedure requires 1–2 days to be performed. Although fascinating in its principle and its application, PCR for diagnosis of tuberculosis is still at the research stage. Major constraints for its routine use are: (1) specific primers should be available, (2) the process of amplification should be conducted under strict conditions of ionic strength, temperature, and primers and nucleotides concentration; (3) the high risk of contamination of the sample by outside DNA; (4) the high cost and sophistication of the method. Despite these presently insurmountable constraints, the combination of nucleic acid amplification in clinical specimens with detection of amplified nucleic acid by specific probes is at present the most exciting development in the field of tuberculosis bacteriology (Brisson-Noël et al., 1989; Hermans et al., 1990).

References

Arloing, S., and Courmont, P. (1904). Serum diagnosis of tuberculosis. *Boston Med. Surg. J.* **151**:617–623.

Barsdale, L., and Kim, K. S. (1977). *Mycobacterium. Bacteriol. Rev.* **41**:217–372.

Bercovier, H., Kafri, O., and Sella, S. (1986). Mycobacteria possess a surprisingly small number of ribosomal RNA genes in relation to the size of their genome. *Biochem. Biophys. Res. Commun.* **136**:1136–1144.

Bönicke, R. (1958). Die differenzierung humaner und boviner tuberkelterien mit hilfe von thiopen-2-carbonsaure-hydrazid. *Naturewissenschaften* **46**: 392–393.

Brisson-Noël, A., Gicquel, B., Lecossier, D., Levy-Frebault, V., Nassif, X., and Hance, A. J. (1989). Rapid diagnosis of tuberculosis by amplification of mycobacteria DNA in clinical samples. *Lancet* **2**:1069–1071.

Brooks, J. B., Daneshvar, M. I., Fast, D. M., and Good, R. C. (1987). Selective procedures for detecting femtomole quantities of tuberculostearic acid in serum and cerebrospinal fluid by frequency-pulsed electron capture gas-liquid chromatography. *J. Clin. Microbiol.* **25**:1201–1206.

Buhler, V. B., and Pollak, A. (1953). Human infection with atypical acid-fast organisms: report of two cases with pathologic findings. *Am. J. Clin. Pathol.* **23**:363–374.

Calmette, A., and Guérin, C. (1908). Sur quelques propriétés du bacille tuberculeux cultivé sur la bile. *CR Acad. Sci.* **147**:1456–1459.

Canetti, G. (1965). Present aspects of bacterial resistance in tuberculosis. *Am. Rev. Respir. Dis.* **92**:687–703.

Canetti, G., Froman, S., Grosset, J., Hauduroy, P., Langerova, M., Mahler, H. T., Meissner, G., Mitchison, D. A., and Sula, L. (1963). Mycobacteria. Laboratory methods for testing drug sensitivity and resistance. *Bull. WHO* **29**:565–578.

Castets, M., Boisvert, H., Grumbach, F., Brunel, P., and Rist, N. (1968). Les bacilles tuberculeux du type africain. *Rev. Tuberc. (Paris).* **32**: 179–184.

Chan, S. L., Reggiardo, Z., Daniel, T. M., Guilling, D. J., and Mitchison, D. A. (1990). Serodiagnosis of tuberculosis using an ELISA with antigen 5 and a hemagglutination assay with glycolipid antigens. *Am. Rev. Respir.* **142**:385–390.

Chaparas, S. D. (1984). Immunologically based diagnostic tests with tuberculin and other mycobacterial antigens. In *The Mycobacteria: A Sourcebook.* Part A. Section 9. Edited by G. P. Kubica and L. G. Wayne. Marcel Dekker, New York, pp. 195–220.

Charpin, D., Herbault, H., Gevaudan, M. J., Saadjian, M., De Micco, P., Arnaud, A., Vervloet, D., and Charpin, J. (1990). Value of ELISA using A60 antigen in the diagnosis of active pulmonary tuberculosis. *Am. Rev. Respir. Dis.* **142**:380–384.

Chester, F. D. (1901). *A Manual of Determinative Bacteriology.* Macmillan, New York.

Clark-Curtiss, J. E. (1990). Genome structure of mycobacteria. In *Molecular Biology of the Mycobacteria.* Section 4. Edited by J. McFadden. Academic Press, London, pp. 77–96.

Crawford, J., and Bates, J. H. (1984). Phage typing of mycobacteria. In *The Mycobacteria: A Sourcebook.* Part A. Section 6. Edited by G. P. Kubica and L. G. Wayne. Marcel Dekker, New York, pp. 123–132.

Daniel, T. M. (1984). Soluble mycobacterial antigens. In *The Mycobacteria: A Sourcebook.* Part A. Section 17. Edited by G. P. Kubica and L. G. Wayne. Marcel Dekker, New York, pp. 417–465.

Draper, P. (1982). The anatomy of mycobacteria. In *The Biology of the Mycobacteria.* Section 2. Vol 1. Edited by C. Ratledge and J. Stanford. Academic Press, London, pp. 9–52.

Edwards, P. Q., and Edwards, L. B. (1960). Story of the tuberculin test from an epidemiologic viewpoint. *Am. Rev. Respir. Dis.* **81**:1–47.

French, G. Y., Cheung, S. W., and Oo, K. T. (1987). Diagnosis of pulmonary tuberculosis by detection of tuberculostearic acid in sputum by using gas chromatography-mass spectrometry with selected ion monitoring. *J. Infect. Dis.* **156**:356–362.

Good, R. C., and Mastro, T. D. (1989). The modern mycobacteriology laboratory: how it can help the clinician. In *Clinics in Chest Medicine.* Vol 10. No. 3. Edited by D. E. Snider. Philadelphia, pp. 315–322.

Grange, J., (1984). The humoral immune response in tuberculosis. Its nature, biological role and diagnostic usefulness. *Adv. Tuberc. Res.* **21**:1–78.

Grosset, J. (1980). Bacteriologic basis of short-course chemotherapy for tuberculosis. *Clin. Chest Med.* **1**:231–241.

Guérin, C. (1957). Early history of BCG. In *BCG Vaccination Against Tuberculosis.* Edited by S. R. Rosenthal. Little, Brown, Boston, pp. 48–53.

Hall, R. M., Sritharan, M., Messenger, A. J. M., and Ratledge, C. (1987). Iron transport in *Mycobacterium smegmatis.* Occurrence of iron-regulated envelope proteins as potentials receptors for iron uptake. *J. Gen. Microbiol.* **133**:2107–2114.

Hawkins, J. E., Wallace, R. J. Jr., and Brown, B. A. (1991). Antibacterial susceptibility tests: Mycobacteria. In *Manual of Clinical Microbiology*, 5th ed. Chapter 114. Edited by W. J. Hausler, Jr., K. L. Herrmann, H. D. Isenberg, and H. J. Shadomy. American Society for Microbiology, Washington, DC, pp. 1138–1153.

Hermans, P. W. M., Schuitema, A. R. J., Van Sooligen, D., Verstynen, C. P. H. J., Bik, E. M., Thole, J. E. R., Kolk, A. H. I., and Van Embden, J. D. A. (1990). Specific detection of *Mycobacterium tuberculosis* complex strains by polymerase chain reaction. *J. Clin. Microbiol.* **28**:1204–1213.

Hirschfield, G. R., McNeil, M., and Brennan, P. J. (1990). Peptidoglycan-associated polypeptides of *Mycobacterium tuberculosis. J. Bacteriol.* **172**:1005–1013.

Jarlier, V., and Nikaido, H. (1990). Permeability barrier to hydrophilic solutes in *Mycobacterium chelonae, J. Bacteriol.* **172**:1418–1423.

Koch, R. (1882). Die Aetiologie der Tuberculose. *Berl. Klin. Wochenschr.* **19**:221–230.

Koch, R. (1891a). Fortsetzung der mittheilung über ein heilmittel gegen tuberculose. *Dtsch. Med. Wochenschr.* **17**:101–102.

Koch, R. (1891b). Weitere mittheilung über das tuberkulin. *Dtsch. Med. Wochenschr.* **17**:1189–1192.

Kubica, G. P. (1984). Clinical Microbiology. In *The Mycobacteria: A Sourcebook.* Part A. Section 7. Edited by G. P. Kubica and L. G. Wayne, Marcel Dekker, New York, pp. 133–175.

Larsson, L., Odham, G., Westerdahl, G., and Olsson, B. (1987). Diagnosis of pulmonary tuberculosis by selected-ion monitoring: improved analysis of tuberculostearate in sputum using negative-ion mass spectrometry. *J. Clin. Microbiol.* **25**:893–896.

Lehmann, K. B., and Neumann, R. (1896). Atlas und Grundis der Bakteriologie und Lehrbuch der speciellen bakteriologischen. *Diagnostik*, 1st ed. J. F. Lehmann, Munich.

McFadden, J., Kunze, Z., and Seechurn, P. (1990). *DNA Probes for detection and identification. In molecular biology of the mycobacteria*. Section 7. Edited by J. McFadden. Academic Press, London, pp. 139–172.

Minnikin, D. E. (1982). Lipids: complex lipids, their chemistry, biosynthesis and roles. In *The biology of the Mycobacteria*. Section 3. Vol 1. Edited by C. Ratledge and J. Stanford. Academic Press, London, pp. 95–184.

Mitchison, D. A., and Dickinson, J. M. (1978). Bactericidal mechanims in short-course chemotherapy. *Bull. Int. Un. Tuberc.* **53**:254–259.

Mitchison, D. A., Allen, B. W., Carrol, L., Dickinson, J. M., and Aber, V. R. (1972). A selective oleic acid albumin agar medium for tubercle bacilli. *J. Med. Microbiol.* **5**:165–175.

Morgan, M. A., Horstmeier, C. D., De Young, D. R., and Roberts, G. D. (1983). Comparison of a radiometric method (BACTEC) and conventional culture media for recovery of mycobacteria from smear-negative specimens. *J. Clin. Microbiol.* **18**:384–388.

Nocard, E., and Roux, E. (1887). Sur la culture du bacille de la tuberculose. *Ann. Inst. Pasteur* **1**:19–29.

Rado, T. A., Bates, J. H., Engel, H. W. B., Mankiewicz, E., Murohashi, T., Mizuguchi, Y., and Sula, L. (1975). World Health Organization studies on bacteriophage typing of mycobacteria. Subdivision of the species *Mycobacterium tuberculosis. Am. Rev. Respir. Dis.* **111**:459–468.

Ratledge, C. (1982). Nutrition, growth and metabolism. In *The biology of the Mycobacteria*. Section 5. Vol 1. Edited by C. Ratledge and J. Stanford. Academic Press, London, pp. 186–271.

Roberts, G. D., Koneman, E. W., Kim, Y. K. (1991). Mycobacterium. In *Manual of Clinical Microbiology*, 5th ed. Chapter 34. Edited by W. J. Hausler Jr, K. L. Herrmann, H. D. Isenberg, and H. J. Shadomy. American Society for Microbiology, Washington, DC, pp. 304–339.

Saiki, R. K., Scharf, S. J., Higusi, G., Faloona, K., Mullis, K. B., Horn, G. T., Erlich, H. A., and Arnheim, N. (1985). Enzymatic amplification of β-globin genomic sequences and restriction site analysis for diagnosis of sickle cell anemia. *Science* **230**:1350–1354.

Schatz, A., Bugie, E., and Waksman, S. A. (1944). Streptomycin: a substance exhibiting antibiotic activity against Gram-positive and Gram-negative bacteria. *Proc. Soc. Exp. Biol. Med.* **55**:66–69.

Shinnick, T. M. (1987). The 65 kilodalton antigen of *Mycobacterium tuberculosis*. *J. Bacteriol.* **169**:1080–1088.

Smith, T. (1898). A comparative study of bovine tubercle bacilli and of human bacilli from sputum. *J. Exp. Med.* **3**:470–511.

Stover, C. K., de la Cruz, V. F., Fuerst, T. R., Burlein, J. E., Benson, L. H., Bennett, L. T., Bansal, G. P., Young, J. F., Lee, M. H., Hatfull, G. F., Snapper, S. B., Barletta, R. G., Jacobs, W. R., Jr., and Bloom, B. R. (1991). New use of BCG for recombinant vaccines. *Nature* **351**:456–460.

Tenover, F. C. (1991). Molecular methods for the clinical microbiology laboratory. In *Manual of Clinical Microbiology*, 5th ed. Chapter 17. Edited by W. J. Hausler Jr, K. L. Herrmann, H. D. Isenberg, and H. J. Shadomy. American Society for Microbiology, Washington, DC, pp. 119–127.

Thierry, D., Brisson-Noël, A., Vincent-Levy-Frebault, V., Nguyen, S., Gueston, J. L., and Gicquel, B. (1990). Characterization of a *Mycobacterium tuberculosis* insertion sequence IS6110 and its application in diagnosis. *J. Clin. Microbiol.* **28**:2668–2673.

Villemin, J. A. (1868). *Etudes expérimentales et cliniques sur la tuberculose.* Baillière, Paris.

Wayne, L. G. (1976). Dynamics of submerged growth of *Mycobacterium tuberculosis* under aerobic and microaerophilic conditions. *Am. Rev. Respir. Dis.* **114**:807–811.

Wayne, L. G. (1984). Mycobacterial speciation. In *The Mycobacteria: A Sourcebook.* Part 1. Section 2. Edited by G. P. Kubica and L. G. Wayne. Marcel Dekker, New York, pp. 25–65.

World Health Organization (1991). Guidelines for tuberculosis treatment in adults and children in National Tuberculosis Programmes. *WHO/ Tub/91.161.*

Ziehl, F. (1882). Zur Färbung des Tuberkelbacillus. *Deutsch. Med. Wochenschr.,* p. 451.

Ziehl, F. (1883). Ueber die Färbung des Tuberkelbacillus. *Deutsch. Med. Wochenschr.,* p. 247.

4

Immunology of Tuberculosis

THOMAS M. DANIEL and JERROLD J. ELLNER

Case Western Reserve University School of Medicine
and University Hospitals of Cleveland
Cleveland, Ohio

I. Introduction

When 39-year-old Robert Koch announced to a stunned audience at the Berlin Physiological Society on March 24, 1882 that he had discovered the cause of tuberculosis (Koch, 1882), he opened a new era in microbiology. Not long thereafter, in 1891, he described what has become known as the Koch phenomenon (Koch, 1891) and in so doing similarly opened a new era in immunology. Koch reported than an animal with prior experience with the tubercle bacillus dealt with the introduction of virulent organisms by walling off and containing the infection, something that naïve animals could not do. Perhaps this observation led him to his ill-conceived recommendation of tuberculin injections for the treatment of tuberculosis. This therapy certainly paved the way for von Pirquet's observation that delayed tuberculin skin reactions were an indicator of tuberculosis infection. The subsequent story of the development of the tuberculin skin test as a well-accepted hallmark of tuberculin cellular hypersensitivity and immunity is familiar to many and has been well recounted in review articles (Edwards and Edwards, 1960; Snider, 1982).

Pathologists had long recognized granulomas as the central histopathological lesions of tuberculosis, and the role of granulomas in containing the spread of disease was recognized from studies of clinical pathological material. Koch's observations provided experimental support for this view. Mackaness and his co-workers demonstrated that tuberculosis immunity depended on the activation of macrophages, the central cells of granulomas, and that some aspects of this macrophage activation were not antigen-specific (Mackaness, 1964). The elegant studies of Warren and his colleagues, who worked primarily with schistosomiasis, demonstrated the immunological nature of infectious tissue granulomas and the dependence of these granulomas on immunologically specific T lymphocytes (Warren et al., 1967).

To Merrill Chase (Chase, 1945) goes credit for observing that delayed hypersensitivity could be transferred by lymphocytes, thus establishing the central memory function of these cells; as noted below, we now recognize diverse subsets of lymphocytes with specific functions in regulating cellular immunity. Subsequent seminal work by David and co-workers (David et al., 1964) led to the demonstration that immunologically competent lymphocytes produce soluble factors—lymphokines—that are responsible for the proliferation and activation of other immunoactive cells, a story that has subsequently unfolded to reveal an extraordinarily complex and highly regulated immune system.

Not only by reason of history but also because of the elegant nature of the clinical model it produces, tuberculosis has become the paradigm for diseases mediated by cellular immunity. In this chapter we will review the immunology of tuberculosis, beginning with the organism that causes tuberculosis and induces the immunity and hypersensitivity characteristic of this infection. We will then move from the organism to the host and the highly regulated cellular immune system responsible for the host's responses to tuberculous infection.

II. Mycobacterial Protein Antigens

Immunologically competent cells of the human host recognize *Mycobacterium tuberculosis* by its antigens, and scores of antigens of this organism have now been described. Indeed, when compared with other pathogens, mycobacteria have an extraordinarily large panoply of antigens. This may be related to the fact that these bacteria are rich in adjuvants, as noted below, so that many minor protein constituents are presented to host cells under circumstances that favor antigenicity. Following the description of an expression library for the entire genome of *M. tuberculosis* by Young and colleagues (Young et al., 1985), there has been a rapid increase in the number of antigenic proteins available for characterization and study. Banks of monoclonal antibodies have provided important reagents facilitating their characterization (Engers et al., 1985, 1986). We will not attempt a comprehensive review of mycobacterial antigens; we will, however, discuss three protein antigens about which a substantial body of knowledge exists.

A. The 65,000-Dalton Heat Shock Protein Antigen

A 65,000-dalton antigen of *M. tuberculosis* and other mycobacteria has been extensively studied and found to be a heat shock protein with substantial homology with other well-known heat shock proteins, including the *Escherichia coli* GroEL protein (Shinnick et al., 1988; Young et al., 1987). Heat shock proteins are widely distributed in nature and highly conserved with substantial structural similarity crossing taxonomic lines. Named because they are produced in increased quantity by cells growing under stressful culture conditions such as high temperature, they are thought to have important functions in maintaining cell integrity and are produced by bacteria under many conditions of culture that are less than optimal. Similar proteins are produced by plant and higher-animal, including mammalian, cells.

The gene for the 65,000-dalton antigen has been cloned (Shinnick, 1987; Thole et al., 1987), and its structure is well known. This protein may exist in polymeric form in mycobacteria. The 65,000-dalton unit contains many helical structures and hydrophobic regions, characteristics typical of highly antigenic proteins. Studies with monoclonal antibodies have demonstrated that this protein has multiple epitopes (Buchanan et al., 1987), many of which are widely shared among mycobacteria, some of which appear to be species specific. Some epitopes appear to be shared with epitopes of mammalian proteins; these have been implicated in adjuvant arthritis and might be related to human autoimmune diseases (Thole et al., 1988).

B. The 38,000-Dalton Species-Specific Antigenic Protein of *M. tuberculosis*

The goal of isolating a species-specific antigenic protein from *M. tuberculosis* has been elusive yet hotly pursued by many investigators. Daniel and Anderson (1978) used immunoabsorbent affinity chromatography to isolate an antigen referred to as antigen 5. With Ellner and others, the immunobiology of this protein was studied extensively, and it was found to be restricted to *M. tuberculosis* and *M. bovis* (Daniel et al., 1979). This antigen elicited T- and B-lymphocyte responses in sensitized guinea pigs and infected humans, and it displayed substantial species specificity in its reactions in guinea pigs. When used to skin-test populations of human subjects, it displayed less species specificity than had been observed in guinea pigs (Daniel et al., 1982). This antigen formed the basis of a serodiagnostic ELISA test with excellent diagnostic test characteristics (Balestrino et al., 1984; Ma et al., 1986), and again patients with nontuberculous mycobacterial disease were found to display reactivity with this antigen (Benjamin and Daniel, 1982). Thus, despite substantial evidence of species specificity, this potent antigen was not completely specific in infected humans.

Ivanyi and his colleagues developed a highly specific serodiagnostic ELISA test based on inhibition of a monoclonal antibody designated TB-72 (Ivanyi et al., 1983; Bothamley et al., 1988). Young used immunoabsorbents prepared from similar monoclonal antibody TB-71 to purify a protein reaction with TB-71 and TB-72, each monoclonal antibody apparently reacting with a distinct epitope (Young et al., 1986). The molecular weight of this protein was found to be 38,000.

Anderson and Hansen (1989) also purified and characterized a 38,000-dalton protein, designating it antigen b. Anderson and co-workers later proposed that this protein is necessary for phosphate metabolism of the organism (Anderson et al., 1990). Haslov and colleagues (Haslov et al., 1990; Ljungqvist, personal communication) demonstrated that protein b and the proteins purified by Daniel and Anderson and by Young were identical, inferring that the original molecular weight estimate of Daniel of 35,000 was in error or that protein b contained a moiety not present on the molecule as prepared by Daniel and Anderson. He and his colleagues considered this protein to be immunodominant in five of seven strains of in-bred guinea pigs (Haslov et al., 1990). Kadival et al. (1987) described preparing a less specific 38,000-dalton antigen by immunoabsorbent affinity chromatography using a monoclonal antibody–derived absorbent, but their product has not been compared with the products of Daniel and Young.

What is currently known about the 38,000-dalton antigen of M. tuberculosis is sufficient to conclude that it is not a major component of this organism but that it is highly antigenic. It is a leading candidate for species specificity, an important characteristic favoring its use for immunodiagnosis and perhaps also for immunization.

C. Antigens of the 85 Complex

Harboe, Wiker, and their colleagues have used elegant crossed immunoelectrophoretic techniques to show close immunologic relationships between three antigens designated by them 85 A, B, and C (Wiker et al., 1986a,b, 1990a,b). While these three antigens share epitopes and have many similar properties, they appear to be encoded by three separate genes (Wiker et al., 1990a,b). The best known of these antigens is 85B, which has been previously described as alpha antigen (Yoneda and Fukui, 1965), antigen a_2 (Daniel and Ferguson, 1970), antigen 6 (Janicki et al., 1972), and MPB-59/MPT-59 (Wiker et al., 1986a,b). With a molecular weight of 30,000 daltons, this antigen is secreted by growing mycobacteria (Wiker et al., 1986a,b; Abou-Zeid et al., 1988a), and it is the predominant antigen in culture medium from growing mycobacteria. It binds fibronectin (Abou-Zeid et al., 1988b), raising the question of whether this property is important in mycobacterial recognition and ingestion by macrophages. The gene for the 30,000-dalton antigen has been cloned from *M. bovis* and *M. kansasii*, and its base sequence and corresponding amino acid sequence are known (Matsuo et al., 1988). This antigen is present in all mycobacteria that have been tested (Yoneda et al., 1965; Daniel, 1980), and there is substantial evidence that the molecule contains both species specific and shared epitopes (Salata et al., 1991).

The 30,000-dalton antigen evokes strong skin test responses in sensitized animals with somewhat more specificity of reactivity than tuberculin purified protein derivative (PPD) (Salata et al., 1991). Measuring IgG antibody to the 30,000-dalton antigen provides the basis for a good serodiagnostic test for active tuberculosis (Sada et al., 1990b). The 30,000-dalton antigen also elicits in vitro correlates of cell-mediated hypersensitivity, and it is of considerable interest that T lymphocytes of healthy *M. tuberculosis*–infected individuals react strongly to this antigen whereas those of patients with active tuberculosis do not (Havlir et al., 1991a,b). This might suggest that decreased T-lymphocyte responsiveness to the 30,000-dalton antigen is a feature of the immune regulation in active tuberculosis, or it might mean that individuals who do not mount T-lymphocyte responses are predisposed to development of disease.

Other members of the 85 complex of antigens are less well studied. The 85A component, also known as antigen P32 (De Bruyn et al., 1987) and MPT44 (Wiker et al., 1990a,b) is also a fibronectin-binding, secreted protein. It has a molecular weight of 31,000–32,000 daltons (Borremans et al., 1989). Its gene has been cloned and has a high degree of homology with the gene of the 85B antigen. This antigen evokes antibodies in patients with tuberculosis (Borremans et al., 1989).

III. The Mycobacterial Cell Wall: Mycobacterial Polysaccharides

The mycobacterial cell wall is a complex structure with many elements of immunologic importance. The external aspect of the cell wall surface comprises unique lipids containing long-chain mycolic aids. These are esterified to arabinogalactan, the principal structural element of the cell wall. Interiorly, linked to the arabinogalactan by phosphodiester bonds, is muramyl dipeptide. Each of these three major elements—mycolic acid lipid, arabinogalactan, and muramyl dipeptide—has importance to the immunology of tuberculosis. Brennan, who has contributed so much to our recent knowledge of the mycobacterial cell wall, has recently provided a very helpful review of this subject (Brennan, 1989).

In early but elegant and historically important studies, Raffel demonstrated that the adjuvant properties of mycobacterial cells resided in their lipids (Raffel et al., 1949). Among these lipids, cord factor, a lipid associated with cording of mycobacterial colonies growing in liquid media and originally thought to be associated with virulence, was found to be of major importance as an adjuvant (Goren, 1982). This activity was further localized to the trehalose esters of mycolic acid, particularly trehalose dimycolate. The immune responses, both cellular and humoral, to any protein antigen are greatly potentiated when the antigen is given in emulsions containing these mycolate adjuvants. Phenolic glycolipid at the surface of the *M. leprae* cell is not antigenic per se (Barrow and Brennan, 1982), but acts as a hapten and contains an epitope that appears to be species specific. In fact, for the complex of *M. avium* and *M. scrofulaceum* strains that can be serotyped, the serovar-specific epitope is that of this glycolipid. Specificity of this epitope is conferred by specific sugar substitution (Brennan, 1981).

A. Arabinogalactan

D-arabino-D-galactan serves as the backbone of the mycobacterial cell wall of mycobacteria and other actinomycetes and corynebacteria. An arabinofuranosyl side chain of arabinogalactan contains a major epitope that is identical among all organisms possessing arabinogalactan (Misaki et al., 1974). This same side chain is also present on cell wall–associated arabinomannan. Arabinogalactan readily elicits antibodies in immunized experimental animals (Misaki et al., 1974; Daniel, 1975), but this polysaccharide induces and elicits few or no cellular immune responses.

Arabinogalactan, together with the underlying peptides phosphodisesterified to it, is a water-soluble adjuvant capable of potentiating a wide variety of immune responses (Adam et al., 1972; Wahl et al., 1979). At the same time, it has major immunosuppressive properties (Kleinhenz, et al., 1981). Cultured peripheral blood mononuclear cells from healthy tuberculin-positive donors had depressed responses to mycobacterial antigens when cocultured with arabinogalactan. This effect was mediated by monocytes, associated with their increased production of prostaglandin E2, and reversible with indomethacin or antibody to arabinogalactan. Immunoabsorption studies provided data suggesting that circulating arabinogalactan, possibly bound in immune complexes, might be responsible for the known immunosuppressive activity of some tuberculous plasma.

The search for the minimal adjuvant unit in the water-soluble adjuvant led to the identification of muramyl dipeptide (*N*-acetylmuramyl-L-alanyl-D-isoglutamine) as an extremely potent adjuvant (Ellouz et al., 1974). This small peptide is phosphodiesterified to cell wall arabinogalactan, with which it forms water-soluble adjuvant. The extensive studies of analogs of muramyl dipeptide by many workers have explored the structural features of this small molecule that confer upon it adjuvant properties. Striking among these studies is the observation of Chedid and co-workers (Chedid et al., 1976) that substitution of the D-isomer for L-alanine created an immunosuppressive compound.

B. Lipoarabinomannan

Phosphorylated lipoarabinomannan has been extensively studied by Hunter, Brennan, and their colleagues and shown to be antigenic (Hunter et al., 1982, 1986; Brennan, 1989). The carbohydrate structure of this polysaccharide was originally elucidated by Misaki, and it was shown to share an epitope-bearing polyarabinose side chain with arabinogalactan, which is the principal structural polysaccharide of the mycobacterial cell wall (Misaka et al., 1977). Circulating antibodies to lipoarabinomannan are easily demonstrated in experimentally immunized animals (Daniel, 1975) and are found in the majority of patients with active tuberculosis (Benjamin and Daniel, 1982; Hunter et al., 1986; Sada et al., 1990a). However, delayed-type hypersensitivity reactions are not induced or evoked by this compound.

Many attributes of lipoarabinomannan may be important to the immunopathogenesis of tuberculosis and other mycobacterial diseases, perhaps functioning as a virulence factor. Ellner and Daniel showed arabinomannan to have immunosuppressive activity (Ellner and Daniel, 1979), and the product they used almost certainly contained the lipid moiety intact and was probably identical to lipoarabinomannan. Lipoarabinomannan inhibits the production of interferon-γ (Chan et al., 1991). It may serve as a scavenger of oxygen free radicals, thus inhibiting a major mechanism for the destruction of intracellular pathogens (Chan et al., 1989).

IV. Granuloma Formation

If one phenomenon can be thought of as central among the multiple manifestations of the immunology of tuberculosis, it is the formation of tubercles—hypersensitivity granulomas. These lesions, which characterize and distinguish the tissue response to mycobacteria, are chiefly composed of macrophages activated in response to mycobacterial antigens and adjuvants. Mackaness demonstrated that macrophages became activated in response to contact with mycobacteria, although this activation lacked the specificity usually associated with immunologic events (Mackaness, 1964). He hypothesized that monocytes, the circulating form of tissue macrophages, entered tissues at the site of tuberculous infection in response to chemotactic cytokines. Once aggregated in granulomas, monocytes transform to become the palisading histiocytes or epithelial cells characteristic of granulomas, and some of these cells fuse to form Langhans giant cells. Current evidence indicates that the most important mediator of these events is tumor necrosis factor (Kindler et al., 1989).

In an elegant set of studies of the pathogenesis of schistosomiasis, Warren and his colleagues (Warren et al., 1967; Boros et al., 1973) demonstrated the essential immune nature of granuloma formation. They showed that granuloma formation is antigen-specific, that it is characterized by anamnesis, that it can be transferred by lymphocytes but not serum, and that it is dependent on intact thymic but not bursal lymphocytes. Having thus firmly established granuloma formation as an immunologic event in schistosomiasis, Boros and Warren extended their studies to tuberculin antigens and confirmed the immunologic nature of the granulomas induced by these mycobacterial antigens (Boros and Warren, 1973).

V. Cell-Mediated Immunity

Mycobacterial infection has been the prototype for the study of the immune response to a facultative intracellular parasite. Passive transfer experiments in experimental animals have demonstrated convincingly that the T lymphocyte is the critical cell for delayed-type hypersensitivity and protective immunity. It has a role in granuloma formation, as well. Clinical observations in patients infected with human immunodeficiency virus likewise indicate a primary role for the CD4 T lymphocyte in protective immunity. Subpopulations of T lymphocytes, identifiable by surface markers, have specific immune and immunoregulatory functions, and interactions between these cells are mediated by soluble lymphokines.

A. T-Cell Subpopulation Mediating Cellular Immune Responses in Experimental Animals

Experimental studies have provided critical insights into the interrelationships of delayed-type hypersensitivity and protective immunity. Different T-cell subpopulations are responsible for these responses. For example, in a murine model, immunization with *M. bovis*, BCG strain resulted in the acquisition by splenic lymphocytes of the ability to transfer immunity against an aerosol challenge with virulent *M. tuberculosis* (Orme and Collins, 1984). Transfers of delayed-type hypersensitivity and protective immunity clearly were dissociable, mediated by different subpopulations of splenic T lymphocytes. In fact, the protective T cells were further separable into three populations on the basis of phenotype, kinetics of emergence, and sensitivity to cyclophosphamide (Orme, 1982). Protective T cells of CD4 and CD8 phenotypes were acquired in the spleen and, on passive transfer, conferred immunity to an aerosol challenge. Kinetic experiments indicated that the CD4 population had a more sustained effect in transfer of protection.

It should be noted that the adoptive immunization of gamma-irradiated T-cell-deficient mice with "memory-immune" lymphocytes from an *M. tuberculosis*-infected animal also conferred resistance against *M. avium*, *M. kansasii*, and *M. simiae* (Orme and Collins, 1986). This observation suggests that the protective immune response is directed against cross-reactive antigens, a notion of potentially signal importance as regards naturally acquired immunity as well as vaccination. Another key precept was added by the observation that immunization with live organisms led to the generation of splenic lymphocytes that transferred protective immunity, whereas killed vaccines transferred only nonspecific resistance and delayed-type hypersensitivity (Orme, 1988). The highest dose of heat-killed organisms, in fact, generated only barely detectable resistance. This finding suggests that protective immunity requires production of antigens by metabolically intact organisms and heightens interest in secreted antigens, as opposed to structural and heat shock proteins.

Recently, the potential role of γδ-T cells in the host response to tuberculosis has excited intensive study. T cells with a γδ receptor were expanded in lymph nodes (Janis et al., 1989) and lung (Augustin et al., 1989) following exposure to mycobacterial antigens. Most γδ-T-cell hybridomas produced from neonatal thymocytes responded to the 65,000-dalton antigen of *M. tuberculosis* (O'Brien et al., 1989), and more specifically, to the 180–196 arthritogenic peptide (Born et al., 1990). Although these data indicate that γδ-T cells infiltrate local tissue sites exposed to mycobacterial antigens, the role of γδ-T cells is not yet resolved. In studies by Orme, mice expressing αβ-T cells only (γδ-T-cell-depleted) acquired resistance to *M. tuberculosis*, whereas γδ-T-cell-expressing (αβ-T-cell-depleted) mice did not (personal communication). In view of the active interest of basic immunologists and mycobacteriologists in this area, additional insights into the role of γδ-T cells in the host immune response to *M. tuberculosis* should be forthcoming shortly. At this time, it appears that the γδ-T cell may be part of a primitive and innate immune response to mycobacterial and other infections reacting to shared antigens, including heat shock proteins, and representing an intermediate between the nonspecific inflammatory and the specific immune response.

B. Phenotype, Antigenic Specificity, and Function of Human *M. tuberculosis*-Reactive T-Cell Subpopulations

M. tuberculosis–infected healthy persons identified on the basis of a positive tuberculin PPD skin test are relatively immune to exogenous reinfection. Blood T cells obtained from these individuals can be used to assess the phenotype, antigenic reactivity, and function of cells responding to *M. tuberculosis* and presumably including "protective T cells." Exposure of peripheral blood mononuclear cells to live *M. tuberculosis* H37Ra leads to selective expansion of γδ-T cells, whereas stimulation with heat-killed organisms or soluble protein antigens leads to expansion of αβ-T cells (Havlir et al., 1991a,b). This observation is of particular interest since live organisms are more efficient at inducing a protective immune response, as discussed above.

Definition of the targets of the human T-cell response has been approached from two directions. Purified native and recombinant antigens, many of which first were identified by reactivity with murine monoclonal antibodies, have been tested for stimulation of peripheral blood mononuclear cells and T-cell lines and clones produced by cyclical restimulation of blood T cells from healthy tuberculin-positive donors. It should be noted that T-cell lines and clones, although enriched for antigen-responsive cells, may no longer reflect the repertoire of the starting population since they have been selected on the basis of favorable growth characteristics. The 12,000-, 14,000-, 19,000-, 38,000-, 65,000-, and 71,000-dalton antigens were among the first to be studied extensively in the era of molecular genetics. Although eliciting and the targets of humoral responses in immunized mice, they do not appear to be major targets of the T-cell response in infected humans. Some degree of reactivity has been reported, however, to each of these antigens (Emmrich et al., 1986; Young et al., 1986; Kingston et al., 1987; Munk et al., 1988; Ottenhoff et al., 1988; Havlir et al., 1991a,b; Mehra et al., 1991). A second group of antigens of considerable interest are the secretory products of *M. tuberculosis*. For example, the 30,000-alpha antigen and the 14,000-dalton MTP40 protein stimulate T-cell responses in tuberculin-positive donors (Havlir et al., 1991a,b; Falla et al., 1991). Of course, interest in secreted antigens is heightened by the importance ascribed to viable mycobacteria in the generation of a protective immune response.

A second approach that may more directly discern the relative contribution of individual antigens to the overall T-cell response is to examine the reactivity of T cells from healthy tuberculin-positive donors to fractions of crude antigens of *M. tuberculosis*. T-cell lines produced by stimulation of peripheral blood mononuclear cells with purified protein-peptidoglycan complex recognized antigens in sonicates of *M. tuberculosis* of molecular weights 10,000, 19,000, 23,000, 28,000, 30,000, 40–50,000, and 65,000 daltons (Barnes et al., 1989a,b). Peripheral blood mononuclear cells from comparable donors responded to culture filtrate antigens of molecular weights 30,000, 37,000, 44,000, 57,000, 64,000, 71,000, and 88,000 daltons (Havlir et al., 1991 a,b); Western immunoblotting showed that the fractions of molecular weights 30,000, 64,000, and 71,000 daltons contained the antigens of these sizes that had been identified previously. It is not clear, however, whether the previously recognized antigens accounted for the reactivity of the respective fractions. The studies to date suggest that the immune response to mycobacterial antigens is complex and heterogeneous and that it represents the sum of responses to a large number of antigens and epitopes, many of which remain unidentified. A number of investigators are exploiting complementary strategies in an attempt to identify the full repertoire of dominant T-cell antigens and epitopes of *M. tuberculosis*.

Another interesting property of mycobacterial antigens concerns their ability to stimulate mononuclear phagocytes directly. PPD stimulates monocytes and alveolar macrophages to increased expression of interleukin-1 (Wallis et al.,

1986) and tumor necrosis factor-α (Valone et al., 1988; Wallis et al., 1990). The active constituents of culture filtrates of *M. tuberculosis* that demonstrate this property are peptides of molecular weights 46,000 and 20,000 daltons. These peptides are of particular interest because the direct stimulation of mononuclear phagocytes may define an adjuvant-like activity or, alternatively, a factor contributory to hypersensitivity and immunosuppression, as discussed below.

The functional properties of T-cell populations reactive to mycobacterial antigens also deserve consideration. Blastogenesis is a readily measured assay of lymphocyte stimulation but may have little to do with in situ immune responses. In general, expression of cytokines such as interleukin-2 and interferon-γ has paralleled blastogenesis of T cells from healthy tuberculin-positive donors stimulated with PPD or purified mycobacterial constituents. Interpretation of such observations is complicated, however, by uncertainty concerning the cytokine or cytokines expressing macrophage-activating factor activity for mycobacteria. In fact, one study has proposed that interferon-γ actually promotes the intracellular replication of *M. tuberculosis* (Douvas et al., 1985). Nonetheless, it seems reasonable to assume that products of stimulated CD4 cells directly or indirectly are essential features of the local immune response to mycobacteria. In this regard, we have recently shown that tumor necrosis factor, which has been ascribed an essential role in granuloma formation (Kindler et al., 1981), also is important as a macrophage-activating factor for *M. tuberculosis* (Yoneda, T., et al., unpublished observations).

Another functional property of CD4 lymphocytes has been described, although its bearing on the interactions of *M. tuberculosis* with the host still is uncertain. CD4 T-cell lines and clones express class II major histocompatibility complex–restricted cytotoxicity for mononuclear phagocytes pulsed with killed *M. tuberculosis*, PPD, or the purified 65,000-dalton antigen (Ottenhoff et al., 1988; Boom et al., 1991). The significance of this phenomenon is uncertain. It is possible to speculate that class II major histocompatibility complex–restricted cytotoxicity is a means for freeing up mycobacteria from overburdened macrophages so that they can be released into an extracellular environment in which they replicate poorly or can be ingested by more potent effector cells such as freshly recruited and activated macrophages. Many alternatives to this scenario exist, however, including a possible role for class II histocompatibility complex–restricted CD4 lymphocytes in autocytotoxicity contributing to the genesis of caseation necrosis or autoimmune phenomena.

The function of γδ-T cells is less certain, although they appear to produce the same group of cytokines and to participate in cytotoxic events. As opposed to CD4 lymphocytes, however, γδ-T cells are restricted at neither the class I nor class II major histocompatibility complex loci in their activation or in their cytotoxicity (Boom, W. H., et al., unpublished observations).

VI. Humoral Immunity

It is important to recognize that the pathogenesis of tuberculosis is almost exclusively determined by host T-lymphocyte-mediated cellular immune responses. At the same time, one must acknowledge that B-lymphocyte-mediated humoral responses to mycobacterial antigens occur in patients with tuberculosis, although these responses have no clearly demonstrated role in disease pathogenesis.

The earliest demonstration of circulating antibody to mycobacterial antigens in patients with tuberculosis was probably the study of Arloing published in 1898. As serology emerged as a laboratory technique and science, most of the classical serological techniques were used to study patients with tuberculosis; antibodies were repeatedly demonstrated, but neither insight into disease pathogenesis nor satisfactory techniques for serodiagnosis emerged. However, following the first use of enzyme-linked immunosorbent assay (ELISA) for the serodiagnosis of tuberculosis by Nassau et al. (1976) and the general availability of conjugated second antibodies specific for individual immunoglobulin isotypes, rapid advances in understanding of humoral immune responses in tuberculosis and in the development of serodiagnostic techniques occurred.

Levels of immunoglobulin-G antibody detectable by ELISA or other immunoassay are usually an indicator of active tuberculous disease. Studies with many antigens using many techniques have found that few control subjects have measurable IgG antibody levels (Daniel and Debanne, 1987). Asymptomatic primary infection (Daniel et al., 1991) and minimal pulmonary disease (Chan et al., 1990) are usually not sufficient to induce a significant antibody response. During the course of treatment, antibody levels rise somewhat for the first 1 or 2 months, falling thereafter but remaining detectable for 1 to several years (Daniel et al., 1985). Patients with remote healed tuberculosis do not have readily detected IgG antibody to mycobacterial antigens.

Immunoglobulin-M responses are directly chiefly at nonspecific polysaccharide antigens. They develop early but never reach high titer, and their level does not correlate well with the presence or absence of active disease (Daniel and Debanne, 1987). Many healthy persons probably develop low levels of IgM antibody in response to contact with environmental mycobacteria.

Immunoglobulin-A antibody has been recognized at low levels in the serum of patients with active tuberculosis but not in control subjects (Daniel and Debanne, 1987). However, IgA antibody to mycobacterial antigens has not been studied adequately in external secretions, and this is an area deserving more attention. One should not exclude a potential role of IgA antibody in mucosal protection immunity to tuberculosis without direct examination of the question.

Many investigators have measured IgG antibody to mycobacterial antigens and proposed serodiagnostic tests based on the identification of such antibody (Daniel and Debanne, 1987). New tests are being proposed almost daily. From the extensive work that has been done, one can state with reasonable confidence that it is possible to devise simple serodiagnostic tests using any of several antigens, but that the choice of antigen is a major determinant of diagnostic test specificity and predictive accuracy. Crude mycobacterial cell lysates and culture filtrates and tuberculin purified protein derivative (PPD) do not provide as satisfactory diagnostic tests as do more highly purified antigens.

Tests with the most consistently favorable diagnostic characteristics have been those employing the 38,000-dalton antigen known as antigen 5 in the Janicki classification system (Ivanyi et al., 1983; Balestrino et al., 1984; Ma et al., 1986; Bothamley et al., 1988). These superior tests include those based on the inhibition of monoclonal antibody TB-72 (Ivanyi et al., 1983; Bothamley et al., 1988). A major limiting factor in the clinical use of these tests has been the unavailability of this antigen, which to date has been purified only in small amounts by immunoaffinity chromatography.

Sada and co-workers have described an ELISA with excellent serodiagnostic test characteristics which employs the 30,000-dalton mycobacterial antigen (Sada et al., 1990b). An antigen designated A-60, which was first prepared by Cocito and Vanlinden (1986) and which probably contains chiefly lipoarabinomannan, provides the basis for a serodiagnostic test now commercially available in Europe. While it provides excellent sensitivity, this test appears to be less specific than desirable (Charpin et al., 1990). Sada has performed a serological study using purified lipoarabinomannan with results that parallel those using the cruder A-60 preparation, finding high sensitivity but low specificity (Sada et al., 1990b). Recent work in our laboratory (Daniel et al., unpublished observations) demonstrates that serodiagnosis of tuberculosis has a decreased sensitivity in human immunodeficiency virus (HIV)-infected patients with tuberculosis.

VII. Immune Spectrum: Immunoregulation

Leprosy is the classical example of a granulomatous disease caused by a facultative intracellular pathogen in which the host immune response shows a predictable linkage to bacterial load in tissues and disease manifestations. At the tuberculoid end of the spectrum, there are vigorous granulomatous hypersensitivity, active T-cell immune reactivity, little in terms of antibody response, few bacilli, and localized disease. At the lepromatous end of the spectrum, there are few and poorly formed granulomas, specific hyporesponsiveness of T cells to mycobacterial antigens, high titers of antibody, and multibacillary disease.

There have been several attempts to define a spectrum of disease manifestations similar to that of leprosy in patients with tuberculosis (Malaviya et al., 1975; Lenzini et al., 1977). These classification schemes have not been entirely convincing, often requiring clinical and pathological distinctions that are not easily made. A few general comments concerning the immune spectrum of tuberculosis are, however, supportable. Healthy tuberculin skin test positive donors express vigorous delayed-type hypersensitivity and have low titers of antibody directed against mycobacterial products. Pulmonary tuberculosis, at least in the United States, usually is characterized by relative hyporesponsiveness to tuberculin; 20–25% of individuals have a negative tuberculin skin test, and hyporesponsiveness to PPD in vitro is 2–3 times more common (Cox et al., 1988). antibody levels are elevated (Havlir et al., 1991a,b), providing the potential basis for serodiagnosis. Miliary tuberculosis and tuberculous meningitis are associated with a greater frequency of skin test anergy and more systemic signs and symptoms than localized disease (Toossi and Ellner, 1991).

The local immune response in tuberculous pleurisy is of some interest since clinical and epidemiological evidence indicates that it is capable of initial self-cure (Ellner et al., 1988). The pleural fluid is enriched in highly antigen-reactive CD4+CDw29+ lymphocytes (Barnes et al., 1989b), apparently the result of in situ expansion rather than sequestration of such cells from the circulating pool (Fujiwara and Tsuyuguchi, 1984). Pleural fluid also contains 5- to 30-fold increased levels of interferon-γ and tumor necrosis factor relative to serum (Barnes et al., 1990).

Based on the data from tuberculous pleurisy, the hyporesponsiveness of peripheral blood mononuclear cells to PPD in pulmonary tuberculosis is not readily explained by shifts in the compartmentalization of antigen-responsive T cells. Likewise, the ratio of CD4/CD8 lymphocytes is preserved in tuberculosis (Kleinhenz and Ellner, 1987; Cox et al., 1988). Active and specific immunosuppression is a factor in the depression of T-cell blastogenic responses and expression of interleukin-2 in response to PPD (Ellner, 1978; Toossi et al., 1986). The mechanism of suppression appears to be unique. Monocytes primed during the course of infection are stimulated directly by PPD or bacterial lipopolysaccharide to increased production of cytokines such as interleukin-1 (Fujiwara et al., 1983), tumor necrosis factor (Takashima et al., 1990; Ogawa et al., 1991), and interleukin-6 (Ogawa et al., 1991), of immunosuppressive factors such as the receptor for interleukin-2 (Toossi et al., 1990), and transforming growth factor-β.

The response to certain protein antigens of *M. tuberculosis* seems to be selectively suppressed in patients with tuberculosis. For example, despite comparable responses to sonicates of *M. tuberculosis*, 84% of healthy household contacts and only 52% of treated and 48% of untreated patients with tuberculosis responded to the MTP40 (14,000 dalton) antigen (Falla et al., 1991). Similarly, tuberculosis patients showed selective hyporesponsiveness to the 30,000-dalton antigen. Seven of eight healthy tuberculin reactors and none of six tuberculosis patients (post 6–20 weeks of treatment) were responsive to the 30,000-dalton antigen (Havlir et al., 1991 a,b). Interpretation of these findings is complicated by the consistent finding that tuberculosis patients in the United States are hyporesponsive to PPD (Havlir et al., 1991a,b). Supportive observations are, however, available from Mexico City. None of 10 patients with newly diagnosed pulmonary tuberculosis and 73% of 21 household contacts showed responses to the 30,000-dalton antigen of *M. tuberculosis*, whereas responses to mycobacterial sonicates were comparable in both groups (Sada, E., et al., personal communication). These results raise two possibilities. First, the absence of response to the 30,000-dalton antigen may be a stable characteristic, perhaps genetically determined, and may predispose individuals to the development of tuberculosis. Second, the 30,000-dalton antigen may activate immunosuppresive pathways, possibly through direct stimulation of monocytes. Distinction between these alternatives is of considerable importance. Serial observations should show whether patients with tuberculosis fail to respond to the 30,000-dalton antigen despite treatment. If this is the case, then lack of response to the 30,000 dalton antigen might be a marker for an individual at increased risk of progressing from infection to disease. Such a discriminatory test, which could be operationalized as a delayed-type hypersensitivity skin test, would provide a tremendous tool for TB control programs. Decisions concerning the application of preventive therapy for healthy *M. tuberculosis*–infected persons would be simplified by the possibility of dichotomizing PPD tuberculin skin test positive individuals based on the projected risk of development of tuberculosis.

The anergy occurring in patients with pulmonary tuberculosis is specific in some and nonspecific in other individuals. In fact, it may be appropriate to assume that patients with pulmonary tuberculosis usually show specific superimposed on nonspecific anergy. Specific anergy has been addressed above; the mechanism of nonspecific anergy is not well understood. It is of interest, therefore, that mycobacterial polysaccharides such as D-arabino-D-mannan and D-arabino-D-galactan stimulate monocyte-dependent suppression of blastogenesis induced by nonspecific mitogens (Ellner and Daniel, 1979; Kleinhenz et al., 1981). Detailed studies, in fact, suggest that the underlying mechanism involves circulating immune complexes containing polysaccharides that stimulate monocyte production of immunosuppressive prostaglandin E2 (Kleinhenz et al., 1981). The finding that a polysaccharide antigen, presumably a major target of the antibody response to tuberculosis, itself suppresses T-cell reactivity is of interest as it may contribute to the inverse and reciprocal relationships between T-cell responses and B-cell responses in tuberculosis as considered above.

VIII. HIV–*M. tuberculosis* Interactions

HIV infection is the strongest known risk factor for the reactivation of a latent tuberculous infection. In a prospective study of a cohort of tuberculin skin test positive intravenous drug users in a methadone-maintenance program in New York, the risk of developing tuberculosis was 7.9% per year during a 2-year period of follow-up (Selwyn et al., 1989). This must be compared to the risk of developing tuberculosis in *M. tuberculosis*–infected, HIV-uninfected persons, which can be estimated to be 5–10% per lifetime. It is also clear that primary infection with *M. tuberculosis* is likely to progress to active tuberculosis in HIV-infected persons. The current outbreaks of multidrug-resistant tuberculosis in HIV-infected persons (Fischl et al., 1991) are clear evidence of this phenomenon.

Several points are beginning to emerge concerning the immunology of dual HIV/*M. tuberculosis* infection. It now is clear that HIV infection increases the likelihood of a negative tuberculin skin test in *M. tuberculosis*–infected persons. For example, HIV-infected postpartum females in Uganda were less likely to show reactions of over 3 mm to Old Tuberculin (48% vs. 82%) and had smaller reaction sizes (7.5 mm vs. 10.6 mm induration) as compared to HIV-negative age-matched postpartum females (Okwera et al., 1990).

The relationship between delayed-type hypersensitivity reactions and CD4 counts in HIV-infected persons has also been studied using panels of nonmycobacterial antigens. Cutaneous anergy was infrequent (< 10%) in individuals with a CD4 count > 500/μl; below this level, however, the frequency of anergy varied inversely with the CD4 count and was 2/3 for CD4 < 200 and 80% for CD4 < 50 (Centers for Disease Control, 1991). Studies in Zaire demonstrated anergy as defined using the CMI-Multitest in 46% of 50 HIV-infected individuals (Colebunders et al., 1989). Importantly, 36% of HIV-infected tuberculin-positive persons had active tuberculosis as compared to 8% of the tuberculin-negative persons. The notion that tuberculosis may boost tuberculin reactivity rather than further depress it in the presence of HIV infection is further supported by recent observations from Uganda. Sixty-eight percent of HIV-positive tuberculosis patients were tuberculin skin test positive with reaction sizes of >10 mm, as compared to 80% in the unmatched cohort of HIV-positive postpartum women discussed above (Vjecha et al., 1991).

Tuberculosis is an early event in the natural history of AIDS, occurring a mean 6–9 months before an AIDS-defining condition (Ellner, 1990). CD4 counts vary according to whether tuberculosis antedates or follows the AIDS-defining condition. In three U.S. series, the mean CD4 counts at the time of diagnosis of tuberculosis were 170, 220, and 367/μl (Modilevsky et al., 1989; Schecter, unpublished observations; Gutierrez, unpublished observations), whereas the mean CD4 count was 552/μl in nine HIV-infected, tuberculin-positive Ugandan tuberculous patients (Wallis, R. S., et al., unpublished observations). These observations strongly suggest that HIV-TB interactions may differ considerably in developing countries with high prevalences of *M. tuberculosis* as compared to developed countries with low prevalences. When tuberculosis occurred more than 2 years before AIDS, 71% of patients were tuberculin skin test positive, as compared to 33% when the diagnoses were concurrent or the AIDS-defining condition preceded tuberculosis (Reider et al., 1989). In the United States, overall, 39–56% of HIV-infected tuberculosis patients are tuberculin skin test positive (Ellner, 1990). In Uganda, 68% of the HIV-infected tuberculosis patients are skin test positive; the skin test negative patients have a poorer prognosis, apparently because of the more advanced state of the HIV infection (Vjecha et al., 1991).

Limited in vitro studies have been conducted in HIV-infected tuberculin-positive tuberculosis patients in Uganda (Wallis, et al., unpublished observations). These patients show an increase in PPD-stimulated blastogenesis and production of interleukin-2, interferon-γ, and tumor necrosis factor compared to HIV-uninfected tuberculin-positive tuberculosis patients. Since tumor necrosis factor is known to promote HIV replication, these observations, as well as theoretical considerations, raise the question of whether tuberculosis might accelerate HIV infection. β_2-microglobulin levels, in fact, were higher in newly diagnosed HIV-infected tuberculosis patients than in a comparable group studied after 2 months of treatment and groups with tuberculosis or HIV infection only. These data, therefore, support the possibility that the immune activation, which is a consistent concomitant of active tuberculosis, activates cells harboring latent HIV infection to promote viral repliation and disease progression. This notion, if substantiated by additional immunological, virological, and epidemiological data would have profound impact on public health policy. Certainly, the potential benefits from preventive therapy of tuberculosis would be enchanced, if, besides preventing tuberculosis, it prolonged the survival from HIV infection.

IX. Conclusions

Although progress toward understanding the immune response to mycobacteria has accelerated in the last decade, this has not been translated into practical advances relevant to the control of tuberculosis. Although existing means of diagnosis and prevention clearly are problematic, new modalities are yet to be developed. It is reasonble to expect the pace of progress to continue to increase, driven by the magnitude of the global problem compounded by the pandemic of HIV infection and outbreaks of multidrug-resistant tuberculosis.

References

Abou-Zeid, C., Ratliff, T. L., Wiker, H. G., Harboe, M., Bennedsen, J., and Rook, G. A. W. (1988a). Characterization of fibronectin-binding antigens released by *Mycobacterium tuberculosis* and *Mycobacterium bovis* BCG. *Infect. Immun.* **56**:3046–3051.

Abou-Zeid, C., Smith, I., Grange, J. M., Ratliff, T. L., Steele, J., and Rook, G. A. W. (1988b). The secreted antigens of *Mycobacterium tuberculosis* and their relationship to those recognized by the available monoclonal antibodies. *J. Gen. Microbiol.* **134**:531–538.

Adam, A., Ciorbaru, R., Petit, J-F., and Lederer, E. (1972). Isolation and properties of a macromolecular, water-soluble, immuno-adjuvant fraction from the cell wall of *Mycobacterium smegmatis*. *Proc. Natl. Acad. Sci. USA* **69**:851–854.

Anderson, A. B., and Hansen, E. B. (1989). Structure and mapping of antigenic domains of protein b, a 38,000-molecular weight protein of *Mycobacterium tuberculosis*. *Infect. Immun.* **57**:2481–2488.

Anderson, A. B., Ljungqvist, L., and Olsen, M. (1990). Evidence that protein antigen b of *Mycobacterium tuberculosis* is involved in phosphate metabolism. *J. Gen. Microbiol.* **136**:477–480.

Arloing, S. (1898). Agglutination de bacille de la tuberculose vraie. *CR Acad. Sci.* **126**:1398–1400.

Augustin, A., Kubo, R. T., and Gek-Kee, S. (1989). Resident pulmonary lymphocytes expressing the γδ T-cell receptor. *Nature* **340**:239–241.

Balestrino, E. A., Daniel, T. M., de Latini, M. D. S., Latini, O. A., Ma, Y., and Scocozza J. B. (1984). Serodiagnosis of pulmonary tuberculosis in Argentina by enzyme-linked immunosorbent assay (ELISA) of IgG antibody to *Mycobacterium tuberculosis* antigen 5 and tuberculin purified protein derivative. *Bull. WHO* **62**:755–761.

Barnes, P. F., Mehra, V., Hirschfield, G. R., Fong, S-J., Abou-Zeid, C., Rook, G. A. W., Hunter, S. W., Brennan, P. J., and Modlin, R. L. (1989a). Characterization of T-cell antigens associated with the cell wall protein-peptidoglycan complex of *Mycobacterium tuberculosis*. *J. Immunol.* **143**:2656–2662.

Barnes, P. F., Misky, S. D., Cooper, C. L., Pirmez, C., Ren, T. N., and Modlin, R. E. (1989b). Compartmentalization of a CD4+ T-lymphocyte population in tuberculous pleuritis. *J. Immunol.* **142**:1114–1119.

Barrow, W. W., and Brennan, P. J. (1982). Immunogenicity of type-specific C-mycoside glycolipids of mycobacteria. *Infect. Immun.* **36**:678–684.

Benjamin, R. G., and Daniel, T. M. (1982). Serodiagnosis of tuberculosis using the enzyme-linked immunoabsorbent assay (ELISA) of antibody to *Mycobacterium tuberculosis* antigen 5. *Am. Rev. Respir. Dis.* **126**:1013–1016.

Benjamin, R. G., Debanne, S. M., Ma, Y., and Daniel, T. M. (1984). Evaluation of mycobacterial antigens in an enzyme-linked immunosorbent assay (ELISA) for the serodiagnosis of tuberculosis. *J. Med. Microbiol.* **18**:309–318.

Boom, W. H., Wallis, R. S., and Chervenak, K. A. (1991). Human *Mycobacterium tuberculosis*-reactive CD4+ T-cell clones: heterogeneity in antigen recognition, cytokine production and cytotoxicity for mononuclear phago-cytes. *Infect. Immun.* **59**:2737–2743.

Born, W., Hall, L., Dallas, A., Boymel, J., Shinnick, T., Young, D., Brennan, P., and O'Brien, R. (1990). Recognition of a peptide antigen by heat-shock reactive γδ T-lymphocytes. *Science* **249**:67–69.

Boros, D. L., and Warren, K. S. (1973). The bentonite granuloma. Character-ization of a model system for infectious and foreign body granulomatous inflammation using soluble mycobacterial, histoplasma and schistosoma antigens. *Immunology* **24**:511–529.

Boros, D. L., Schwartz, H. J., Powell, A. E., and Warren, K. S. (1973). De-layed hypersensitivity, as manifested by granuloma formation, dermal re-activity, macrophage migration inhibition and lymphocyte transformation, induced and elicited in guinea pigs with soluble antigens of Schistosoma mansoni eggs. *J. Immunol.* **110**:1118–1125.

Borremans, M., De Wit, L., Volkaert, G., Ooms, J., De Bruyn, J., Huygen, K., Van Vooren, J. P., Stelandre, M., Verhofstadt, R., and Content, J. (1989). Cloning, sequence determination, and expression of a 32-kilodalton-protein gene of *Mycobacterium tuberculosis*. *Infect. Immun.* **57**:3123–3130.

Bothamley, G., Udani, P., Rudd, R., Festenstein, F., and Ivanyi, J. (1988). Humoral response to defined epitopes of tubercle bacilli in adult pul-monary and child tuberculosis. *Eur. J. Clin. Microbiol. Infect. Dis.* **7**:639–645.

Brennan, P. J. (1981). Structure of the typing antigens of atypical mycobacteria. A brief review of present knowledge. *Rev. Infect. Dis.* **3**:905–913.

Brennan, P. J. (1989). Structure of mycobacteria: Recent developments in de-fining cell wall carbohydrates and proteins. *Rev. Infect. Dis.* **11**(Suppl): S420–S430.

Buchanan, T. M., Nomaguchi, H., Anderson, D. C., Young, R. A., Gillis, T. P., Britton, W. J., Ivanyi, J., Kolk, A. H. J., Closs, O., Bloom, B. R., and Mehra, V. (1987). Characterization of antibody-reactive epitopes on the 65-kilodalton protein of *Mycobacterium leprae*. *Infect. Immun.* **55**:1000–1003.

Centers for Disease Control (1991). Purified protein derivative (PPD)-tuberculin anergy in HIV infection: guidelines for anergy testing and management of anergic persons at risk of tuberculosis. *MMWR* **40**(No RR-5):27–32.

Chan, J., Fujiwara, T., Brennan, P. J., McNeil, M., Turco, S. J., Sibille, J-C., Snapper, M., Aisen, P., and Bloom, B. R. (1989). Microbial glycolipids: possible virulence factors that scavenge oxygen radicals. *Proc. Natl. Acad. Sci. USA* **86**:2453–2457.

Chan, J., Fan, X., Hunter, S. W., Brennan, P. J., and Bloom, B. R. (1991). Lipoarabinomannan, a possible virulence factor involved in persistence of *Mycobacterium tuberculosis* within macrophages. *Infect. Immun.* **59**:1755–1761.

Chan, S. L., Reggiardo, Z., Daniel, T. M., Girling, D. J., and Mitchison, D. A. (1990). Serodiagnosis of tuberculosis using an enzyme-linked immunosorbent assay (ELISA) with antigen 5 and a hemagglutination assay with glycolipid antigens. Results in patients with newly diagnosed pulmonary tuberculosis ranging in extent of disease from minimal to extensive. *Am. Rev. Respir. Dis.* **142**:385–390.

Charpin, D., Herbault, H., Gevaudan, M. J., Saadjian, M., De Micco, P., Arnaud, A., Vervloet, D., and Charpin, J. (1990). Value of ELISA using A60 antigen in the diagnosis of active pulmonary tuberculosis. *Am. Rev. Respir. Dis.* **142**:380–384.

Chase, M. W. (1945). The cellular transfer of cutaneous hypersensitivity to tuberculin. *Proc. Soc. Exp. Biol. Med.* **59**:134–135.

Chedid, L., Audibert, F., Lefrancier, P., Choay, J., and Lederer, E. (1976). Modulation of the immune response by a synthetic adjuvant and analogs. *Proc. Natl. Acad. Sci. USA* **73**:2472–2475.

Cocito, C. and Vanlinden F. (1986). Preparation and properties of antigen 60 from *Mycobacterium bovis* BCG *Clin. Exp. Immunol.* **66**:262–272.

Colebunders, R. L., Lebughe, I., Nzila, N., Kalunga, D., Francis, H., Ryder, R., and Piot, P. (1989). Cutaneous delayed-type hypersensitivity in patients with human immunodeficiency virus infection in Zaire. *J. Acq. Immunodeficien. Syndr.* **2**:576–578.

Cox, R. A., Downs, M., Neimes, R. E., Ognibene, A. J., Yamashita, T. S., and Ellner, J. J. (1988). Immunogenetic analysis of human tuberculosis. *J. Infect. Dis.* **158**:1302–1308.

Daniel, T. M. (1975). The antigenicity in guinea pigs and monkeys of three mycobacterial polysaccharides purified by affinity chromatography with concanavalin A. *Am. Rev. Respir. Dis.* **111**:787–793.

Daniel, T. M. (1980) The immunology of tuberculosis. *Clin. Chest Med.* **1**:189–201.

Daniel, T. M. and Anderson, P. A. (1978). The isolation by immunoabsorbent affinity chromatography and physicochemical characterization of *Mycobacterium tuberculosis* antigen 5. *Amer. Rev. Respir. Dis.* **117**:533–539.

Daniel, T. M. and Debanne, S. M. (1987). The serodiagnosis of tuberculosis and other mycobacterial diseases by enzyme-linked immunosorbent assay. *Am. Rev. Respir. Dis.* **135**:1137–1151.

Daniel, T. M. and Ferguson, L. E. (1970). Purification and characterization of two proteins from culture filtrates of *Mycobacterium tuberculosis* H37Ra strain. *Infect. Immun.* **1**:164–168.

Daniel, T. M., Ellner, J. J., Todd, L. S., McCoy, D. W., Payne, V. D. N., Anderson, P. A., and Bhe, F. T. (1979). Immunobiology and species distribution of *Mycobacterium tuberculosis* antigen 5. *Infect. Immun.* **24**:77–82.

Daniel, T. M., Balestrino, E. A., Balestrino, O. C., Davidson, P. T., Debanne, S. M., Kataria, S., Kataria, Y. P., and Scocozza, J. B. (1982). The tuberculin specificity in humans of *Mycobacterium tuberculosis* antigen 5. *Am. Rev. Respir. Dis.* **126**:600–606.

Daniel, T. M., Debanne, S. M., and van der Kuyp, F. (1985). Enzyme-linked immunosorbent assay using *Mycobacterium tuberculosis* antigen 5 and PPD for the serodiagnosis of tuberculosis. *Chest* **88**:388–392.

Daniel, T. M., McDonough, J. A., and Huebner, R. E. (1991). Absence of IgM or IgG antibody response to *Mycobacterium tuberculosis* 30,000-Da antigen after primary tuberculous infection (letter). *J. Infect. Dis.* **164**:821.

David, J. R., Al-Askari, S., Lawrence, H. S., and Thomas, L. (1964). Delayed hypersensitivity in vitro. I. The specificity of inhibition of cell migration by antigens. *J. Immunol.* **93**:264–273.

De Bruyn, J., Huygen, K., Bosmans, R., Fauville, M., Lippens, R., Van Vooren, J. P., Falmagne, P., Weckx, M., Wiker, H. G., Harboe, M. and Turneer, M. (1987). Purification, characterization and identification of a 32 kDa protein antigen of *Mycobacterium bovis* BCG. *Microbial. Pathogen.* **2**:351–366.

Douvas, G. S., Looker, D. L., Vatter, A. E., and Crowle, A. J. (1985). Gamma-interferon activates human macrophages to become tumoricidal and leishmanicidal but enhances replication of macrophage-associated mycobacteria. *Infect. Immun.* **50**:1–8.

Edwards, P. Q. and Edwards, L. B. (1960). Story of the tuberculin test from an epidemiologic viewpoint. *Am. Rev. Respir. Dis.* **81**(Suppl):1–47.

Ellner, J. J. (1978). Suppressor adherent cells in human tuberculosis. *J. Immunol.* **121**:2573–2578.

Ellner, J. J. (1990). Tuberculosis in the time of AIDS. The facts and the message. *Chest* **98**:1051–1052.

Ellner, J. J. and Daniel, T. M. (1979). Immunosuppression by mycobacterial arabinomannan. *Clin. Exp. Immunol.* **35**:250–257.

Ellner, J. J., Barnes, P. F., Wallis, R. S., and Modlin, R. L. (1988). The immunology of tuberculous pleurisy. *Semin. Respir. Med.* **3**:335–342.

Ellouz, F., Adam, A., Cirobaru, R., and Lederer, E. (1974). Minimal structure requirements for adjuvant activity of bacterial peptidoglycan derivatives. *Biochem. Biophys. Res. Commun.* **59**:1317–1325.

Emmrich, F., Thole, J., van Embden, J., and Kaufmann, S. H. E. (1986). A recombinant 64 kilodalton protein of *Mycobacterium bovis* Bacillus Calmette-Guérin specifically stimulates human T4 clones reactive to mycobacterial antigens. *J. Exp. Med.* **163**:1024–1029.

Engers, H. D., Bloom, B. R., Godal, T. (1985). Monoclonal antibodies against mycobacterial antigens. *Immunol. Today* **6**:345–347.

Engers, H. D., Houba, V., Bennedsen, J., Buchanan, T. M., Chaparas, S. D., Kadival, G., Closs, O., David, J. R., van Embden, J. D. A., Godal, T., Mustafa, S. A., Ivanyi, J., Young, D. B., Kaufmann, S. H. E., Khomenko, A. G., Kolk, A. H. J., Kubin, M., Louis, J. A., Minden, P., Shinnick, T. M., Trnka, L., and Young, R. A. (1986). Letter to the editor. Results of a World Health Organization-sponsored workship to characterize antigens recognized by Mycobacterium-specific monoclonal antibodies. *Infect. Immun.* **51**:718–720.

Falla, J. C., Parra, C. H., Mendoza, M., Franco, L. C., Guzman, F., Forero, J., Orozco, O., and Patarroyo, M. E. (1991). Identification of B- and T-cell epitopes within the MPT 40 protein of *Mycobacterium tuberculosis* and their correlation with the course of disease. *Infect. Immun.* **59**:2265–2273.

Fischl, M., Uttamchandani, R., Reyes, R., Cleary, T., Otten, J., Breeden, A., Bigler, W., Valdez, H., Cacciatore, R., Witte, J., Hoskins, R. S., Grieco, M. H., Williams, J., Sordillo, E., Rivera, P., Pitta, A., Mullen, M. P., Gordon, M. T., Busillo, C. P., Boyle, J. F., Adler, J., Ong, K. R., DiFerdinando, J. F., Jr., and Morse, D. L. (1991). Nosocomial transmission of multidrug resistant tuberculosis among HIV-infected persons—Florida and New York, 1988–1991. *MMWR* **40**:585–591.

Fujiwara, H. and Tsuyuguchi, I. (1984). Frequency of tuberculin-reactive T-lymphocytes in pleural fluid and blood from patients with tuberculous pleurisy. *Chest* **89**:530–532.

Fujiwara, H., Kleinhenz, M. E., and Ellner, J. J. (1983). Defective interleukin-2 production and responsiveness in human pulmonary tuberculosis. *Am. Rev. Respir. Dis.* **133**:73–77.

Goren, M. B. (1982). Immunoreactive substances of mycobacteria. *Am. Rev. Respir. Dis.* **125**(Suppl):50–69.

Haslov, K., Anderson, A. B., Ljungqvist, L., Weis and Bentzon, M. (1990). Comparison of the immunological activity of five defined antigens of *Mycobacterium tuberculosis* in seven inbred guinea pig strains. The 38-kDa antigen is immunodominant. *Scand. J. Immunol.* **31**:503–514.

Havlir, D. V., Ellner, J. J., Chervenak, K. A., and Boom, W. H. (1991a). Selective expansion of human γδ T-cells by monocytes infected with live *Mycobacterium tuberculosis. J. Clin. Invest.* **87**:729–733.

Havlir, D. V., Wallis, R. S., Boom, W. H., Daniel, T. M., Chervenak, K., and Ellner, J. J. (1991b). Human immune response to *Mycobacterium tuberculosis* antigens. *Infect. Immun.* **59**:665–670.

Hunter, S. W., Fujiwara, T., and Brennan, P. J. (1982). Structure and antigenicity of the major specific glycoplipid antigen *Mycobacterium leprae. J. Biol. Chem.* **257**15072–15078.

Hunter, S. W., Gaylord, H., and Brennan, P. J. (1986). Structure and antigenicity of the phosphorylated lipopolysaccharide antigens from the leprosy and tubercle bacilli. *J. Biol. Chem.* **261**:12345–12351.

Ivanyi, J., Krambovitis, E., and Keen, M. (1983). Evaluation of a monoclonal antibody (TB72) based serological test for tuberculosis. *Clin. Exp. Immunol.* **54**:337–345.

Janicki, B. W., Chaparas, S. D., Daniel, T. M., Kubica, G. P., Wright, G. L., Jr., and Yee, G. S. (1972). A reference system for antigens of *Mycobacterium tuberculosis*. *Am. Rev. Respir. Dis.* **104**:602–604.

Janis, E. M. Kaufmann, S. H. E., Schwartz, R. M., and Pardoll, D. M. (1989). Activation of δ T-cells in the primary immune response to mycobacteria. *Science* **244**:713–716.

Kadival, G. V., Chaparas, S. D., and Hussong, D. (1987). Characterization of serologic and cell-mediated reactivity of a 38-kDa antigen isolated from *Mycobacterium tuberculosis*. *J. Immunol.* **139**:2447–2451.

Kindler, V., Sappino, A. P., Grau, G. E., Piguet, P. F., and Vassali, P. (1989). The inducing role of tumor necrosis factor in the development of bactericidal granulomas during BCG infection. *Cell* **56**:731–740.

Kingston, A. E., Salgame, P. R., Mitchison, N. A., and Colston, M. J. (1987). Immunological activity of a 14-kilodalton recombinant protein of *Mycobacterium tuberculosis* H37Rv. *Infect. Immun.* **55**:3149–3154.

Kleinhenz, M. E. and Ellner, J. J. (1987). Antigen responsiveness during tuberculosis: Regulatory interaction of T-cell subpopulations and adherent cells. *J. Lab. Clin. Med.* **110**:31–40.

Kleinhenz, M. E., Ellner, J. J., Spagnuolo, P. J., and Daniel, T. M. (1981). Suppression of lymphocyte responses by tuberculous plasma and mycobacterial arabinogalactan. Monocyte dependence and indomethacin reversibility. *J. Clin. Invest.* **68**:153–162.

Koch, R. (1932). Die aetiologie der tuberculose, a translation by Berna Pinner and Max Pinner with an introduction by Allen K. Krause. *Am. Rev. Tuberc.* **25**:285–323.

Koch, R. (1891). Weitere mitteilungen uber ein heilmittel gegen tuberculose. *Deutsch Med. Wochenschr.* **17**:101–102.

Lenzini, L., Rottoli, P., and Rottoli, L. (1977). The spectrum of human tuberculosis. *Clin. Exp. Immunol.* **27**:230–237.

Ma, Y., Wang, Y. M., and Daniel, T. M. (1986). Enzyme-linked immunosorbent assay using *Mycobacterium tuberculosis* antigen 5 for the diagnosis of pulmonary tuberculosis in China. *Am. Rev. Respir. Dis.* **134**:1273–1275.

Mackaness, G. B. (1964). The immunological basis of acquired cellular resistance. *J. Exp. Med.* **120**:105–120.

Malaviya, A.N., Sehgal, K. L., Kumar, R., and Dingley, H. B. (1975). Factors of delayed hypersensitivity in pulmonary tuberculosis. *Am. Rev. Respir. Dis.* **112**:49–52.

Matsuo, K., Yamaguchi, R., Yamazaki, A., Tasaka, H., and Yamada, T. (1988). Cloning and expression of the *Mycobacterium bovis* BCG gene for extracellular a antigen. *J. Bacteriol.* **170**:3847–3854.

Misaki, A., Seto, N., and Azuma, I. (1974). Structure and immunological properties of D-arabino-D-galactans isolated from cell walls of *Mycobacterium* species. *J. Biochem.* **76**:15–27.

Misaki, A., Azuma, I., and Yamamura, Y. (1977). Structural and immunchemical studies on D-arabino-D-mannans and D-mannans of *Mycobacterium tuberculosis* and other *Mycobacterium* species. *J. Biochem.* **82**:1759–1770.

Modilevsky, T., Suttler, F. R., and Barnes, P. F. (1989). Mycobacterial disease in patients with human immunodeficiency virus infection. *Arch. Intern. Med.* **149**:2201–2205.

Munk, M. E., Schoel, B., and Kaufmann, S. H. E. (1988). T cell responses of normal individuals towards recombinant protein antigens of *Mycobacterium tuberculosis. Eur. J. Immunol.* **18**:1835–1838.

Nassau, E., Parsons, E. R., and Johnson, G. D. (1976). The detection of antibodies to *Mycobacterium tuberculosis* by microplate enzyme-linked immunosorbent assay (ELISA). *Tubercle* **57**:67–70.

O'Brien, R. L., Happ, M., Dallas, A., Palmer, E., Kubo, R., and Born, W. K. (1989). Stimulation of a major subset of lymphocytes expressing T-cell receptor γδ by an antigen derived from *M. tuberculosis. Cell* **57**:667–674.

Ogawa, T., Uchida, H., Kusumoto, Y., Mori, Y., Yamamura, Y., and Hamada, S. (1991). Increase in tumor necrosis factor alpha and interleukin-6-secreting cells in peripheral blood mononuclear cells from subjects infected with *Mycobacterium tuberculosis. Infect. Immun.* **59**:3021–3025.

Okwera, A., Eriki, P. P., Guay, L. A., Ball, P., and Daniel, T. M. (1990). Tuberculin reactions in apparently healthy HIV-seropositive and HIV-seronegative women—Uganda. *MMWR* **39**:638–646.

Orme, I. M. (1982). The kinetics of emergence and loss of mediator T-lymphocytes acquired in response to infection with *Mycobacterium tuberculosis. J. Immunol.* **138**:293–298.

Orme, I. M. (1988). Induction of nonspecific acquired resistance and delayed-type hypersensitivity but not specific acquired resistance in mice inoculated with killed mycobacterial vaccines. *Infect. Immun.* **56**:3310–3312.

Orme, I. M. and Collins, F. M. (1984). Adoptive protection of the *Mycobacterium tuberculosis*-infected lung. Dissociation between cells that passively transfer protective immunity and thos that transfer delayed-type hypersensitivity to tuberculosis. *Cell Immunol.* **83**:113–120.

Orem, I. M. and Collins, F. M. (1986). Cross protection against nontuberculous mycobacterial infection by *Mycobacterium tuberculosis* memory immune T-lymphocytes. *J. Exp. Med.* **163**:203–208.

Ottenhoff, T. H. M., Kale, B., van Embden, J. D. A., Thole, J. E. R., and Kiessling, R. (1988). The recombinant 65-kD heat-shock protein of *Mycobacterium bovis* Bacillus Calmette-Guerin/*M. tuberculosis* is a target molecule for CD4+ cytotoxic T-lymphocytes that lyse human monocytes. *J. Exp. Med.* **168**:1947–1952.

Raffel, S., Arnaud, L. E., Dukes, C. D., and Huang, J. S. (1949). The role of the "wax" of the tubercle bacillus in establishing delayed hypersensitivity. II. Hypersensitivity to a protein. *J. Exp. Med.* **90**:53–71.

Reider, H. L., Cauthen, G. M., Bloch, A. B., Cole, C. H., Holtzman, D., Snider, D. E. Jr., Bigler, W. J., and Witte, J. J. (1989). Tuberculosis and acquired immunodeficiency syndrome—Florida. *Arch. Intern. Med.* **149**:1268–1273.

Sada, E., Brennan, P. J., Herrera, T., and Torres, M. (1990a). Evaluation of lipoarabinomannan for the serological diagnosis of tuberculosis. *J. Clin. Microbiol.* **28**:2587–2590.

Sada, E. D., Ferguson, L. E., and Daniel, T. M. (1990b). An ELISA for the serodiagnosis of tuberculosis using a 30,000-Da native antigen of *Mycobacterium tuberculosis*. *J. Infect. Dis.* **162**:928–931.

Salata, R. A., Sanson, A. J., Malhotra, I. J., Wiker, H. G., Harboe, M., Phillips, N. B., and Daniel T. M. (1991). Purification and characterization of the 30,000 dalton native antigen of *Mycobacterium tuberculosis* and characterization of six monoclonal antibodies reactive with a major epitope of this antigen. *J. Lab. Clin. Med.* **118**:589–598.

Selwyn, P. A., Hartel, D., Lewis, V. A., Schoenbaum, E. E., Vermund, S. H., Klein, R. S., Walker, A. T., and Friedland, G. H. (1989). A prospective study of the risk of tuberculosis among intravenous drug users with human immunodeficiency virus infection. *N. Engl. J. Med.* **320**: 545–550.

Shinnick, T. M. (1987). The 65-kilodalton antigen of *Mycobacterium tuberculosis*. *J. Bacteriol.* **169**:1080–1088.

Shinnick, T. M., Vodkin, M. H., and Williams, J. C. (1988). The *Mycobacterium tuberculosis* 65-kilodalton antigen is a heat shock protein which corresponds to common antigen and to the *Escherichia coli* GroEL protein. *Infect. Immun.* **56**:446–451.

Snider, D. E., Jr. (1982). The Tuberculin skin test. *Am. Rev. Respir. Dis.* **125**(Suppl):108–118.

Takashima, T., Ueta, C., Tsuyugushi, I., and Kishimoto, S. (1990). Production of tumor necrosis factor alpha by monocytes from patients with pulmonary tuberculosis. *Infect. Immun.* **58**:3286–3292.

Thole, J. E. R., Keulen, W. J., de Bruyn, J., Kolk, A. H. J., Groothius, D. G., Berwald, L. G., Tiesjema, R. H., and van Embden, J. D. A. (1987). Characterization, sequence determination, and immunogenicity of a

64-kilodalton protein of *Mycobacterium bovis* BCG expressed in *Escherichia coli* K-12. *Infect. Immun.* **55**:1466–1475.

Thole, J. E. R., Hindersson, P., de Bruyn, J., Cremers, F., van der Zee, J., de Cock, H., Tommassen, J., van Eden, W., and van Embden, J. D. A. (1988). Antigenic relatedness of a strongly immunogenic 65 kDa mycobacterial protein with a similarly sized ubiquitous bacterial common antigen. *Microbial. Pathogen.* **4**:71–83.

Toossi, Z. and Ellner, J. J. (1991). Tuberculosis. In *Textbook of Internal Medicine, 2nd ed.* Edited by W. N. Kelley. JB Lippincott, Philadelphia, pp. 1426–1434.

Toossi, Z., Kleinhenz, M. E., and Ellner, J. J. (1986). Defective interleukin-2 production and responsiveness in human pulmonary tuberculosis. *J. Exp. Med.* **163**:1162–1172.

Toossi, Z., Sedor, J. R., Lapurga, J. P., Ondash, R. J., and Ellner, J. J. (1990). Expression of functional interleukin 2 receptors by peripheral blood monocytes from patients with active pulmonary tuberculosis. *J. Clin. Invest.* **85**:1777–1784.

Valone, S. E., Rich, E. A., Wallis, R. S., and Ellner, J. J. (1988). Expression of tumor necrosis factor in vitro by human monomuclear phagocytes stimulated with whole *Mycobacterium bovis* BCG and mycobacterial antigens. *Infect. Immun.* **56**:3313–3315.

Vjecha, M., Okwera, A., Nyold, S., Byekwaso, F., Okot-Nwang, M., Mugerwa, R. D., Eriki, P., Aisu, T., Ellner, J., Huebner, R., Hom, D., Daniel, T. M., Edmonds, K., and Wallis, R. (1991). Association between anergy, prior complications of HIV-1 infection, and increased mortality in HIV-1 infected patients with active tuberculosis in Uganda (abstract). *Proc. Seventh Internat. Conf. AIDS* WB 2346.

Wahl, S. M., Wahl, L. B., McCarthy, J. B., Chedid, L., and Mergenhagen, S. E. (1979). Macrophage activation by mycobacterial water soluble compounds and synthetic muramyl dipeptide. *J. Immunol.* **122**:2226–2231.

Wallis, R. S., Fujiwara, H., and Ellner, J. J. (1986). Direct stimulation of monocyte release of interleukin-1 by mycobacterial protein antigens. *J. Immunol.* **136**:193–196.

Wallis, R. S. Amir-Tahmasseb, M., and Ellner, J. J. (1990). Induction of interleukin-1 and tumor necrosis factor by mycobacterial proteins: the monocyte western blot. *Proc. Natl. Acad. Sci. USA* **87**:3348–3352.

Warren, K. S., Domingo, E. O., and Cowan, R. B. T. (1967). Granuloma formation around schistosome eggs as a manifestation of delayed hypersensitivity. *Am. J. Pathol.* **51**:735–756.

Wiker, H. G., Harboe, M., and Lea, T. E. (1986a). Purification and characterization of two protein antigens from the heterogeneous BCG85 complex in *Mycobacterium bovis* BCG. *Int. Arch. Allergy Appl. Immunol.* **81**:298–306.

Wiker, H. G., Harboe, M., Nagai, S., Patarroyo, M. E., Ramirez, C., and Cruz, N. (1986b). MPB59, a widely cross-reacting protein of *Mycobacterium bovis* BCG. *Int. Arch. Allergy Appl. Immunol.* **81**:307–314.

Wiker, H. G., Harboe, M., Nagai, S., and Bennedsen, J. (1990a). Quantitative and Qualitative studies on the major extracellular antigen of *Mycobacterium tuberculosis* H37Rv and *Mycobacterium bovis* BCG *Am. Rev. Respir. Dis.* **141**:830–838.

Wiker, H. G., Sletten, K., Nagai, S., and Harboe, M. (1990b). Evidence for three separate genes encoding the proteins of the mycobacterial 85 complex. *Infect. Immun.* **58**:272–274.

Yoneda, M. and Fukui, Y. (1965). Isolation, purification, and characterization of extracellular antigens of *Mycobacterium tuberculosis. Am. Rev. Respir. Dis.* **92**(Suppl):9–18.

Yoneda, M., Fukui, Y., and Yamanouchi, T. (1965). Extracellular proteins of tubercle bacilli V. Distribution of α and β antigens in various mycobacteria. *Biken J.* **8**:201–223.

Young, D., Kent, L., Rees, A., Lamb, J., and Ivanyi, J. (1986). Immunological activity of a 38-kilodalton protein purified from *Mycobacterium tuberculosis. Infect. Immun.* **54**:177–183.

Young, D. B., Ivanyi, J., Cox, J. H., and Lamb, J. R. (1987). The 65kDa antigen of mycobacteria—a common bacterial protein? *Immunol. Today* **8**:215–219.

Young, R. A., Bloom, B. R., Grosskinsky, C. M., Ivanyi, J., Thomas, D., and Davis, R. W. (1985). Dissection of *Mycobacterium tuberculosis* antigens using recombinant DNA. *Proc. Natl. Acad. Sci. USA* **82**:2583–2587.

5

Pathogenesis of Tuberculosis

EDWARD A. NARDELL

Harvard Medical School
The Cambridge Hospital
Cambridge, Massachusetts and
Massachusetts Department of Public Health
Boston, Massachusetts

I. Introduction

Much has been written on the pathogenesis of tuberculosis since Robert Koch reported his discovery of the causative organism in 1882. By the middle of this century, as streptomycin and isoniazid were dramatically improving the prognosis of the disease, Arnold Rich published the thousand-page, second edition of his treatise on pathogenesis (Rich, 1951). But by the centennial of Koch's publication, as tuberculosis eradication was being discussed in many developed countries, and control was being considered a plausible goal in countries of the developing world, the acquired immunodeficiency syndrome (AIDS) had just been recognized, fundamentally changing the pathogenesis of the disease and dimming the prospects for tuberculosis eradication and control in rich and poor countries alike.

In central Africa and other areas with a high prevalence of both human immunodeficiency virus (HIV) and tuberculosis infections, their combined mortality is predicted to result in population changes of historic proportions (Stanford et al., 1991). In developed countries such as the United States, less profound effects are anticipated, with high mortality and morbidity rates limited to certain high-risk populations and their contacts. In New York City in particular, a soaring tuberculosis case rate, together with outbreaks of HIV-associated, multidrug-resistant tuberculosis in hospitals, clinics, shelters for the homeless, prisons, and drug treatment facilities, has highlighted several interrelated aspects of transmission and pathogenesis: accelerated progression from infection to disease in immunocompromised persons, widespread transmission under a variety of environmentally favorable conditions, and accelerated epidemic propagation of the disease among HIV-infected persons. HIV coinfection, for example, alters the clinical presentation of tuberculosis, making the diagnosis more difficult, facilitating transmission in health care facilities, and increasing the need for environmental precautions (Nardell, 1990). The worldwide resurgence of tuberculosis has stimulated increased basic research, especially in the application of molecular and cellular biology to long-standing problems in prevention, pathogenesis, diagnosis, and therapy. Whereas Chapter 4 focuses on the immunologic interactions of humans and tubercle bacilli, emphasizing mycobacterial protein antigens, cell wall polysaccharides, and T-cell subpopula-

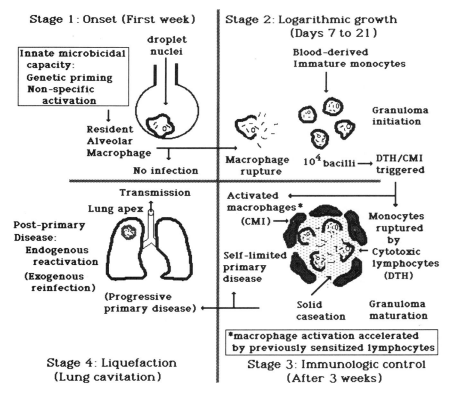

Figure 1 Four stages in the pathogenesis of tuberculosis in the normal host. See text for detailed description. (Based on Dannenberg, 1991.)

tions, the present chapter provides a descriptive overview of the interactions of host and tubercle bacilli from the perspective of the clinician, the epidemiologist, and the experimental pathologist, fully recognizing that many details of pathogenesis remain to be elucidated, and that some conclusions based on animal work may ultimately be found not to apply to humans. Because of its importance, the impact of HIV infection on tuberculosis in developed and developing countries is mentioned throughout this chapter and discussed again in two subsequent chapters.

Based largely on the classic animal studies of Lurie (Lurie, 1964), with whom he worked for many years, Dannenberg has described four stages in the pathogenesis of tuberculosis: onset, symbiosis, immunologic control, and liquefaction (Dannenberg, 1991). This chapter follows the same convenient organization, summarized in Figure 1, drawing heavily on Dannenberg's analysis.

II. Stage 1 (First Week): Onset—Innate Macrophage Resistance, Virulence, and the Infecting Dose of Tubercle Bacilli

To begin infection, virulent tubercle bacilli must reach the alveolar surface. Although tuberculosis infections occur by ingestion, direct inoculation, and other unusual routes, inhalation is by far the most important mode of transmission. Bacilli landing on the ciliated respiratory epithelium are usually carried up the mucocililary escalator, swallowed, and, in the normal host, rendered harmless. As noted in Chapter 6, the 1- to 2-μm droplet nuclei that reach the alveoli contain no more than than two or three tubercle bacilli, far short of the 10^3 to 10^4 bacilli required to initiate cell-mediated immunity (CMI) and delayed-type hypersensitivity (DTH) (Dannenberg, 1992; Smith and Wiengeshaus, 1989; Balasubramanian et al., 1992) The first defense against infection at the alveolar level, therefore, is the resident alveolar macrophage. This initial contest between host and parasite is in many ways crucial to all subsequent events, determining whether infection will occur at all, and if it does, initiating recruitment to the focus of both cytotoxic cells (DTH) and macrophages (CMI). Derived from circulating monocytes, alveolar macrophages scavenge the alveolar surface, ingesting organisms and other inhaled particulates, becoming nonspecifically activated in the process. Depending on host genetic factors and the degree of nonspecific activation, alveolar macrophages ingesting tubercle bacilli have variable, innate microbicidal capacity. However, tubercle bacilli have also evolved variable, innate resistance mechanisms to counter the host's defenses.

A. Virulence and the Infecting Dose of Tubercle Bacilli

Whereas rabbit macrophages (from blood) offered little resistance to the early replication of virulent H37Rv *Mycobacterium tuberculosis*, they were able to inhibit replication of the avirulent H37Ra strain (Lurie, 1964). These and other observations raised the possibility that virulent tubercle bacilli were somehow toxic for macrophages. The factors determining virulence are not fully understood, but experimental evidence suggests that virulent bacilli impair innate macrophage antimicrobial mechanisms by: (1) inhibiting lysosome-phagosome fusion, and (2) destroying the phagosome membrane (Myrvik et al., 1988). Virulence mechanisms appear to be effective against nonactivated macrophages, but not against fully activated macrophages. The identity of the mycobacterial components responsible for these mechanisms remains controversial despite decades of research. Cord factor (6,6′-trehalose dimycolate, TDM) and sulfur-containing lipids (sulfolipids) on the surface of mycobacteria are the leading biochemical candidates. Thus, both the virulence of inhaled tubercle bacilli and the innate resistance of the ingesting alveolar macrophage determine whether the initial inoculum of tubercle bacilli is destroyed, or whether bacilli replicate, ultimately leading to destruction of the macrophage.

The concept of infecting dose is different for tuberculosis than for many other respiratory infections. Thousands of potentially pathogenic mouth bacteria are routinely aspirated without causing pneumonia, apparently having been cleared by lung defenses. In guinea pigs and susceptible strains of inbred rabbits, however, experimental exposure studies using dilute aerosols (confirmed by culture) have shown that a single inhaled droplet nucleus carrying no more than one to three virulent organisms is sufficient to cause infection, manifest by a tuberculin skin test conversion and a single peripheral lung lesion (Ratcliffe, 1952; Lurie, 1950). In humans, resistance to initial tuberculosis infection appears to be variable, leading to the assumption that inhalation of more than one droplet nucleus, possibly many, may be necessary to cause infection in resistant individuals. Because the concentration of droplet nuclei in air under ordinary exposure conditions is believed to be extremely low, averaging 1 in 11,000 ft^3 in air exhausted from a tuberculosis ward over a 4-year period, multiple or recurrent inhalations are unlikely unless exposure is prolonged or the source case is unusually infectious (Riley et al., 1962). The dose of droplet nuclei required to cause infection depends on the probability of success by alveolar macrophages in each encounter with tubercle bacilli, that is, their microbicidal capacity relative to the virulence of inhaled tubercle bacilli (Dannenberg, 1989). The infecting dose will be high in persons whose macrophages generally have great innate microbicidal capacity, where bacilli are of low virulence. In persons whose macrophages generally have relatively low innate microbicidal capacity, where bacilli are fully virulent, the infecting dose will be low, probably a single droplet nucleus. Chance plays an important role because of the low likelihood of inahaling even one droplet nucleus during most exposures, the variable innate microbicidal capacity of alveolar macrophages that happen to be near the implantation site, and the relatively low probability that inhaled droplet nuclei will reach the especially vulnerable apical or subapical region of the lung. The last factor is considered more important for reinfection than for initial infection (see below).

B. Innate Resistance and Racial Susceptibility to Tuberculosis

Blacks have long been known to suffer disproportionately from tuberculosis. Greater exposure to infection due to poor socioeconomic conditions and greater progression to active disease have been the presumed causes (Rich, 1951, pp. 126–148). Youmans (1979) devoted a short chapter of his monograph to the subject of innate resistance, arguing against any substantial natural resistance to tuberculosis infection: "It can be stated categorically that in a person who has never had a previous experience with mycobacteria, none of the internal defense mechanisms will be very effective in preventing the growth and multiplication of virulent tubercle bacilli." He suggests that Rich and other writers may have been misled by epidemiological evidence suggesting racial differences in resistance, and that experimental evidence indicating species and genetic differences may actually reflect acquired immunity. Although mice and rats appear to be much more resistant to tuberculosis infection than are humans, monkeys, or guinea pigs, mice, hamsters, and guinea pigs reacted similarly histologically to inhaled virulent or avirulent strains of tubercle bacilli during the first 3 weeks, exhibiting differences only as acquired resistance developed during the fourth week of infection (Ratcliffe and Palladino, 1953). In both resistant and susceptible inbred rabbits, bacillary growth was logarithmic (stage 2 of pathogenesis, Fig. 1) during the first 3 weeks after infection, until about 10^4 organisms were reached, and local, cell-mediated responses were triggered (Lurie, 1964). In both immunized and nonimmunized guinea pigs, bacillary growth was unimpeded for about 2 weeks, until approximately 10^3 organisms were reached, at which point growth was inhibited in vaccinated animals while growth in nonvaccinated animals continued until a larger antigenic stimulus triggered a cell-mediated response (Smith and Harding, 1977). In rats, examination of thoracic duct lymphocytes showed that CMI developed as early as 4 days after infection, much sooner than expected, supporting the notion that CMI accounts for their apparent innate resistance compared to some other species (Lefford et al, 1973).

Increased susceptibility to initial tuberculous infection among blacks has recently again been reported (Stead et al., 1990). On repeat testing of 25,398 initially tuberculin-negative nursing home residents, Stead found 13.8% of blacks and only 7.2% of whites were recently infected under conditions where exposure was believed to be equal. However, of those infected, 11.5% of blacks and 10.6% of whites went on to clinical tuberculosis without therapy. The authors concluded that blacks were more readily infected with *M. tuberculosis* than whites, and that resistance to tuberculosis infection appeared to be handled separately from resistance to progression to clinical disease. Although this report has sparked controversy (Rosenman, 1990; Aoki, 1990; Felton et al., 1990), mainly over the inability to separate out other potential risk factors associated with race, there is also experimental support for Stead's observations, as follows.

In an established in vitro model, unstimulated macrophages from blacks permitted more intracellular replication of tubercle bacilli than those of whites, an effect that was accentuated by autologous serum in the culture medium (Crowle and Elkins, 1990). While 1,25-D_3, a hormonally active form of vitamin D, corrected the permissiveness of macrophages from blacks, its protective effect on macrophages from whites was even greater. The role of vitamin D in the pathogenesis of tuberculosis has recently been reviewed in view of the speculation that vitamin D deficiency might explain recent epidemiological evidence of increased susceptibility to tuberculosis of dark-skinned residents of Asiatic origin in the United Kingdom (Rook, 1988; Davies, 1989, 1990).

In the mouse model, susceptibility to mycobacterial infections has been found to be determined by a single, dominant, autosomal gene, *Bcg*, located on the centromeric portion of chromosome 1 (Skamene, 1989). Mice with the resistant allele of the gene have macrophages capable of responding very early in the course of mycobacterial infection by activation without priming by specifically sensitized T lymphocytes. This genetic shortcut gives the appearance of innate resistance without involving the immune process. Mice with the susceptible allele have macrophages that are also capable of achieving full activation, but they require more intensive or prolonged stimulation by mycobacteria and the full T-cell-dependent macrophage activation sequence of events. Assuming that these observations are relevant to humans and to animals infected via the airway rather than by the experimental intravenous route, there may be a biological basis in macrophage function for the long-observed species, racial, and individual variation in susceptibility to tuberculosis infection. However, species differences have been reported at the cellular level, for example, the activation of mouse but not human macrophages by gamma interferon (Douvas et al., 1985). Moreover, the very notion of innate resistance in humans is complicated by aging, concomitant illnesses, and numerous environmental influences, including variable exposure to tubercle bacilli, nutrition, sunlight-associated vitamin D metabolism, and sensitization by environmental mycobacteria. The possible contributions of historical, socioeconomic, and demographic factors on the evolution of genetic differences in resistance to tuberculosis have recentlly been explored (Stead, 1992).

C. Initial Infection Among HIV-Infected Persons

There is strong epidemiological evidence that HIV infection markedly predisposes persons already infected with tuberculosis to reactivation (Selwyn et al., 1989). It also evident that some persons immunocompromised by HIV infection who secondarily become infected with tuberculosis progress rapidly to clinical disease, often with multiorgan involvement (DiPerri et al., 1989; Daley et al., 1992). Whether HIV infection also makes initial tuberculosis infection more likely is an important, but unanswered, question. The pathophysiological basis for the development of tuberculosis in HIV-infected persons was the subject of a recent review (Rose, 1991). If CMI and DTH have no role during the first several weeks of mycobacterial replication, and if HIV primarily impairs immunity by infecting lymphocytes directly involved in CMI and DTH, then HIV might not reduce innate resistance. However, a number of institutional outbreaks of HIV-associated tuberculosis, especially outbreaks where transmission has been proven by multidrug resistance patterns and genetic bacteriological markers, have had attack rates suggesting increased susceptibility to infection as well as rapid progression to active disease. In Italy, for example, a 28-year-old HIV-infected man with no signs of pulmonary tuberculosis, a normal chest X-ray, and negative bronchoscopy specimens by acid-fast stain ultimately had a positive culture (DiPerri et al., 1989). Within 60 days of the diagnosis of the index case, seven additional active cases were identified among 20 HIV-infected patients who had been on the ward before the diagnosis was made and the index case isolated, all with the same drug susceptibility pattern. This extraordinarily rapid rate of progression to active disease diverts attention from an equally remarkable infection rate, especially if it is presumed that additional infections occurred that did not progress to active disease, and that some infections may have been undetectable owing to skin test anergy. Although it is possible that exposure was unusually intense, the normal chest X-ray and the negative smears of the index case would not have predicted an exceptional transmitter. Increased susceptibility to new infection as well as prompt progression to active disease is a more likely explanation.

An outbreak in a housing facility for HIV-infected persons was analyzed using restriction-fragment-length polymorphism (RFLP) of cultured tubercle bacilli to prove transmission within the facility (Daley et al., 1992). Among 30 residents exposed to possible infection, active tuberculosis developed in 11 (37%), and four others (13%) had newly positive skin tests. Of 28 staff members with possible exposure, at least six had documented skin test conversions and eight others were positive of unknown duration. At the time of the most recent published report, one staff member had developed active tuberculosis, but the RFLP pattern was not yet known. While the accelerated progression from infection to disease was the most striking feature of the outbreak, the extent of transmission was also remarkable. Again, the intensity of exposure was unknown, but it was probably greater than in the hospital in Italy, given the transmission to staff.

In a Florida hospital where 29 patients developed tuberculosis with organisms resistant to both isoniazid and rifampin, a case-control analysis indicated recent nosocomial transmission (CDC, 1990). In the initial report of the outbreak, 27 of 29 patients were HIV infected, and nine (31%) had evidence in their medical records of prior tuberculosis or a positive tuberculin skin test, making exogenous reinfection with drug-resistant organisms highly likely. As discussed below, exogenous reinfection requires repeated exposure, but it also requires a breach in the local macrophage defense system, which ordinarily effectively halts growth of bacilli through rapidly recalled CMI. Therefore, HIV infection apparently somehow reduced the effectiveness of clones of T lymphocytes that were previously sensitized by exposure to tubercle bacilli. In addition, HIV virus may be able to impair the innate resistance of alveolar macrophages acquired by previous experience with environmental microorganisms and other nonspecific stimulants.

In these and other HIV-associated outbreaks, the intensity of exposure has been unknown, and one can only speculate on the contribution of impaired resistance to the rates of new infection. The rapid progression to active disease observed among HIV-infected persons complicates the issue in that a single index case may rapidly lead to multiple secondary transmitters, greatly increasing exposure. It is possible that a careful case-control analysis of HIV-positive and HIV-negative persons exposed under similar conditions might answer the question of whether susceptibility to new infection is increased. However, preliminary, unpublished in vitro experiments with macrophages and lymphocytes from HIV-infected persons have shown impaired microbicidal capacity (A. J. Crowle, personal communication, 1992). Although lung macrophages may also be infected and impaired by the HIV virus, bronchopulmonary lavage material (predominantly macrophages) from HIV-infected subjects contained HIV-1 DNA in amounts consistent with infection of approximately 1 in 10^5 cells (Rose et al, 1991). Any impairment in resistance to tuberculosis infection, therefore, is most likely mediated indirectly by lymphocytes, presumably through lymphokines, or through unidentified mechanisms.

III. Stage 2 (Weeks 2 and 3): Logarithmic Bacillary Growth and the Early Tuberculous Lesion

When innate macrophage microbicidal capacity is inadequate to destroy the initial few tubercle bacilli of the droplet nucleus, they replicate within the macrophage, causing it to rupture. Monocytes derived from the circulation are attracted to the focus by various chemotactic factors, initiating granuloma formation. Although immature monocytes readily ingest the released tubercle bacilli, they appear to have no capacity to destroy or inhibit their growth, which proceeds exponentially. The cytoplasm of immature monocytes from both Lurie's resistant and susceptible rabbits were equally permissive, as reflected in the parallel growth curves in Figure 2. Like aveolar macrophages, blood-derived monocytes acquire microbicidal capacity only upon activation, nonspecifically, or specifically through T lymphocytes as CMI develops. The influence of ge-

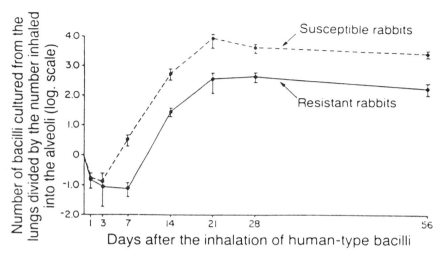

Figure 2 Changes in the number of human-type tubercle bacilli in the lungs of naturally resistant and naturally susceptible rabbits at different intervals after infection by quantitative airborne inhalation. (Reproduced with permission from Lurie et al., 1955; see Dannenberg, 1991.)

netic priming suggested by studies in mice has already been mentioned (Skamene, 1989). Mice with the allele for resistance have macrophages capable of activation very early in the course of mycobacterial infection without priming by specifically sensitized T lymphocytes. As discussed below, a more prominent role of cytotoxic T cells in limiting the stage of logarithmic growth has recently been postulated. The ''stage of logarithmic growth'' may be a better name than ''symbiotic stage,'' the term used by Lurie, since the uncontrolled growth of bacilli during this stage, while apparently not highly toxic for macrophages, conveys no obvious benefits to the host other than producing the antigenic stimulus necessary to trigger DTH and CMI.

IV. Stage 3 (After Week 3): Control by CMI and DTH

As depicted in Figure 2, after 21 days of uninhibited growth within immature monocytes, growth of tubercle bacilli in both Lurie's susceptible and resistant rabbits rather suddenly ceased. Although the onset of control over bacillary growth had traditionally been thought to coincide with the development of enhanced macrophage killing (CMI), Kaufmann (1989) has recently emphasized a cooperative role for cytotoxic (DTH) lymphocytes. Dannenberg (1991) supports a primary role for DTH initially, noting that CMI was poorly developed in Lurie's susceptible rabbits at the time that logarithmic bacillary growth was inhibited. Both Rich and Youmans devoted chapters to the question of whether hypersensitivity is entirely harmful or a beneficial response to tuberculoproteins (Rich, 1951; Youmans, 1979). Immunity and hypersensitivity were first shown to be separable experimentally when tuberculous guinea pigs that were desensitized by daily injections of tuberculin retained their resistance to exogenous reinfection (Rothchild et al., 1934). Fifty years later, CMI and DTH in the mouse model were convincingly shown by adoptive transfer studies to be due to two distinct cell lines, corresponding in humans to CD4 (CMI) and CD8 (DTH) lymphocytes (Orme and Collins, 1984). Kaufmann (1989) views the various potential interactions between T lymphocytes and macrophages as potentially protective or harmful to the host, depending on specific local circumstances, as illustrated in Figure 3. Cytotoxic cells (DTH) apparantly benefit the host by destroying immature macrophages, which provide an environment conducive to bacillary growth (Fig 3C).

Although tubercle bacilli survive for many years in solid caseous material, they are unable to multiply owing to unfavorable local conditions and the presence of inhibitors. Bacilli released from immature macrophages may be taken up and controlled by T-cell-activated macrophages (Fig. 3A,F). After control is established, mature macrophages accumulate around the periphery of the caseous lesion (epithelioid cells), preventing further extension (Crowle, 1988; Dannenberg, 1991). Tuberculin-like products derived from intracellular bacilli are thought to be important early stimulants to caseous necrosis, which involves several poorly defined processes in addition to DTH (Dannenberg, 1991). Later in the course of tuberculosis, DTH may indeed be more harmful to the host than helpful, causing the tissue damage characteristic of tuberculosis, especially lung cavitation. Lung cavities are largely responsible both for the transmission of tuberculosis and for the development of drug resistance. In the HIV-immunocompromised patient, once tuberculosis infection is established, the absence of adequate DTH (evidenced by a negative tuberculin reaction), and CMI may allow early progression of the infection, altering both the characteristic histopathology and the radiographic presentation (Barnes et al., 1991).

In the normal host, the bacillary population is stable during the third stage of pathogenesis, as growth in counterbalanced by bacillary destruction and inhibition. Before weeks 4 or 5, caseous granulomas in the lung are microscopic or barely visible. In Lurie's resistant rabbits, lung lesions contained relatively few bacilli, many activated macrophages (mature epithelioid cells), and rela-

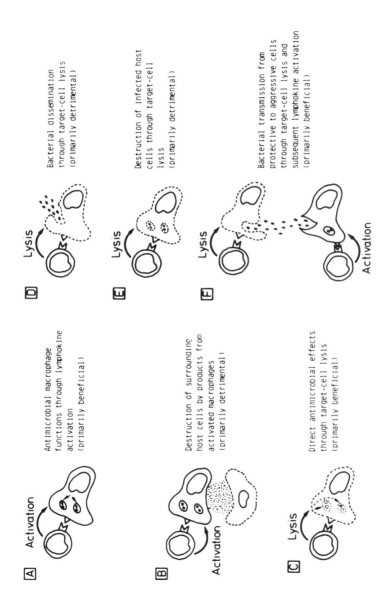

Figure 3 Possible sequelae of T cell–macrophage interactions in tuberculosis. See text for detailed description. (Reproduced with permission from Kaufmann, 1989.)

tively little necrosis, whereas in the susceptible rabbits, many bacilli, few activated macrophages, and more necrosis were found (Lurie, 1964; Dannenberg, 1991). At the sites of lymphohematogenous dissemination, accelerated tubercle formation (CMI) in resistant rabbits rapidly destroyed foci with minimal necrosis, whereas in susceptible animals bacillary growth led to progressive caseous foci. Ultimately, susceptible rabbits died of disseminated tuberculosis, not unlike tuberculosis patients with AIDS. In humans, as discussed below, hematogenous foci in the apical region of the lung, Medlar's "vulnerable region" (Medlar, 1948), are thought to be incompletely sterilized by CMI, leaving behind bacilli that may later reactivate (Smith and Wiengeshaus, 1989; Balasubramanian et al., 1992).

A. Primary and Progressive Primary Tuberculosis

Stages 1–3 (Fig. 1) comprise the pathogenesis of primary tuberculosis in the immunologically normal host. Depending on the immunocompetence of the host, primary tuberculosis is most often a subclinical, or mild, self-limited illness. In high-prevalence populations, primary infection is likely early in life, often the result of household exposure to parents or grandparents with infectious, cavitary, postprimary tuberculosis. Under low-prevalence conditions, however, the majority of the population reaching adulthood have not been infected. When tuberculosis infection occurs for the first time in adults, the disease resembles primary tuberculosis in childhood, with nonspecific lung infiltrates and lymphadenopathy, sometimes followed by tuberculous pleuritis. These "atypical" patterns of tuberculosis in adults were first recognized in the United States in the 1960s as the national case rate fell (Stead et al., 1968). Although human primary tuberculosis is usually self-limited, the infection can progress locally or systemically when host defenses are inadequate. An apical or subapical primary site, undernutrition, concomitant illnesses, immunosuppressive therapy, and, most important, HIV coinfection are factors predisposing to progressive primary tuberculosis. The profound public health consequences of rapid progression from initial infection to communicable case among HIV-infected persons in institutions have already been stressed in relation to three recent examples of outbreaks (DiPerri et al., 1989; Daley et al. 1992; CDC, 1990). Whereas, among otherwise normal hosts under endemic conditions, one active, communicable case usually results, on average, in less than one new communicable secondary case, in group settings where HIV coinfection is prevalent, new cases appear to rapidly and regularly produce many secondary cases, each with the potential for further transmission. Thus, accelerated progression from tuberculosis infection to active disease in individual immunocompromised patients can lead to accelerated epidemic propogation among susceptible persons in group settings.

V. Stage 4: Liquefaction and Lung Cavity Formation (Endogenous Reactivation, Exogenous Reinfection, and the Importance of the Apical-Subapical Location)

Although immunocompetent persons in whom CMI fails to control primary tuberculosis may progress to cavitary tuberculosis (progressive primary disease), this final stage of pathogenesis usually results from a second (postprimary) phase of disease activity, occurring months to decades after apparent recovery from the initial process. As discussed below, cavitary disease may also result from exogenous reinfection. The lifetime risk of postprimary (reactivation) disease for otherwise healthy persons with tuberculosis infection is usually estimated at 5–10%, with the higher figure applicable to persons with less resistance in developing countries. For HIV-infected persons, however, the risk of reactivation disease is considerably higher, estimated at approximately 7% per year in a 2-year study of patients in an ambulatory drug treatment program (Selwyn et al., 1989). The risk should be even higher for more immunocompromised patients.

Lurie (1964) and Dannenberg (1976, 1991) have called attention to the public health significance of liquefaction necrosis, the incompletely understood process leading to lung cavitation, which has been largely responsible for transmission and perpetuation of tuberculosis in the pre-HIV era. Moreover, they have noted that the large numbers of tubercle bacilli in cavities, estimated at greater than 10^8, also increase the probability of mutations to drug resistance, a growing obstacle to tuberculosis control worldwide. In HIV-infected patients cavitation is less common, but because resistance is diminished, bacilli apparently reach large numbers in lung and other tissues, and transmission has been amply documented (DiPerri et al., 1989; Daley et al., 1992). While the exact causes of liquefaction are unknown, hydrolytic enzymes and DTH to tuberculin-like proteins are thought to be important factors. Presumably, reduced or absent DTH in advanced, HIV-immunocompromised patients precludes cavity formation. In normal hosts, however, uncontrolled growth of tubercle bacilli in macrophages stimulates DTH, leading to caseation and liquefaction, both of which are deadly to macrophages. When a liquefied caseous lesion discharges its contents into a nearby bronchus, a cavity is formed, the characteristic radiographic and pathological presentation of tuberculosis and other chronic, granulomatous infections (Canetti, 1955). The local inflammatory response to the sudden spillage of necrotic, highly antigenic, infectious liquid within the lungs is recognized clinically as a tuberculous pneumonitis. Although tubercle bacilli are disseminated within the lung, the most important consequence of liquefaction occurs in the cavities themselves. Within cavities, host defenses are ineffectual, and in this unique extracellular milieu, tubercle bacilli multiply to great numbers. The patient with cavitary tuberculosis characteristically has persistent coughing and may have hemoptysis. Systemic symptoms of fever, weight loss, and anorexia are also associated with cavitary disease. In the prechemotherapy era, both local and systemic symtoms often responded to collapse therapy, procedures that attempted to close cavities mechanically, thereby restoring conditions in the lung that were less favorable for rapid bacillary multiplication (Gaensler, 1982).

A. Endogenous Reactivation and Exogenous Reinfection

Whether chronic, cavitary tuberculosis in adult humans results from exogenous reinfection or endogenous reactivation was once a subject of considerable debate. As noted by Stead in a recent essay on the subject: "When the prevalence and incidence of tuberculosis are both high, study of pathogenesis of disease is difficult. It is impossible in this situation to distinguish reinfection from new infection or from recrudescence of old infection because everyone is exposed and reexposed frequently" (Stead, 1989). However, as the U.S. case rate fell, an analysis of epidemiological data led Stead to conclude that reactivation was the etiology of sporadic cases under low-prevalence conditions (Stead, 1967). Stead's "unitary" concept was supported by the decreasing probability of recurrent airborne infection and by a growing understanding of the ability of antigen-specific (memory) T cells to rapidly activate macrophages, destroying foci of potential reinfection. Although resistance is long-lasting, some patients apparently outlive their antigen-specific, T-cell resistance to reinfection. Stead and To (1987) showed that reinfection after exposure occurred in nonanergic, elderly nursing home residents whose tuberculin test had reverted from positive to negative over the years. These reinfected persons had the same small chance of clinical disease as persons never previously infected. However, skin test reversion is not required for reinfection. In high-prevalence countries, epidemiological data have continued to support reinfection as an important pathogenic pathway to chronic, cavitary tuberculosis. Styblo (1978, 1984) concluded that exogenous reinfection had a major role in tuberculosis among Alaskan Eskimos before 1950, because the introduction of treatment for active cases resulted in a sharp decrease in new disease in all age groups, including adults previously infected in childhood. He suggested that prior to Word War II, exogenous reinfection may have been an important mechanism in most developed countries, just as it appears to be important in developing countries today. In India, for example, the failure of the most recent BCG vaccination trial has been attributed, in part, to a high prevalence of exgenous reinfection (ten Dam and Pio, 1982).

In low-prevalence countries, reactivation of latent foci undoubtedly accounts for most sporadic cases of chronic tuberculosis. However, epidemiological tracing together with bacteriological markers has permitted documentation of exogenous reinfection in several case reports (Raleigh and Wichelhausen,

1973; Raleigh et al., 1975; Omerod and Skinner, 1980). More widespread rein-fection has been documented under epidemic conditions in a 350-bed shelter for the homeless (Nardell et al., 1986). The epidemiological clue to exogenous re-infection was a cluster of new, cavitary cases in one shelter, many of whom had resistance to both isoniazid and streptomycin. Phage testing confirmed that at least 22 of 42 cases were the result of recent transmission, and further investi-gation revealed that four of the cavitary cases had evidence of previous tuber-culosis infection or disease. Another three cases of exogenous reinfection were later added to the series, for a total of at least 7 of 25 (28%) recently transmitted cases. Others among the bacteriologically linked cases may have been rein-fected, given the high prevalence of tuberculosis infection among the homeless, but medical records were often unavailable to document previous infection.

The factors that permitted exogenous reinfection in at least seven shelter residents are unclear. None of the reinfection cases were known to have had, or subsequently acquire, HIV infection. In the mid-1980s at the time of this out-break, HIV coinfection was an uncommon tuberculosis risk factor among the homeless of Boston. While tuberculin skin test reactivity was not known at the time of reinfection, most cases were known to be tuberculin positive in the past, and the presence of prominent lung cavitation in all seven cases indicated a strong DTH response, despite inadequate CMI. Like many of the homeless, however, those who were reinfected were not healthy, well-nourished individu-als. Most were chronic alcoholics and heavy smokers with severe underlying ob-structive lung disease by chest X-ray. While chronic bronchitis and emphysema have not been recognized as risk factors for tuberculosis, the association of ob-structive lung diseases with the environmental mycobacterioses and with chronic histoplasmosis raises the possibility that impaired respiratory clearance may be sufficient to tip the balance in favor of exogenous reinfection under con-ditions of high exposure. If this is true, the steep rise in tobacco consumption occurring in developing countries may further hinder the success of underfunded tuberculosis control programs already struggling against such obstacles as HIV infection, malnutrition, and concomitant disease.

The one definite prerequisite for reinfection is repeated exposure. As dis-cussed below, repeated exposure is necessary because only bacilli inhaled into the vulnerable apical or subapical regions of the lung are likely to successfully overcome established CMI (Smith and Wiengeshaus, 1989; Balasubramanian et al., 1992). In the homeless outbreak, the rapid progression from reinfection to cavitary disease resulted in several highly contagious cases residing in the shel-ter at any given time, assuring the high levels of exposure necessary to reinfect yet others, with a multiplier effect. This accelerated propagation of tuberculosis resembled the recent HIV-associated institutional outbreaks already cited (DiPerri et al., 1989; Daley et al., 1992). Not only were large percentages of contacts infected in each of these different situations, but many rapidly progressed to an infectious stage—owing to exogenous reinfection in the case of the shelter outbreak and to HIV coinfection in the other settings.

B. The Importance of the Apical/Subapical Location

All seven of the reinfection cases discussed above had upper lung cavitation, the characteristic radiographic presentation of postprimary, reactivation tuberculosis. Medlar (1948) first raised the possibility that foci in the apical region of the lung, what he had called the "vulnerable" region," may be incompletely sterilized by lung defenses (Smith and Wiengeshaus, 1989; Balasubramanian et al., 1992). Whereas primary lesions occur throughout the lungs, with a predominance in the lower lobes due to the distribution of ventilation, postprimary disease is strikingly an upper lung phenomenon (Sweany et al, 1931). In the view of Smith and his co-workers, bacilli reach the upper lung either through lymphohematogenous dissemination occuring during primary infection or through the airways in instances of exogenous reinfection. If bacilli are of low virulence, or if CMI is enhanced by cross-reactive epitopes (BCG or environmental mycobacteria), bacillemia is reduced, and upper lobe implantatation is less likely (Smith and Wiengeshaus, 1989; Balasubramanian et al., 1992). However, if bacilli are fully virulent, or if CMI is relatively weak, apical foci with a potential for future reactivation are more likely to occur. In developed countries, fully virulent tubercle bacilli are usually required to cause infection and lymphohematogenous dissemination in otherwise healthy subjects, and the cavitary disease resulting from reactivation favors propagation of virulent strains. In developing countries, however, where host resistance may be impaired by undernutrition and concomitant illness, full virulence may not be necessary to cause infection. In fact, if fully virulent bacilli greatly shorten the lives of human hosts, thereby reducing the opportunities for transmission, it may be disadvantagious for the survival of the microorganism. Moreover, under conditions where recurrent exposures occur, exogenous reinfection of the upper lobes through the airways is a plausible alternative pathway to the cavitary disease necessary for propogation. In Madras, India, for example, about 70% of patients entering chemotherapy trials have had sputum isolates showing low virulence for guinea pigs (Mitchison et al., 1960). While apical foci have been considered essential for the propagation of tuberculosis in the pre-HIV era, the relative importance of the reactivation and reinfection pathways to cavitary disease may vary under different conditions around the world. This analysis is consistent with the principle of *balanced pathogenicity* espoused by Mims (1987). Whereas vertebrates slowly evolve defenses against microbial infections over thousands of years, the rapid generation time of microorganisms permits more rapid adaptation to changing conditions. The most successful pathogens appear to balance their virulence to the susceptibility of their obligate hosts.

References

Aoki, S. K. (1990). Racial differences in susceptibility to infection by Mycobacterium tuberculosis (letter). *N. Engl. J. Med.* **322**:1670.

Balasubramanian, V., Wiegeshaus E., Taylor, B., and Smith D. W. (1992). Pathogenesis of tuberculosis: historical perspective and current understanding and there meaning for tuberculosis control strategies. *Tubercle Lung Dis.* (in press).

Barnes, P. F., Bloch, A. B., Davidson, P. T., and Snider, D. E. (1991). Tuberculosis in patients with human immunodeficiency virus infection. *N. Engl. J. Med.* **324**:1644–1650.

Canetti, G. (1955). *The Tubercle Bacillus in the Pulmonary Lesion of Man.* Springer, New York.

Centers for Disease Control. (1990). Nosocomial transmission of multidrug-resistant tuberculosis to health-care workers and HIV-infected patients in an urban hospital—Florida. *MMWR* **39**:718–722.

Crowle, A. J. (1988). The tubercle bacillus—human macrophage relationship studied in vitro. In Mycobacterium tuberculosis: *Interactions with the Immune System.* Edited by M. Bendinelli and H. Friedman. Plenum Press, New York, pp. 99–136.

Crowle, A. J., and Elkins, N. (1990). Relative permissiveness of macrophages from black and white people for virulent tubercle bacilli. *Infect. Immun.* **58**:632–638.

Daley, C. L., Small, P. M., Schecter, G. F., Schoolnik, G. K., McAdam, R. A., Jacobs, W. R., and Hopewell, P. C. (1992). An outbreak of tuberculosis with accelerated progression among persons infected with the human immuonodeficiency virus: an analysis using restriction-fragment-length polymorphism. *N. Engl. J. Med.* **326**:231–235.

Dannenberg, A. M. (1989). Immune mechanisms in the pathogenesis of pulmonary tuberculosis. *Rev. Infect. Dis.* **11**:S369–S378.

Dannenberg, A. M. (1991). Delayed-type hypersensitivity and cell-mediated immunity in the pathogenesis of tuberculosis. *Immunol. Today* **12**:228–233.

Dannenberg, A. M. (1992). Pathogensis of pulmonary tuberculosis: host-parasite interactions, cell-mediated immunity, and delayed-type hypersensitivity. In *Basic Principles in Tuberculosis.* 3rd ed. Edited by D. Schlossberg. Springer-Verlag, New York (in press).

Dannenberg, A. M. and Sugimoto, M. (1976). Liquifaction of caseous foci in tuberculosis. *Am. Rev. Respir. Dis.* **113**:257–259.

Davies, P. D. (1989). The role of vitamin D in tuberculosis (letter). *Am. Rev. Respir. Dis.* **139**:1571.

Davies, P. D. (1990). Racial differences and *Mycobacterium tuberculosis* infection (letter). *N. Engl. J. Med.* **322**:1672.

DiPerri, G., Danzi, M. C., DeChecchi, G, Pizzighella, S., Solbilati, M., Cruciani, M., Luzzati, R., Malena, M., Mazzi, R., Concia, E., and Bassetti, D. (1989). Nosocomial epidemic of active tuberculosis among HIV-infected patients. Lancet **2**:1502–1504.

Douvas, G. S., Looker, D. L., Vatter, A. E., and Crowle, A. J. (1985). Gamma interferon activates human macrophages to become tumoricidal and leishmanicidal but enhances replication of macrophage-associated mycobacteria. *Infect. Immun.* **50**:1–8.

Felton, C. P., Smith, J. A., and Ehrlich, M. H. (1990). Racial differences in susceptibility to infection by Mycobacterium tuberculosis. *N. Engl. J. Med.* **322**:1670–1671.

Gaensler, E. A. (1982). The surgery for pulmonary tuberculosis. *Am. Rev. Respir. Dis.* **125**(Suppl):85–94.

Kaufmann, S. H. E. (1989). In vitro analysis of the cellular mechanisms involved in immunity to tuberculosis. *Rev. Infect. Dis.* **11**(Suppl):S448–454.

Lefford, M. J., McGregor, D. D., and Mackaness, G. B. (1973). Immune respnse to Mycobacterium tuberculosis in rats. *Infect. Immun.* **8**:182–189.

Lurie, M. B. (1964). *Resistance to Tuberculosis: Experimental Studies in Native and Acquired Defensive Mechanisms.* Harvard University Press, Cambridge, MA.

Lurie, M. B., Heppleston, S. A., Swartz, I.B. (1950). An evaluation of the method of quantitative airborne infection and its use in the study of the pathogenesis of tuberculosis. *Am. Rev. Tuberc.* **61**:765–797.

Lurie, M. B., Zappasodi, P., and Tickner, C. (1955). On the nature of genetic resistance to tuberculosis in the light of the host-parasite relationships in natively resistant and susceptible rabbits. *Am. Rev. Tuberc. Pulm. Dis.* **72**:297.

Medlar, E. M. (1948) The pathogenesis of minimal pulmonary tuberculosis: a study of 1225 necropsies in cases of sudden and unexpected death. *Am. Rev. Tuberc.* **58**:583–611.

Mims, C.A. (1987). *The Pathogenesis of Infectious Disease*, 3rd ed. Academic Press, London, pp. 1–7.

Mitchison, D. A., Wallace, J. G., Bhatia, A. L., Selkon, J. B., Subbaiah, T. V., and Lancaster, M. C. (1960). A comparison of the virulence in guinea pigs of south Indian and British tubercle bacilli. *Tubercle* **41**:1–22.

Myrvik, Q. N., Leake, E. S., and Goren, M. B. (1988). Mechanisms of toxicity of tubercle bacilli for macrophages. In Mycobacterium tuberculosis:

Interactions with the Immune System. Edited by M. Bendinelli and H. Friedman. Plenum Press, New York, pp. 305–325.

Nardell, E. A. (1990). Dodging droplet nuclei: reducing the risk of tuberculosis transmission in the AIDS era. *Am. Rev. Respir. Dis.* **142**:501–503.

Nardell, E., Mcinnis, B., Thomas., and Weidhaas, S. (1986). Exogenous rininfection with tuberculosis in a shelter for the homeless. *N. Engl. J. Med.* **315**:1570–1575.

Omerod, P., and Skinner, C. (1980). Reinfection tuberculosis two cases in a family of a patient with drug-resistant disease. *Thorax* **35**:56–59.

Orme, I. M., and Collins, F. M. (1984). Adoptive protection of the *Mycobacterium tuberculosis*–infected lung. *Cell. Immunol.* **84**:113–120.

Raleigh, J. W., and Wichelhausen R. (1973). Exogenous reinfection with *Mycobacterium tuberculosis* confirmed by phage typing. *Am. Rev. Respir. Dis.* **108**:639–642.

Raleigh, J. W., Wichelhausen R. H., Rado, T. A., and Bates, J. H. (1975). Evidence for infection by two distinct strains of *Mycobacterium tuberculosis* in pulmonary tuberculosis: report of 9 cases. *Am. Rev. Respir. Dis.* **112**:497–503.

Ratcliffe, H. L. (1952). Tuberculosis induced by droplet nuclei infection: pulmonary tuberculosis of predeterminded initial intensity in mammals. *Am. J. Hyg.* **55**:36–48.

Ratcliffe, H. L., and Palladino, V. S. (1953). Tuberculosis induced by droplet nuclei infection. Initial homogeneous response of small mammals (rats, mice, guinea pigs, and hamsters) to human and to bovine bacilli, and rate and pattern of tubercle development. *J. Exp. Med.* **97**:61.

Rich, A. R. (1951). *The Pathogenesis of Tuberculosis*, 2nd ed. Charles C Thomas, Springfield, IL.

Riley, R. L., Mills, C. C., O'Grady, F., Sultan, L. U., Wittstadt, F., and Shivpuri, D. N. (1962). Infectiousness of air from a tuberculosis ward. *Am. Rev. Respir. Dis.* **85**:511–525.

Rook, G. A. (1988). The role of vitamin D in tuberculosis. *Am. Rev. Respir. Dis.* **138**:768–770.

Rose, R. M. (1991). Immunology of the lung in HIV infection: the pathophysiologic basis for the development of tuberculosis in the AIDS setting. *Bull. Int. Union. Tuberc. Lung Dis.* **66**:15–20.

Rose, R. M., Krivine, A., Pinkston P., Gillis, J. M., Huang, A., and Hammer, S. M. (1991). Frequent identification of HIV-1 DNA in bronchoalveolar lavage cells obtained from individuals with the acquired immunodeficiency syndrome. *Am. Rev. Respir. Dis.* **143**:850–854.

Rosenman, K. D. (1990). Racial differences in susceptibility to infection by *Mycobacterium tuberculosis* (letter). *N. Engl. J. Med.* **322**:1670.

Rothchild, H., Friedenwald, J. S., and Bernstein, C. (1934). The relationship of allergy to immunity in tuberculosis. *Bull. Johns Hopkins Hosp.*, **63**:232–257.

Selwyn, P. A., Hartel, D., Lewis, V. A., Schoenbaum, E. E., Vermund, S. H., Klein, R. S., Walker, A. T., and Friedland, G. H. (1989). A prospective study of the risk of tuberculosis among intraveneous drug users with human immunodefeficiency virus infection. *N. Engl. J. Med.* **320**:545–550.

Skamene, E. (1989). Genetic control of susceptibility to mycobacterial infections. *Rev. Infect. Dis.* **11**(Suppl. 2):S394–S399.

Smith, D. W., and Harding, G. E. (1977). Animal model: experimental airborne tuberculosis in the guinae pig. *Am. J. Pathol.* **89**:273–276.

Smith, D. W., and Wiengeshaus E. H. (1989). What animal models can teach us about the pathogenesis of tuberculosis in humans. *Rev. Infect. Dis.* **11**:S385–S393.

Stanford, J. L., Grange, J. M., and Pozniak, A. (1991). Is Africa lost? *Lancet* **338**:557–558.

Stead, W. W. (1967). Pathogenesis of the sporadic case of tuberculosis. *N. Engl. J. Med.* **277**:1008–1012.

Stead, W. W. (1989). Pathogenesis of tuberculosis: clinical and epidemiologic perspective. *Rev. of Infect. Dis.* **11**:S366–S368.

Stead, W. W. (1992) Genetics and resistance to tuberculosis. Could resistance be enchanced by genetic engineering? *Ann. Intern. Med.* **116**:937–941.

Stead, W. W., and To, T. (1987). The significance of the tuberculin skin test among elderly persons. *Ann. Intern. Med.* **107**:837–842.

Stead, W. W., Kerby, G. R., Schlueter, D. P., and Jordahl, C. W. (1968). The clinical spectum of primary tuberculosis in adults. Confusion with reinfection in the pathogenesis of chronic tuberculosis. *Ann. Intern. Med.* **68**:731–745.

Stead, W. W., Senner, J. W., Reddick, W. T., and Lofgren, J. P. (1990). Racial differences in susceptibility to infection by Mycobacterium tuberculosis. *N. Engl. J. Med.* **322**:422–427.

Styblo, K. (1978). Etat actuel de la question. I. Epidemiologie de la tuberculose. *Bull. Int. Union. Tuberc.* **53**:153–156.

Styblo, K. (1984). *Epidemiology of Tuberculosis.* VEB Gustav Fischer, Jena, pp. 119–120.

Sweany, H. C., Cook, C. E., and Kegerreis, R. (1931). A study of the position of primary cavities in pulmonary tuberculosis. *Am. Rev. Tuberc.* **24**:558–582.

ten Dam, H. G., and Pio, A. (1982). Pathogenesis of tuberculosis and effectiveness of BCG vaccination. *Tubercle* **63**:225–233.

Youmans, G. P. (1979). *Tuberculosis.* WB Saunders, Philadelphia, pp. 202–208.

6

Transmission and Environmental Control of Tuberculosis

RICHARD L. RILEY*

Petersham, Massachusetts

I. Transmission of Tuberculosis

In 1934, William F. Wells studied the bacterial contamination of the air of textile mills in Massachusetts (Wells and Riley, 1937). Previous experiments had shown "that humidification by the atomization of water produces, by evaporation, droplet nuclei which are exceedingly minute and which settle with extreme slowness as compared with the coarser airborne dust with which we are more familiar" (Wells, 1934). Wells' mind was thus prepared to make the distinction, in the mill study, between organisms associated with dust and organisms associated with droplet nuclei arising from humidification by atomization of contaminated water. His genius lay in visualizing, from this nonhuman evidence, the epidemiological significance of infectious droplet nuclei produced in the respiratory tract of humans.

Wells went on to demonstrate by animal exposure experiments that droplet nuclei could carry a tubercle bacillus directly from room air to deep lung tissue. If a rabbit or guinea pig was infected by the airborne route and sacrificed after about 4 weeks, individual lesions, arising from individual infective droplet

---

*Professor Emeritus, The Johns Hopkins University, Baltimore, Maryland.

nuclei, appeared as pearly white, 3-mm tubercles, easily seen and counted on inspection of the surface of the lung lobes. If the animal inhaled a given number of tubercle bacilli in the form of a fine particle aerosol, approximately the same number of tubercles subsequently developed in the lungs. Thus a susceptible animal could become a quantitative sampler of tubercle bacilli attached to droplet nuclei (Wells, 1955).

Wells designed an experiment using guinea pigs to sample human tubercle bacilli. The air of a tuberculosis ward would be breathed continuously by a large colony of guinea pigs under conditions that eliminated the possibility of transmission by direct contact, respiratory droplets as such, or ordinary house dust. Only droplet nuclei would be buoyant enough to be carried out of the patients' rooms through vents in the ceiling and wafted gently through large ventilating ducts and a riser leading to the floor above where the guinea pigs would be housed. The basic design would eliminate particles with appreciable settling tendency, and the upper respiratory tracts of the guinea pigs would serve as final filters for dust-borne organisms.

By dint of extraordinary cooperation between the Veterans Administration Central Office and the administrators, physicians and staff at the Veterans Administration Hospital in Baltimore, this experiment was in fact carried out during the 1950s and 1960s (Riley et al., 1957, 1959, 1962). Approximately 130 guinea pigs were exposed for a total of 4 years. All animals were tuberculin-tested at monthly intervals, and an average of approximately three per month converted to positive. Converters were removed from the colony and were replaced by fresh animals, keeping the census constant. The infected animals were sacrificed and autopsied. The characteristic lesion was the single pulmonary tubercle, assumed to have developed from a single infectious droplet nucleus.

Over the 4-year period, 134 guinea pigs were infected. Since each guinea pig breathes about 240 ft^3 of air per month, over 48 months the colony of 130 breathed collectively about 1,500,000 ft^3 of air. If, in this huge volume, there were 134 infectious doses of tuberculosis, then there was one infectious dose in about 11,000 ft^3 of air. This figure is consistent with the estimated average amount of air breathed by a student nurse working on a tuberculosis ward in the prechemotherapy era, before converting the tuberculin test to positive (Riley, 1957). The comparison betweeen guinea pigs and a student nurse makes use of the same assumption in both cases: when a single infectious droplet nucleus is implanted on deep lung tissue, infection occurs and the tuberculin test converts to positive a month or two later.* The data suggested that the susceptibility of

*The actual volume of air that would have to be breathed to implant a single infectious droplet nucleus in the lung would have to be somewhat larger than the volume containing a single droplet nucleus. Because of the respiratory dead space, some of the

both guinea pigs and healthy young people to initial infection approaches the ultimate—the single infectious droplet nucleus.

The average values dealt with so far mask the extraordinary variation in infectivity between different patients (Riley et al., 1962). Among 61 untreated patients with drug-susceptible organisms, only eight infected any guinea pigs, and among six untreated patients with drug-resistant organisms, only two proved infectious for the guinea pigs. From a total of 40 patients under chemotherapy, only two infected guinea pigs. Thus, the infectivity of many tuberculosis patients with positive sputum was too low to be detected in the Veterans Administration study. On the other hand, one patient with laryngeal tuberculosis infected 15 guinea pigs in 3 days. By calculation, the concentration of infectious particles in the air at that time was about 1 in 200 ft^3, or more than 50 times the average concentration of 1 in 11,000 ft^3 of air.

A sharp outbreak of tuberculosis abroad the naval vessel "Richard E. Byrd" provided evidence of airborne transmission between people and added further insight into the relative importance of airborne transmission and direct contact (Houk et al., 1968). Sixty-six men shared one bunking compartment with the index case, who had a large cavity in his lung. Eighty-one men, with minimal direct contact with the others, shared a second compartment in which three-quarters of the ventilation came through interconnecting ducts from the first compartment. Eighty percent of the men in the first compartment converted the tuberculin test from negative to positive, and 54% of the men in the second compartment converted. The rate of conversion in the second compartment was nearly the same as the expected rate based on the proportion of ventilation coming from the first compartment (¾ × 80%, or 60%, vs. 54%). In this inadvertent experiment, the men in the two compartments were infected roughly in proportion to the amount of contaminated air from the first compartment that they breathed. But direct contact with the index case occurred only in the first compartment. Thus, close personal contact did not greatly increase the likelihood of infection. Airborne droplet nuclei constituted the predominant mechanism of infection.

In a report on a measles outbreak in a suburban elementary school, the quantitative assessment of airborne infection was further refined (Riley et al.,

---

inspired air, with its contained organisms, never reaches the deep lung tissue, and because some droplet nuclei are filtered out in the upper respiratory tract, some organisms, otherwise destined for deep lung deposition, never get there. There may also be differences in susceptibility (Stead et al., 1990). Wells ignored these specific mechanisms, apparently considering them to be subsumed under his definition of a "quantum" of infection (see footnote, p. 126).

1978). Since the number of infectious droplet nuclei required to infect a person is generally unknown, Wells defined a "quantum" of infection as an infectious dose, which could be one or more infectious particles.* In the following derivation, let q = quanta of airborne infection produced by an infectious person (infector) per unit of time. Let I = number of infectors. Let Q = rate of room ventilation with germ-free air (outdoor or disinfected air). Iq/Q = equilibrium concentration of quanta in room air. Let S = number of susceptible people exposed, and p = pulmonary ventilaion rate per susceptible. The symbol t = duration of exposure to infection, and pt = the volume of potentially infected air breathed. If quanta were evenly dispersed throughout the air, the number breathed by a susceptible person would be the concentration in the air (Iq/Q) times the volume of air breathed (pt), or $Iqpt/Q$. Since, in fact, quanta are discrete, randomly distributed, and in very low concentration, the probability, P, that a susceptible, S, will breathe one or more quanta and become a case, C, is better approximated by:

$$P = 1 - e^{-Iqpt/Q} \tag{1}$$

and the number of new cases will be:

$$C = S\left(1 - e^{-Iqpt/Q}\right) \tag{2}$$

This formulation applies to a single room or enclosed space, but it has been applied, with less validity, to spaces served by the same heating, ventilating, or air-conditioning (HVAC) system.

In analyzing successive generations of the measles epidemic, C, S, I, p, t, and Q were either known or estimated for each room throughout the school, and the value of q was calculated. The infectiousness, q, of the index case was found to be 5,580 quanta per hour, about 10 times that of secondary cases appearing in the next generation. Measles patients thus showed the same variability in infectiousness that was seen in tuberculosis patients in the Veterans Administration study, but the rate of production of infectious airborne particles was much higher.

The mathematical model developed to analyze the measles epidemic was applied to an outbreak of tuberculosis in an office building (Nardell et al., 1991). A 30-year-old woman returned to her office from vacation with cough, fever, and fatigue. After 4 weeks she sought medical attention, was found to have sputum-positive tuberculosis, and was removed from her job. Thus, during 40 hr/week for 4 weeks the patient's tubercle bacilli were put into the air by cough-

---

*More specifically, with reference to bovine tubercle bacilli in rabbits: "Since 36.8 per cent of the rabbits will escape infection when one bacillus, on the average, has been breathed per rabbit, the dose per animal which infects 63.2 per cent of the animals is called a *quantum of infection*" (Wells, 1955, pp. 143–144).

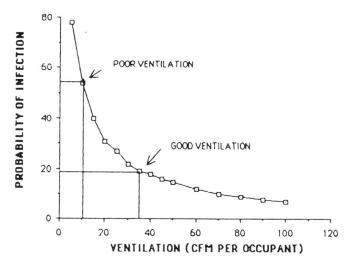

Figure 1 The effect of room ventilation on the probability of infection. (Reprinted from Nardell, 1991.)

ing and other respiratory activities. They were distributed through the single HVAC system by recirculation. The average value of fresh-air makeup was estimated from carbon dioxide measurements to be 15 ft³/min (cfm) per occupant. There was inadequate information to deal with exposures on a room-by-room basis. Thus, the 13,000 ft² of office space on two floors was treated as a single enclosed space with equal airborne exposure throughout.*

There were 27 conversions of the tuberculin test to positive among 67 workers with documented negative tuberculin tests before the outbreak, a conversion rate of 40%. Equation (2) was applied as follows: $C = 27$, $S = 67$, $I = 1$, p estimated as 0.353 cfm, $t = 160$ hr, and $Q = 15$ cfm/person × 93 total occupants of the space, or 1395 cfm. The remaining unknown factor, q, was calculated by Eq. (2) to be 12.7 quanta per hour (qph), the rate at which the index case put infectious doses of tubercle bacilli into the air.

A graph of the probability of infection versus fresh-air ventilation per occupant shows the importance of adequate ventilation and the diminishing effectiveness of high levels of ventilation (Fig. 1). Figure 1 was plotted using Eq. (1) and refers to the outbreak of tuberculosis in an office building described above. A similar plot (not shown) for an outbreak of tuberculosis resulting from a brief

---

*People occupying the same room as the index case would actually be much more heavily exposed than those in other rooms breathing recirculated organisms. The index case moved around too much to permit room-by-toom analysis.

but intense exposure during bronchoscopy (Catanzaro, 1982) yields a curve of similar shape, but the probability of infection is approximately doubled at levels of ventilation above 20 cfm/occupant and increased by a lesser amount below 20 cfm/occupant. The similarity of the curves under two such different types of outbreak leads us to conclude that Figure 1 is a fairly representative curve for tuberculosis outbreaks and suitable for use in designing control measures (see below).

The advent of AIDS in the last decade has caused a resurgence of tuberculosis, particularly in HIV-positive people (CDC, 1989). As discussed earlier, healthy people are highly susceptible to initial infection with the tubercle bacillus, but their infection seldom progresses to active disease and seldom becomes a hazard to others (CDC, 1990). By contrast, those whose immune system is damaged by HIV infection progress rapidly from primary infection to active tuberculosis (DiPerri et al., 1989; Daley et al., 1992) HIV infection also causes reactivation and rapid progression of old tuberculosis (Selwyn et al., 1989; Nardell, 1991). These developments, accentuated by the recent spread of organisms resistant to all known chemotherapeutic agents, have created a demand for environment measures to interrupt the transmission of tuberculosis and thus prevent infection (CDC, 1991).

II. Environmental Control of Tuberculosis

A. Control at the Source

The most efficient place to stop airborne transmission is at the source, the infected person. It is easier to trap infectious particles before they disperse throughout rooms and HVAC systems. Ideally they should be trapped at the mouth by covering the mouth and nose when coughing or sneezing. This is more effective than might be imagined because respiratory droplets can be caught by impingement on the hand or tissue before they evaporate and become extremely elusive droplet nuclei. Face masks represent an attempt to apply this principle, but guaze masks become saturated and ineffective. Bacteria-tight masks that can be fitted snugly are available but require careful use. The continuous wearing of masks by patients is not feasible, but use in hazardous situations is helpful. The wearing of bacteria-tight masks by well people in contact with infectious patients provides a degree of protection that is desirable but inadequate.

A booth has been developed in which cough-producing procedures can be performed safely. Although particles reach the droplet nucleus stage, they are trapped by a high-efficiency particle (HEPA) filter or vented to the outdoors, thus preventing dispersal throughout indoor spaces. Aerosolized pentamidine for *Pneumocystis carinii* infection or aerosolized saline to induce sputum should be administered in a booth or similar apparatus to trap droplet nuclei. Such control at the source is more efficient and cheaper than high rates of fresh-air ventilation to vent organisms from the entire treatment room.

B. Control by Air Disinfection

Air disinfection is designed to interrupt transmission from patient to victim. Ultraviolet (UV) radiation of 254 nm wavelength has long been known to kill or inactivate organisms in airborne droplet nuclei with great efficiency (Wells and Fair, 1935). Test organisms, such as *Escherichia coli* or *Serratia marcescens*, are easily inactivated, but the germicidal effect drops off sharply at relative humidities above 60% (Wells, 1955, p. 66; Riley and Kaufman, 1972). Tubercle bacilli are not as easily inactivated, but UV maintains its effectiveness at least as high as 65% relative humidity (Riley et al, 1976). Studies at higher humidities have not been done. Excessive exposure of people to germicidal (254 nm) UV gives painful superficial irritation of skin and eyes but is devoid of serious long-term effects (Blum and Lippincott, 1942; Riley and Nardell, 1989). The National Institute for Occupational Safety and Health (NIOSH) has set a limit of $0.2 \ \mu W/cm^2$ for continuous 8-hr exposure (NIOSH, 1972)

Germicidal UV is usually directed to the upper air of a room, above people's heads, in order to prevent excessive personal exposure (California Indoor Air Quality Program, 1990). Disinfection of the lower air, where prople breathe, depends on mixing relatively germ-free upper air with air in the lower part of the room. This is accomplished by convection and by forced air movement (Riley and Permutt, 1971). Figure 2 shows the disappearance curve of tubercle bacilli (BCG) from the lower room air with approximately half the recommended UV wattage applied to the upper air (Riley et al, 1976). A good UV installation can reduce airborne tubercle bacilli by an amount equivalent to about 20 air changes per hour (AC/hr) or 100 cfm/person of outside air (Riley, 1988; Riley and Nardell, 1989). Adding 100 cfm to 10 cfm/occupant (Fig. 1, "poor ventilation") gives a total of 110 cfm and, under the stated conditions of exposure, reduces the probability of infection from 54% to less than 10%. Even starting with 35 cfm/occupant (Fig. 1, "good ventilation"), one finds the probability of infection at 135 cfm to be less than half that at 35 cfm. The effect of UV is so predominant that high rates of outside air ventilation can be dispensed with, at considerable saving in energy.

Intense UV radiation can be applied in ventilating ducts at low cost and without hazard to room accupants. In this way, recirculated air can be made germ-free, and the distribution of airborne organisms throughout the HVAC system prevented. If, for example, total room ventilation were 25 cfm/occupant and 80% were recirculated, the remaining outside air makeup available to dilute

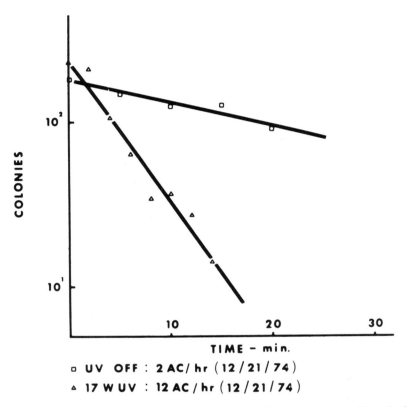

○ **UV OFF** : **2 AC/ hr** (**12 / 21 / 74**)
△ **17 W UV** : **12 AC / hr** (**12 / 21 / 74**)

Figure 2   Disappearance of bacille Calmette-Guérin (BCG) from room with and without upper air ultraviolet (UV) irradiation using one fixture with a 17-watt (W) tube. Based on experiments of this type, one suspended 29-W UV tube is expected to produce the air-disinfecting equivalent of approximately 20 air changes per hour (AC/hr). (Reprinted from Riley et. al., 1976.)

airborne organisms would be only 5 cfm/occupant. This is dangerously low, leading to 80% probability of infection under the conditions on which Figure 1 is based. UV irradiation of recirculated air would make the total ventilation of 25 cfm/occupant germ-free and reduce the probability of infection to 27%. In general, the effectiveness of duct irridation is at its best, and the need greatest, when the percentage of recirculated air is high, outside air makeup low, and the steep part of the probability curve applicable.

Room air can be passed through an enclosed container in which it is intensely irradiated with UV or passed through a HEPA filter, or both. One such self-contained apparatus on the market is designed to add about 3 AC/hr of germ-free air to the ventilation of the room. Other devices have larger capacity, but the amount of air blown through the apparatus is limited by noise, energy, and comfort constraints. The chief advantage of enclosed apparatus is that people cannot be exposed to UV. The amount of room air disinfection accomplished is small compared to upper air irradiation. As with duct irradiation, the effectiveness is greatest when outside air ventilation is low and the steep part of the probability curve is applicable (Fig. 1).

Upper air irradiation in each room is more effective than central duct irradiation or self-contained units in the room because the volume of relatively germ-free air diluting organisms in the lower part of each room is greater. With duct irradiation, germ-free ventilation in each room is limited to the amount entering through supply ducts, say 5 AC/hr or 25 cfm/occupant. With upper air irradiation, partly disinfected upper air exchanges with lower room air across the entire boundary between irradiated and unirradiated zones, which in the room where much experimental work was done was about 200 ft^2. Calculated rates of air movement across this boundary, unassisted by fans, averaged about 100 AC/hr, or 3333 cfm (Riley and Permutt, 1971). Because of the large boundary area, 3333 cfm can be accomplished without high velocity of air movement. The resulting dilution of tubercle bacilli in the lower room air is equivalent to about 20 AC/hr when a 30-watt suspended fixture is operating in a 200 ft^2 room (Riley et al., 1976). This is four times the postulated 5 AC/hr accomplished by duct irradiation and is in addition to actual outside air makeup. The efficacy of upper-air irradiation also outdistances that of self-contained units in the room.

The quantitative advantage of upper air irradiation must be balanced against the possibility of exposing people to UV if the fixtures are poorly designed. In older buildings without a central HVAC system, duct irradiation is not an option, and if ceilings are high, overhead UV, using suspended fixtures, provides a safe, effective solution. However, when ceilings are low, louvered wall fixtures must be employed, and these must control both downward radiation that would strike occupants and upward radiation that would ''bounce'' off the ceiling and overexpose occupants. Fixtures that collimate UV in a horizontal beam require carefully designed and constructed louvers. Furthermore, upper air irradiation, whether by wall-mounted or suspended fixtures, cannot effectively disinfect lower room air unless there is adequate mixing between upper and lower parts of the room. Studies under various conditions indicate that supplemental fans may be needed, since air mixing can be poor under unfavorable weather conditions or when HVAC systems are poorly designed (Riley and Permutt, 1971; Riley et al., 1971a,b, 1976). Upper air irradiation is thus a more difficult undertaking than duct irradiation or self-contained units but provides much more protection from airborne infection.

One can expect air disinfection to be most effective in places where the sources of infection congregate or are confined, such as shelters for the

homeless, prisons, hospitals, clinics, drug-abuse treatment centers, and microbiology laboratories. These are the places where the current need is most urgent.

Examples of Control by Air Disinfection

The classic example of control by UV air disinfection was Wells' control of a
measles epidemic in grade schools in Germantown and Swarthmore, Pennsylvania, in the early 1940s (Wells et al., 1942). Here there were few exposures
outside of school and these were traced. Efforts to repeat Wells' results have
been unsuccessful, primarily because of large numbers of untraced outside exposures (Perkins et al, 1947; Medical Research Council, 1954).

Since air disinfection is not of benefit when the people to be protected are
heavily exposed elsewhere, its maximum benefit is to be expected when uniquely
high-risk spaces can be identified. For example, a reference laboratory in Albany,
New York, where sputum specimens were processed was involved in a outbreak
of tuberculosis that involved workers throughout the building. The workers were
unlikely to be exposed elsewhere. The source of the airborne organisms was attributed to faulty laboratory techniques, and distribution throughout the building
was facilitated by open pipe chases. Both were corrected, but UV air disinfection was added to make doubly sure there would be no recurrence.

An outbreak of tuberculosis occurred in a large shelter for the homeless in
Boston. Many cases were linked to the index case by identity of phage type of
their organisms. This indicated that they were probably infected in the shelter,
the only place where they were crowded together indoors (Nardell et al., 1986;
Nardell, 1988). Suspended fixtures for upper air irradiation were installed. In
subsequent years there was reduction in the tuberculin conversion rate among
the staff, but quantification of the effectiveness of air disinfection has not been
possible because the degree of exposure varies unpredictably depending on the
presence or absence of disseminators of infection.

UV air disinfection was employed over a 12-year period in a tuberculosis
ward in Milwaukee. None of the medical and nursing students, tuberculin-tested
before and after a 6-week tour of duty, converted to positive, suggesting protection by air disinfection (Stead, 1989).

In a clinic in Florida, where many conversions of the tuberculin test occurred in the staff, the air was found to be almost totally recirculated (CDC,
1988, 1989; Brundage et al., 1988). Tubercle bacilli were distributed throughout
the building and infected even staff members who had no direct contact with
patients. Administration of aerosolized pentamidine without special precautions
created an additional hazard. Along with other measures, UV tubes were installed in air-handling units to disinfect air supplied by the HVAC system
(Bromberger-Barnea, 1988). The combined effect has been a sharp reduction in

tuberculin conversions among the staff during a 3-year follow-up (James Jolley, personal communication).

The need for air disinfection arises in many medical settings where there is a high probability that patients with undiagnosed tuberculosis will be present (NTA, 1967). The need also exists in spaces where instrumentation of the respiratory tract is carried out, such as bronchoscopy rooms and intensive care units (Malasky et al., 1990; Catanzaro, 1982). Such procedures often produce cough and therefore airborne droplet nuclei. When least expected, these invisible particles may transmit tuberculosis and other airborne diseases.

References

Blum, H. F., and Lippincott, S. W. (1942). Carcinogenic effectiveness of ultraviolet radiation of wave length 2537A. *J. Natl. Cancer. Inst.* **3**:211–216.

Bromberger-Barnea B. (1988). Report to J. Howell, Director, Palm Beach County Department of Health.

Brundage, J. D., Scott, R. McN., Lednar, W. M., Smith, D. W., and Miller, R. N. (1988). Building-associated risk of febrile acute respiratory diseases in army trainees. *JAMA* **259**:2108–2112.

California Indoor Air Quality Program (1990). *Using Ultraviolet Radiation and Ventilation to Control Tuberculosis.* California Department of Health Services.

Catanzaro, A. (1982). Nosocomial tuberculosis. *Am. Rev. Respir. Dis.*, **123**:559–562.

Centers for Disease Control (1988). Report to Palm Beach County Health Department by Kubica, G. P., and Cieseilski, C. A., Atlanta.

Centers for Disease Control (1989). *Mycobacterium tuberculosis* transmission in a health clinic—Florida 1988. *MMWR* **38**:256–264.

Centers for Disease Control (1990). Guidelines for preventing the transmission of tuberculosis in health-care settings, with special focus on HIV-related issues. *MMWR* **39**:1–29.

Centers for Disease Control (1991). Nosocomial transmission of multi-drug resistant tuberculosis among HIV-infected persons—Florida and New York, 1988–1991. *MMWR* **40**:585–559.

Daley, C. L., Small, P. M., Schecter, G. F., Schoolnik, G. K., McAdam, R. A., Jacobs, W. R., and Hopewell, P. C. (1992). An outbreak of tuberculosis with accelerated progression among persons infected with the human immuonodeficiency virus: an analysis using restriction-fragment-length polymorphism. *N. Engl. J. Med.* **326**:231–235.

DiPerri, G., Danzi, M. C., DeChecchi, G, Pizzighella, S., Solbiati, M., Cruciani, M., Luzzati, R., Malena, M., Mazzi, R., Concia, E., and Bassetti, D. (1989). Nosocomial epidemic of active tuberculosis among HIV-infected patients. *Lancet* **2**:1502–1504.

Houk, V. N., Kent, D. C., Baker, J. H., and Sorensen, K. (1968). The epidemiology of tuberculosis infection in a closed environment. *Arch. Environ. Health* **16**:26–35.

Malasky, C., Potulski, F., Jordan, T., and Reichman, L. B. (1990). Occupational tuberculosis infections among pulmonary physicians in training. *Am. Rev. Respir. Dis.* **142**:505–507.

Medical Research Council (1954). Air disinfection with ultraviolet irradiation: its effect on illness among school children. Her Majesty's Stationery Office, Special Report Series No. 283, London.

Nardell, E. A. (1988) Ultraviolet air disinfection to control tuberculosis in a shelter for the homeless. In *Architectural Design and Indoor Microbial Pollution*. Edited by R. B. Kundsin. Oxford University Press, New York, pp. 296–308.

Nardell, E. A. (1991) Nosocomial tuberculosis in the AIDS era: strategies for interrupting transmission in developed countries. *Bull. Int. Union Tuberc. Lung Dis.* **66**:107–111.

Nardell, E., Mcinnis, B., Thomas, B., and Weidhaas, S. (1986). Exogenous reinfection with tuberculosis in a shelter for the homeless. *N. Engl. J. Med.* **315**:1570–1575.

Nardell, E. A., Keegan, J., Cheney, S. A., and Etkind, S. C. (1991). Airborne infection: theoretical limits of protection achievable by building ventilation. *Am. Rev. Respir. Dis.* **144**:302–306.

National Institute of Occupational Safety and Health (1972). *Occupational Exposure to Ultraviolet Radiation*. U.S. Government Printing Office, Washington, DC.

National Tuberculosis Association (1967). Infectiousness of tuberculosis: a report of the NTA ad hoc committee on treatment of TB patients in general hospitals. *Am. Rev. Respir. Dis.* **96**:836–837.

Perkins, J. E., Bahlke, A. M., and Silverman, H. F. (1947). Effect of ultraviolet radiation of classrooms on the spread of measles in large rural central schools. *Am. J. Public Health* **38**:529–537.

Riley, E. C., Murphy, G., and Riley, R. L. (1978). Airborne spread of measles in a suburban elementary school. *Am. J. Epidemiol.* **107**:421–432.

Riley, R. L. (1957). The J. Burns Amberson Lecture: Aerial dissemination of pulmonary tuberculosis. *Am. Rev. Tuberc. Pulm. Dis.* **76**:931–941.

Riley, R. L. (1988) Ultraviolet air disinfection for control of respiratory contagion. In *Architectural Design and Indoor Microbial Pollution*. Edited by R. B. Kundsin. Oxford University Press, New York, pp. 174–197.

Riley, R. L., and Kaufman, J. E. (1972). Effect of relative humidity on the inactivation of airborne Serratia marcescens by ultraviolet radiation. *J. Appl. Microbiol.* **23**:1113–1120.

Riley, R. L., Nardell, E. A. (1989) Clearing the air: the theory and application of ultraviolet air disinfection. *Am. Rev. Respir. Dis.* **139**:1286–1294.

Riley, R. L., and Permutt, S. (1971). Room air disinfection by ultraviolet irradiation of upper air: air mixing and germicidal effectiveness. *Arch. Environ. Health* **22**:208–219.

Riley, R. L., Wells, W. F., Mills, C. C., Nyka, W., and McLean, R. L. (1957). Air hygiene in tuberculosis: quantitative studies of infectivity and control in a pilot ward. *Am. Rev. Tuberc. Pulm. Dis.* **75**:420–431.

Riley, R. L., Mills, C. C., Myka, W., Weinstock, N., Storey, P. B., Sultan, L. V., Riley, M. C., and Wells, W. F. (1959). Aerial dissemination of pulmonary tuberculosis: a two year study of contagion in a tuberculosis ward. *Am. J. Hyg.* **80**:185–196.

Riley, R. L., Mills, C. C., O'Grady, F., Sultan, L. U., Wittstadt, F., and Shivpuri, D. N. (1962). Infectiousness of air from a tuberculosis ward. *Am. Rev. Respir. Dis.* **85**:511–525.

Riley, R. L., Permutt, S., and Kaufman, J. E. (1971a). Convection, air mixing and ultraviolet air disinfection in rooms. *Arch. Environ. Health* **22**:200–207.

Riley, R. L., Permutt, S., and Kaufman, J. E. (1971b). Room air disinfection by ultraviolet irradiation of upper air: further analysis of convective air exchange. *Arch. Environ. Health* **23**:35–39.

Riley, R. L., Knight, M., and Middlebrook, G. (1976). Ultraviolet susceptibility of BCG and virulent tubercle bacilli. *Am. Rev. Respir. Dis.* **113**:413–418.

Selwyn, P. A., Hartel, D., Lewis, V. A., Schoenbaum, E. E., Vermund, S. H., Klein, R. S., Walker, A. T., and Friedland, G. H. (1989). A prospective study of the risk of tuberculosis among intravenous drug users with human immunodefeficiency virus infection. *N. Engl. J. Med.* **320**:545–550.

Stead, W. W. (1989). Letter to the editor concerning "Clearing the air: the theory and application of ultraviolet air disinfection." *Am. Rev. Respir. Dis.* **140**:1832.

Stead, W. W., Lofgren, J. P., Senner, J. W., and Reddick, W. T. (1990). Racial differences in susceptibility to infection with *M. tuberculosis. N. Engl. J. Med.* **322**:422–427.

Wells, W. F. (1934). On air-borne infection. II. Droplets and droplet nuclei. *Am. J. Hyg.* **20**:611–618.

Wells, W. F. (1955). *Airborne Contagion and Air Hygiene: An Ecological Study of Droplet Infections.* Harvard University Press., Cambridge, MA, Chapter XII.

Wells, W. F., and Fair, G. M. (1935). Viability of *E. colil* exposed to ultraviolet radiation in air. *Science* **82**:280–281.

Wells, W. F., and Riley, E. C. (1937). An investigation of the bacterial contamination of the air of textile mills with special reference to the influence of artificial humidification. *J. Indust. Hyg. Toxicol.* **19**:513–561.

Wells, W. F., Wells, M. W., and Wilder, T. S. (1942). The environmental control of epidemic contagion. I. An epidemiologic study of radiant disinfection of air in day schools. *Am. J. Hyg.* **35**:97–121.

Part Two

PRACTICAL ASPECTS

7

The Tuberculin Test

JOHN B. BASS, JR.

University of South Alabama College of Medicine
Mobile, Alabama

> There may be nostalgia for the days when all tuberculin reactions meant tuberculous infection, and no nonsense.
>
> —Edwards and Edwards, 1960

I. Introduction

Following his discovery of the tubercle bacillus, Robert Koch continued his work in tuberculosis. He found that a concentrated filtrate from cultures of *Mycobacterium tuberculosis*, which had been killed by heat, protected guinea pigs from experimental tuberculosis. He believed that this material, which he called tuberculin, could also cure human patients with tuberculosis (Koch, 1890). Koch's reports were uncharacteristically vague and consisted of superficial descriptions of his methods and anecdotal reports of cures in patients with extrapulmonary tuberculosis such as lupus vulgaris. Some of this secrecy was probably due to Koch's position as an employee of the German government, which presumably would have profited greatly from a genuine cure for tuberculosis. Despite the vagueness of his reports, Koch's reputation brought rapid support for his claims from medical journals such as *The Lancet* (Editorial, 1890a) and the *Journal of the American Medical Association* (Editorial, 1890b), as well

139

as from scientists such as Sir Joseph Lister. Detractors, however, were equally prominent and included Billroth, Virchow, and Sir Arthur Conan Doyle, who correctly recognized that patients with pulmonary tuberculosis were not cured and that the reported "cures" were due to severe local tissue reactions with necrosis and sloughing. Koch continued his work, but within a few years his claims were widely discredited.

Koch's method of therapy involved the intrascapular subcutaneous injection of increasing graduated doses of tuberculin. Local reaction at the site of injection was minimal, but patients with tuberculosis had a generalized systemic reaction, with fever, generalized aches, abdominal discomfort, nausea, and vomiting several hours following the injection. People without tuberculosis did not develop this reaction, and the possibility of using tuberculin as a diagnostic test occurred to a number of investigators. Methods of application of tuberculin tests included a cutaneous scratch (Von Pirquet), a percutaneous patch (Moro), and direct application to the conjuctiva (Calmette). At about the same time, Mantoux described the intracutaneous test that remains the standard today. The Mantoux test became popular because of its precision despite the fact that it requires specialized equipment and skill.

II. Tuberculins

When Koch fully disclosed his method of preparing tuberculin (Koch, 1891), it was clear that the secrecy surrounding his previous reports was unwarranted since his extraction methods were in common use. The crude extraction methods resulted in a material containing a large number of carbohydrate and protein antigens. Koch's original material also contained some foreign antigens from the beef broth that was used as a culture medium. Old Tuberculin (OT) is still produced using methods almost identical to Koch's original description, with the exception that beef broth is no longer used. For a number of years, tuberculins were manufactured without much attempt at standardization. This situation was well described by Green:

> It would surely simplify life for manufacturers if O.T. were plainly described as 'any witches' brew derived by evaporation of any unspecified fluid medium in which any unspecified strain of mammalian *M. tuberculosis* had been grown, provided its potency matched that of another witches' brew kept in Copenhagen and called international standard, or any allegedly equivalent sub-standard thereof, when tested on an unspecified number of guinea-pigs without worrying too much about statistical analysis of results (Green, 1951).

The most important alteration in the manufacture of tuberculin came in the early 1930s when Florence Seibert prepared precipitates of OT, first with trichloracetic acid and later with ammonium sulfate. She called this precipitated material purified protein derivative (PPD) (Seibert, 1934). PPD has been studied by a variety of techniques and has been shown to contain a number of antigenic components, most of which are low- and medium-weight proteins. PPD contains les carbohydrate than OT and there are fewer nonspecific immediate reactions with PPD. In 1941, Seibert and Glenn prepared a large batch of PPD (PPD-S) that has served as the standard reference material in the United States since that time (Seibert and Glenn, 1941). Other important improvements in tuberculin include the addition of Tween, a detergent that prevents the adsorption of tuberculin to glass and plastic syringes (Magnus et al., 1958; Landi et al., 1966; Zack and Fulkerson, 1970), and the requirement in 1978 by the Federal Drug Administration that all PPD lots be bioassayed in humans and demonstrate equal potency to PPD-S (Sbarbaro, 1978).

"Tuberculins" and "PPDs" have been prepared from other mycobacterial species, but these materials appear to be less sensitive and specific than materials prepared from *M. tuberculosis*. They have been useful epidemiologically (Edwards et al., 1969), but have not been widely used or recommended as diagnostic tests.

III. Dose of Tuberculin

At the turn of the century, about 90% of the population reacted in some way to tuberculin. The earliest use in humans was as a diagnostic test to rule out tuberculosis in patients. Tuberculin was administered in graduated doses and all visible reactions were considered positive. The decreasing prevalence of tuberculosis in the 1920s and 1930s resulted in decreased transmission of infection to younger age groups and led to the use of tuberculin to diagnose the infected state rather than the disease. However, the use of a series of skin tests with graduated doses of tuberculin was impractical on a large scale. In 1941, Furcolow reported that a dose of 0.0001 mg was best to discriminate patients with tuberculosis from those unlikely to have tuberculosis (Furcolow et al., 1941). This dose was five times as large as the usual starting dose with a graduated regimen and was, therefore, said to contain five tuberculin units (5 TU). A 5-TU dose became the standard for use in the United States. It should be noted that newly manufactured batches of tuberculin are bioassayed as stated previously, and the standard 5-TU dose is that dose which produces a reaction equivalent to the standard regardless of the exact amount of material contained.

Other doses of tuberculin, such as "first strength" (1 TU) and "second strength" (250 TU), are remnants of the old graduated system of administration and represent the smallest and largest doses of tuberculin that were administered. These strengths of tuberculin are not commonly available and, even if available, are not standardized by bioassay. The clinical utility of these strengths of tuberculin is essentially nil at the current time.

IV. Measuring Results

Although erythema is usually present with a positive Mantoux skin test, the results using erythema as a criterion are imprecise, and results have been standardized based on the amount of induration at the site of injection. The test is usually administered on the forearm and induration is measured after 48–72 hr. Reactions are slightly larger at 72 hr than at 48 hr and on the dorsal surface of the forearm as compared to the volar surface, but the differences are small (Palmer and Bates, 1952). Host variation as determined by measurement of induration in tests simultaneously applied to both arms averages about 15%, and variability in measuring induration among experienced observers is similar. Interobserver variability may be decreased by using the ballpoint pen method of Sokal to measure induration (Sokal, 1975). Although multiple puncture devices are convenient and may be better tolerated by children, results from these devices are less sensitive and specific than results from the Mantoux method (Sbarbaro, 1978). The issue of specificity is of particular importance in low-prevalence populations (such as most children today), and the Mantoux method is preferred.

V. Interpretation of Results

As expected with a biological test, results from tuberculin testing demonstrate normal variability. The utilization of tuberculin testing requires a thorough understanding of those characteristics which are inherent in the test itself (sensitivity and specificity) and those characteristics which influence the interpretation of the results based on the likelihood of the condition in the person or population being tested (the effect of prevalence or prior probability on the predictive value of a positive and a negative test).

The sensitivity of a test is the percentage of people with the condition who have a positive test. If false-negatives are uncommon, sensitivity is high. Early studies in tuberculosis sanitoria demonstrated an extremely high sensitivity, and negative results to graduated skin testing with tuberculin were thought to rule out tuberculosis as a diagnostic possibility for many years. More recent studies have reported false-negative rates of 25% during the initial evaluation of persons with tuberculosis (Holden et al., 1971; Nash and Douglass, 1980). False-negative rates of 50% or more may be seen in patients critically ill with disseminated tuberculosis. These high false-negative rates appear to be due to a combination of poor nutrition and general health, overwhelming acute illness, and specific immunosuppression, which may be seen early during disease. An important cause of a false-negative tuberculin test is immunosuppression due to human immunodeficiency virus (HIV) infection. Because of the low sensitivity

Table 1 Causes of a False-Negative Tuberculin Reaction

Host factors
  Acute or overwhelming tuberculosis
  HIV infection
  Other immunosupressive diseases (lymphoma, etc.)
  Viral infections (measles, mumps, varicella)
  Live virus vaccination
  Renal failure
  Malnutrition

Factors related to testing procedure
  Improper storage of PPD
  Improper dilution
  Delayed injection after filling syringe
  Subcutaneous injection
  Lack of experience in interpretation
  Bias in interpretation

in acutely ill patients and those who are infected with HIV, the tuberculin test cannot be used in these circumstances to eliminate the possibility of tuberculosis. Other factors that may cause false-negative results are listed in Table 1. Although testing for generalized anergy has been recommended in HIV-infected persons (Centers for Disease Control, 1991), it has not been demonstrated that this will improve the sensitivity of the test, and specific anergy to tuberculin without generalized anergy has been reported (Nash and Douglass, 1980).

The specificity of a test is the percentage of people without the condition who have a negative test. False-positive results decrease the specificity. False-positive results in tuberculin testing occur because of antigens that appear in PPD which are shared with other mycobacteria (Harboe, 1981; Daniel and Janicki, 1978). These cross-reactions tend to result in smaller amounts of induration than reactions due to *M. tuberculosis*, but the overlap may be considerable in areas of the world where other mycobacteria are common.

Large skin-testing studies have demonstrated a spectrum of results (Edwards et al., 1969). At one end of the spectrum there are some populations whose results from tuberculin testing resemble the distribution in Figure 1. These results demonstrate a normally distributed response with a mean reaction size of 16–18 mm and a very small number of measurable reactions less than 10 mm. This distribution is essentially identical to that obtained when patients with tuberculosis are skin-tested and suggests that populations demonstrating these results have a very low number of false-positive results and the tuberculin test is highly specific. At the other end of the spectrum, some

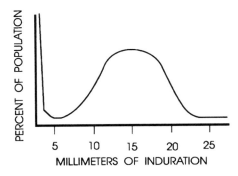

Figure 1 Distribution of tuberculin reactions in a population with few cross-reactions.

populations demonstrate results shown in Figure 2. Here there is no clear-cut unimodal distribution, there are many more reactions smaller than 10 mm, and no clear separation of positive and negative tests is possible. In populations such as this, the specificity of the test is highly dependent on the criterion used to determine a positive result. The specificity of the test can be improved progressively by increasing the cut point for positivity from 5 mm to 15 mm.

In the United States there is a tendency for results to resemble those shown in Figure 2 with progression from west to east and north to south. There may be considerable variability, however, even within a single state, and it is difficult to estimate the specificity of a tuberculin reaction in the absence of recent local results from large-scale skin-testing surveys. These results are generally unavailable for most populations in this country.

For any given population, the likelihood that a positive test represents a true infection is influenced by the prevalence of infection. Table 2 shows how the prevalence of infection influences the predictive value of a positive tuberculin test. Populations that demonstrate a clear-cut unimodal distribution of tuberculin reactions (Fig. 1) may be assumed to have approximately a 99%

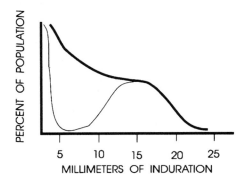

Figure 2 Distribution of tuberculin reactions in a population with an increased number of cross-reactions. A hypothetical subpopulation of true tuberculin reactors with a distribution similar to that of Figure 1 is indicated by the thin line.

Table 2 Predictive Value of a Positive Tuberculin Test

Prevalence of infection (%)	Specificity	
	0.95	0.99
90	0.99	0.999
50	0.95	0.99
25	0.86	0.97
10	0.67	0.91
5	0.50	0.83
1	0.16	0.49
0.1	0.03	0.10
0.01	0.002	0.09

specificity. In populations whose distribution of reactions is more like that in Figure 2, the specificity may be 95% or less depending on the cut point used to define a positive reaction. With 95% specificity, the predictive value of a positive reaction is poor at a prevalence below 25%. Even in areas likely to have 99% specificity, the test becomes poor when less than 5% of the tested population are likely to be infected.

To put these prevalences in perspective, about 90% of adults were infected at the turn of the century. At that time the tuberculin test had a very high positive predictive value. There continue to be a number of countries where the adult population has an infection rate of 25–50%, and many people from these countries immigrate to the United States. Close contacts to cases of active tuberculosis are also 25–50% likely to be infected. Tuberculin testing remains a useful test in such populations. The general adult population of the United States at this time has an infection rate of 5–10%, and the tuberculin test begins to have a decreasing positive predictive value when applied to this population, especially in areas where cross-reactions are common. Children entering school in many areas of the country have 0.1–1% likelihood of being infected. Even in areas with few cross-reactions, tuberculin testing has a poor positive predictive value in such populations. The yearly incidence of new tuberculosis infection in the general population without known exposure to tuberculosis is 0.01–0.1%. Yearly skin testing of such a population would obviously be foolish.

Based on the above considerations, the American Thoracic Society and Centers for Disease Control have recently recommended three cut points for defining a positive tuberculin reaction (American Thoracic Society, 1990).

A cut point ≥5 mm is suggested for populations with a high likelihood of being infected with *M. tuberculosis*. These populations include persons who have had close recent contact with infectious tuberculosis cases and persons who have chest radiographs consistent with old healed tuberculosis. In addition, a cut point of ≥5 mm is suggested for persons with HIV infection because of the suppressive effects of HIV on the tuberculin reaction.

A cut point of ≥10 mm is suggested for persons who are moderately likely to be infected with *M. tuberculosis*. These include foreign-born persons from high-prevalence countries in Asia, Africa, and Latin America, intravenous drug users, medically underserved, low-income populations, residents of long-term care facilities, and persons with medical conditions that increase the risk of tuberculosis, such as silicosis and diabetes mellitus. In addition, other high-prevalence populations may be identified in local areas.

Persons who are not likely to be infected with *M. tuberculosis* should generally not be skin-tested since the predictive value of a positive test in low-risk populations is poor. If a tuberculin skin test is performed on a person without a defined risk factor for tuberculosis infection, a cut point of ≥15 mm is suggested to improve the specificity of the test.

VI. Boosted Reactions and Serial Tuberculin Testing

Although skin testing with tuberculin will not induce a positive reaction on subsequent tests, small reactions due to waned hypersensitivity to *M. tuberculosis* or to cross-reactions to antigens from other mycobacteria can be boosted or enhanced. A larger reaction may occur on subsequent tuberculin tests given 1 week to 1 year after the initial test (Thompson et al., 1979). Boosting is particularly common in populations resembling the one shown in Figure 2 and is a significant cause of false conversion in serial skin-testing programs. Many of these false conversions can be eliminated by applying a second tuberculin test 1 week following a negative initial test to persons enrolled in serial skin-testing programs (Bass and Serio, 1981). Perhaps because of problems with continued cross-reactions, the specificity of the tuberculin test is less with serial skin testing than with a single test. Serial skin-testing programs, therefore, tend to overestimate the incidence of new tuberculosis infection in the population being tested (Bass et al., 1985; De March-Ayuela, 1990). Because of this, serial skin-testing programs should be targeted to populations who are at high risk for transmission of tuberculosis infection.

References

American Thoracic Society (1990). Diagnostic standards and classification of tuberculosis. *Am. Rev. Respir. Dis.* **142**(3):725–735.

Bass, J. B., Jr., and Serio, R. A. (1981). The use of repeat skin tests to eliminate the booster phenomenon in serial tuberculin testing. *Am. Rev. Respir. Dis.* **123**:394–396.

Bass, J. B., Sanders, R. V., and Kirkpatrick, M. B. (1985). Choosing an appropriate cutting point for conversion in annual tuberculin skin testing. *Am. Rev. Respir. Dis.* **132**:379–381.

Centers for Disease Control (1991). Purified protein derivative (PPD)-tuberculin anergy and HIV infection: guidelines for anergy testing and management of anergic persons at risk of tuberculosis. *MMWR* **40**:27–33.

Daniel, T. M., and Janicki, B. W. (1978). Mycobacterial antigens:a review of their isolation, chemistry, and immunological properties. *Microbiol. Rev.* **42**(1):84–113.

De March-Ayuela, P. (1990). Choosing an appropriate criteria for true or false conversion in serial tuberculin testing. *Am. Rev. Respir. Dis.* **141**:815–820.

Editorial (1890a). Koch and his critics. *JAMA* **15**:902.

Editorial (1890b). The nature of Dr. Koch's liquid. *Lancet* **2**:1233.

Edwards, P. Q., and Edwards, L. B. (1960). Story of the tuberculin test. *Am. Rev. Respir. Dis.* **81**:1–49.

Edwards, L. B., Acquaviva, F. A., Livesay, V. T., Cross, F. W., and Palmer, C. E. (1969). An atlas of sensitivity to tuberculin, PPD-B, and histoplasmin in the United States. *Am. Rev. Respir. Dis.* **99**:1–132.

Furcolow, M. L., Hewell, B., Nelson, W. E., and Palmer, C. E. (1941). Quantitative studies of the tuberculin reaction:I. Titration of tuberculin sensitivity and its relation to tuberculous infection. *Public Health Rep.* **56**:1082.

Green, H. H. (1951). Discussion on tuberculins in human and veterinary medicine. *Proc. Roy. Soc. Med.* **44**:1045.

Harboe, M. (1981). Antigens of PPD, old tuberculin, and autoclaved *Mycobacterium bovis* BCG studied by crossed immunoelectrophoresis. *Am. Rev. Respir. Dis.* **124**:80–87.

Holden, M., Dubin, M. R., and Diamond, P. H. (1971). Frequency of negative intermediate-strength tuberculin sensitivity in patients with active tuberculosis. *N. Engl. J. Med.* **285**:1506–1509.

Koch, R. (1890). Uber bacteriologische Forschung. *Deutsche Med. Wochnschr.* **16**:756 (translated in *Lancet* 1890; **2**:673).

Koch, R. (1891). Fortsetzung der Mittheilungen uber ein Heilmittel gegen Tuberculose. *Deutsche Med. Wochnschr.* **17**:101 (translated in *Lancet* 1891; **1**:168).

Landi, S., Held, H. R., Houschild, A. H. W., et al. (1966). Adsorption of tuberculin PPD to glass and plastic surfaces. *Bull. WHO* **35**:593–602.

Magnus, K., Guld, J., Waaler, H., et al. (1958). Stability of purified tuberculin in high dilution. *Bull. WHO* **19**:765–782.

Nash, D. R., and Douglass, J. E. (1980). A comparison between positive and negative reactors and an evaluation of 5 TU and 250 TU skin test doses. *Chest* **77**:32–37.

Palmer, C. E., and Bates, L. E. (1952). Tuberculin sensitivity of tuberculous patients. *Bull. WHO* **7**:171.

Sbarbaro, J. A. (1978). Skin test antigens: an evaluation whose time has come. *Am. Rev. Respir. Dis.* **118**:1–5.

Seibert, F. B. (1934). The isolation and properties of the purified protein derivative of tuberculin. *Am. Rev. Tuberc.* **30**:713.

Seibert, F. B., and Glenn, J. T. (1941). Tuberculin purified protein derivative: preparation and analyses of a large quantity for standard. *Am. Rev. Tuberc.* **44**:9.

Sokal, J. E. (1975). Measurement of delayed skin-test responses. *N. Engl. J. Med.* **293**:501–502.

Thompson, N. J., Glassroth, J. L., Snider, D. E., Jr., and Farer, L. S. (1979). The booster phenomenon in serial tuberculin testing. *Am. Rev. Respir. Dis.* **119**:587–597.

Zack, M. B., and Fulkerson, L. L. (1970). Clinical reliability of stabilized and nonstabilized tuberculin PPD. *Am. Rev. Respir. Dis.* **102**:91–93.

8

Diagnosis of Tuberculosis

JEFFREY GLASSROTH

Northwestern University Medical School
Chicago, Illinois

I. Introduction and Approach to Diagnosis

Diagnosis, with respect to *Mycobacterium tuberculosis*, may be viewed as having two general components: the diagnosis of tuberculous infection with or without concomitant disease and the diagnosis of disease due to the organism (i.e., tuberculosis). The diagnosis of tuberculous infection has traditionally been accomplished by means of tuberculin skin testing, a topic covered in Chapter 7. The diagnosis of tuberculosis, on the other hand, has used a variety of clinical and microbiological methods, which, until recently, had changed very little since the discovery of the tubercle bacillus over a century ago. Recent developments in the epidemiology of tuberculosis have tended to make diagnosing this disease even more challenging and urgent than it has previously been. Technological developments are creating new tools for meeting this challenge.

Tuberculosis is a disease of protean manifestations. In the United States, about 18–19% of new tuberculosis cases have extrapulmonary disease (Centers for Disease Control, 1991). Among tuberculosis patients who are coinfected by human immunodeficiency virus (HIV), about one-third will have extrapulmonary disease with or without a pulmonary component (Small et al., 1991). Thus, tuberculosis should be viewed as a systemic condition that can be expected to manifest itself increasingly outside the lung as HIV-infected persons constitute a growing proportion of new tuberculosis cases. Clinicians who are aware of this situation will maintain a high index of suspicion of tuberculosis when confronted by a wide variety of symptoms.

Most tuberculosis patients will be symptomatic. Although some signs and symptoms will help to localize the disease to a particular organ system (e.g., cough, localized lymphadenopathy, or localized bone pain), other patients will present with nonlocalizing, "constitutional" complaints or findings. Typically, the approach to diagnosis in all these patients will begin with a thorough history and physical examination and then proceed to a variety of "tests" as directed by the initial evaluation. These tests may be grouped into two categories, general or staging tests, which identify potential sites and extent of involvement, and specific or confirmatory studies, which identify tubercle bacilli as the cause of the disease process. The former tests are often rapidly performed but provide only circumstantial evidence about tuberculosis, whereas the latter, more definitive, studies may take substantially longer to complete.

II. Traditional Diagnostic Techniques

A. Indirect Tests

Tuberculin Skin Testing

As noted, skin testing is discussed in detail in Chapter 7; however, several issues concerning skin testing with respect to diagnosis of tuberculosis will be considered here. Since all patients with tuberculosis are, by definition, infected by *M. tuberculosis*, a test that can exclude or confirm the presence of such infection would be quite useful in the initial evaluation of many patients. If infection could be excluded, tuberculosis could likewise be eliminated as a diagnostic consideration. If infection were confirmed, the presence of tuberculous disease, while not also confirmed, would at least be possible and tuberculosis would have to be considered as the evaluation proceeded. Indeed, this is a way in which skin testing has been used for many years. Nonetheless, there are limitations to such an approach, particularly with respect to the negative predictive value of the skin test (i.e., its ability to exclude infection). Problems with unresponsiveness, anergy, have been appreciated for many years. Twenty percent or more of debilitated or malnourished patients with extensive disease will have falsely negative skin tests (Rooney et al., 1976). Skin test anergy may be particularly problematic in certain forms of tuberculosis, such as pleural disease with effusion, where suppressor adherent monocytes depress the ability of lymphocytes to respond to tuberculin with consequent anergy (Ellner et al., 1978). It is also well appreciated that HIV-coinfected tuberculosis patients are prone to the development of anergy and that such unresponsiveness becomes more frequent as the HIV infection progresses. Thus, whereas most HIV-coinfected tuberculosis patients have been noted to respond to tuberculin tests when their tuberculosis was diagnosed 2 or more years prior to their developing an AIDS-defining event, only about two-thirds had positive reactions when tuberculosis occurred less than 2 years prior to AIDS, and this declined to about one-third of patients whose tuberculosis was diagnosed simultaneously or subsequent to their AIDS-defining illness (Rieder et al., 1989). Clinicians must recognize these and other limitations. Although a positive skin test supports the possibility that the condition under evaluation could be tuberculosis, a negative test by no means excludes that possibility. Particular care must be taken when considering negative reactions in the context of certain forms of disease or with certain comorbidities.

Imaging Procedures

Chest Radiographs

Because the majority of tuberculosis patients will have a pulmonary component to their disease, chest X-ray films and, to a lesser degree, newer imaging procedures such as computed tomography of the chest (chest CT) have played an important role in differential diagnosis and determining extent of tuberculosis. Despite the fact that no chest radiographic pattern is unique to tuberculosis and that an abnormality does not prove the presence of active disease, certain configurations have traditionally been viewed as highly suggestive of tuberculosis. Thus, fibronodular changes involving the apical or posterior segments of the upper lobes and/or superior segments of the lower lobes have been viewed as "highly suggestive" of postprimary tuberculosis. The presence of cavitation would generally add support to that conclusion. The manifestations of primary tuberculosis in the chest (i.e., disease arising soon after initial infection) have been less specific and have included hilar and mediastinal adenopathy, pleural effusions, and infiltrates in the lower lung zones. In fact, these generalizations will not be helpful in a substantial proportion of patients. In the pre-HIV era, as many as one-third of newly diagnosed pulmonary tuberculosis patients were found to have "atypical" findings on chest radiograph, including the changes of primary tuberculosis, single or multiple pulmonary nodules (i.e., tuberculomas), and miliary disease (Khan et al., 1977). Other atypical patterns, such as adult respiratory distress syndrome (Huseby and Hudson, 1976), have also been reported, albeit more rarely. The occurrence of tuberculosis among HIV-coinfected persons has produced an even larger proportion of patients with unusual chest radiographic findings. Thus, in one study contrasting chest radiographic manifestations of tuberculosis in AIDS patients with a group of tuberculosis patients without AIDS, adenopathy was seen in 59% and 3%, lower lung filed infiltrates in 29% and 3% and diffuse infiltrates in 18% and none of the AIDS patients and non-AIDS patients, respectively. Cavitary disease was not present in any of the AIDS patients but was noted in over two-thirds of the non-AIDS group. One-third of the AIDS patients were noted to have no parenchymal infiltrates despite the identification of *M. tuberculosis* in respiratory secretions (Pitchenik and Robinson, 1985). Thus, thoughtful clinicians will maintain a broad view of how pulmonary tuberculosis may present on the chest X-ray film. Among HIV-coinfected persons, virtually any radiographic presentation may be encountered, including a "normal" film.

Computed Tomography

CT, using "rapid" scan times of 1–2 sec, provides an elegant means of assessing the lung parenchyma, mediastinum, and pleura. Although typically CT cannot provide more definitive diagnostic information than conventional chest radiography, there are situations in which it may be helpful. Because CT scans provide a cross-sectional view of the chest, overlying shadows (e.g., ribs) do not obscure the field of interest as they sometimes do on conventional films. Similarly, the greater sensitivity of CT for mediastinal abnormalities favors that technology when questions of disease in that anatomical region arise. Similarly CT, particularly when performed as high-resolution CT and reconstructed with a high-frequency resolution algorithm, appears to be a very sensitive technique for identifying parenchymal disease (Muller and Miller, 1990). Moreover, these high-resolution scans may provide information that can suggest specific diagnostic considerations. Thus, chest CT, either conventional or high resolution, may be useful for evaluating occasional patients with subtle or confusing clinical findings.

Other Imaging Techniques

With the increasing importance of extrapulmonary disease, a variety of additional imaging modalities, such as ultrasound and magnetic resonance imaging (MRI), are occasionally useful. Clearly, conventional radiographic procedures and CT can also be used. In general, results of such testing, while useful in identifying specific organ system involvement, rarely provide definitive diagnostic information. Rather, such results may help narrow the differential diagnosis and direct subsequent diagnostic procedures.

Fluid and Secretion Analysis

Tuberculosis, particularly extrapulmonary disease, frequently produces aberrations in normally present body fluids or causes effusions to form. Analysis of these fluids may be helpful in suggesting the diagnosis.

Hematological changes of a wide variety have been reported in association with TB. Though occasionally severe, these abnormalities are rarely diagnostic.

Thus, isolated cytopenias, mono- or lymphocytosis, and findings of intravascular coagulation have all been attributed to tuberculosis (Glasser et al., 1970; Maartens et al., 1990). Abnormalities of serum calcium have also been observed and attributed to enhanced vitamin D metabolism by activated monocytes/macrophages.

Because pulmonary tuberculosis is the most common form of the disease, sputum and other respiratory secretions are important diagnostic specimens in many patients. The yield of sputum typically correlates with the extent of pulmonary disease. When patients cannot spontaneously raise sputum, induction with inhaled saline mist can produce diagnostic specimens in up to two-thirds of patients. Lavage of gastric secretions to retrieve swallowed tubercle bacilli can provide a diagnosis in up to one-third of patients. However, in patients who are unable to produce a specimen, bronchoscopy with lavage can be a highly effective procedure for obtaining diagnostic material (Jett et al., 1981).

Pleural, peritoneal, cerebrospinal, and joint fluid abnormalities associated with tuberculosis share several characteristics. Protein is usually elevated and the glucose reduced, although a wide range of values, including normal ones, have been observed. A leukocytosis of varying degree is common. Polymorphonuclear cells predominate early in all these fluids and remain the predominant cell in joint effusions. In the other sites, lymphocytes generally come to predominate over the first several days of involvement. Mesothelial cells, common in most pleural fluid specimens, are said to account for less than 2% of the cells in tuberculous effusions (Light et al., 1973). Eosinophilia is, likewise, uncommon (Adelman et al., 1984).

Tuberculosis involving the genitourinary (GU) tract produces a sterile (on "conventional" bacterial culture) pyuria, often with microscopic hematuria and a reduced pH. These findings, particularly sterile pyuria, should always prompt consideration of tuberculosis. It should be noted that a substantial proportion of patients with pulmonary tuberculosis and no signs or symptoms of GU disease, including a normal urine sediment, will have positive urine cultures for *M. tuberculosis*, presumably because the organism is cleared through the kidney. With disseminated forms of tuberculosis and in the setting of HIV coinfection, as many as 20% of patients will have positive urine cultures (Bentz et al., 1975; Chaisson et al., 1987). Thus, urine may be a very useful specimen for culture purposes even in the absence of abnormalities of the sediment.

Therapeutic Trial

A patient whose clinical picture is consistent with tuberculosis should not be denied appropriate therapy simply because the diagnostic data to confirm tuberculosis are lacking. When the managing clinician believes *M. tuberculosis* is the cause of a clinical problem, appropriate therapy should be started. The response to that therapy may, in some cases, be the most important factor supporting a final diagnosis of tuberculosis and should not be ignored.

B. Confirmatory Tests (Direct Tests)

Stains for Acid-Fast Bacilli

Acid-fast bacilli (AFB) stains are not truly confirmatory of tuberculosis in that other species of mycobacteria as well as unrelated organisms, such as the weakly acid-fast *Nocardia*, may produce a "positive" stain. However, in the appropriate clinical context, such a result substantially narrows the differential diagnosis and allows the clinician to focus on a rather circumscribed set of options. A great deal has been written about "falsely positive" AFB smears (Boyd and Marr, 1975; Strumpf et al., 1979). In general, this problem reflects the prevalence of *M. tuberculosis* in a population to be tested. The relationship between the rate of false-positive test results, the prevalence of the condition being tested for, and the intrinsic characteristics of the test used are described by Baye's theorem (Daniel and DeBanne, 1987). In essence, this analysis indicates that as the prevalence of the condition and the ability of the test to exclude the condition when it is not present (i.e., test specificity) decline, the proportion of falsely positive results increases. With respect to a test such as the AFB stain, it is essential that clinicians screen patients carefully and submit specimens for AFB staining only when there is a reasonable likelihood that tuberculosis is present. This type of screening will serve to increase the prevalence of tuberculosis in the population being tested and thereby reduce the rate of false-positive tests. Patients with tuberculosis and "true positive" sputum AFB smears have clinical and radiographic evidence of disease, whereas "false positive" sputum AFB results are typically obtained from persons who were tested despite few or no clinical findings to suggest tuberculosis (Boyd and Marr, 1975). Nontuberculous mycobacteria are legitimately acid fast and, therefore, positive AFB stains for these organisms are "true positives." The clinical significance and management implications of their possible presence must also be considered when a specimen stains positive for AFB.

Several techniques have been used to stain for AFB. These include fluorochrome (e.g., auramine/rhodamine) and traditional (e.g., Ziehl-Neelsen) techniques. All staining techniques share the advantages of being relatively rapid and inexpensive to perform. The fluorochrome stains require somewhat more sophistication on the part of the laboratory and a fluorescence microscope but allow the microscopist to quickly screen slides for the presence of AFB. All fluorochrome-positive specimens should be confirmed by traditional techniques. One additional advantage of the AFB sputum smear is its close correlation with infectiousness; persons who are sputum smear positive/culture positive are far more likely to be infectious than persons who are culture positive but smear negative (Narain et al., 1971). Despite their advantages, AFB staining is limited. Sensitivity of staining is at least a log order of magnitude less than that of culture. Thus, it has been estimated that for stains to reliably identify AFB, at least 10^4 AFB must be present per milliliter of specimen. Stains do not speciate organisms and are, therefore, less specific than other technologies. Finally, AFB stains do not distinguish between dead and live mycobacteria. This is a particular limitation when evaluating patients who are receiving antimycobacterial therapy.

Biopsy Procedures

A variety of biopsy specimens are potentially available depending on the anatomical involvement of the tuberculous process. The need for invasively obtained specimens is inversely related to the ease of obtaining specimens through less aggressive means. Thus, pulmonary and genitourinary tuberculosis, situations in which tubercle bacilli are frequently shed into easily sampled body fluids, generally do not require biopsy for diagnosis. Isolated involvement of the pleura or other tissues that do not communicate externally may best be diagnosed through examination of tissue. It should be noted, however, that the finding of histologically compatible tissue changes, most notably granuloma formation within the specimens, does not conclusively prove a diagnosis of tuberculosis. Other conditions, including those caused by nontuberculous mycobacteria and fungi as well as inflammatory diseases such as sarcoidosis, may produce similar tissue changes. In some immunocompromised patients, such as those with advanced HIV infection, minimal tissue reaction may occur despite extensive disease.

In the setting of disseminated or miliary disease, multiple organs may be seeded with tubercle bacilli. Although organs such as the lung and kidney are frequently involved in such a setting, sputum and urine specimens are found to contain tubercle bacilli in perhaps only 20–25% of such patients. Tissue examination may be very helpful in such situations. Transbronchial biopsy has been reported to be diagnostic or highly suggestive of tuberculosis in up to 85% of patients with miliary changes on chest X-ray film and negative sputum studies (Burk et al., 1978). The yield of liver and bone marrow biopsy has also been evaluated in the setting of miliary tuberculosis. Both these sites provide important diagnostic opportunities and may yield information suggesting tuberculosis in 40–90% of patients. Thus, in a review of 36 patients with miliary tuberculosis, liver biopsy showed granulomas in 91% of patients, with 52% having caseation; 40% were culture positive. In contrast, only 50% of bone marrow biopsies showed granulomas (most noncaseating) and only 25% were culture positive (Cucin et al., 1973).

Percutaneous biopsy of pleura, peritoneum, and synovium can also be pursued in the appropriate setting. The yield of granulomata in these tissues has typically ranged from 40 to 80%. Culture of these specimens and associated fluids can increase this yield. New technology has facilitated the performance of such procedures under direct vision and is likely to maximize the diagnostic yield from these tissues. Finally, open biopsy may be useful when more limited procedures are inadequate or when technical considerations make such an approach safer, as with pericardial tuberculosis.

Conventional Culture Techniques

Culture remains the "gold standard" for diagnosis of tuberculosis. Culture is more sensitive than AFB staining and can reliably find mycobacteria when they are present in a concentration of about 10^3 organisms/ml of specimen. Growing cultures also permit speciation and drug susceptibility testing. The major drawbacks of conventional culture techniques are that they are slow, requiring weeks before a positive culture for *M. tuberculosis* can be identified, and they require at least a moderately well-equipped laboratory. Virtually any specimen can be considered for culture. In recent years even blood cultures, using lysis centrifugation systems, have been useful, particularly with disseminated disease.

The conventional culture process usually involves the use of an egg-potato-base (e.g., Lowenstein-Jensen) and/or an agar-base (e.g., Middlebrook 7H-11) medium. Specimens that are not sterile (e.g., sputum) and/or combined with other cellular material or debris must first be subjected to a digestion and decontamination process. When properly done, this process prevents the overgrowth of more rapidly growing bacteria and also concentrates of the mycobacteria within the specimen. If this step is too vigorous, however, *M. tuberculosis* in the specimen may also be killed. Proper quality control in the laboratory includes the monitoring of the contamination rate of mycobacterial cultures. A rate of about 1% suggests that the decontamination procedures are appropriate. The rate of growth, physical characteristics, and results of a series of standard biochemical tests permit the speciation of the growing mycobacterial culture.

III. New or Experimental Technologies

A variety of new methods and technologies have been applied in recent years to the diagnosis of tuberculosis. The impetus for their application has generally been a desire to make a more rapid diagnosis. However, the potential for more sensitive tests as well as for tests that can be adapted for use with minimal equipment under so-called "field conditions" also seems to exist. As with more traditional techniques, experimental and emerging technologies may be viewed as those which indirectly identify tuberculosis and those which identify tubercle bacilli directly.

A. New Indirect Techniques

Serological Testing

Serodiagnosis of tuberculosis is not really new. However, technological developments, particularly the enzyme-linked immunosorbent assay (ELISA) and the development of more purified antigens has renewed interest in this diagnostic approach. Many studies of the sensitivity and specificity of serological diagnosis of tuberculosis have been published. An elegant review by Daniel and DeBanne (1987) summarizes many of these. The reported sensitivity of these assays ranges from about 60 to 80%. In general, higher sensitivities have been reported by studies of populations from less well-developed countries endemic for tuberculosis. It has been assumed that disease is more chronic in these populations and results in higher levels of serum antibody. Reported specificities have also varied widely, probably reflecting the many different mycobacterial antigens used as well as the types of control populations studied. Crude antigen preparations have resulted in specificities of up to 1.00. A provocative study by Zeiss and colleagues (Zeiss et al., 1984) combined ELISA results with the results of first fluorochrome sputum stain and attained a sensitivity of 86%. When both tests were negative, there was a 97% predictive value that tuberculosis was not present. It should be noted that while most studies have applied serodiagnosis to the diagnosis of pulmonary tuberculosis, its application to extrapulmonary disease has also been promising. Preliminary studies among AIDS patients have suggested that the serological response in HIV/TB-coinfected persons is complex, with an initial high antibody titer following infection with *M. tuberculosis* followed by declining titers as tuberculosis progresses. This raises the possibility that serodiagnosis in that setting might be most useful as an adjunct to identifying tuberculous infection.

At the present time, it appears that serological testing for tuberculosis is technically possible but most likely to be positive among patient populations with advanced disease, a setting where conventional tests (e.g., AFB stain) are also quite sensitive. The currently attained serodiagnostic test specificities suggest that a substantial proportion of positive tests will be falsely positive among low-prevalence populations. Further study is needed to see whether serological testing can be enhanced by use of more purified antigens or adapted in such a way as to make testing possible with minimal training or equipment. Finally, assessment of the utility of serodiagnosis as an adjunct for the diagnosis of extrapulmonary tuberculosis or for the evaluation of special populations, such as HIV-infected persons, seems warranted.

Adenosine Deaminase

Adenosine deaminase (ADA), a purine-degrading enzyme, is necessary for the maturation and differentiation of a variety of cells, including monocytes, macrophages, and, most particularly, T lymphocytes. High serum levels of this enzyme have been reported in a number of disease states. With respect to tuberculosis, several laboratories have reported that ADA concentrations in pleural, pericardial, and cerebrospinal fluid (CSF) may be elevated when tuberculosis involves those sites. In general, ADA levels have not correlated well with serum ADA levels or fluid cell counts in these studies. Thus, Martinez-Vazquez and colleagues reported 66 patients with ascites due to various etiologies, including tuberculosis, septic peritonitis, malignancy, and trasudative conditions. The 10 tuberculosis patients had peritoneal ADA concentrations that did not overlap with any of the other groups; ADA concentration was also more useful that absolute lymphocyte count or lymphocyte proportion (Martinez-Vazquez et al., 1986). Pettersson and co-workers studied pleural fluid specimens resulting from a variety of disease states. Although ADA levels tended to be elevated in the 14 specimens from tuberculous patients, there was considerable overlap with levels obtained in the nontuberculous patients (Pettersson et al., 1984). These same investigators also found elevated ADA concentrations in CSF specimens from 32 patients with tuberculosis. There was minimal overlap between those levels and those found in the CSF of 213 patients without tuberculosis. Moreover, the sensitivity and specificity of ADA concentration met or exceeded the sensitivity and specificity of conventional diagnostic tests such as tuberculin skin test, CSF glucose content, and culture (Ribera et al., 1987).

The ultimate role of ADA for the diagnosis of tuberculosis awaits further clarification. Additional studies will provide more patients and, particularly, a wider array of control and allow a better definition of the sensitivity and specificity of this test.

Lysozyme

This bacteriolytic protein, also known as muramidase, is normally found in serum, activated macrophages and monocytes, and granulocytes. Pleural tuberculosis has been reported to cause elevations in the absolute concentration of this enzyme and increases in the ratio of pleural fluid to serum lysozyme. The reported accuracy and predictive value of this test have been impressive, and it has been used to enhance the predictive accuracy of ADA (Bueso et al., 1988). However, experience with this test is limited, and it should be regarded as experimental at the present time.

B. Direct Tests

Because conventional tests are relatively slow, there has been great interest in developing techniques that could identify tubercle bacilli more rapidly. To be useful, such tests should be at least as sensitive and specific as existing techniques.

Table 1   Microbiological Identification of *M. tuberculosis*

Test	Sensitivity	Species specificity	Time for performance
AFB smear	Low	No	Hours
Conventional culture	Moderate	Yes	Weeks
Radiometric culture	Moderate	Yes	Days to weeks
HPLC	Low to moderate	Yes	Weeks[a]
DNA probe	Moderate to high	Yes	Weeks[a]
RNA probe	Moderate to high	Yes	Weeks[a]
PCR + DNA probe	High	Yes	Days

[a]Currently require growing culture although test itself requires hours to perform.

Ideally, these new procedures would not be excessively expensive to perform and could be used in the "field" or in laboratories not dedicated to mycobacteria. As shown in Table 1, there are promising developments in this area.

Radiometric Assays

Radiometric systems, of which BACTEC (Becton Dickinson, Towson, MD) is perhaps the most widely available, have been used for almost 20 years for the detection of mycobacteria (Middlebrook et al., 1977). The principle behind such systems involves the incorporation of a radiolabeled substrate, typically ^{14}C-palmitic acid, by the growing mycobacterial inoculum with the consequent release of $^{14}CO_2$. It is the detection of this gas that allows the early detection of mycobacterial growth prior to the presence of visible growth. Such systems can indicate the presence of mycobacteria weeks before conventional culture systems. Moreover, by application of the NAP (*p*-nitro-alpha-acetylamino-beta-hydroxypropiophenone) growth inhibition test, *M. tuberculosis* can be distinguished from nontuberculous mycobacteria (NTM). This test relies on the ability of NAP, a chloramphenicol intermediate, to inhibit the growth of *M. tuberculosis* but not the NTM. The test can be accomplished in several days. Using such a system, it is possible to identify the presence of growing mycobacteria in 1 week or less and to identify the mycobacteria as *M. tuberculosis* or other species (i.e., NTM) in several additional days. The speed of identification in this system, as in conventional systems, is dependent on the concentration of the initial inoculum. Thus, the average time required to classify 88 mycobacterial cultures in one report was 6.4 days, with a range from 3 to 12 days (Siddiqui et al., 1984). Smear-positive (i.e., high-concentration) specimens may be expected to be identified most rapidly. Drug susceptibility tests can also be adapted to such a system with additional savings in time (Siddiqui et al., 1981). Because of their cost, technical sophistication, and use of radioisotopes, such systems are most appropriate for large clinical microbiology laboratories. However, since these systems can be used for the rapid identification of other bacteria, their utility in the laboratory is enhanced. Modification of the measured end-points to nonradioactive indicators should further enhance the attractiveness of the rapid culture systems.

Nucleic Acid Probes

It is now possible to identify chromosomal DNA or ribosomal RNA from my-cobacteria growing in culture. These tests involve the use of complementary DNA (cDNA) or RNA (cRNA) probes that are highly specific for nucleic acid within certain species of mycobacteria. If the appropriate nucleic acid sequences are present in sufficient amounts within the specimen being probed, the cDNA or cRNA will hybridize with them, producing a radioisotopic or other signal, depending on the system in use. The major advantage of such probes is their high degree of specificity. However, the probes require that nucleic acid be present in relatively high concentration in the tested specimen and that mycobacteria be lysed to provide the probe access to the free nucleic acid. Because ribosomal RNA is present in concentrations that are at least several logs greater than is DNA, the most commonly used probes have been directed at ribosomal RNA, thus maximizing the sensitivity of the test system. Nonetheless, to obtain adequate mycobacterial nucleic acid, perhaps 10^5 to 10^6 bacilli must be present, and application has generally been limited to the probing of growing cultures. Thus, although the probing itself can be performed in several hours, the culture process requires days or weeks. Nucleic acid probes are quite sensitive within the limits of the procedure and they are exquisitely specific (Drake et al., 1987). Their widest use to date has been to expedite the identification of growing cultures of *M. tuberculosis*, *M. avium*, and *M. intracellulare*. Using these probes with radiometric culture systems can provide further time savings, as demonstrated by Ellner and colleagues, who used a cDNA probe of BACTEC grown cultures to identify 66% of *M. tuberculosis* cultures within 2 weeks (Ellner et al., 1988). Application of other new technology is permitting the use of these elegant procedures with native specimens.

Polymerase Chain Reaction plus Nucleic Acid Probes

This technology has been widely applied to other bacteria and other viruses and is now being used with mycobacteria. Polymerase chain reaction (PCR) requires first that DNA from the test specimen be exposed and dissociated. Highly specific nucleic acid probes known as "primers" are then used to attach to a segment of the targeted mycobacterial DNA. Because the primer attaches only to complementary DNA sequences, this attachment process is highly specific. By selecting sequences common only to a particular species of mycobacteria (e.g., *M. tuberculosis*), attachment will occur only in the presence of that species. In the presence of DNA polymerases and other substrates and at the proper temperature, two copies of double-stranded DNA segments identified by the primers will be formed. By repeating the process over a number of cycles, the amount of genetic material present in the original specimen is copied or "amplified." A variety of detection systems can then be used to identify this material. In essence, PCR can amplify the specimen and raise it to the sensitivity of the detection system being used. PCR is now being applied to specimens such as sputum with dramatic results. In a recent report of 162 sputum specimen assays, 51 were culture positive for *M. tuberculosis* and all 51 were PCR positive. An additional 42 specimens were positive for nontuberculous mycobacteria and only one produced a positive PCR result. Tests were completed within 48 hr (Eisenach et al., 1991). It is estimated that PCR can detect mycobacteria in suspensions of as few as 10–100 cells, making this technology at least as sensitive as culture. Although PCR, or a variant of the technology known as ligase chain reaction (LCR), could be used in many clinical microbiology laboratories, experience in its application to mycobacteria is still limited.

Chromatography

Mycobacteria contain large amounts of lipid material within their cell wall. The detection of certain forms of lipid by means of various chromatographic techniques has received considerable interest as an investigational approach to diagnosis of tuberculosis.

Gas-liquid chromatography (GLC) coupled with a mass spectrometer has been used to detect minute amounts of indolic-type compounds in CSF from patients with tuberculous meningitis, thereby distinguishing them from patients with other forms of lymphocytic meningeal disease (Craven et al., 1977). More recently, GLC has been directed at the detection of tuberculostearic acid, a fatty acid present in virtually all species of mycobacteria. The detection of this material in CSF and serum has been proposed as a relatively rapid and highly sensitive method for the diagnosis of tuberculous meningitis (Brooks et al., 1987). High-performance liquid chromatography (HPLC) and GLC are rapid and can be performed in a matter of hours. Although they appear to be highly sensitive and, indeed, GLC may be the most sensitive technique for detecting tuberculosis in such sites as the meninges, there are drawbacks to their general use. The equipment required for their application is costly and sophisticated. HPLC currently requires the presence of around 10^7 to 10^8 tubercle bacilli, so growing cultures several weeks in age must be available for its use. In addition, because tuberculostearic acid is present in other mycobacteria, detection of this material would be of limited usefulness for tuberculosis diagnosis in areas where nontuberculous mycobacteria are common.

Detection of Mycobacterial Antigens

Systems using antibody raised against *M. tuberculosis* or BCG have been used to detect tubercle bacilli. These test systems have been applied directly to clinical specimens and have also been used in conjunction with culture systems as a means of accelerating identification of the organism (Raja et al., 1988). When applied to CSF or sputum specimens, these assays have typically had sensitivities of about 50% and specificities of only about 90% (Kardival et al., 1986; Yanez et al., 1986). Nonetheless, the potential of such assays for automation, as well as the possibility that definition of more well-defined epitopes could render these tests more specific, makes antigen assays attractive candidates for additional study.

DNA Fingerprinting

Although not a diagnostic test, DNA fingerprinting using restriction endonuclease fragment analysis is becoming an important epidemiological tool. This technique involves fragmenting mycobacterial DNA with highly specific enzyme endonucleases. This results in a series of fragments which, together, constitute the DNA "fingerprint" of the strain under study. Fragments or fingerprints from one specimen can be compared to others (Cave et al., 1991). This technique, also known as restriction fragment length polymorphism (RFLP), has been applied to other bacteria and is now being used in the study of tuberculosis outbreaks.

IV. Summary

Ultimately, the diagnosis of tuberculosis begins by suspecting the disease. Given the protean manifestations of the disease, particularly in the immunocompromised host, the clinician's threshold for such suspicion should be low. Based on the potential sites of involvement, a diagnostic plan can be developed. Usually this involves selecting several "indirect" tests that can provide supporting or circumstantial evidence of tuberculosis and also help to define the extent of disease. Definitive diagnosis is then pursued by the application of direct tests for the tubercle bacillus. With rapid technological development, the armamentarium of diagnostic tests for this disease is greater than ever before, providing new opportunities for sensitive and rapid diagnosis of tuberculosis.

References

Adelman, M., Albelda, S. M., Gottlieb, J., and Haponic, E. F. (1984). Diagnostic utility of pleural fluid eosinophilia. *Am. J. Med.* **77**:915–920.

Bentz, R. R., Dimcheff, D. G., Nemiroff, M. J., Tsang, A., and Weg, J. G. (1975). The incidence of urine cultures positive for *Mycobacterium tuberculosis* in a general patient population. *Am. Rev. Respir. Dis.* **111**:647–650.

Boyd, J. C., and Marr, J. J. (1975). Decreasing reliability of acid-fast smear techniques for detection of tuberculosis. *Ann. Intern. Med.* **92**:489–492.

Brooks, J. B., Daneshvar, M. I., Fast, D. M., and Good, R. C. (1987). Selective procedures for detecting femtomole quantities of tuberculostearic acid in serum and cerebrospinal fluid by frequency-pulsed electron capture gas-liquid chromatography. *J. Clin. Microbiol.* **25**:1201–1206.

Bueso, J. F., Hernando, H. V., Garcia-Buela, J. P., et al. (1988). The diagnostic value of simultaneous determination of pleural adenosine deaminase and pleural lysozyme/serum lysozyme ratio in pleura effusions. *Chest* **93**:303–311.

Burk, J. R., Viroslav, J., and Bynum, L. J. (1978). Miliary tuberculosis diagnosed by fiberoptic bronchoscopy and transbronchial biopsy. *Tubercle* **59**:107–109.

Cave, M. D., Eisenach, K. D., McDermott, P. F., et al. (1991). Conservation of sequence in the *Mycobacterium tuberculosis* complex and its utilization in DNA fingerprinting. *Mol. Cell Probes* **5**:73–80.

Centers for Disease Control (1991). *1989 Tuberculosis Statistics in the United States*. U.S. Department of Health and Human Services, HHS Pub. No (CDC)91-8322, Atlanta, pp. 6–7.

Chaisson, R. E., Schecter, G. F., Theur, C. P., Rutherford, G. W., Echenberg, D. F., and Hopewell, P. C. (1987). Tuberculosis in patients with the acquired immunodeficiency syndrome: clinical features, response to therapy, and survival. *Am. Rev. Respir. Dis.* **136**:570–574.

Craven, R. B., Brooks, J. B., Edman, D. C., Converse, J. D., Greenlee, J., et al. (1977). Rapid diagnosis of lymphocytic meningitis by frequency-pulsed electron capture gas-liquid chromatography: differentiation of tuberculous, cryptococcal, and viral meningitis. *J. Clin. Invest.* **6**:27–32.

Cucin, R. L., Coleman, M., Eckardt, J. J., and Silver, R. T. (1973). The diagnosis of miliary tuberculosis: utility of peripheral blood abnormalities, bone marrow and liver needle biopsy. *J. Chronic Dis.* **22**:355–361.

Daniel, T. M., and DeBanne, S. M. (1987). The serodiagnosis of tuberculosis and other mycobacterial diseases by enzyme-linked immunosorbent assay. *Am. Rev. Respir. Dis.* **135**:1137–1151.

Drake, T. A., Hindler, J. A., Berlin, O. G. W., and Bruckner, D. A. (1987). Rapid identification of *Mycobacterium avium* complex in culture using DNA probes. *J. Clin. Microbiol.* **25**:1442–1445.

Eisenach, K. D., Sifford, M. D., Cave, M. D., Bates, J. H., and Crawford, J. T. (1991). Detection of *Mycobacterium tuberculosis* in sputum samples using a polymerase chain reaction. *Am. Rev. Respir. Dis.* **144**:1160–1163.

Ellner, J. J. (1978). Pleural fluid and peripheral blood lymphocyte function in tuberculosis. *Ann. Intern. Med.* **89**:932–933.

Ellner, P. D., Kiehn, T. E., Cammarata, R., and Hosmer, M. (1988). Rapid detection of pathogenic mycobacteria by combining radiometric and nucleic acid probe methods. *J. Clin. Microbiol.* **26**:1349–1352.

Glasser, R. M., Walker, R. I., and Herion, J. C. (1970). The significance of the blood in patients with tuberculosis. *Arch. Intern. Med.* **125**:691–695.

Huseby, J. S., and Hudson, L. D. (1976). Miliary tuberculosis and adult respiratory distress syndrome. *Ann. Intern. Med.* **85**:609–611.

Jett, J. R., Cortese, D. A., and Dines, D. E. (1981). The value of bronchoscopy in the diagnosis of mycobacterial disease. A five-year experience. *Chest* **80**:575-578.

Kardival, G. V., Mazarelo, T. B. M. S., and Chaparas, S. D. (1986). Sensitivity and specificity of enzyme-linked immunosorbent assay in the detection of antigen in tuberculous meningitis cerebrospinal fluids. *J. Clin. Microbiol.* **23**:901–904.

Khan, M. A., Kovnat, D. M., Bachus, B., et al. (1977). Clinical and roentgenographic spectrum of pulmonary tuberculosis in adults. *Am. J. Med.* **62**:31–38.

Light, R. W., Erozan, Y. S., and Ball, W. C. (1973). Cells in pleural fluid: their value in differential diagnosis. *Arch. Intern. Med.* **132**:854–860.

Maartens, G., Wilcox, P. A., and Benatar, S. R. (1990). Miliary tuberculosis: rapid diagnosis, hematologic abnormalities and outcome in 109 treated adults. *Am. J. Med.* **89**:291–296.

Martinez-Vazquez, J. M., Ocana, I., Ribera, I., Segura, R. M., and Pascual, C. (1986). Adenosine deaminase activity in the diagnosis of tuberculous peritonitis. *Gut* **27**:1049–1053.

Middlebrook, G., Reggiardo, Z., and Tigert, W. D. (1977). Automatable radiometric detection of growth of *Mycobacterium tuberculosis* in selective media. *Am. Rev. Respir. Dis.* **115**:1066–1069.

Muller, N. L., and Miller, R. R. (1990). Computed tomography of chronic diffuse infiltrative lung disease. *Am. Rev. Respir. Dis.* **142**:1206–1215.

Narain, R., Rao, M. S., Chandrasekhar, P., et al. (1971). Microscopy positive and microscopy negative cases of pulmonary tuberculosis. *Am. Rev. Respir. Dis.* **103**:761–773.

Pettersson, T., Ojala, K., and Weber, T. H. (1984). Adenosine deaminase in the diagnosis of pleural effusions (1984). *Acta Med. Scand.* **215**:299–304.

Pitchenik, A. E., and Robinson, H. A. (1985). The radiographic appearance of tuberculosis in patients with the acquired immunodeficiency syndrome (AIDS) and preAIDS. *Am. Rev. Respir. Dis.* **131**:393–396.

Raja. A., Machicao, A. R., Morrissey, A. B., et al. (1988). Specific detection of *Mycobacterium tuberculosis* in radiometric cultures by using an immunoassay for antigen 5. *J. Infect. Dis.* **158**:468–470.

Ribera, E., Martinez-Vazquez, J. M., Ocana, I., Seguar, R. M., and Pascular, C. (1987). Activity of adenosine deaminase in cerebrospinal fluid for the diagnosis and follow-up of tuberculous meningitis in adults. *J. Infect. Dis.* **155**:603–607.

Rieder, H. L., Cauther, G. M., Block, A. B., et al. (1989). Tuberculosis and acquired immunodeficiency syndrome—Florida. *Arch. Intern. Med.* **149**:1268–1273.

Rooney, J. J., Crocco, J. A., Kramer, S., et al. (1976). Further observations on tuberculin reactions in active tuberculosis. *Am. J. Med.* **60**:517–522.

Siddiqui, S. H., Libonati, J. P., and Middlebrook, G. (1981). Evaluation of a rapid radiometric method for drug susceptibility testing of *Mycobacterium tuberculosis. J. Clin. Microbiol.* **13**:908–912.

Siddiqui, S. H., Hwangbo, C. C., Silcox, V., Good, R. C., Snider, D. E., Jr., and Middlebrook, G. (1984). Rapid radiometric methods to detect and differentiate *Mycobacterium tuberculosis/bovis* from other mycobacterial species. *Am. Rev. Respir. Dis.* **130**:634–640.

Small, P. M., Schecter, G. F., Goodman, P. C., Sande, M. A., Chaisson, R. E., and Hopewell, P. C. (1991). Treatment of tuberculosis in patients with advanced human immunodeficiency virus infection. *N. Engl. J. Med.* **324**:289–294.

Strumpf, I. J., Tsang, A. Y., and Sayre, J. W. (1979). Re-evaluation of sputum staining for the diagnosis of pulmonary tuberculosis. *Am. Rev. Respir. Dis.* **119**:599–602.

Yanez, M. A., Coppola, M. P., Russo, D. A., et al. (1986). Determination of mycobacterial antigens in sputum by enzyme immunoassay. *J. Clin. Microbiol.* **23**:822–825.

Zeiss, C. R., Kalish, S. B., Erlich, K. S., Levitz, D., Metzger, E., Radin, R., and Phair, J. P. (1984). IgG antibody to purified protein derivative by enzyme-linked immunosorbent assay in the diagnosis of pulmonary tuberculosis. *Am. Rev. Respir. Dis.* **130**:845–848.

9

Case Finding

HANS L. RIEDER

Federal Office of Public Health
Liebefeld-Berne, Switzerland

I. Introduction

In order to ultimately reduce the incidence of tuberculosis in a community, the primary epidemiological aim of tuberculosis control is to reduce the pool of persons with tuberculous infection. Without intervention, future cases of tuberculosis will emerge from this pool.

Principally, there are two supplementary lines of action to accomplish this objective. The first is the use of appropriate chemotherapy to interrupt transmission from newly occurring infectious cases of tuberculosis as rapidly as possible after their occurrence. What stands between onset of transmissibility and its arrest is the delay of the patient to seek medical attention and the delay of health care providers to make the diagnosis and to commence appropriate chemotherapy. (Fig. 1). This delay is variably attributable to patients' attitudes toward symptoms and health care providers' ability to rapidly diagnose tuberculosis. The second line of action is the prevention of tuberculosis cases before they occur with preventive therapy of infected persons (Fig. 1). The first line of action will reduce the incidence of infection and the second will reduce the incidence of disease.

The term ''case finding'' in its narrowest use refers to all activities that aim at reducing the interval between the onset of clinically and/or bacteriologically

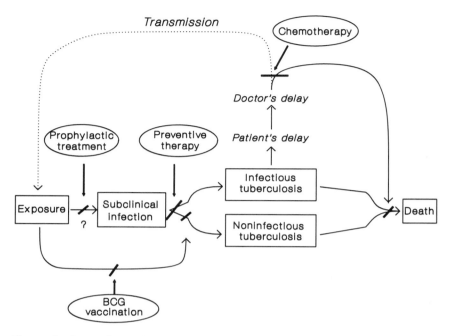

Figure 1 Prevention and chemotherapy of tuberculosis.

active tuberculosis and the arrest of transmission. Patient's and doctor's delay are the two major factors that determine the length of uncontrolled transmission of tubercle bacilli in the community and thus the incidence of infection.

In its wider sense "case finding" may also be understood as the identification of population segments infected with tubercle bacilli, who are at high risk of developing tuberculosis and who may benefit from preventive intervention. Such preventive treatment will reduce the incidence of disease.

The emphasis here will be placed on case-finding activities in the narrower sense, because it is apparent that failure to prevent uncontrolled transmission from infectious sources has much larger implications on the epidemiological situation than failure to identify subclinically infected persons (Sutherland, 1981).

II. Sources of Transmission and Other Cases

It has been recognized for some time and documented in several large studies (Shaw and Wynn-Williams, 1954; Meijer et al., 1971) that the major sources of infection in the community are patients with tuberculosis of the respiratory tract who are excreting such large numbers of tubercle bacilli that they can be seen by direct microscopic examination of their sputum. Patients with sputum smear-negative culture-only positive tuberculosis are far less efficient transmitters. Epidemiologically, the rapid discovery of infectious cases is of higher priority than that of other cases. However, through reduction of unnecessary morbidity and fatality, the identification of the latter group also carries individual and public health benefits.

III. Identification of Sources of Transmission

A. Active Case-Finding Methods

The term "active case finding" is used here to describe methods for the identification of tuberculosis cases, where the first initiative for an individual patient/provider contact is taken by health care providers.

Mass Radiography

Hypothetically, periodic radiographic screening of the entire population could help in identifying tuberculosis patients at a point when their disease has not yet progressed to high infectiousness. Mass radiography campaigns became an important component of tuberculosis control activities in the 1940s and 1950s in the United States (United States Public Health Service, 1958) and many other industrialized countries (Meijer et al., 1971; Horwitz and Darrow, 1976; Toman, 1976).

In a series of studies conducted between 1960 and 1973 (Meijer et al., 1971; Křivinka et al., 1974; Toman, 1976), it was shown that in places with active case-finding programs between 54 and 66% of sputum smear-positive patients were discovered because of their symptoms. Only some 20% of new cases were found through indiscriminate mass radiography alone (Meijer et al., 1971). This is explained by the relative rapidity with which infectious cases develop, faster than repeat screening can logistically be accomplished and economically be justified (Styblo et al., 1967). Because of the relatively low yield of cases through indiscriminate mass radiography, the method has generally become recognized as an inefficient tool in tuberculosis control (Meijer et al., 1971; Křivinka et al., 1974; World Health Organization, 1974; Toman, 1976; Styblo and Meijer, 1980; United States Public Health Service, 1983; American Thoracic Society/Centers for Disease Control, 1983; Snider et al., 1984).

Involvement of Community Leaders

In three studies jointly conducted by the Respiratory Diseases Research Centre, Nairobi, and the British Medical Research Council, approaches to improve case finding by involving community leaders have been evaluated in Kenya (Nsanzumuhire et al., 1977, 1981; Aluoch et al., 1978).

In the first study, the efficiency of case finding by community leaders was investigated in a district in Kenya (Nsanzumuhire et al., 1977) describing a house-to-house investigation and random sampling methods. Suspects were defined as having any of the following: (1) cough $\geq$ 1 month, (2) hemoptysis at any time, (3) confined to home on account of illness, or (4) diagnosed previously with tuberculosis. The study showed that almost three-quarters of cases were among those who fit the case definition and that the suspects' segment made up 6.5% of the 29,508 eligible population aged 6 years and older in the district. The authors interpreted the efficiency of community leaders in tuberculosis case finding as disappointing. Nevertheless, among the total eligible population, the utilization of community leaders led to six (29.6%) of the expected 20.3 cases by pointing at just 363 (1.2%) suspects among the total population. Most important was the finding that slightly more than 80% of newly diagnosed cases claimed that they had attended a medical facility for treatment of their symptoms but had not been investigated for tuberculosis.

In the second study (Aluoch et al., 1978) the efficiency of requestioning community leaders about 1 year later was evaluated. Of the 421 suspects named, 129 (30.6%) were new suspects, among whom three culture positive (including two smear-positive) cases were identified. Among 189 spontaneously renamed suspects, five cases were now culture-positive and both smear-positive cases among them had become registered. Active follow-up yielded only 0.7 case per 100 contacts of all cases, but 2.3 contact cases per 100 newly registered cases. Again, the yield was considered disappointing. However, because reinterrogation yielded several new cases with relatively little workload, a third study was undertaken to evaluate the usefulness of requestioning community leaders at shorter intervals.

The third study (Nsanzumuhire et al., 1981) showed that interrogation of household heads on a single occasion produced more than two-thirds of all the bacteriologically confirmed cases found in the community by several case-finding methods combined. However, the yield from interrogation of community leaders was almost double per 100 suspects. Interrogation of household heads was naturally much more cumbersome than interrogation of community leaders. Although the yield by requestioning community elders increased, the yield of repeated questioning was disproportionately lower.

A further important finding of the third study was that among 37 cases who were registered 1 or more years earlier and could be examined, four (10.8%) were found to be sputum smear-positive.

In the three studies, the number of cases per 100 suspects identified by community elders was between 1.7 and 2.8. As in previous studies, the most important finding was the confirmation that about 80% of new smear-positive cases claimed to have attended a health care facility because of their respiratory symptoms, but had not been investigated for tuberculosis.

B. Identification of Population Segments at High Risk of Having or Developing Tuberculosis

HIV Infection

Among the numerous factors that are recognized to increase the risk of progression from subclinical infection with *Mycobacterium tuberculosis* to active tuberculosis, infection with the human immunodeficiency virus (HIV) has been identified as the strongest (Rieder et al., 1989a). The annual risk of tuberculosis among dually infected persons might be some 8% (Selwyn et al., 1989). It appears that at least 30% of patients with the acquired immunodeficiency syndrome (AIDS) who are also infected with tubercle bacilli develop tuberculosis at some time, and very commonly before the appearance of other AIDS-defining conditions (Rieder et al., 1989b). While preventive therapy of asymptomatically dually infected persons appears to be quite efficacious (Wadhawan et al., 1991), the identification of tuberculous infection among HIV-infected persons may pose serious problems (Robert et al., 1989).

As among other population groups, failure to make a diagnosis in this group of patients is not uncommon and may lead to unnecessary morbidity and fatality (Flora et al., 1990; Kramer et al., 1990). Because HIV-associated tuberculosis often has radiologically unusual pictures (Pitchenik and Rubinson, 1985) and may be commonly found at any extrapulmonary site (Barnes et al., 1991), a high index of suspicion is warranted and specimens from numerous sites may be required to establish the diagnosis (Centers for Disease Control, 1989).

Although extrapulmonary tuberculosis and sputum smear-negative pulmonary tuberculosis among patients with HIV infection or AIDS is more common than among tuberculosis patients without (Barnes et al., 1991), a considerable increase in sputum smear-positive tuberculosis is observed in several populations that are heavily affected by HIV (International Union Against Tuberculosis and Lung Disease and Tanzania National Tuberculosis/Leprosy Programme, 1991; Styblo, 1990). Such excess infectious cases that are attributable to HIV infection will necessarily lead to a deterioration of the epidemiological situation by increasing the risk of infection in the community. In population groups such as in large metropolitan areas of the United States (Rieder et al., 1989c) and in many sub-Saharan countries, the potential for excess transmission of tubercle bacilli is large. In many areas, the health care facilities for patients who present with symptoms have become so stretched (International Union against Tuberculosis and Lung Disease and Tanzania National Tuberculosis/Leprosy Programme, 1991) that little hope remains for active case-finding activities.

Recent Infection

It is well recognized that newly acquired tuberculous infection is an important risk factor for the progression to tuberculosis disease (Rieder et al., 1989a). The effectiveness of active case finding among contacts is undisputed because it is logistically almost always practical and provides a relatively high yield of new cases (Aluoch et al., 1978). Furthermore, active follow-up of contacts of new cases can identify a large proportion of high-risk, asymptomatically infected persons who might benefit from preventive therapy.

Fibrotic Lesions

Patients with fibrotic lesions resulting from previous, spontaneously healed tuberculosis without adequate treatment are at high risk of recurrence (International Union Against Tuberculosis Committee on Prophylaxis, 1982). In a first-time-prevalence survey of a population group, the prevalence of fibrotic lesions might be severalfold higher than that of bacteriologically active disease (Styblo et al., 1967; Grzybowski et al., 1987). For this reason, a large proportion of preventable cases might be identified by a single radiographic examination of a high-risk population, such as alcoholics and drug addicts (Friedman et al., 1987), other persons living in socially depressed inner-city areas (Grzybowski et al., 1987), or immigrants and refugees from high-incidence countries (Ormerod et al., 1990; Sutter and Haefliger, 1990).

Other Risk Factors

Numerous other factors have been identified that increase the risk from subclinical infection to active tuberculosis (Rieder et al., 1989a). Accordingly, persons with such factors (diabetes, silicosis, malignancies, hemodialysis, etc) may be at an increased risk of having or developing tuberculosis while being treated for their underlying condition. In industrialized countries, screening for tuberculosis or tuberculous infection is often recommended for such patients (Centers of Disease Control, 1990a).

C. Passive Case-Finding Methods

The term "passive case finding" is used here to describe methods for the identification of tuberculosis cases, where the first initiative for an individual patient/provider contact is taken by the patient.

Methods Aiming at Reducing Patient's Delay

Patients seek medical care when their symptoms are subjectively sufficiently severe for them to consult a health care provider despite its disadvantages (costs, interruption of normal activities). It is conceivable that in different societies, among different population segments, and between individuals, different forces are at work that influence the patient's delay from the first occurrence of symptoms to the seeking of medical attention.

In the studies that evaluated the role of mass miniature radiography, it has been shown that more than 90% of sputum smear-positive patients have symptoms, predominantly cough (Toman, 1976; Meijer et al., 1971; Banerji and Andersen, 1963).

In industrialized countries with a dense network for health care provision, the distance between residence or workplace and health care facilities may be an unimportant factor to a patient's delay in seeking medical attention (Aoki et al., 1985). In contrast, it is conceivable that in resource-poor countries the distance to the next health care provider may influence the patient's attitude toward seeking medical attention (Nagpaul et al., 1970; Aluoch et al., 1984).

In Japan, the median interval between the occurrence of symptoms and the first contact with a health care provider was 17 days, but varied remarkably between individual patients (Aoki et al., 1985). Patient's delay was also influenced by profession and location of residence. In Hong Kong, an intensive campaign using mass media failed to attract significant numbers of tuberculosis patients and failed to attract older subjects more likely to have the disease (Girling, 1985).

Methods Aiming at Reducing Doctor's Delay

In a series of studies in Kenya it became clear that a large proportion of cases found through interrogation of community leaders and heads of households (Nsanzumuhire et al., 1977, 1981; Aluoch et al., 1978;) had actually attended health care facilities with complaints, but had not been examined bacteriologically or radiographically. Similarly, in Bangalore City in India, where both general health institutions and specialized tuberculosis clinics exist, it was observed that patients do not bypass the general city health institutions (Gothi et al., 1970).

The problem thus seems to be not so much that patients do not develop symptoms or do not seek medical attention, but *when* the proper diagnosis is made. In the Japanese study (Aoki et al., 1985), the median patient's delay was 17 days, and the median doctor's delay 31 days. The authors found that the most influential factor for the doctor's delay was whether a radiographic examination was done or not done at the first visit. The median delay was only 13 days for patients who had a chest radiograph done at the first visit, but 50 days for those who were not examined.

There is little doubt that with decreasing incidence of tuberculosis in most industrialized countries, physicians will think less of tuberculosis as a differential diagnosis. It is appalling that in the United States the diagnosis of tuberculosis is missed in a large proportion of patients (Rieder et al., 1991). Among all cases reported to the Centers for Disease Control, the proportion of cases who did not receive treatment and in whom the diagnosis was made after death was 5%. This proportion increased to 11% among those aged 65 years and older and was 18% among those with meningeal, peritoneal, or miliary tuberculosis.

In other studies jointly conducted by the Respiratory Disease Research Center, Nairobi, and the British Medical Research Council, approaches to improve case finding by more thoroughly examining patients attending health care facilities have been evaluated (Aluoch et al., 1982, 1984, 1985, 1987). In the fourth study (Aluoch et al., 1982), similar to the previous three studies, 90% of suspects without a history of tuberculosis claimed they had attended a health care facility for an average of more than 5 times, yet 65% had neither a chest radiograph nor their sputum examined bacteriologically.

In the fifth study (Aluoch et al., 1984), careful screening for patients with a cough of 1 month or more duration in outpatients attending a district hospital identified 601 (2.9%) suspects among 20,756 new outpatients. Among the suspects, 5.6% had bacteriologically or radiographically active tuberculosis. An additional 2.2% were considered to have inactive tuberculosis. The authors found that the method was uniformly effective within a radius of about 9 miles of the hospital, but became less effective in increasing distance from the hospital. The study demonstrated the need for considerable improvement in the infrastructure of the primary health care system in the periphery.

In the sixth study (Aluoch et al., 1985), the effectiveness of careful screening of patients attending as general outpatients at four different district hospitals for the first time was examined. A suspect was defined as in the earlier studies (Nsanzumuhire et al., 1977, 1981; Aluoch et al., 1978). Among the general outpatient population, 2.6% fit the definition of a suspect. Among suspects, 4.7% had culture-positive pulmonary tuberculosis (including 3.6% who were also positive on sputum smear examination). A history of cough for between 1 and 12 months was the most predictive factor for tuberculosis, and would have identified 92% of the smear-positive cases by examining 70% of the suspects. An important observation was, similar to the previous study (Aluoch et al., 1984), that the proportion of cases decreased with increasing distance of their homes, but that the proportion of cases among suspects increased with increasing distance of the home from the hospital.

In the seventh study (Aluoch et al., 1987), the effectiveness of case finding among attendants of maternity and child welfare clinics was examined, by questioning them about suspects in their households. The results were disappointing because only 4% of the estimated total annual incidence were undiscovered by this method.

The authors concluded from their series of studies in Kenya that a substantial yield of tuberculosis cases can be obtained from the area surrounding district hospitals. The major detriment to discovering a larger proportion of cases lay, however, with the complacency of health staff in the periphery. Unless primary health care facilities in the periphery were improved, the proportion of identified cases among all actually newly occurring cases would remain disappointing. Furthermore, it might be added, the failure to interrupt transmission by definitively curing the patients was clearly documented in the third study (Nsanzumuhire et al., 1981) showing that more than 10% of previously treated patients were alive and smear-positive.

What stands behind the vicious circle of transmission in both resource-poor and industrialized countries is the failure to undertake appropriate examinations in patients who present themselves with relevant symptoms referable to the respiratory tract. Second, in resource-poor countries, a strengthening of the primary health care services must be implemented. Third, if patients are diagnosed but not cured, and do not die, the primary objective to curtail transmission in the community cannot be achieved (Grzybowski and Enarson, 1978).

IV. Factors Modifying the Choice of Case-Finding Methods

A. Availability of Resources

Where resources are scarce, case-finding methods are limited to those activities which have been shown to bring the highest rewards. In most resource-poor countries, passive case finding for infectious cases, active case finding among contacts, and simultaneously raising the awareness of the community and the medical profession have become the method of choice for their tuberculosis control programs (International Union Against Tuberculosis and Lung Disease, 1991). In these countries, the emphasis in tuberculosis control lies first with achieving an increase in the proportion of cures (Murray et al., 1990) and then expanding case finding (Kochi, 1991).

In countries with more resources, targeted screening activities among population groups at high risk of tuberculosis are commonly advocated. In low-incidence countries, a common group that is often required to submit to an initial radiographic screening are immigrants and refugees (Centers for Disease Control, 1990b), and screening is recommended particularly for immigrants from high-prevalence countries (Ormerod, 1990).

B. Prevalence of Disease

For tuberculosis screening to be justified, the prevalence of tuberculosis must be high in the target population and/or the population has a high prevalence of tuberculous infection and is at high risk of progression to tuberculosis.

Population segments that fit one or both these conditions in industrialized countries are immigrants and refugees from high-prevalence countries (Rieder et al., 1989c), inner-city marginalized populations (Grzybowski et al., 1987; Friedman et al., 1987), miners (Burke et al., 1979), inmates of correctional facilities (Anderson et al., 1986), professions that are chosen by high-prevalence groups (Judson et al., 1983), and many other groups (Centers for Disease Control,

1990a), including indigenous peoples especially in the Americas. Individuals who meet one or both conditions notably include persons with HIV infection, recent infection, and a multitude of clinical conditions (Centers for Disease Control, 1990a).

In industrialized countries where resources are available, active case finding is often expanded to these groups. In resource-poor countries, most active case-finding activities that go beyond contact examination are prohibitively expensive in relation to the yield.

V. The Role of Case Finding in Tuberculosis Control

Although the logical sequence in tuberculosis control is discovery of cases, followed by treatment, it cannot be concluded that the basis for the documented inefficiency of tuberculosis control programs in many developing countries (Murray et al., 1991) lies primarily with deficiencies in case finding. In contrast, there is much evidence that the failure to cure those sources of infection which are discovered by one or the other activity is the major problem. The introduction of chemotherapy has greatly reduced case fatality, but many programs testify that epidemiologically little has been accomplished, because the proportion of cases that remain infectious has remained largely unchanged with or without chemotherapy (Grzybowski and Enarson, 1978). It has been clearly recognized that there is an urgent need to increase the proportion of cures, if the risk of infection in the community is to be reduced (Murray et al., 1991). The hypothesis has been offered that indeed low cure ratios may even lead to a deterioration of the epidemiological situation, because prolongation of infectiousness may ensue beyond the natural course of untreated disease (Styblo and Bumgarner, 1991). Mutual Assistance Programmes of the International Union against Tuberculosis and Lung Disease have shown that higher cure ratios can be achieved with cost-effective short-course chemotherapy (Murray et al., 1990, 1991). The World Health Organization has set the target for a cure ratio of 85% in low-income countries and for 95% in high-income countries (Kochi, 1991).

In numerous studies, notably in those in Kenya (Nsanzumuhire et al., 1977, 1981; Aluoch et al., 1978), India (Gothi et al., 1970), and Japan (Aoki et al., 1985), it has been demonstrated that the problem of delay between onset of symptoms and initiation of appropriate treatment lies less with the patient than with the medical system. This in itself would seem to be sufficient reason to put scarce resources into improving the skills and training of health care providers to pursue appropriate diagnostic action in patients who spontaneously present themselves to health care facilities rather than into active case-finding methods and screening outside the system. In most low-income, high-incidence countries, the primary health care system is too underdeveloped to appropriately identify and diagnose tuberculosis patients who seek medical attention for symptoms referable to the respiratory tract. In high-income, low-incidence countries, it is not the unavailability of diagnostic services that prevents rapid diagnosis, but the failure to include tuberculosis in the differential diagnosis (Aoki et al., 1985; Flora et al., 1990; Kramer et al., 1990; Rieder et al., 1991).

If cure cannot be guaranteed for a large majority of patients, expanding case-finding activities does not make sense. This is true not only for low-income countries, but also for high-income countries. In New York City, for example, a study has clearly shown that active case finding among deprived inner-city population segments can be very rewarding (Friedman et al., 1987). Such yield may be, however, of little benefit to the program because of the high attrition ratio before patients complete an adequate course (Sbarbaro, 1987). Only when cure of a large proportion of cases can be assured is it appropriate to consider case-finding activities. The World Health Organization has set the target for case finding at 65% for low-income countries and at 85% for middle-income countries (Kochi, 1991).

VI. Conclusions

There is little doubt that passive case finding coupled with efficient treatment is the most rewarding activity in tuberculosis control. In both resource-poor and resource-rich countries, the problem of delay in diagnosis does not lie so much with the patient's failure to seek medical attention as with the failure of the medical system to properly and timely diagnose tuberculosis. In resource-poor countries, tremendous efforts will need to be made to improve the cure of patients, to expand the primary health care system, and to educate health care providers to react appropriately to patients who complain about prolonged respiratory tract symptoms. Similarly, in high-income countries the most important conclusion that can be drawn from available studies is that although targeted active case finding in high-risk population segments is giving a high yield, the emphasis must be placed on continuously educating health care providers and physicians in particular that the diagnosis of tuberculosis can usually easily be made if it is only thought of. Most important for both low-income and high-income countries is the lesson that all case-finding activities, even if they are successful, are in vain if patients' compliance can not be assured. In addition to the failure of improving the epidemiological situation with inadequate treatment, the threat of losing rather than winning the battle against tuberculosis looms with the emergence of drug resistance (Manalo et al., 1990) to which the noncompliance of the medical system may contribute more than is openly accepted.

References

Aluoch, J. A., Karuga, W. K., Nsanzumuhire, H., Edwards, E. A., Stott, H., Fox, W., and Sutherland, I. (1978). A second study of the use of community leaders in case-finding for pulmonary tuberculosis in Kenya. *Tubercle* **59**:233–243.

Aluoch, J. A., Edwards, E. A., Stott, H., Fox, W., and Sutherland, I. (1982). A fourth study of case-finding methods for pulmonary tuberculosis in Kenya. *Trans R. Soc. Trop. Med. Hyg.* **79**:679–691.

Aluoch, J. A., Swai, O. B., Edwards, E. A., Stott, H., Darbyshire, J. H., Fox, W., and Sutherland, I. (1984). Study of case-finding for pulmonary tuberculosis in outpatients complaining of a chronic cough at a district hospital in Kenya. *Am. Rev. Respir. Dis.* **129**:915–920.

Aluoch, J. A., Swai, O. B., Edwards, E. A., Stott, H., Darbyshire, J. H., Fox, W., Stephens, R. J., and Sutherland, I. (1985). Studies of case-finding for pulmonary tuberculosis in outpatients at 4 district hospitals in Kenya. *Tubercle* **66**:237–249.

Aluoch, J. A., Oyoo, D., Swai, O. B., Kwamanga, D., Agwanda, R., Edwards, E. A., Stott, H., Darbyshire, J. H., Fox, W., and Sutherland, I. (1987). A study of the use of maternity and child welfare clinics in case-finding for pulmonary tuberculosis in Kenya. *Tubercle* **68**:93–103.

American Thoracic Society/Centers for Disease Control (1983). Control of tuberculosis. *Am. Rev. Respir. Dis.* **128**:336–342.

Anderson, K. M., Keith, E. P., and Norsted, S. W. (1986). Tuberculosis screening in Washington State male correctional facilities. *Chest* **89**:817–821.

Aoki, M., Mori, T., and Shimao, T. (1985). Studies on factors influencing patient's, doctor's and total delay of tuberculosis case-detection in Japan. *Bull. Int. Union Tuberc.* **60**:128–130.

Banerji, D., and Anderson, S. (1963). A sociological study of awareness of symptoms among persons with pulmonary tuberculosis. *Bull. WHO* **29**:665–683.

Barnes, P. F., Bloch, A. B., Davidson, P. T., and Snider, D. E., Jr. (1991). Tuberculosis in patients with human immunodeficiency virus infection. *N. Engl. J. Med.* **324**:1644–1650.

Burke, R. M., Schwartz, L. P., and Snider, D. E., Jr. (1979). The Ottawa County project: a report of a tuberculosis screening project in a small mining community. *Am. J. Public Health* **69**:340–347.

Centers for Disease Control (1989). Tuberculosis and human immunodeficiency virus infection: Recommendations of the Advisory Committee for the Elimination of Tuberculosis (ACET). *MMWR* **38**:236–250.

Centers for Disease Control (1990a). Screening for tuberculosis and tuberculous infection in high-risk populations. Recommendations of the

Advisory Committee for Elimination of Tuberculosis. *MMWR* **39**(no. RR-8):1–7.

Centers for Disease Control (1990b). Tuberculosis among foreign persons entering the United States. Recommendations of the Advisory Committee for Elimination of Tuberculosis. *MMWR* **39**(No. RR-18):1–21.

Flora, G. S., Modilevsky, T., Antoniskis, D., and Barnes, P. F. (1990). Undiagnosed tuberculosis in patients with human immunodeficiency virus infection. *Chest* **98**:1056–1059.

Friedman, L. N., Sullivan, G. M., Bevilaqua, R. P., and Loscos, R. (1987). Tuberculosis screening in alcoholics and drug addicts. *Am. Rev. Respir, Dis.* **136**:1188–1192.

Girling, D. J. (1985). Hong Kong Chest Service / British Medical Research Council survey of patients presenting to the Government Chest Service and the effects of active case-finding by a publicity campaign. *Bull. Int. Union Tuberc.* **60**:121.

Gothi, G. D., Savíc, D., Baily, G. V. J., and Samuel, R. (1970). Cases of pulmonary tuberculosis among the out-patients attending general health institutions in an Indian city. *Bull. WHO* **43**:35–40.

Grzybowski S., and Enarson, D. A. (1978). The fate of cases of pulmonary tuberculosis under various treatment programmes. *Bull. Int. Union Tuberc.* **53**:70–75.

Grzybowski, S., Allen, E. A., Black, W. A., Chao, C. W., Enarson, D. A., Isaac-Renton, J. L., Peck, S. H. S., and Xie, H. J. (1987). Inner-city survey for tuberculosis: evaluation of diagnostic methods. *Am. Rev. Respir. Dis.* **135**:1311–1315.

Horwitz, O., and Darrow, M. M. (1976). Principles and effects of mass screening: Danish experience in tuberculosis screening. *Public Health Rep.* **91**:146–153.

International Union Against Tuberculosis Committee on Prophylaxis. (1982). Efficacy of various durations of isoniazid preventive therapy for tuberculosis: five years of follow-up in the IUAT trial. *Bull. WHO* **60**:555–564.

International Union Against Tuberculosis and Lung Disease. (1991). *Tuberculosis Guide for High Prevalence Countries*, 2nd ed. International Union Against Tuberculosis and Lung Disease / Misereor, Paris.

International Union Against Tuberculosis and Lung Disease and Tanzania National Tuberculosis / Leprosy Programme (1991). International Union Against Tuberculosis and Lung Disease progress report No. 26.

Judson, F. N., Sbarbaro, J. A., Tapy, J. M., and Cohn, D. L. (1983). Tuberculosis screening. Evaluation of a food handlers' program. *Chest* **83**:879–882.

Kochi, A. (1991). The global tuberculosis situation and the new control strategy of the World Health Organization (leading article). *Tubercle* **72**:1–6.

Kramer, F., Modilevsky, T., Waliany, A. B., Leedom, J. M., and Barnes, P. F. (1990). Delayed diagnosis of tuberculosis in patients with human immunodeficiency virus infection. *Am. J. Med.* **89**:451–456.

Křivinka, R., Drápela, J., Kubík, A., Daňková, D., Křivánek, J., Ruzha, J., Miková, Z., and Hejdová, E. (1974). Epidemiological and clinical study of tuberculosis in the district of Kolín, Czechoslovakia. Second report (1965–1972). *Bull. WHO* **51**:59–69.

Manalo, F., Tan, F., Sbarbaro, J. A., and Iseman, M. D. (1990). Community-based short-course treatment of pulmonary tuberculosis in a developing nation. *Am. Rev. Respir. Dis.* **142**:1301–1305.

Meijer, J., Barnett, G. D., Kubík, A., and Stýblo, K. (1971). Identification of sources of infection. *Bull. Int. Union Tuberc.* **45**:5–50.

Murray, C. J. L., Styblo, K., and Rouillon, A. (1990). Tuberculosis in developing countries: burden, intervention and cost. *Bull. Int. Union Tuberc. Lung Dis.* **65**:6–24.

Murray, C. J. L., Styblo, K., and Rouillon, A. (1991). Health sector priorities review: tuberculosis. In D. T. Jamison, and W. H. Mosley, editors. Oxford University Press for the World Bank, New York.

Nagpaul, D. R., Vishwanath, M. K., and Dwarakanath, G. (1970). A socio-epidemiological study of outpatients attending a city tuberculosis clinic in India to judge the place of specialized centres in a tuberculosis control programme. *Bull. WHO* **43**:17–34.

Nsanzumuhire, H., Lukwago, E. W., Edwards, E. A., Stott, H., Fox, W., and Sutherland, I. (1977). A study of the use of community leaders in case-finding for pulmonary tuberculosis in the Machakos District of Kenya. *Tubercle* **58**:117–128.

Nsanzumuhirc, H., Aluoch, J. A., Karuga, W. K., Edwards, E. A., Stott, H., Fox, W., and Sutherland, I. (1981). A third study of case-finding methods for pulmonary tuberculosis in Kenya, including the use of community leaders. *Tubercle* **62**:79–94.

Ormerod, L. P. (1990). Tuberculosis screening and prevention in new immigrants 1983–88. *Respir. Med.* **84**:269–271.

Pitchenik, A. E., and Rubinson, H. A. (1985). The radiographic appearance of tuberculosis in patients with the acquired immune deficiency syndrome (AIDS) and pre-AIDS. *Am. Rev. Respir. Dis.* **121**:393–396.

Rieder, H. L., Cauthen, G. M., Comstock, G. W., and Snider, D. E., Jr. (1989a). Epidemiology of tuberculosis in the United States. *Epidemiol. Rev.* **11**:89–95.

Rieder, H. L., Cauthen, G. M., Bloch, A. B., Cole, C. H., Holtzmann, D., Snider, D. E., Jr., Bigler, W. J., and Witte, J. J. (1989b). Tuberculosis and acquired immunodeficiency syndrome—Florida. *Arch. Intern. Med.* **149**:1268–1273.

Rieder, H. L., Cauthen, G. M., Kelly, G. D., Bloch, A. B., and Snider, D. E., Jr. (1989c). Tuberculosis in the United States. *JAMA* **262**:385–389.

Rieder, H. L., Kelly, G. D., Bloch, A. B., Cauthen, G. M., and Snider, D. E., Jr. (1991). Tuberculosis diagnosed at death in the United States. *Chest* **100**:678–681.

Robert, C.-F., Hirschel, B., Rochat, T., and Deglon, J.-J. (1989). Tuberculin skin reactivity in HIV-seropositive intravenous drug addicts (correspondence). *N. Engl. J. Med.* **321**:1268.

Sbarbaro, J. A. (1987). To seek, find, and yet fail (editorial). *Am. Rev. Respir. Dis.* **136**:1072–1073.

Selwyn, P. A., Hartel, D., Lewis, V. A., Schoenbaum, E. E., Vermund, S. H., Klein, R. S., Walker, A. T., and Friedland, G. H. (1989). A prospective study of the risk of tuberculosis among intravenous drug users with human immunodeficiency virus infection. *N. Engl. J. Med.* **320**:545–550.

Shaw, J. B. and Wynn-Williams N. (1954). Infectivity of pulmonary tuberculosis in relation to sputum status. *Am. Rev. Tuberc.* **69**:724–732.

Snider, D. E., Jr., Anderson, H. R., and Bentley, S. E. (1984). Current tuberculosis screening practices. *Am. J. Public Health* **74**:1353–1356.

Styblo, K. (1990). The global aspects of tuberculosis and HIV infection. *Bull. Int. Union Tuberc. Lung Dis.* **65**:28–32.

Styblo, K., and Bumgarner, J. R. (1991). Tuberculosis can be controlled with existing technologies: evidence. In *Tuberculosis Surveillance Research Unit of the International Union Against Tuberculosis and Lung Disease.* Vol. 2. K.N.C.V., The Hague, pp. 60–72.

Styblo, K., and Meijer, J. (1980). The quantified increase of the tuberculosis infection rate in a low prevalences country to be expected if the existing MMR programme were discontinued. *Bull. Int. Union Tuberc.* **55**:3–8.

Styblo, K., Daňková, D., Drápela, J., Galliová, J., Ježek, Z., Křivánek, J., Kubík, A., Langerová, M., and Radkovský, J. (1967). Epidemiological and clinical study of tuberculosis in the District of Kolín, Czechoslovakia, Report of the first 4 years of the study (1961–64). *Bull. WHO* **37**:819–874.

Sutherland, I. (1981). The epidemiology of tuberculosis—is prevention better than cure? *Bull. Int. Un. Tuberc.* **56**:127–134.

Sutter, R. W., and Haefliger, E. (1990). Tuberculosis morbidity and infection in Vietnamese in Souteast Asian refugee camps. *Am. Rev. Respir. Dis.* **141**:1483–1486.

Toman, K. (1976). Mass radiography in tuberculosis control. *WHO Chronicle* **30**:51–57.

United States Public Health Service (1958). X-ray case-finding programs in tuberculosis control. *Public Health Rep.* **73**:83–85.

United States Public Health Service (1983). *The Selection of Patients for X-Ray Examinations: Chest X-Ray Screening Examinations*. Department of Health and Human Services HHS Publication No. (FDA) 83-8204.

Wadhawan, D., Hira, S., Mwansa, N., Tembo, G., and Perine, P. (1991). Preventive tuberculosis chemotherapy with isoniazid among persons infected with human immundodeficiency virus. VII International Conference on AIDS, Florence, 16–21 June 1991. Abstract W.B.2261.

World Health Organization. WHO Expert Committee on Tuberculosis, Ninth Report. (1974). *WHO Tech. Rep. Ser.* No. 552.

10

Case Holding

ERIC BRENNER

EPI Resources
Columbia, South Carolina

CAROL POZSIK

Tuberculosis Control Division
South Carolina Department of Health
and Environmental Control
Columbia, South Carolina

I. Introduction

A. The Problem of Case Holding

For any tuberculosis control program (TBCP), the objectives of treatment are not only to diagnose and institute a proper course of treatment for every new case of tuberculosis, but also to take all possible and necessary means to ensure regularity of drug intake for a duration adequate to achieve a cure (Chaulet, 1983). The term "case holding" refers to activities and techniques that can be used to meet this objective. Paradoxically, case holding is so difficult because modern chemotherapy is so potent that patients usually recover their sense of well-being after only a few weeks of treatment. At this time they may often, and quite naturally, lose the subjective need to continue taking medications. However, controlled clinical trials have shown that even modern chemotherapy regimens must be maintained for 6–12 months to assure the patient, and the community, of a lasting cure. No matter the setting, the problems of case holding are therefore among the most challenging in tuberculosis. This is true in the office of a private physician who may be approaching the patient primarily in terms of *diagnosis and treatment*; in the TBCP of a developed country where control strategy is based on *surveillance and containment*; or in the program of a developing country where the focus is on *case finding and treatment*.

Nonetheless the problem of case holding has been relatively neglected. One reason is that those on the "frontlines" of TBCPs (public health nurses, community outreach workers, and others), who shoulder the daily responsibilities for case holding, do not usually have the opportunity to contribute to the medical literature. A second reason is that a rigorous approach to the subject requires skills and knowledge not only in the clinical sciences and epidemiology, but also in behavioral and social disciplines, such as psychology and anthropology. A final reason may lie in an older model of medical care under which it was understood by physicians that their responsibility was to diagnose and prescribe treatment for a particular disease. After that, it was up to the patient to comply with the physician's advice and take the medications. However, in the case of tuberculosis, failure to comply with therapy can lead not only to individual treatment failure, disability, and death, but also to perpetuation of the cycle of transmission, infection, and disease in the community. In the era of human immunodeficiency virus (HIV), this cycle can be accelerated by transmission to individuals who are (or soon will be) immunoincompetent (Daley et al., 1992). Recent experience has also shown that the transmission cycle can be maintained even by drug-resistant organisms leading to outbreaks that can only be controlled by intensive and costly public health measures (Edlin et al., 1992; CDC, 1991a). The fact that many of these outbreaks can be traced back to failure of case holding underscores the importance of this subject.

B. Case Holding in the United States

To what extent do TBCPs in the United States fail to hold cases until therapy is complete? In a report from a major North American tuberculosis symposium, a 1979 article termed patient compliance "the most serious remaining problem in the control of tuberculosis in the United States" (Addington, 1979), and other presentations at the same meeting echoed the theme and proposed various approaches to the problem (Sbarbaro, 1979; Dudley, 1979). Ten years later, in 1989, the U.S. Public Health Service's Advisory Committee for Elimination of Tuberculosis (ACET) stated: "More than 25% of sputum-positive patients are *not* known to have converted from positive to negative sputum cultures within 6 months. In addition, almost 12% of patients are *not* known to be currently receiving therapy, and more than 17% of tuberculosis patients do *not* take their medications continuously" (CDC, 1989a).

Finally, the Division of Tuberculosis Elimination of the Centers for Disease Control (CDC) reports, based on standardized program evaluation forms received from state and large-city TBCPs, that about 22% of patients currently fail to complete therapy within a 12-month period and that in some areas the figure is as high as 55% (CDC, 1991b). These data make it clear that weaknesses in the quality of case-holding efforts in the United States are common. This situation presents a formidable public health challenge, especially in light of the recently launched initiative to eliminate tuberculosis from the United States by 2010. This initiative (CDC, 1989a) proposes, as the first of the three steps in its strategic plan, to make "more effective use of existing prevention and control methods." There is no doubt that improved case holding, essential to successful containment through chemotherapy, will be a basic prerequisite to a successful elimination effort. In the rest of this chapter we will discuss the problem of case holding from several points of view. We will present:

1. A simple numerical model illustrating the epidemiological importance of case holding
2. Brief summaries from recent publications dealing with compliance
3. Selected experiences with case-holding activities from the state of South Carolina
4. Remarks regarding the use of microcomputer tools for evaluating case-holding activities

II. Modeling the Importance of Case Holding

The public health goal of a modern TBCP program is to reduce the prevalence of individuals who are excreting tubercle bacilli and who thus serve as points of infection for the community. Broadly speaking, this can be accomplished through two types of measures: (1) those which reduce the incidence of new cases of pulmonary tuberculosis, and (2) those which reduce the average duration of infectiousness of those cases which do occur. The magnitude of the reduction that can be achieved through a chemotherapy program will depend on four parameters, all of which reflect TBCP effectiveness:

1. The proportion of incident cases that are detected
2. The proportion of detected cases begun on chemotherapy
3. The biological efficacy of the prescribed drug regimens
4. The proportion of those beginning therapy who successfully complete their prescribed course

The combined effect of these four factors can be obtained by simple multiplication, as is shown in the schema presented in Table 1. Examples 1 and 2 illustrate the situation as it might exist in a developed country where most cases are reported, where essentially all detected cases will have access to care and be placed on medications, and where the financial means exist to prescribe the most

Table 1 Contribution of Case Holding to the Overall Reduction in Sources of Infection

Measure of →	Overall impact		Case finding or surveillance		Access to care		Biology of drugs and tuberculosis		Case holding
			Operationally equivalent to						
	Reduction in sources of infection		Proportion of cases detected		Proportion beginning therapy		Efficacy of drug regimen		Proportion completing therapy
Example no.[a]									
1	88%	=	95%	×	99%	×	96%	×	98%
2	72%	=	95%	×	99%	×	96%	×	80%
3	38%	=	70%	×	80%	×	85%	×	80%

[a]See text.

potent regimens containing INH and rifampin supplemented as necessary by pyrazinamide, streptomycin, and ethambutol. It is easy to see that in such circumstances case holding is likely to be the weak link in the calculation chain. In example 2 where case holding is only 80%, over one-quarter of cases could become long-term excreters of tubercule bacilli, a proportion not much different from that observed in the prechemotherapy era! Of course, in the poorest countries where case-finding activities may not yet cover the entire population, where access to treatment and drugs may not be universal, and where only less efficacious (because less costly) chemotherapy regimens are available, the relative impact of failure of case holding per se may be different. This is illustrated in example 3.

Because it is so straightforward and easy to understand, this model can be presented even to a relatively nontechnical audience. It can help health workers appreciate the context in which case holding takes place and illustrate how the four presented aspects of the TBCP combine, through simple multiplication of effect, to produce a particular outcome for the community.

In 1991 the 44th World Health Assembly passed a resolution concerning tuberculosis, which included a request to the Director-General:

> to intensify collaboration with Member States in strengthening national control programmes in order to improve case-finding and treatment and *attain a global target of cure of 85% for sputum-positive patients under treatment and detection of 70% of cases* by the year 2000, taking care to ensure that these activities are integrated as far as possible into primary health care activities (WHO, 1991).

This resolution shows that the limits of the case-finding and case-holding goals as they are formulated on a global basis remain relatively modest compared to those formulated by developed countries. The fact that the goal for case holding and cure is placed first and has a higher target is also consistent with the current emphasis by WHO on the importance, for less developed programs, to increase case-holding rates before attempts are made to improve detection of cases for whom treatment cannot yet be assured even if they were found.

III. Patient Compliance with Prescribed Medications

The literature on patient compliance with medical prescriptions is extensive. A particularly useful recent review article (Sbarbaro, 1990), written in the context of what is known about compliance in developed countries, emphasizes the following points:

1. The health behavior of most individuals is quite unpredictable and does not conform with our expectations that patients will follow our professional advice.

2. It may be expected that about 33% of patients will fail to follow medical recommendations, and that in some settings, this percentage may approach 100%.

3. Numerous studies confirm (contrary to the "naïve" or "common sense" view) that it is *not* possible to predict noncompliance on the basis of age, sex, race, marital status, educational achievement, or socioeconomic situation.

4. Health beliefs and behaviors are not necessarily altered by mastery of technical or factual information about the disease being treated.

5. Many "educational sessions," which superficially appear to be serving a useful purpose, are only stylized rituals in which the provider first lectures the patient, then questions him about whether he understands all he has been told, and finally receives the reassuring answers he wishes to hear—after which the patient goes out and does exactly what he pleases.

Given these conclusions, carefully drawn from the published literature, the author ends with a plea for the establishment of strong patient-provider relationships as a means to overcome the problems suggested by these observations:

. . . only through a relationship with a health professional truly concerned with the patient's entire health, in fact, concerned with the patient as a whole individual, as a member of a family and a community, and willing to remain a concerned friend, can we hope to influence a patient's behavior.

Related points have also been made by the World Health Organization (WHO) in a document somewhat more oriented toward developing countries (Chaulet, 1983) but which remain universally applicable. Stressed are operational points including the need for:

1. Prescribed regimens to be supplied free of charge

2. Emphasis in a treatment program on an operation that is convenient for the patient and not just for the health staff

3. Health education of the patient and his family, which should be systematic, repeated, and conducted by staff, and which is punctual, conscientious, and kind in a setting that is welcoming, clean, and accessible

The Division of Tuberculosis Elimination of the Centers for Disease Control (CDC) has prepared a 20-page booklet, *Improving Patient Compliance in Tuberculosis Treatment Programs* (CDC, 1989b), which presents a clear, well-structured, and practical approach to the problem of compliance. It begins by pointing out that a patient will be more compliant with a prescribed course of medication if he or she:

Perceives it as important

Is capable of performing the task

Perceives benefits from performing the task

Can easily assimilate the task into his/her life-style

From this viewpoint a line of reasoning is developed to the effect that the responsibility for dealing with the problem of noncompliance does *not* belong solely to the patient, but is shared by the health care provider, who must:

Assure that the patient has the knowledge and skills necessary for compliant behavior

Maintain an awareness of the "signs and symptoms" of noncompliance

Help the patient identify and remove obstacles to compliant behavior

The approach, developed in detail in the text, is outlined in modified form in Table 2, which draws on extensive experience gained from the frontlines of tuberculosis control activities.

An appendix is devoted to the subject of urine tests for the presence of antituberculous drugs or their metabolites. The technical references cited on this subject are included in Appendix I.

Given the case-holding failures that are invariably observed wherever staff operate strictly under a traditional biomedical approach to case management, it is essential for all TBCP staff (including physicians, nurses, and others responsible for case-holding activities) to become familiar with the concepts presented either in the publications cited above or in others like them. Program directors can sensitize their staffs either by distributing literature, or better, through experiential workshops. This admonition is all the more important for programs in areas where tuberculosis is found in conjunction with poverty, unemployment, drug use, homelessness, or AIDS/HIV infection, all of which can tax the case-holding capacity of even the best programs.

IV.   Approach to Case Holding in South Carolina

This section summarizes in an anecdotal manner observations concerning case holding by public health nurses in our program. Our aim here is to communicate some of the feel or flavor of the subject as it is experienced on the frontlines of tuberculosis control in our state.

South Carolina is a relatively poor and largely rural state in the Southeastern United States with a population of about 3,500,000. In most years it ranks among the top 5–10 states in the country as ranked according to

Table 2 Approach to the Problem of Noncompliance in Tuberculosis Treatment Programs

I. Measuring compliance
   A. Direct measures: Measuring
       drugs or metabolites
       1. In urine
       2. In blood
   B. Indirect measures:
       1. Following response to therapy
           a. Clinical improvement
           b. Bacteriological
               improvement
           c. Radiological improvement
       2. Interview technique
       3. Regularity in keeping appoint-
           ments and filling prescrip-
           tions; pill counts
       4. Medication monitors
       5. Subjective judgment of the
           provider

II. Factors affecting compliance
   A. Features of the health care
       system
       1. Efficiency of the referral
           process
       2. Clinical setting
       3. Demographic features of the
           provider
   B. Features of the regimen
       1. Duration of treatment
       2. Number of medicines
           prescribed
       3. Frequency of dosing
       4. Prescription labeling
       5. Side effects
       6. Cost
       7. Safety lock containers
       8. Parenteral medications
   C. Features of the patient
       1. Life-style
       2. Social support
       3. Locus of control

       4. Demographic features of the
           patient
       5. Degree of disability
       6. Health beliefs regarding:
           a. His/her susceptibility to
               the disease
           b. The seriousness of the
               disease
           c. The benefits to be gained
               from health actions
           d. The barriers to the
               action
   D. Features of the patient-health
       care provider relationship

III. Predicting compliance
   A. Attitudes as predictors
   B. Compliance barriers as
       predictors

IV. Strategies for improving
    compliance
   A. Patient education
       1. Be specific
       2. Discuss desired behaviors
           first
       3. Elicit feedback and
           questions
       4. Provide written instructions
   B. Appointment reminders (letters
       and phone calls)
   C. Open discussion with the
       patient
   D. Enlist social support
   E. Formal written contract (com-
       pliance agreement)
   F. Behavior modification (tailor
       the regimen)
   G. Enablers and incentives
   H. Prompt home visits for missed
       appointments

Table 2 (*continued*)

I. Daily DOT therapy in the clinic	initial visit. Emphasize the need
J. Twice-weekly DOT in the clinic	to take medications and continue
K. Twice-weekly DOT at home, at work, or in the community	taking them for the entire duration of therapy.
L. Court-ordered DOT (any setting)	D. Collect information to assess the
M. Court-ordered confinement for DOT	likelihood of adherence to recommended therapy. If probability of
V. Tips on getting started	noncompliance judged to be
A. Assign one staff member (e.g., a nurse or outreach worker) the responsibility for monitoring the progress of each patient.	high, consider immediate institution of DOT.
B. Agree on the treatment plan as a team.	E. Reassess situation within first 2 weeks through an interview with the patient and a home visit.
C. Lay the groundwork for good compliance at the time of the	Modify treatment plan if necessary.

Source: Adapted from CDC, 1989b.

tuberculosis case rates. Throughout the 1980s, an average of about 500 new cases were diagnosed each year. Care for most patients is provided through a single TBCP, which operates in all 46 county health departments, which in turn are grouped into 13 health districts. All districts and counties follow uniform procedures under the technical guidance of a central TBCP directed from the State Health Department. Technical guidelines usually follow very closely official recommendations promulgated by the CDC and by the American Thoracic Society. Public health nurses carry most of the responsibility for day-to-day work in the program. They are assisted by physicians, by X-ray technicians, by the state laboratory, and by a central computerized state tuberculosis registry. As few other outreach workers are available, nurses are responsible for tuberculosis work in the field, including investigation of contacts, home visits, and administration of directly observed therapy. They also work in the health department clinics where most patients pick up medications and are monitored during their course of therapy. All nurses working with the TBCP attend an intensive 1-week orientation course, which is offered every year. The course was initially modeled after CDC's "TB Today" course, but over the years portions of the training have been adapted to local needs. Nurses receive supervision and support from District Adult Health Program Nurse Specialists and from nursing consultants from the TBCP. Technical updates are provided through periodic workshops and at an annual meeting, which features nationally recognized tuberculosis experts. The tuberculosis nurses are trained not only regarding all key biomedical aspects of tuberculosis, but also in a full range of strategies relating to case holding.

A. Patients Who Are Hard to Hold

In our experience, no one group or social class can be identified as being at risk for noncompliance with a prescribed tuberculosis treatment regimen. Even well-educated, relatively affluent, and seemingly concerned individuals have been found to fall short when it comes to taking medications. Conversely, many of the poor and uneducated have been models of cooperation. In general, our experience thus confirms the central message reported in the literature (Sbarbaro, 1990), namely that there is no easy way to predict true patient compliance. We have found, however, that certain characteristics may suggest, albeit imperfectly, that a patient may require extra attention to be able complete a course of therapy.

Patients Who Complied Poorly with Previous Treatment

As modern chemotherapy is so potent, the greatest risk factor for relapse is now noncompliance. Thus, we pay special attention to patients whom we are seeing "for the second time." Patients who, as a result of past noncompliance, developed acquired drug resistance are also in this category, as are for that matter persons who have histories of failing to take other important prescribed medications such as antihypertensives or oral contraceptives.

Abusers of Alcohol

Many of these patients forget to take their medications when they are under the influence of the substance they abuse. As a result of disorganized life-styles, they may also be unreliable in submitting sputum specimens, picking up medication, or keeping clinic appointments.

Patients with Mental, Emotional, and Physical Impairments

Patients in this category include those with dementia; the mentally retarded and mentally ill; those who have a fear of swallowing pills; and those with physical problems such as esophageal strictures, peptic ulcer disease, severe arthritis, quadriplegia, or cerebrovascular insufficiency.

Patients Who "Openly Resist"

Ironically, it is sometimes easier to work through problems with patients who may initially frankly state that they have no intention of following through with the proposed treatment plan. As one of our nurses has explained: "At least in this situation you know where you stand right from the start and you can then select a strategy appropriate to the situation."

The Least Expected

We experience our greatest frustrations with patients for whom the probability of noncompliance had initially, but incorrectly, been assessed as being low. This group includes individuals who are cooperative and pleasant, who want to be educated about their disease, and who from all appearances are going to be the best patients. In South Carolina this group has included respected members of the community, such as ministers, teachers, and health professionals. One pattern we have observed with this group is that in order to maintain appearances consonant with their position, they keep appointments, pick up their medications on time, and assure the nurses that they are taking them regularly. However, as we have at times later learned, at home they would either take medications when they "felt so inclined" or would simply stop taking them altogether after a certain point. We have also observed, as reported by others (Geisler et al., 1987; Miller and Snider, 1987; Fox 1983a, b), that health care workers themselves tend to be difficult tuberculosis patients.

Persons Entrusted with Giving Medicines to Others

This group includes mothers who give medicines to their children, wives to their husbands, or adults to their elderly parents. The concept of deputizing a responsible adult to supervise therapy in the family setting is attractive in theory, but care must be taken to "supervise this supervisor," as intrafamilial dynamics can lead to special problems. In one instance an unusual situation developed when a child began to resist her mother's attempts to give her daily medications. Not wanting to appear unreliable to the visiting nurse, the mother daily decanted just the proper amount of pediatric suspension so that the volume of medications remaining would match the amount expected by the nurse at each home visit. This enabled the mother to maintain a facade of responsibility. Some caregivers find such behavior so repugnant that they refuse to recognize that it might even occur. Our experienced nurses, especially if they have previously lived through such situations and the serious medical and public health consequences that can result, have learned to be more realistic. In many instances, therefore, to be fair to the family, we have found it best *not to assign professional responsibility*. In this way the integrity of family relationships can be maintained and unnecessary conflicts avoided.

Poor Nurse-Patient Relationship

As mentioned above, a significant cause of nonadherence can be the relationship between the health worker and the patient. If the client sees the provider as noncaring, then the patient has less reason to care about the therapy. If the provider is too aggressive or too forceful, a power struggle may ensue. If the provider appears to be naïve, and without convictions about the treatment plan, the patient may simply take control of his own program.

Cases Presumed to Be Preventive Treatment Failures

We have seen a number of tuberculosis patients whose records indicate that they had previously taken a full course of preventive treatment with isoniazid (INH). The inexperienced health worker may assume these cases represent treatment failures. Seasoned tuberculosis workers know that each of these such supposed "biological failures" should be evaluated critically. For example, patients may pick up their INH tablets faithfully each month, yet fail to take them. Thus it is always important to ask such patients not only whether they *picked up* their INH (information that may be available from the patient record in any case), but also whether they *took* the INH. If the question is posed in a nonthreatening manner, the answer may well reveal that the problem is in the patient and *not* in the medication. Many patients do not wish to be considered "unreliable" and they will thus make the necessary effort to pick up medications though they may not intend to swallow them.

One such case, involving a teacher's aide who gave a history of having completed 1 year of preventive therapy, ended dramatically. A chart review showed that the 12 months of treatment had extended over 24 months. The patient repeatedly failed to pick up his medication and required repeated reminders by the nurse to resume his treatment. This scenario was repeated several times. In retrospect, the fact that so many reminders were needed and that the course of treatment took so long should have been a clue. When the patient finally developed tuberculosis several years later, he admitted that he had taken very few of the pills but had picked them up to maintain appearances. The result of this charade was a school outbreak in which 14 children were found to have disease and over 90 others were found to have been infected.

B. Strategies to Improve Case Holding

Directly Observed Therapy

Other than through chemical monitoring of blood and urine, the only way to be certain that a patient has received his scheduled dose of medications is through direct observation. Although an official joint statement of the Centers for Disease Control (CDC) and American Tuberculosis Society had endorsed supervised intermittent therapy (SIT) as long ago as 1974 (Sbarbaro et al., 1974), it is only within the past few years that this intervention has been implemented on a wide scale. After specialized tuberculosis hospitals were closed, many TBCPs arranged a system of regional hospitals with which the TBCP would contract for care whenever inpatient services were needed. Programs quickly found that treatment failures were ultimately very costly in every way. They also realized just how many of patients had failed to take medicines on their own regularly under previous outpatient treatment programs. At the same time, numerous chemotherapy trials showed that after an initial intensive phase of daily therapy, a continuation phase of treatment could be continued with administration of twice-weekly medications. In recent years, therefore, increased use of twice-weekly directly observed therapy (DOT) by nurses and outreach workers has greatly facilitated case holding. It has been estimated that about 17% of tuberculosis patients in the United States currently receive directly observed therapy. Where staffing permits, preventive treatment with isoniazid can now also be administered on a twice-weekly DOT regimen (CDC, 1990), although in practice such use of resources is justified only in selected high-risk situations.

While DOT is now routinely administered by health departments and in institutional settings, this form of treatment can rarely be offered by a private practitioner. We have found, therefore, that cooperative relationships need to be built between health departments and private physicians who diagnose and treat tuberculosis. For example, it is usually possible to arrange matters so that the TBCP can administer DOT even though the patient will be returning to the private physician for periodic medical evaluation.

We have found that a subset of patients receiving DOT present special problems and require even more than the usual close attention. For example, we have observed patients who keep appointments for DOT therapy but still attempt to avoid taking medications. Techniques used include palming medicines, spitting them into an opaque cup, holding them under the tongue or in the cheeks, vomiting them shortly after administration, and sliding them into pockets or underwear. Such situations demand extreme vigilance on the part of the public health nurse. When such stratagems are detected, they usually require an honest confrontation and a negotiated solution.

Supervised intermittent therapy (SIT) was initially considered an appropriate means to treat noncompliant patients at home, at work, or at any other locale in the community (e.g., bars, pool halls, fishing holes, etc.) where arrangements for a twice-weekly encounter could be negotiated. However, we have found that SIT and DOT can also be used right in the clinic, which results in a substantial economy of travel and outreach time. We often make such arrangements in conjunction with the use of enablers and incentives, as discussed below.

In the United States, because of recent trends in tuberculosis related to the HIV epidemic and because of the emergence of multidrug-resistant tuberculosis (MDRTB) as a public health problem (CDC, 1991a; Edlin et al., 1992), it is likely that use of SIT and DOT will continue to increase. In fact, it can be argued that every patient with pulmonary tuberculosis ought to have every dose of therapy observed directly, and if sufficient resources are made available to TBCPs, SIT and DOT should become part of the accepted standard of care.

Use of Communicable Disease Laws

Some patients for whom DOT is proposed avoid our public health nurses even though every reasonable effort is made to show sensitivity to their individual problems, needs, and life-style. Such patients cause nurses to waste precious time and money traveling to appointments that are not kept. These resources are then lost to other patients who also require special attention. In most states laws require that persons with communicable disease conduct themselves so as not to be a threat to the public health. Health departments are also usually required by law to protect the public from communicable disease. In fact, such laws make it clear that TBCPs not only *should* concern themselves with patient compliance, but *must* do so (Sbarbaro, 1979) to protect the public health. In most states, court hearings for recalcitrant patients can thus be held, and if the court so rules, the patient can subsequently be quarantined in a secure facility. In South Carolina, in the mid-1980s, an average of five patients per year (1% of our cases) were quarantined under court order in a state hospital under such circumstances. These measures were used only for patients with bacteriologically confirmed pulmonary tuberculosis for whom it had proven impossible to provide treatment in any other way. Since 1986, in an attempt to decrease the number of such quarantine cases to the absolute minimum, we have found a way to refine our interaction with the judicial system. Because we have gained so much experience in directly observed therapy, we are now able to obtain court orders for DOT rather than for enforced quarantine. In effect, in these cases, the courts, after reviewing the details of the case, have told each patient: "Thou shalt faithfully meet the public health nurse at the appointed time for thy directly observed antituberculous chemotherapy." In almost all instances we have found that the solemnity of the court proceedings has sufficed to make such an impression on our patients that SIT is successful and that subsequent forced confinement is not necessary. As a result of this approach, we now resort to court-ordered quarantine only about once a year (an 80% reduction). We have also estimated that this more subtle use of the judicial system has saved the state $440,000 in institutionalization costs over the past 5 years alone. Of course, this has also enabled our patients in question to remain in their homes, on their jobs, and in the community during the rest of their treatment.

Using Incentives and Enablers

The concept of incentives is very simple, and it is not a new idea. The principle is that a thoughtfully planned gift can provide satisfaction both to the donor and to the recipient and can help build a bond between them. The use of incentives, with less sentimental objectives, has certainly been widely adopted in the commercial world where the most rigorous cost-benefit evaluations of generous acts are certainly made. A familiar example is that of banks providing small gifts to entice new depositors. However, the formal use of incentives in disease control programs does seem to be new. One possible exception: the cash rewards that were offered in the declining days of the WHO global smallpox eradication campaign to anyone who could assist surveillance efforts by reporting a (subsequently confirmed) case of smallpox. In any case, our program has now accumulated over 10 years of experience using incentives and enablers as a means to enhance patient compliance. Further, the practice appears to be spreading as, according to the CDC, this approach is now used in some form in 23 states.

Enablers are used to help, or, literally, to enable, the patient to complete his treatment. Without the enabler, it would, essentially by definition, be difficult or impossible for him to do so. Examples of enablers we have used are provision of bus tokens, gasoline, assistance in obtaining driver's licenses, coats for cold weather, thrift-shop shoes without holes in the soles, and even, on an occasion or two, a new car battery.

Using incentives requires more subtlety. Incentives are used primarily to motivate patients to take their medicine and keep appointments. They must be specially tailored for the individual. What motivates one person may not motivate another. The key is finding that "something special" that appeals and has meaning for the patient.

Because not everyone is in philosophical agreement with the concept, our nurses feel that only caregivers who really believe in incentives should use this tool. Feelings of moral or ethical ambivalence transmit a message of half-heartedness to the patient and cancel the desired beneficial effect. The point made by our nurses who use incentives successfully is that it is *not* the incentive in itself which is so important. Rather, the incentive is a symbol of commitment and communicates to the patient that he is important to the caregiver and therefore deserving of the gift. Such feelings require genuine human commitment and cannot be bluffed.

A carefully tailored choice of incentives is also required. The point is certainly not to hand out a dollar bill to every patient—an empty and impersonal gesture at best. What is important is to make a gesture that expresses sensitivity to the patient's individual situation. Simple examples would be finding a warm sweater at a church sale or a thrift shop for a patient who lives in a shack with no heat or arranging a birthday party in clinic for a lonesome child. A patient who has no running water would be happy to receive a canned soft drink or even a jug of bottled water at each home visit. For an elderly couple on a limited income, a weekly chicken from the market might be a wonderful gift. A young child who might otherwise balk at taking bitter medicines from a stranger might look forward to having the visiting nurse read him a story for a few minutes at each visit. Incentives may be given routinely or when milestones are reached. For example, for the child mentioned above, the gift of the picture book when treatment was successfully completed would be a treasure to look forward to.

Recently we have expanded use of incentives and provide them also to selected patients whom we feel are at high risk of defaulting even though they are, for the time being, still adhering to the therapeutic contract. (This approach might be thought of as roughly analogous to that of providing AZT to HIV-positive patients *before* they have their first episode of *Pneumocystis* pneumonia.) For some, incentives can serve to maintain interest in the course of chemotherapy. For others, especially for those receiving supervised twice-weekly therapy, incentives serve as an insurance policy that they will be waiting for the nurse at the appointed time and place. For all, the incentive is experienced as an expression of care and concern by the public health nurse.

Despite our experience, we have found that there are no easily generalizable rules about incentives. The approach seems to work wonders, especially for certain nurses. One of them summarized her philosophy as follows:

> Often an incentive isn't what you buy, an incentive is what you are. If you go by with a birthday cake that you made for somebody, that says: "You're special to me." You take them to a doctor's appointment, that says: "You're worth the time." Everything that you do for a patient that says you care about them is an incentive. It's your personal involvement with that patient that's important. That is very different from having the patient walk in the clinic to pick up a package of pills. (ALASC, 1989)

Public health professionals certainly recognize that few taxpayers in most states are ready to hear that $2.30 of state monies allocated to tuberculosis control have been spent for tulip bulbs, or that 75 cents were spent for a birthday card (for a patient who has never received one). In South Carolina, therefore, money for enablers and incentives comes from our constituent chapter of the American Lung Association. Each county tuberculosis nurse receives a renewable petty-cash allowance of $25.00, which she can spend at her discretion. In other states funding has come from other sources, including churches, civic groups, and other benevolent donors or groups anxious to do "something nice" for their fellow human beings but who do not know how to go about it.

In our program, it is expected that tuberculosis nurses will understand how to use enablers and incentives just as they understand how to administer and read tuberculin skin tests, monitor patients for adverse reactions to medications, or carry out a contact investigation. The American Lung Association of South Carolina has recently published a 35-page booklet, *Enablers and Incentives*, which includes formal guidelines for their use as well as the transcript of a discussion on the subject held by 10 of our most experienced nurses (ALASC, 1989).

We believe that thoughtful use of enablers and incentives can make a substantial contribution to case holding and thus become a major tool in current tuberculosis control and eradication efforts in the United States. We are not aware of reports concerning the use of enablers and incentives from developing countries, and we recognize that their use would necessarily vary in different circumstances according to economic and cultural realities. It is even likely that in some settings, they might be considered inappropriate. Nonetheless, in settings where their use can be considered, we suggest that their impact should to be evaluated just as would any other new tuberculosis control methodology. Incentives and enablers should be evaluated in programmatic terms, regarding their effectiveness in increasing the proportion of patients who successfully complete therapy, and in economic terms, regarding their cost-effectiveness. If it can be shown that incentives and enablers provide a cost-effective method to improve case holding, then we may see them used much more widely in the future.

V. Microcomputers and Evaluation of Case Holding

Modern tuberculosis programs require accurate current information to assist decision making and evaluation at all levels. Fortunately, progress made in the field of electronics during the past decade has led to microcomputer technologies that are easy to use, affordable, and of immense value to communicable disease control programs.

The practical consequence of this technology is that it has now become relatively easy to computerize tuberculosis case registries. Microcomputer tuberculosis registries are usually run on IBM-compatible personal computers. In the United States, this type of hardware has become a de facto standard for city, county, state, and federal public health programs. In the international arena, WHO, UNICEF, and ministries of health in most developing countries also depend primarily on IBM-compatible systems.

A tuberculosis registry software package called TBDS (Tuberculosis Data Base System) has recently been developed by the Division of Tuberculosis Elimination of the CDC. TBDS is based on Clipper, which produces compiled DBASE-compatible code and which maintains data in a the widely used DBF file format.

The TBDS permits computerization of the individual tuberculosis case report form currently used by all 50 states to report new cases to the CDC. Data concerning additional laboratory reports and radiological examinations can also be entered. Single computerized records can be used as a tool for making clinical decisions concerning individual patients in much the same way as a paper clinical chart is currently used. The real interest for a TBCP, however, lies in the software technology, which permits a rapid review of totality of the computerized records. It thus becomes possible for program managers to obtain essentially instantly and on demand a variety of useful reports such as lists of delinquent patients, statistical summaries of various types, and program evaluation indices.

On the international scene, the software of choice for computerized tuberculosis case registries is likely to become EPI INFO, a program that has been developed CDC and WHO (Dean et al., 1990). EPI INFO has been translated into French and Arabic, and printed guides are available in several other languages as well. Of special interest for the international community is the fact that EPI INFO lies in the public domain. It may thus be legally and freely copied and distributed. (Information about ordering EPI INFO is given in Appendix II.)

On screen, a simple EPI INFO entry form for use in a developing country might look something like this:

TUBERCULOSIS REGISTER

DATE REG: CASE No: SEX: AGE:

ADDR1:
ADDR2:
CITY: PROVINCE:

HLTH UNIT: DATE BEG RX: REGIMEN: PT CATEG:

SUPTUM EXAMINATIONS   SMEARS   CULTURES
                        SM MO 0:   CLT MO 0:
                        SM MO 2:   CLT MO 2:
                        SM MO 5:
                        SM MO 8:   CLT MO 8:
                        SM M 12:

DATE END RX: OUTCOME:
REMARKS:

The names and meanings for the computerized variables that would be produced from this questionnaire are shown in Table 3. Although this data entry screen appears simple, it includes the essential information suggested by the *Tuberculosis Guide for High Prevalence Countries* published by the International Union Against Tuberculosis and Lung Disease (IUATLD).

As EPI INFO was written with an eye toward the needs of practical field epidemiology and of disease control surveillance systems, it incorporates routines that permit the user, by means of extremely simple and absolutely intuitive commands (see Table 4) to obtain summary information in the form of line listings, frequency distributions, cross-tables, comparisons of means and proportions, and pie, bar, histogram, and line graphics. Analyses can easily be carried out either for all records or for any user-selected subset thereof. EPI INFO can analyze datasets maintained in its own REC file format, but can also read

DBASE DBF files directly. This means that study data entered and maintained in DBASE can be analyzed directly with EPI INFO. In the context of this chapter, the best example of EPI INFO's utility is that it would permit a program director to have instant information about the success of his program in case holding. For example, if the variable OUTCOME in the registry form shown above were coded with values for the various possible outcomes for patients registered in treatment centers, the two-word command FREQ OUTCOME could give a summary table containing the frequency of outcomes that looked like this:

One-Year Posttreatment Outcome Evaluation for Patients Enrolled in the Utaral Tuberculosis Treatment Center Between Jan. 1, 1993, and March 31, 1993

OUTCOME	Freq	Percent	Cum.
CURED BACT NEGATIVE	115	76.7%	76.7%
RX COMPLETED NO BACT	10	6.7%	83.4%
DIED	5	3.3%	86.7%
BACT POSITIVE	12	8.0%	94.7%
DEFAULTED	5	3.3%	98.0%
TRANSFERRED OUT	3	2.0%	100.0%
Total	150	100.0%	

It would be an easy task to evaluate the quality of case holding for specific subgroups, such as for patients belonging to different age groups, residing in different cities, or being followed at different health centers. If the program had the policy of assigning primary responsibility for each case to a single person, it would even be possible to evaluate the case-holding success of individual staff members!

VI. Conclusion

To have an impact on the epidemiology of tuberculosis in a population, tuberculosis control programs must not only detect incident cases of pulmonary tuberculosis, but must hold on to each case until a proper chemotherapy regimen has cured the patient. Currently most tuberculosis programs have deficiencies in their case-holding activities. Improvements can be made through a variety of measures, including (1) increased sensitivity and training regarding often overlooked psychological and behavioral issues, (2) expanded use of directly observed therapy so that as many patients as possible will take every dose of

Table 3 Variables Computerized in a Hypothetical EPI INFO–based Tuberculosis Registry for a Developing Country

Variable name	Meaning
DATEREG	Date patient was registered
CASENO	Case number
SEX	Sex
AGE	Age
ADDR1	First line of address
ADDR2	Second line of address
CITY	City
PROVINCE	Province
HLTHUNIT	Name of the health unit
DATEBEGRX	Date of beginning of treatment
REGIMEN	Regimen used (coded by number)
PTCATEG	Patient category (coded by number)
SMMO0	Smear at month 0 (pretreatment)
CLTMO0	Culture at month 0 (pretreatment)
SMMO2	Smear after 2 months
CLTMO2	Culture after 2 months
SMMO5	Smear after 5 months
SMMO8	Smear after 8 months
CLTMO8	Culture after 8 months
SMM12	Smear after 12 months
DATEENDRX	Date of end of therapy
OUTCOME	Outcome of treatment (coded by number)
REMARKS	Miscellaneous remarks

medication under direct supervision, (3) application of modern microcomputer technology at all program levels to provide timely evaluation of case-holding and other priority program activities.

Appendix I: References Regarding Methods of Testing for Presence of Antituberculous Drugs or Their Metabolites in Urine

Burkhardt, K. R., and Nel, E. E. (1990). Monitoring regularity of drug intake in tuberculosis patients by means of simple urine tests. *S. Afr. Med. J.* **57**:981–985.

Eidus, L., and Ling, G. M. (1969). Tests for the detection of antituberculous drugs or their metabolites in the urine. *WHO Tech. Bull.* **76**:1–9.

Table 4 Selected EPI INFO Commands as They Would Be Used to Obtain Summary Information from a Computerized Tuberculosis Case Registry

Command	Meaning
LIST NAME AGE SEX	Obtain a line listing of all patients showing their name, age, and sex
SELECT AGE<5	Select only those patients whose age is less than 5
SORT CITY	Sort all cases according to the name of the city in which they live
FREQ SMMO2	Obtain a frequency distribution of results of smears obtained at the end of 2 months of therapy
HISTOGRAM AGE	Produce a histogram showing the age distribution of patients
PIE PROVINCE	Create a pie chart showing distribution of patients according to province
TABLES OUTCOME SEX	Obtain a cross-table showing outcome of therapy according to sex (chi-square test is also automatically performed)

Ellard, G. A., and Greenfield, C. A. (1977). Sensitive urine test for monitoring the ingestion of isoniazid. *J. Clin. Pathol.*, **30**:84–87.

Henderson, W. T. (1986). The development and use of the Potts-Cozart tube test for the detection of isoniazid (IHN) metabolites in urine. *J. Arkansas Med. Soc.* **82**(10):445–446.

Kilburn, J. O., Beam, R. E., David, H. L. Sanches, E., Corpe, R. F., and Dunn, R. F. (1972). Reagent impregnated paper strip for detection of metabolic products of isoniazid in urine. *Am. Rev. Respir. Dis.* **106**:923–924.

Kirsten, C., Armstrong, C., and Gatner, E. (1980). A simple test for the identification of ethambutol in urine. *S. Afr. Med. J.* **58**:992, 1980.

Appendix II: Ordering EPI INFO

In the United States, EPI INFO may be ordered through:

USD Incorporated
2075A West Park Place
Stone Mountain, GA 30087
Tel: (404)-469-4098

A French version may be ordered through:

Editions de l'ENSP
Ave Professeur Leon Bernard
35043 Rennes Cedex
France

The program is also distributed by WHO through:

Distribution and Sales
World Health Organization
1211 Geneva 27
Switzerland

References

Addington, W. (1979). Patient compliance: the most serious remaining problem in the control of tuberculosis in the United States. *Chest* **76**(6) (Suppl):741–743.

ALASC (1989). *Using Incentives and Enablers in The Tuberculosis Control Program* (booklet). American Lung Association of South Carolina, Columbia, SC.

Centers for Disease Control (1989a). A strategic plan for the elimination of tuberculosis in the United States. *MMWR* (Suppl 38):S-3.

Centers for Disease Control (1989b). *Improving Patient Compliance in Tuberculosis Treatment Programs*. Division of Tuberculosis Elimination.

Centers for Disease Control (1990). Use of preventive therapy for tuberculous infection in the United States. *MMWR* RR-8.

Centers for Disease Control (1991a). Nosocomial transmission of multidrug-resistant tuberculosis among HIV infected persons—Florida and New York, 1988–1991. *MMWR* **40**:585–591.

Centers for Disease Control (1991b). Unpublished data, Division of Tuberculosis Elimination, CDC.

Chaulet, P. (1983). *Treatment of Tuberculosis: Case Holding Until Cure*. WHO/TB/83.141. World Health Organization, Geneva.

Daley, C., Small, P., Schechter, G., Schoolnik, G., McAdam, R., Jacobs, W., and Hopewell, P. (1992). An outbreak of tuberculosis with accelerated progression among persons infected with the human immunodeficiency virus. *N. Engl. J. Med.* **326**:231–235.

Dean. A., Dean, J., Burton, A., and Dicker, R. (1990). EPI INFO, Version 5: a word processing data base, and statistics program for epidemiology on microcomputers. USD Inc., Stone Mountain, GA.

Dudley, D. (1979). Why patients don't take pills. *Chest* **76**(6)(Suppl):744–749.

Edlin, B., Tokars, J., Grieco, M., Crawford, J., Williams, J., Sordillo, E., Ong, K., Kilburn, J., Dooley, S., Castro, K., Jarvis, W., and Holmberg, S. (1992). An outbreak of multidrug-resistant tuberculosis among hospitalized patients with the acquired immunodeficiency syndrome. *N. Engl. J. Med.* **326**:1514–1521.

Fox. W. (1983a). Compliance of patients and physicians: experience and lessons from tuberculosis. I. *Br. Med. J.* **287**:33.

Fox, W. (1983b). Compliance of patients and physicians: experience and lessons from tuberculosis. II. *Br. Med. J.* **287**:101.

Geisler, P., Nelson, K., and Crispen, R. (1987). Tuberculosis in physicians. Compliance with preventive measures. *Am. Rev. Respir. Dis.* **135**:3.

IUATLD. *Tuberculosis Guide for High Prevalence Countries*, 2nd ed. International Union Against Tuberculosis and Lung Disease, Paris.

Miller, B., and Snider, D. (1987). Physician noncompliance with tuberculosis preventive measures. *Am. Rev. Respir. Dis.* **135**:1.

Sbarbaro, J., Barlow, P., and Craig, M. (1974). Intermittent chemotherapy for adults with tuberculosis. *Am. Rev. Respir. Dis.* **110**:374.

Sbarbaro, J. (1979). Compliance: inducements and enforcements. *Chest*, **76**(6)(Suppl):750–756.

Sbarbaro, J. (1990). The patient-physician relationship: compliance revisited. *Ann. Allergy* **64**:325.

WHO (1991). Resolutions of the 44th World Health Assembly. World Health Organization, Geneva.

11

The Treatment of Tuberculosis

RICHARD J. O'BRIEN

Tuberculosis Programme
World Health Organization
Geneva, Switzerland

I. Introduction

There are few diseases of such global importance for which the standards of treatment have been so rigorously defined and recommendations so universally accepted as for tuberculosis. A large number of randomized, controlled clinical trials conducted over the past four decades first established the effectiveness of chemotherapy for tuberculosis and then refined therapy regimens leading to what is generally know as "short-course" chemotherapy, the modern standard used throughout the world (D'Esopo, 1982). Furthermore, there is virtual international consensus concerning appropriate therapy, so that nearly uniform treatment guidelines have been issued by expert groups in developed countries with low rates of tuberculosis such as the United States (American Thoracic Society, 1986) and Great Britain (British Thoracic Society, 1990) and by international bodies such as the World Health Organization (WHO Tuberculosis Unit, 1991) and the International Union Against Tuberculosis and Lung Disease (IUATLD, 1988), groups targeting their recommendations toward developing countries where tuberculosis is most prevalent.

This chapter will summarize the theoretical basis for chemotherapy, review in some detail the drugs used for the treatment of tuberculosis, provide specific recommendations on treatment regimens and monitoring response to treatment, give guidelines on the treatment of tuberculosis in special clinical situations, and conclude with a section on the problem of nonadherence with therapy.

II. Theoretical Basis for Chemotherapy

With the first randomized clinical trials of tuberculosis therapy to assess the efficacy of streptomycin, two important principles of treatment were discovered. The first principle is that successful therapy requires the administration of a minimum of two drugs to which the organisms are susceptible; at least one of these drugs should be bactericidal. Because of the spontaneous emergence of drug resistance in a small number of tubercle bacilli, monotherapy with even the most potent bactericidal drug (e.g., isoniazid) may select a resistant bacterial population and lead to treatment failure with the development of acquired drug resistance (Ferebee et al., 1960). This is more likely in persons having forms of disease in which the bacterial population is large, e.g., cavitary pulmonary tuberculosis. This occurs because a small number of tubercle bacilli spontaneously develop drug resistance (e.g., estimated to be 1 organism per 1,000,000 bacilli for isoniazid). Because the probability that a single bacillus may develop spontaneous resistance to two drugs is the product of the probabilities of resistance to the individual drugs, the use of two active drugs generally prevents the development of acquired resistance. The number of bacilli required to produce a spontaneous mutant resistant to two drugs is much larger than the bacterial population in most patients with tuberculosis.

Tuberculosis drugs vary in their ability to prevent the emergence of resistance to a companion drug. Isoniazid and rifampin are the most effective agents, ethambutol and streptomycin are intermediate, and pyrazinamide and thiacetazone are the least effective (Mitchison, 1985).

The second principle of therapy is that curing tuberculosis requires treatment well after the amelioration of clinical disease. Prolonged drug therapy is required to eliminate ''persistent'' bacilli, which are comprised of a small population of metabolically inactive organisms. Inadequate treatment leads to the increased possibility of relapse months to years after apparent cure. With the treatment regimens used in the 1950s and 1960s, 18–24 months of therapy were required to ensure cure. However, with the multidrug therapy used today, the majority of tuberculosis patients successfully complete treatment in as short a period as 6 months. Failure to complete even this duration of prescribed therapy is the most common cause of relapse cases of tuberculosis.

From these principles, tuberculosis therapy may be divided into an initial bactericidal phase and a subsequent sterilizing phase. Antimycobacterial agents that are actively bactericidal may not be the most active sterilizing drugs, and those which are particularly effective in the sterilizing phase may not be the most active bactericidal agents. Studies of the early bactericidal activity of various tuberculosis drugs in newly diagnosed patients have shown that isoniazid is the most potent bactericidal drug available (Jindani et al., 1980). Laboratory studies and data from clinical trials have suggested that rifampin and pyrazinamide are the most effective sterilizing drugs (Grosset, 1978; Fox, 1979). More recent animal studies have also suggested that isoniazid may inhibit the sterilizing activities of these two drugs (LeCoeur et al., 1989).

Based on data from the laboratory and from clinical trials, Mitchison has explained the effect of drugs used in modern short-course therapy on the basis of differing actions on separate populations of tubercle bacilli (Mitchison, 1985) (Fig. 1). The largest population consists of metabolically active, extracellular organisms that are rapidly killed by bactericidal drugs, especially isoniazid. Rifampin is particularly effective against bacilli that are dormant and undergo periodic bursts of activity. A third population consists of those organisms in an acid environment (e.g., intracellular bacilli and those in caseous material), which are particularly susceptible to the action of pyrazinamide. Finally, there

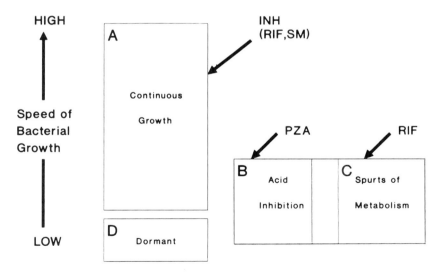

Figure 1 Special bacterial populations hypothesis. Parts of the bacterial population at the start of treatment that are killed by particular drugs: (A) actively growing organisms killed mainly by isoniazid, (B) semidormant organisms inhibited by an acid environment, killed mainly by pyrazinamide, (C) semidormant organisms with spurts of active metabolism, killed preferentially by rifampin, (D) completely dormant organisms not killed by drugs. (From Mitchison, 1985.)

may be a population of metabolically inactive organisms that are not affected by any agents but are eliminated over time by the host's immune system.

III. Drugs Used for the Treatment of Tuberculosis

Drugs used for the treatment of tuberculosis are generally divided into "first-line" and "second-line" drugs. The first-line drugs—isoniazid, rifampin, pyrazinamide, ethambutol, and streptomycin—are bactericidal (except for ethambutol), are relatively free of toxicity, and are quite effective when used in combination (World Health Organization, 1991). Furthermore, they may be adapted to intermittent therapy given two or three times weekly. Table 1 lists these drugs together with dosages for adults and children and their major toxicities. Second-line agents—cycloserine, ethionamide, kanamycin, capreomycin, and para-aminosalicylic acid (PAS)—are more toxic and less well tolerated and are reserved for the treatment of drug-resistant tuberculosis. Furthermore, with the exception of PAS, their adaptation to intermittent therapy has not been well studied. Table 2 gives dosages and toxicities of these drugs. Information is also provided about thiacetazone, a drug frequently used in combination with isoniazid throughout the developing world. Finally, in this section, new drugs which have not yet been widely studied in therapy trials but which may have some usefulness, particularly in the treatment of drug-resistant tuberculosis, are mentioned.

A. First-Line Drugs

Isoniazid

Isoniazid is the most widely used of the antituberculosis drugs. It is highly active against *Mycobacterium tuberculosis*, most strains being inhibited in vitro by concentrations of 0.05–0.20 µg/ml. Absorption from the gastrointestinal tract is nearly complete, with peak blood concentrations occurring 1–2 hr after administration. A usual dose of 3–5 mg/kg body weight produces a peak concentration of approximately 5 µg/ml. The drug penetrates well into all body fluids and cavities, producing concentrations similar to those found in serum.

Hepatitis is the major toxic effect of isoniazid. In a study of 13,838 patients being given isoniazid alone as preventive therapy, the rate of hepatitis increased directly with increasing age to 65, being 0% for those younger than 20 years of age; 0.3%, for those 20–34 years of age; 1.2%, for those 35–49 years of age; 2.3% for those 50–64 years of age (Kopanoff et al., 1978). Alcohol consumption and hepatitis B infection also increase the probability of isoniazid hepatotoxicity (Cross et al., 1980; Wu et al., 1990).

Peripheral neuropathy, most likely caused by interference with metabolism of pyridoxine, is associated with isoniazid administration but is uncommon at a

Table 1 Recommended Drugs for the Initial Treatment of Tuberculosis in Children and Adults

Drug	Dosage forms	Daily dose[a]		Maximal daily dose in children and adults	Twice-weekly dose	
		Children	Adults		Children	Adults
Isoniazid[d]	Tablets: 100mg, 300 mg[b]; Syrup: 50 mg/ml; Vials: 1 g	10–15 mg/kg PO or IM	5 mg/kg PO or IM	300 mg	20–40 mg/kg Max. 900 mg	15 mg/kg Max. 900 mg
Rifampin[d]	Capsules: 150 mg, 300 mg[b]; Syrup: formulated from capsules 10 mg/ml	10–20 mg/kg PO	10 mg/kg PO	600 mg	10–20 mg/kg Max. 600 mg	10 mg/kg Max. 600 mg
Pyrazinamide[d]	Tablets: 500 mg	20–40 mg/kg PO	15–30 mg/kg PO	2 g	50–70 mg/kg	50–70 mg/kg
Streptomycin	Vials: 1 g, 4 g	20–40 mg/kg IM	15 mg/kg[c] IM	1 g[c]	20–40 mg/kg IM	25–30 mg/kg IM
Ethambutol	Tablets: 100 mg, 400 mg	15–25 mg/kg PO	15–25 mg/kg PO	2.5 g	50 mg/kg	50 mg/kg

[a]Doses based on weight should be adjusted as weight changes.
[b]Isoniazid and rifampin are available as a combination capsule containing 150 mg of isoniazid and 300 mg of rifampin.
[c]In persons older than 60 years, the daily dose of streptomycin should be limited to 10 mg/kg, with a maximal dose of 750 mg.
[d]Fixed-dose combinations of isoniazid, rifampin, and pyrazinamide are available and should be used if of demonstrated bioavailability.
PO = perorally; IM = intramuscularly.
Source: American Thoracic Society (1986).

Table 2 Second-Line Antituberculosis Drugs[a]

Drug	Dosage forms	Daily dose in children and adults[b]	Maximal daily dose in children and adults	Major adverse reactions	Recommended regular monitoring
Capreomycin	Vials: 1 g	15–30 mg/kg IM	1 g	Auditory, vestibular, and renal toxicity	Vestibular function, audiometry, blood urea nitrogen, and creatinine
Kanamycin	Vials: 75 mg 500 mg 1 g	15–30 mg/kg IM	1 g	Auditory and renal toxicity, rarely vestibular toxicity	Vestibular function, audiometry, blood urea nitrogen, and creatinine
Ethionamide	Tablets: 250 mg	15–20 mg/kg PO	1 g	Gastrointestinal disturbance, hepatotoxicity, hypersensitivity	Hepatic enzymes
Para-aminosalicylic acid	Tablets: 500 mg 1 g Bulk Powder	150 mg/kg PO	12 g	Gastrointestinal disturbance, hypersensitivity, hepatotoxicity, sodium load	
Cycloserine	Capsules: 250 mg	15–20 mg/kg PO	1 g	Psychosis, convulsions, rash	Assessment of mental status

[a]These drugs are more difficult to use than drugs listed in Table 1. They should be used only when necessary and should be given and monitored by health providers experienced in their use.
[b]Doses based on weight should be adjusted as weight changes.
For definition of abbreviations, see Table 1.
Source: American Thoracic Society (1986).

dose of 5 mg/kg/day. In persons with conditions in which neuropathy is common (diabetes, uremia, alcoholism, malnutrition), pyridoxine, at a dose of 10 mg/day, should be given with isoniazid (Snider, 1980). It is also advisable to give pyridoxine with isoniazid to persons who are pregnant or who have a seizure disorder. Mild central nervous system effects are common with isoniazid and may necessitate adjustments in the timing of administration of the drug to enhance adherence.

The interaction of isoniazid and phenytoin increases the serum concentration of both drugs (Miller et al., 1979). When these drugs are given concomitantly, the serum level of phenytoin should be monitored, and the phenytoin dosage decreased if necessary.

Rifampin

Rifampin is bactericidal for *M. tuberculosis*. It is readily absorbed from the gastrointestinal tract, with peak serum concentrations of 6–7 µg/ml occurring 1.5–2 hr after ingestion. Most strains of *M. tuberculosis* are inhibited in vitro by concentrations of 0.5 µg/ml. Although approximately 75% of the drug is protein-bound, it penetrates well into tissues and cells. Penetration through noninflamed meninges is poor, but therapeutic concentrations are achieved in cerebrospinal fluid when the meninges are inflamed.

The most common adverse reaction to rifampin is gastrointestinal upset. Other reactions include pruritus, skin eruptions, and hepatitis (Grosset and Leventis, 1983). Mild jaundice in the absence of evidence of hepatocellular damage may also occur. Rarely, thrombocytopenia, hemolytic anemia, and acute renal failure occur, the latter complications being more frequent when rifampin is given intermittently and in doses exceeding 10 mg/kg. Intermittent administration (particularly once weekly) may also be associated with an influenza-like syndrome. However, these reactions are uncommon at the recommended dose of 10 mg/kg/day up to a maximum dose of 600 mg. In general, the frequency of these reactions is quite low.

Because rifampin induces hepatic microsomal enzymes, it may accelerate clearance of drugs metabolized by the liver. These include methadone, coumadin derivatives, glucocorticoids, estrogens, sulfonylureas, digitoxin, antiarrhythmic agents (quinidine, verapamil, mexiletine), theophylline, anticonvulsants, ketoconazole, and cyclosporin (Baciewicz et al., 1987). By accelerating estrogen metabolism, rifampin may interfere with the effectiveness of oral contraceptives. Rifampin may also precipitate Addisonian crisis among those with marginal adrenal function (Wilkins et al., 1989)

Rifampin is excreted in urine, tears, sweat, and other body fluids, and it colors them orange. Patients should be advised of discoloration of body fluids and of possible permanent discoloration of soft contact lenses.

Pyrazinamide

Pyrazinamide is bactericidal for *M. tuberculosis* in an acid environment. The drug is active against organisms in macrophages, presumably because of the acid environment within the cell. Absorption from the gastrointestinal tract is nearly complete, with peak serum concentrations occurring approximately 2 hr after ingestion. Serum concentrations generally range from 30 to 50 μg/ml with doses of 20–25 mg/kg. Pyrazinamide penetrates well into most tissues, including the cerebrospinal fluid. At a pH of 5.5, the minimal inhibitory concentration of pyrazinamide for *M. tuberculosis* is 20 μg/ml.

The most important adverse reaction to pyrazinamide is liver injury, and high rates of serious hepatoxicity were seen when the drug was first introduced in the United States in the 1950s and given in doses of 50 mg/kg/day. However, there does not appear to be a significant increase in hepatotoxicity when pyrazinamide in a dose of 15–30 mg/kg is added to a regimen of isoniazid and rifampin and administered only during the initial 2 months of therapy (Girling, 1978).

Pyrazinamide is metabolized to pyrazinoic acid, which inhibits renal secretion of uric acid. Thus, hyperuricemia occurs frequently, occasionally accompanied by arthralgia; however, acute gout is uncommon. Skin rash and gastrointestinal intolerance are also seen.

Ethambutol

Ethambutol in usual doses is generally considered to have a bacteriostatic effect on *M. tuberculosis*. It may have a bactericidal effect when given in the higher dosage used for intermittent therapy. Peak plasma concentrations occur 2–4 hr after ingestion. With doses of 15 mg/kg, the peak concentration is approximately 4 μg/ml. In persons with normal renal function, serum half-life is approximately 4 hr. The half-life is prolonged and the drug accumulates in persons with renal insufficiency. Ethambutol is water-soluble with a limited volume of distribution. Therefore, for grossly overweight persons, it is appropriate to use ideal body weight to calculate drug dosage. Some authorities recommend adding 20% of obese weight (weight over ideal body weight) to the ideal body weight for this calculation (Peloquin, C., personal communication).

Most strains of *M. tuberculosis* are inhibited in vitro by concentrations of the drug in a range from 1 to 5 μg/ml. Cerebrospinal fluid concentrations of ethambutol are low even in the presence of meningeal inflammation, averaging 1–2 μg/ml after a dose of 25 mg/kg.

Retrobulbar neuritis is the most frequent and serious adverse effect of ethambutol (Citron and Thomas, 1986). Symptoms include blurred vision, central scotomata, and red-green color blindness. This complication is dose-related, occurring in less than 1% of persons given a daily dose of 15 mg/kg and increasing with a daily dose of 25 mg/kg. The frequency of ocular effects is increased in patients with renal failure, presumably because of increased serum concentrations of the drug. Visual symptoms commonly precede a measurable decreased visual acuity. Patients should be informed to report any change in vision. In children who are too young for assessment of visual acuity and red-green color discrimination, ethambutol should be used with particular caution, and consideration should be given to the use of possible alternative drugs.

Streptomycin

Streptomycin is bactericidal in an alkaline environment. Because the drug is not absorbed from the gut, it must be given parenterally. Peak serum concentrations occur approximately 1 hr after an intramuscular dose. With a dose of 15 mg/kg, the peak concentration is in the range of 40 μg/ml. Most strains of *M. tuberculosis* are inhibited in vitro at a concentration of 8 μg/ml. The half-life in blood is approximately 5 hr. Excretion is almost entirely renal. The drug should be used in reduced dosage and with extreme caution in patients with renal insufficiency. The drug has good tissue penetration, but because of poor cell membrane penetration, intracellular concentration is low. The drug enters the cerebrospinal fluid only in the presence of meningeal inflammation.

The most common serious adverse effect of streptomycin is ototoxicity. This usually results in vertigo, but hearing loss may also occur. Ototoxicity, often irreversible, is more likely if other ototoxic drugs are given concomitantly. Streptomycin has less adverse effect on the kidneys than kanamycin and capreomycin, but nephrotoxicity occasionally occurs; it is usually reversible after the drug has been discontinued. Renal toxicity may be increased in patients with preexisting renal insufficiency or with simultaneous use of other nephrotoxic drugs. The risks of ototoxicity and nephrotoxicity are related both to cumulative dose and to peak serum concentrations and are more common in persons older than 60 years of age. A total dose of more than 120 g should not be given unless other therapeutic options are not available.

B. Second-Line Drugs

Cycloserine

Cycloserine, a broad-spectrum antibiotic produced by a strain of *Streptomyces*, is used almost exclusively for the treatment of drug-resistant tuberculosis and susceptible strains of nontuberculous mycobacteria. The drug is readily absorbed from the gastrointestinal tract with peak serum levels at 4–8 hr; serum concentration following conventional twice-daily doses are generally maintained at 25–30 μg/ml, somewhat in excess of the usual minimal inhibitory concentration (MIC) for susceptible strains of *M. tuberculosis*. The drug penetrates well into most tissues and fluids, including cerebrospinal fluid and breast milk, with concentrations similar to serum levels. Excretion is primarily by the renal route.

The most frequent and serious adverse reactions to cycloserine are dose-related central nervous system effects, such as depression, psychosis, seizures, headache, peripheral neuropathy, and vertigo. These effects are more common in patients receiving doses in excess of 500 mg/day and in alcoholic patients. Anticonvulsant drugs or sedatives may be effective in controlling these symptoms.

The drug is given orally in divided doses, with a total dose of 500 mg to 1 g/day. It is advisable, especially for patients receiving more than 500 mg/day and those with impaired renal clearance, to monitor blood levels, with the dosage adjusted to keep levels below 30 µg/ml.

Ethionamide

Ethionamide is bacteriostatic against *M. tuberculosis* and is used for the treatment of drug-resistant disease. Ethionamide is readily absorbed from the gastrointestinal tract with peak serum level of 9 µg/ml 3 hr after ingestion of a 1-g dose. However, because of intolerance, patients are generally not able to ingest more than 500 mg at a single time. The drug is widely distributed throughout the body, with tissue levels and cerebrospinal fluid levels approximating those in the serum.

The most common adverse reaction is gastrointestinal intolerance, with abdominal pain, nausea, and vomiting. The drug is also hepatotoxic and teratogenic in animals. Management of diabetes mellitus may be more difficult in diabetic patients receiving the drug. The drug may also potentiate the central nervous system effects of cycloserine.

The average adult dose is 500 mg to 1 g/day in divided doses, with the total dose commonly limited by gastrointestinal side effects. Some authorities have found that administration by rectal suppository reduces these side effects, but the drug is not approved for administration by this route. Children tolerate the drug much better than adults at the usual pediatric dose of 15–20 mg/kg/day.

Capreomycin

Capreomycin is a polypeptide antibiotic isolated from *Streptomyces capreolus*. The drug is not absorbed from the gastrointestinal tract and must be given parenterally. Excretion is primarily renal. Peak serum levels averaging 30 µg/ml occur 1–2 hr following intramuscular administration of 1 g in adults; this is well in excess of the usual MIC of susceptible strains of *M. tuberculosis*. Most streptomycin-resistant strains of *M. tuberculosis* are susceptible to capreomycin.

Nephrotoxicity is the most common serious side effect seen with administration of this drug; ototoxicity manifested by hearing loss occurs less frequently.

The usual adult dose of capreomycin is 1 g/day, not exceeding 20 mg/kg/day, by intramuscular injection. The drug is usually given daily during the first

2–4 months of treatment and then reduced to two to three times weekly. The dosage must be reduced in patients with renal impairment. Monitoring of renal function should be done periodically during treatment.

Kanamycin (and Amikacin)

Kanamycin is an aminoglycoside antibiotic produced by *Streptomyces kanamyceticus*. It also must be administered parenterally. Cross-resistance with capreomycin to *M. tuberculosis* is common. The major adverse effects are nephrotoxicity, ototoxicity, and neuromuscular blockade. The usual adult dosage is 15 mg/kg/day (with a maximum dose of 1 g/day), given either intramuscularly or intravenously. The later route of administration may be useful for patients who cannot receive intramuscular therapy and must be treated with an aminoglycoside antibiotic. The same precautions relating to the use of capreomycin must also be exercised when kanamycin is administered.

Amikacin has also achieved the status of a second-line antimycobacterial drug, commonly used for the treatment of disseminated *M. avium* complex infections in patients with human immunodeficiency virus (HIV) infection. However, it has not been evaluated in the treatment of tuberculosis and has no particular advantage over capreomycin or kanamycin for the treatment of streptomycin-resistant tuberculosis.

Para-aminosalicylic Acid

PAS was the first drug used orally for the treatment of tuberculosis. It is bacteriostatic against *M. tuberculosis* and its primary use has been to prevent the emergence of drug resistance when administered with other agents. However, with the discovery of other antimycobacterial drugs, it is much less frequently used, and it has become difficult to obtain supplies of the drug in the United States.

The drug is well absorbed orally, with a peak serum level of 75 μg/ml (well in excess of the MICs of sensitive strains) 1–2 hr following a dose of 4 g. Administration of PAS is associated with a high frequency of gastrointestinal upset, and hypersensitivity reactions occur in 5–10% of patients. In addition, the usual dose of 10–12 g/day requires ingestion of 20–24 tablets.

Thiacetazone

Thiacetazone is bacteriostatic and may help prevent the emergence of resistance to other drugs, such as isoniazid. It is inexpensive, but its usefulness is limited to developing countries with insufficient resources to provide more effective drugs. It is not available in the United States or Canada.

Thiacetazone is always given with isoniazid at a dose of 2.5 mg/kg (up to 150 mg) for both adults and children. Intermittent doses have not been established. Gastrointestinal intolerance is the most common side effect. Vestibular disturbances are also common, and the drug potentiates streptomycin ototoxicity. Rashes, often trivial, also occur frequently. However, more severe hypersensitivity reactions, including exfoliative dermatitis, Stevens-Johnson syndrome, and toxic epidermal necrolysis with death, do occur. Because skin pathology appears to be especially common in HIV-infected patients, thiacetazone should not be used in persons known to be (or suspected of being) infected with HIV (World Health Organization, 1992). Other serious toxicities include hepatitis and bone marrow depression with thrombocytopenia and agranulocytosis. Unacceptably high rates of toxicity have been reported from Asian countries, although no clear racial difference in tolerance has been demonstrated.

C. New Drugs

Quinolones: Ciprofloxacin and Ofloxacin

Many of the new 4-fluoroquinolone antibiotics have in vitro activity against *M. tuberculosis*; of those currently marketed, ciprofloxacin and ofloxacin are most active (Leysen et al., 1989). These agents act by inhibiting DNA gyrase, and there is no cross-resistance with other antimycobacterial drugs. However, the treatment of mycobacterial diseases, including tuberculosis, is not among the approved indications for ciprofloxacin or ofloxacin, and no randomized clinical trials have demonstrated their efficacy in tuberculosis. Based on limited clinical data, these drugs' effects are limited and resistance to quinolones develops frequently.

Ciprofloxacin and ofloxacin are well absorbed orally, with peak serum levels 1–2 hr following administration. Although food does not interfere with absorption, time-to-peak concentrations are lowered by meals. Therefore, it is preferable to give these drugs on an empty stomach. Antacids containing aluminum hydroxide or magnesium hydroxide substantially reduce absorption and should not be given concomitantly.

The elimination of ofloxacin is impaired in patients with renal failure, and the drug is not dialyzable. Therefore, reduced dosages should be used in patients with a creatinine clearance of 50 ml/min or less. On the other hand, ciprofloxacin is eliminated in part by nonrenal routes, so it may be given in the usual dosage to patients with mild renal failure. Unlike ofloxacin, ciprofloxacin prolongs the elimination half-life of theophylline, leading to theophylline toxicity when both drugs are used.

These drugs should be restricted to use in patients with multidrug-resistant tuberculosis for which there are no other satisfactory treatment options, including in the treatment regimen at least two other drugs to which the organism is susceptible, and directly supervising treatment. Ofloxacin's pharmacokinetic characteristics and antimycobacterial activity suggest that it would be a more effective antituberculosis drug than ciprofloxacin. Therefore, ofloxacin may be preferable to ciprofloxacin for the treatment of patients with multidrug-resistant tuberculosis.

When ofloxacin is used to treat tuberculosis, the maximal adult dosage (400 mg twice daily) is preferred. For ciprofloxacin, the maximal adult dose of 750 mg twice daily is recommended. These drugs are generally well tolerated. Of reported side effects, gastrointestinal complaints are most frequent. Patients experiencing gastric upset can take the drug with food. Hypersensitivity reactions and mild central nervous symptoms are less frequently associated.

Rifamycin Derivatives

Several new derivatives of rifamycin B have been developed and are of potential usefulness in treating patients with tuberculosis. Most of these derivatives have longer half-lives than rifampin and, on an equimolar basis, are more active against *M. tuberculosis* than is rifampin. Most of the derivatives show cross-resistance with rifampin, so their major usefulness may be to replace rifampin in the sterilizing phase of therapy, perhaps being given at more widely spaced intervals during intermittent therapy.

Among those compounds studied, rifabutin has been most widely tested and may soon be available (O'Brien et al., 1987). Strains of *M. tuberculosis* with low-level rifampin resistance may be susceptible to rifabutin, but the clinical efficacy of rifabutin in rifampin-resistant tuberculosis has not been clearly demonstrated. Nonetheless, it may be used when in vitro studies suggest it may be active, and other therapeutic options are limited. The usual adult dose for the drug is 300–450 mg/day in a single oral dose. Its toxicities are similar to those seen for rifampin, although dose-related leukopenia may be more commonly seen.

Macrolide Antibiotics

Several new macrolide compounds have demonstrated in vitro activity against mycobacteria. Of those available, clarithromycin has been of greatest interest because of its activity against *M. avium* complex and potential for the treatment of disseminated disease in patients with HIV infection (Dautzenberg et al., 1991). However, it does not appear to have substantial activity against *M. tuberculosis*, and no reports of the clinical use of macrolides for the treatment of tuberculosis have yet appeared.

Beta-Lactam Antibiotics

Combinations of clavulanic acid and beta-lactam antibiotics (e.g., amoxicillin) have been shown to have some in vitro activity against *M. tuberculosis*. A recent report suggests that this combination may be useful for the treatment of multidrug-resistant tuberculosis when combined with other active agents

(Nadler et al., 1991). However, none of these compounds has been evaluated clinically for the treatment of tuberculosis.

IV. Standard Treatment Regimens for Pulmonary Tuberculosis

As noted above, treatment is divided into the initial or bactericidal phase of 2 months and the continuation or sterilizing phase of 4 months or longer. In the most effective regimens, isoniazid and rifampin are given throughout for a total of 6 months. (See Table 3 for a listing of recommended treatment regimens.) Pyrazinamide is given during the initial 2-month phase, commonly with a fourth drug such as ethambutol or streptomycin (Combs et al., 1990). Because pyrazinamide has comparatively poor ability to prevent the emergence of resistance to a companion drug, the fourth drug should be given for the initial 2 months or until patients are shown to have fully susceptible tuberculosis. In those patients with little chance of having primary drug resistance, the fourth drug may be omitted from the initial phase. However, because it is difficult to precisely predict primary drug resistance, it is prudent to give routinely four drugs during the initial phase.

Treatment during the initial phase is usually daily; however, regimens given three times weekly from the start have been shown to be effective (Hong Kong Chest Service, 1987). For fully intermittent therapy, all four drugs have usually been given throughout treatment. Treatment during the continuation phase is either daily or intermittent (two or three times weekly). In all but unusual circumstances, when treatment is given intermittently, it should be directly supervised. A fully supervised regimen of only 62 doses administered under program conditions in the United States has given excellent results (Cohn et al., 1990).

When, because of cost considerations, rifampin cannot be given throughout, it may be replaced by ethambutol in the continuation phase, which is given for 6 months (i.e., 8 months total). Programs with limited resources may elect to given isoniazid and thiacetazone during the continuation phase, also for 6 months. Isoniazid given alone for 6 months during the continuation phase is also effective (East and Central African/British Medical Research Council Fifth Collaborative Study, 1986). These substitutions also help to avoid the unsupervised use of rifampin, making the development of rifampin drug resistance unlikely.

When pyrazinamide is not used, isoniazid and rifampin must be given for at least 9 months (Dutt et al., 1984). In this regimen, a third drug (e.g., ethambutol) is added to the initial phase unless there is little chance of initial drug resistance. This regimen should be given daily for at least the first month. Thereafter, therapy may be either daily or twice weekly.

Table 3 Recommended Treatment Regimens[a]

Pulmonary tuberculosis
  Preferred treatment: 2IRZ/4IR[b]
  Alternative treatment: 9IR[b]
  Variations for directly observed therapy:
    $2IRZ/4I_2R_2$[b]
    $2wkIRZS/6wkI_2R_2Z_2S_2/18wkI_2R_2$
    $6I_3R_3Z_3S_3$ or $6I_3R_3Z_3E_3$
    $2IR/7I_2R_2$[b]

Extrapulmonary tuberculosis
  Same as for pulmonary tuberculosis—corticosteroids are included for tuberculous meningitis and pericardial tuberculosis.

Tuberculosis in children
  Pulmonary tuberculosis—same as for adults, except that primary tuberculosis with hilar adenopathy may be treated with 6IR if organisms are fully susceptible.

  Extrapulmonary tuberculosis—same as for pulmonary tuberculosis, except that some authorities recommend longer periods of therapy for bone/joint, miliary, and meningeal forms.

Special clinical situations
  Tuberculosis in HIV infection—same as for pulmonary tuberculosis except that treatment period should be extended to at least 9 months and a fourth drug should be added initially for severe disease.

  Silicotuberculosis—same as for pulmonary tuberculosis except that the treatment period should be extended by at least 2 months.

Isoniazid-resistant tuberculosis
  Preferred treatment: 2REZ/7RE (if Z not used, RE must be given for a minimum of 12 months)

---

[a]Abbreviation are given for the regimens, using the letters to indicate the drugs, preceded by a number to indicate the duration in months of treatment. Subscripts are used following the individual drugs to indicate that the drugs are given intermittently during the week. When drugs are given daily, no subscripts are used. For example, $2IRZE/4I_2R_2$ is used to designate the regimen of 2 months of daily isoniazid, rifampin, pyrazinamide, and ethambutol, followed by 4 months of twice-weekly isoniazid and rifampicin.
[b]Add E (or S) until drug susceptibility results are available.

When isoniazid is omitted from the regimen (e.g., for drug intolerance or because of known isoniazid resistance), the optimal therapy is with rifampin and ethambutol throughout for 15–18 months. The addition of pyrazinamide to the initial phase of therapy permits reduction of the duration of treatment to 9–12 months (Swai et al., 1988).

When rifampin is not included in the regimen, treatment with isoniazid and ethambutol is given for 18–24 months. Generally, a third drug such as streptomycin is included in the initial phase of treatment. The addition of both streptomycin and pyrazinamide to the initial phase may permit reducing treatment to as short a period as 12 months; however, this regimen has not been evaluated in a clinical trial. Nine-month regimens of isoniazid, streptomycin, and pyrazinamide given two or three times weekly throughout have been shown to be effective (Hong Kong Tuberculosis Treatment Service, 1977).

V. Monitoring Treatment

A. Treatment Response/Treatment Failure

The best measure of response to treatment of pulmonary tuberculosis is the disappearance of tubercle bacilli from the patient's sputum. This is best assessed by serial collection of sputum for AFB microscopy and culture. Ideally, specimens are collected every 2 weeks during the initial therapy until the sputa are AFB smear negative. Thereafter, sputa should be collected monthly during the remainder of therapy or at least until sputum culture conversion is documented, and a final specimen should be obtained at the end of treatment. Sputa should also be collected at any time that treatment failure is suspected. When patients are unable to spontaneously produce sputum, induction by ultrasonic nebulization of isotonic saline is often effective.

Patients' response to therapy is also measured by change in clinical status. Cough frequency and intensity will diminish and patients will begin to regain lost weight. Failure of improvement in the clinical status may signal treatment failure or the presence of another medical condition. Serial chest radiographs are not a sensitive or efficient method of monitoring response (Lordi and Reichman, 1985). Radiographic resolution of disease is often slow, lagging behind sputum culture conversion and amelioration of clinical symptoms of tuberculosis. Furthermore, subtle changes in radiographic status may be masked by differences in radiographic technique, and occasionally disease may appear to be worsening when no change or even improvement has occurred. However, a chest radiograph should be obtained at the time of completion of therapy for future comparison.

With short-course therapy, virtually all patients with initially susceptible bacilli will have become sputum culture negative at the end of the third month of treatment. Failure of sputum culture conversion by the third month or reappearance of viable bacilli in the sputum following negativization may signal failure of therapy.

Patient nonadherence with unsupervised therapy is the most common cause of treatment failure. Patients may take medication irregularly or completely stop treatment after clinical symptoms have improved. Selective monotherapy on the part of the patient may result not only in treatment failure, but also in the development of acquired drug resistance. This may occur when a patient discontinues one of the medications because of actual or perceived toxicity without notifying the treating physician.

Physician error in prescribing inappropriate therapy (i.e., the wrong drugs or the wrong drug dosages) is also a common cause of treatment failure. An all-too-frequent example is the failure to recognize the possibility of initial drug resistance, leading the physician to prescribe a regimen in which only one of the drugs is truly active. This can have disastrous consequences, leading to the development of multdrug-resistant disease.

When failure is suspected, additional sputa should be collected for culture and drug susceptibility studies. If a change in the treatment regimen is indicated before the results of current susceptibility studies are available, it is mandatory that a minimum of two new bactericidal drugs that have not yet been used and to which the organisms were previously susceptible be given. The most common cause of continued failure and further drug resistance is the addition of a single drug to a failing regimen.

Following successful completion of therapy, routine follow-up assessments are not generally indicated. Most relapses occur during the first year following therapy. In general, patients who have received short-course therapy with isoniazid and rifampin and who had fully susceptible bacilli initially and who had an appropriate response to therapy will have susceptible organisms should they relapse (Snider et al., 1984). Thus, reinitiation of therapy with the standard 6-month regimen is sufficient for such patients. However, patients who did not receive short-course therapy or whose compliance during initial therapy was doubtful are at increased risk of having drug-resistant disease. For these patients a retreatment regimen should contain two new drugs.

B. Toxicity

Many of the commonly associated side effects have been mentioned above. In most cases of minor drug intolerance, patients can be persuaded to continue therapy, or the side effect may be managed symptomatically. Thus, antihistamines may be effective in reducing the pruritus associated with rifampin, and salicylates may control arthralgia associated with pyrazinamide. However, allopurinol is not effective in controlling pyrazinamide-induced arthralgia, because despite its effect of decreasing uric acid synthesis, it increases concentrations of pyrazinoic acid, which in turn inhibits renal urate secretion (Lacroix et al., 1988). In other cases, a temporary interruption of therapy with the gradual reintroduction of the drugs may indicate that the symptoms were not related to drug therapy.

The most common and most serious toxicity seen with tuberculosis therapy is drug-induced hepatitis. This is more frequent among older patients, among those with preexisting liver disease, and among those who abuse alcohol (Kopanoff et al., 1978; Wu et al., 1990; Cross et al., 1980). For these patients, pretreatment assessment of liver function, periodic biochemical monitoring during therapy, and monthly questioning about signs and symptoms of hepatotoxicity are indicated. For other patients at lower risk of hepatotoxicity, monthly clinical assessment is required, but routine biochemical monitoring during therapy is not needed.

Many patients with asymptomatic increases in hepatic transaminases do not require a change in therapy. For significant increases, e.g., an AST value exceeding three times the upper limit of normal, isoniazid might be temporarily discontinued and restarted when the transaminases return to normal. During this period it is not usually necessary to substitute another drug, unless the patient would otherwise receive monotherapy for more than 1 week. Should rechallenge with isoniazid result in a recurrence of the hepatitis requiring that isoniazid be permanently discontinued, ethambutol should be substituted for isoniazid. In most cases, this change would necessitate a longer period of treatment.

Rifampin alone uncommonly causes true hepatotoxicity but may potentiate isoniazid hepatotoxicity (Steele et al., 1991). However, if the picture is that of cholestatic jaundice, i.e., an increase in bilirubin with normal or minimally increased transaminases, rifampin is a likely cause. Depending on the degree of abnormality, rifampin may be stopped.

Should the clinical picture be that of more serious hepatotoxicity, e.g., high transaminases and symptoms of hepatitis, all drugs should be stopped. Should the clinical condition require continued tuberculosis treatment, ethambutol and streptomycin should be given, until the offending drug is identified by rechallenge and the other drugs added back.

When rechallenging patients who have developed hepatotoxicity, one drug should be introduced at a time. Because rifampin is uncommonly the cause of toxicity, that drug may be given first. Isoniazid may then be restarted, followed by pyrazinamide. Because pyrazinamide hepatotoxicity is dose-related, the lower range of the recommended dosage (20 mg/kg/day) should be given. During the period of rechallenge, the patient should be carefully monitored with frequent measurement of liver function.

Hypersensitivity reactions are also common. While desensitization schedules have been devised that utilize frequent and increasing doses of the offending drug, with the availability of satisfactory alternative regimens, this is infrequently required. Finally, several types of adverse reactions, such as thrombocytopenia or renal failure associated with rifampin, are absolute contraindications to resumption of rifampin therapy.

VI. Special Clinical Situations

A. Smear- and Culture-Negative Pulmonary Tuberculosis

Shorter treatment is possible in persons with sputum smear- and culture-negative pulmonary tuberculosis. Four months of isoniazid and rifampin, preferably with pyrazinamide for the first 2 months, yields results equivalent to those for patients with culture-positive disease treated with longer regimens (Hong Kong Chest Service, 1989a; Dutt et al., 1989). However, when this therapy is given, it is essential that at least three adequate pretreatment sputa are obtained and are processed in a competent mycobacteriology laboratory to ensure that the patients are indeed sputum culture negative. If any doubt exists about the adequacy of sputum examination, treatment for the standard period is more prudent.

B. Drug Resistance

In the United States, the prevalence of primary drug-resistant tuberculosis has been low, with single-drug resistance to isoniazid being most frequent (Centers for Disease Control, 1983). Recently, however, outbreaks of multidrug resistance (i.e., resistance to at least isoniazid and rifampin) have been documented in the United States, suggesting the possibility that drug resistance may increasing (Centers for Disease Control, 1991). Furthermore, in some developing countries where therapy is not supervised, high rates of primary isoniazid resistance have been found. In settings where rifampin has been indiscriminately used, primary rifampin resistance may also be quite high. This is of quite serious consequence because the loss of rifampin as an effective drug would be disastrous for tuberculosis control. Thus, when rifampin is given, its use should be supervised or the drug given as a combination tablet.

Fortunately, for the more common problem of primary isoniazid resistance, the use of short-course therapy with four drugs given initially results in the cure of the majority of patients (Mitchison and Nunn, 1986). However, when multidrug resistance is present, the response is poor, and only approximately 50% of persons with combined isoniazid-and-rifampin-resistant disease respond favorably (Iseman and Madsen, 1989).

The basic principle of managing patients whose organisms are resistant to one or more drugs is administration of at least two agents to which there is demonstrated susceptibility. For patients with isolated isoniazid resistance, supervised treatment with rifampin, ethambutol, and pyrazinamide for 2 months, followed by 7 months of rifampin and ethambutol, gives excellent results (Swai et al., 1988). When pyrazinamide is not included, treatment with rifampin and ethambutol should be given for a minimum of 12 months (Zierski, 1977). Isoniazid may be included if studies show incomplete or low-level isoniazid resistance, but there is no advantage to adding the drug if the organisms are fully resistant.

Unfortunately, good data are not available on the relative effectiveness of various regimens and the necessary duration of treatment for patients with isoniazid-and-rifampin-resistant disease. Moreover, many such patients will have resistance to other first-line drugs (e.g., ethambutol and pyrazinamide) when drug resistance is discovered. Because of the poor outcome in such cases, it is preferable to give at least three new drugs, including an injectable agent (e.g., ethionamide, cycloserine, and capreomycin), to which the organism is susceptible. Treatment should be fully supervised, and this regimen should be continued at least until bacteriological sputum conversion is documented, followed by at least 12 months of two-drug therapy. Often, a total of 24 months of therapy is given empirically. The role of new agents such as the quinolones and amikacin in the treatment of multidrug-resistant disease is not known, although these drugs are being used in such cases. Finally, surgery appears to offer considerable benefit and significantly improved cure rate for those patients in whom the bulk of disease can be resected (Iseman et al., 1990).

C. Extrapulmonary Tuberculosis

Although much less common than pulmonary tuberculosis, extrapulmonary forms of tuberculosis are increasing being seen, especially among persons with HIV infection. The basic principles that underlie the treatment of pulmonary tuberculosis also apply to extrapulmonary forms of the disease. Although there have not been the same kinds of carefully conducted controlled trials of treatment for extrapulmonary tuberculosis as for pulmonary disease, increasing clinical experience is indicating that 6- to 9-month short-course regimens are effective (Dutt and Stead, 1989).

Bacteriological evaluation of extrapulmonary tuberculosis may be limited by the relative inaccessibility of the sites of disease. Thus, response to treatment often must be judged on the basis of clinical and radiographic findings.

The use of adjunctive therapies such as surgery and corticosteroids is more commonly required in extrapulmonary tuberculosis than in pulmonary disease. Surgery may be necessary to obtain specimens for diagnosis and to treat such processes as constrictive pericarditis and spinal cord compression from Pott's disease. Corticosteroids have been beneficial in the treatment of some forms of extrapulmonary tuberculosis, such as tuberculous pericarditis and tuberculous meningitis.

Lymphatic Tuberculosis

Short-course regimens appear to be quite satisfactory for the treatment of lymphatic tuberculosis. Prospective studies of regimens of 9 months' duration (isoniazid and rifampin with initial ethambutol) in adults (British Thoracic Society Research Committee, 1988) and 6 months' duration of fully intermittent therapy in children (Jawahar et al., 1990) give excellent results compared to longer treatment with the same drugs or longer, substandard regimens. Occasionally, fresh lymph nodes will appear and previous nodes will increase in size during therapy, and a substantial proportion of patients (up to one-third) may have significant residual adenopathy following completion of treatment. Neither of these is a sign of treatment failure, and nearly all patients with residual adenopathy will continue to experience regression of nodes after completion of treatment.

Pleural Tuberculosis

Several studies have demonstrated the efficacy of 9-month short-course therapy with isoniazid and rifampin and initial ethambutol for the treatment of pleural tuberculosis (Dutt et al., 1986; Malik et al., 1987). It is believed that 6-month therapy with pyrazinamide initially would be equally efficacious. One study has demonstrated the usefulness of corticosteroids in hastening the resolution of effusion (Lee et al., 1988), but this adjunct treatment is not generally recommended.

Renal Tuberculosis

Although no randomized clinical trials of short-course therapy for genitourinary tuberculosis have been reported, studies have shown that most patients with this form of disease respond well to regimens as short as 4 months in duration (Gow and Barbosa, 1984). However, most authorities recommend the use of standard 6- to 9-month regimens. Surgical intervention is frequently necessary with advanced disease, and consultation with a urological specialist during therapy is recommended.

Bone and Joint Tuberculosis

A number of studies have shown that short-course treatment of 6–9 months' duration is quite effective in the treatment of bone and joint tuberculosis (Working Group on Osteo-articular Tuberculosis in Algeria, 1988). Spinal involvement (Pott's disease), especially in adults, may require surgical intervention for optimal treatment, although the need for surgical treatment and immobilization appears to be infrequent (Medical Research Council Working Party on Tuberculosis of the Spine, 1986).

Meningeal Tuberculosis

A number of prospective studies have shown that short-course regimens of 6–12 months' duration are effective for the treatment of tuberculous meningitis (Ramachandran et al., 1986; Alarcon et al., 1990), although one recent report has called into question the adequacy of short-course therapy (Goel et al., 1990). Consequently, some authorities recommend a longer period of treatment, such as 12 months. Recent studies have also indicated significant benefit from the inclusion of corticosteroids during the initial phase of treatment (Girgis et al., 1991). Prognosis appears most closely related to the stage of central nervous system dysfunction at the time treatment is initiated, with those patients with stage III disease experiencing high rates of mortality and neurological dysfunction. Treatment with corticosteroids during the initial phase of therapy appears to improve results, especially for those with disease stages I and II.

Miliary Tuberculosis

Although there are several recent retrospective reports in the literature (Maartens et al., 1990; Kim et al., 1990), no prospective assessment of treatment for miliary tuberculosis has been conducted. In the pre-AIDS era, most cases of miliary tuberculosis occurred among the elderly and those with immunosuppression related to medical conditions and/or immunosuppressive drug therapy. Diagnosis may be difficult and mortality is high. An aggressive approach to diagnosis and early presumptive treatment with standard short-course regimen are recommended. The value of initial streptomycin has been suggested but is not proven (Kim et al., 1990).

Pericardial Tuberculosis

Uncommon in the pre-AIDS era, this form of extrapulmonary tuberculosis is now frequently observed among persons with HIV infection. Although no prospective comparison of various therapeutic regimens has been reported, a recent study confirms the benefits of adjunct corticosteroid treatment in reducing death and the need for surgical intervention (Strang et al., 1987). In this study all patients were given standard short-course tuberculosis therapy.

D. Tuberculosis in Children

The basic principles of treatment of tuberculosis in children are essentially the same as for adults. Nine-month regimens containing isoniazid and rifampin have been demonstrated to have a high rate of success in children (Abernathy et al., 1983), and hilar adenopathy in children has been successfully treated with only 6 months of this combination (Jacobs and Abernathy, 1985). More recent studies of 6-month regimens containing pyrazinamide have also produced excellent results with minimal toxicity (Starke, 1990). Therefore, the short-course regimens recommended for adults are also the regimens of choice for children with pulmonary tuberculosis. However, some authorities recommend longer periods of therapy for bone and joint, miliary, and meningeal forms of disease (American Academy of Pediatrics, 1992).

E. Complicating Medical Conditions

HIV Infection

HIV infection has been shown to be among the most potent factors facilitating the progression of tuberculosis infection to active tuberculosis. The risk of tuberculosis among persons with both HIV and tuberculous infections was estimated to be 15% in a 2-year period (Selwyn et al., 1989), and this association has been a prime factor in the increase in tuberculosis in the United States beginning in 1986.

Tuberculosis in HIV-infected persons usually precedes or coincides with the diagnosis of AIDS but may occur at any time during the course of HIV disease. Most clinical series of HIV-infected tuberculosis patients have indicated that extrapulmonary tuberculosis and atypical forms of pulmonary disease (e.g., hilar adenopathy, middle- and lower-zone infiltrates without cavitary formation) are more common than among persons without HIV infection (Sunderam et al., 1986). HIV-infected persons with pulmonary tuberculosis may be as infectious as similar patients without HIV infection, and the sputum culture may be positive in persons with normal chest radiographs. Thus, the diagnosis of tuberculosis in the setting of HIV infection may be difficult and requires careful evaluation of any person with HIV infection who develops symptoms consistent with tuberculosis.

Available information indicates that most tuberculosis patients with HIV infection respond well to standard short-course therapy and that adherence to the prescribed regimen is a more important determinant of success than duration of therapy (Small et al., 1991). Treatment regimens which do not include rifampin and which are commonly used in developing countries give distinctly inferior results and are not recommended (Perriens et al., 1991). Because the optimal duration of therapy has not been established, authorities in the United States have recommended that HIV-infected patients be treated for a minimal period of 9-12 months (Centers for Disease Control, 1989). Others, however, have recommended standard, short-course regimens (World Health Organization Tuberculosis Programme, 1991). Therapy should consist of isoniazid, rifampin, and pyrazinamide for 2 months, followed by isoniazid and rifampin for the remainder of the treatment period. Patients with severe forms of tuberculosis (miliary and meningeal disease) and those with an increased likelihood of primary drug resistance should receive a fourth drug (streptomycin and ethambutol, respectively) for the first 2 months of therapy or until susceptibility results are available. Prolonged suppressive therapy with isoniazid following successful completion of therapy has been suggested. However, a preliminary report from a clinical trial does not indicate that additional treatment with isoniazid improves the results of therapy (Prignot, J., personal communication).

Side effects from antituberculosis drugs, especially rifampin, may be common (Small et al., 1991). High rates of hypersensitivity reactions to thiacetazone, at times fatal, have been reported from several African countries; consequently, this drug is contraindicated in patients with HIV infection unless other treatment options are not available (World Health Organization, 1992).

Renal Failure

Of the first line antituberculosis drugs, isoniazid, rifampin, and pyrazinamide may be given at the usual dosages in mild to moderate renal failure. In severe renal failure, both isoniazid and pyrazinamide should be given at slightly reduced dosages unless maintenance hemodialysis is being given (Bowersox et al., 1973; Stamatakis et al., 1988). The renal clearance of both ethambutol and streptomycin is reduced in renal failure, and potentially toxic serum levels of ethambutol occur with standard doses (Varughese et al., 1986). Thus, when either drug is required for the treatment of tuberculosis in patients with renal failure, it is mandatory to reduce the drug dose and closely monitor serum levels. Of the second-line drugs, doses of PAS, cycloserine, kanamycin, and capreomycin must be reduced in renal failure, and the latter two drugs should be used with great caution because of the potential for further renal impairment.

Hepatic Disease

Patients requiring treatment for tuberculosis often have underlying liver disease. This is especially common among alcoholic patients and injecting drug users. In these cases, the underlying liver disease may increase the risk of hepatotoxicity from isoniazid, rifampin, and/or pyrazinamide. Furthermore, isoniazid and rifampin depend on hepatic mechanisms for metabolism and clearance, so increased drug levels may occur when these drugs are given to patients with severe hepatic impairment (Acocella et al., 1972).

In such cases, the severity of tuberculosis and the degree of hepatic impairment must be considered in deciding what drugs to give. Patients with relatively mild forms of tuberculosis and severe hepatic disease may be treated with ethambutol and streptomycin until the hepatic dysfunction is lessened. In those with more severe forms of tuberculosis requiring more aggressive therapy, rifampin and/or isoniazid may be included, with careful monitoring of hepatic function. In severe hepatic insufficiency, the dosages of both drugs may be reduced. Pyrazinamide is best avoided in these cases, as serum levels and half-life are markedly increased in the presence of hepatic insufficiency (Lacroix et al., 1990), and the drug's contribution to the bactericidal phase of therapy is modest.

Silicosis

Silicosis is a potent risk factor for the development of tuberculosis in persons infected with the tubercle bacillus. This occurs because of impairment of pulmonary macrophage function by silica crystals leading to the development of active tuberculosis. There is also evidence that standard, 6-month short-course therapy may be inadequate for patients with silicotuberculosis (Hong Kong Chest Service, 1991). In these patients the sterilizing phase of therapy must be prolonged and patients treated for a minimum of 9 months. If pyrazinamide is not included in the initial phase, treatment with isoniazid and rifampin should be given for at least 12 months. Tuberculosis occurring in association with other pneumoconioses, such as coal workers' pneumoconiosis, can be treated with standard short-course regimens (Jones, 1982).

Immunosuppression (Other than HIV)

Another risk factor for the development of tuberculosis is immunosuppression, induced iatrogenically through immunosuppressive drugs or related to diseases such as reticuloendothelial neoplasms. There are data suggesting that these patients respond well to standard tuberculosis therapy, although mortality from the underlying disease process may be substantial (Dautzenberg et al., 1984). However, these patients may be at increased risk for relapse if therapy has not been taken as recommended. Thus, if it cannot be assured that these patients have been fully compliant with therapy, it may be prudent to prolong therapy (e.g., an additional 3 months) to ensure cure.

Pregnancy/Lactation

Of the first-line drugs, isoniazid, rifampin, and ethambutol can be given safely in pregnancy, and the rifampin-isoniazid regimen with or without ethambutol is the treatment of choice in the United States (Snider et al., 1980). Streptomycin may cause ototoxicity in the fetus and is contraindicated in pregnancy. Although there are no data indicating that pyrazinamide is teratogenic, it has not been recommended in the United States. However, both the International Union Against Tuberculosis and Lung Diseases and the World Health Organization recommend that pyrazinamide be included in the treatment regimen given to pregnant women (World Health Organization, 1991; International Union Against Tuberculosis and Lung Disease, 1988). With the exception of aminoglycosides, which are teratogenic, little is known about the teratogenicity of the second-line drugs.

Most antituberculosis drugs appear in small concentrations in breast milk. However, these levels do not produce toxicity in the nursing infants. Therefore, breast feeding is not contraindicated (Snider and Powell, 1984). However, the levels of these drugs in breast milk do not provide adequate therapy or preventive therapy for infants.

VII. Adherence to Treatment (See Chapter 10)

It is axiomatic that patient nonadherence to therapy is the major unsolved problem in tuberculosis treatment (Addington, 1979). Surveys have indicated that serious nonadherence is present in up to 20% of tuberculosis patients in developed countries with good tuberculosis control services. In programs in some developing countries using outmoded and lengthy therapy with poor or little patient follow-up services, over 50% of patients fail to complete therapy. Thus, worldwide, nonadherence is believed to be responsible for the majority of instances of treatment failure and relapse. Improving patient adherence is the single most important factor in improving tuberculosis treatment.

A. Predicting Nonadherence

Although it is difficult to predict which patients may be nonadherent, there are both patient (internal) and provider (external) factors that are associated with an increased likelihood of nonadherence (Blackwell, 1973). Patient factors include complicating illnesses (particularly substance abuse and mental illness), homelessness, and lack of a social support system (e.g., a ''significant other''). Education and social class have not been associated with nonadherence.

Provider factors include the complexity of treatment (i.e., the number of drugs that must be taken and the schedule with which they should be taken), the accessibility of the provider (e.g., distance from home, convenient hours, short waiting periods), and the setting of the provider (e.g., adequate waiting rooms).

B. Monitoring Adherence

Measuring or screening for noncompliance should be routinely done. This is accomplished by asking patients about pill taking, performing pill counts, urine screening for the red color of rifampin or isoniazid metabolites, and home visits. Patients should be asked in a nonthreatening, nonjudgmental way about their medication taking, stressing both the importance of optimal adherence and the necessity of accurate assessment of medication taking in determining when therapy may be stopped.

Pill counts may be helpful, but patients may discard untaken medication to avoid being identified as nonadherent. Medication monitors are being developed that provide increased information about medication taking, but these are not completely reliable and are expensive. Their use in routine practice has not been studied. Screening for the urine for isoniazid metabolites (Schraufnagel et al., 1990) or for the orange-red color of rifampin is useful, although nonadherent patients can avoid being detected by taking medication just before visits to the health care provider. During the initial phase of therapy, an elevated serum uric acid is generally evidence of adherence with pyrazinamide. Unannounced home visits by clinic staff, at which time pill counts are made and urine specimens obtained, are probably the best means of assessing compliance. However, this requires additional resources for making the home visits. When this is being done, patients' consent for unannounced home visits should be obtained before any visits are made.

C. Improving Adherence

Measures to improve patient adherence include reminding patients about scheduled appointments, providing accessible services (e.g., clinic hours suited to patients' schedules, short waiting times, availability of transportation, interpreters for patients who do not speak English), and simplifying treatment as much as possible (e.g., combination tablets rather than individual drugs) (Snider and Hutton, 1989). Combination, fixed-dose tablets of isoniazid, rifampin, and pyrazinamide have been evaluated in several controlled clinical trials and gave results comparable to those achieved when the drugs were given as individual tablets, either daily (Geiter et al., 1987) or three times weekly (Hong Kong Chest Service, 1989b). However, other studies of the combination products have shown that rifampin bioavailability may be poor in certain formulations (Fox, 1990). Thus, careful assessment of rifampin bioavailability is required to ensure that these combination tablets are satisfactory.

Providing special patient incentives has also improved adherence in a variety of settings (Pozsik, 1989). However, these incentives probably work by helping to foster relationships between patients and staff. The provision of special residential treatment facilities has also improved the outcome of tuberculosis treatment for homeless patients.

Nonadherence is best managed by providing directly observed therapy. This is greatly facilitated by using treatment regimens proven to be effective when given on an intermittent basis (e.g., twice or three times weekly). Not only has this approach proven to be highly effective, but it results in significant savings compared to the cost of hospitalizing these patients and the cost of treating advanced drug resistance, which is a frequent consequence of noncompliance (Judd et al., 1989). Although routine hospitalization for tuberculosis patients was abandoned several decades ago, in some programs in developing countries, supervised therapy by hospitalization during the initial phase of therapy has greatly improved adherence and treatment success (Styblo and Chum, 1987). This may be especially important for patients living in rural areas distant from treatment facilities. However, the decision to institute routine hospitalization must be based on careful assessment of costs and outcomes and probably is not commonly justified. Finally, as a last resort when all reasonable efforts to foster and ensure adherence have failed, enforced incarceration and treatment may be an option in areas where this is legally permitted. In such cases the balance between individual rights of the patient and the welfare of the public must be carefully considered.

References

Abernathy, A. S., Dutt, A. K., Stead, W. W., and Moers, D. J. (1983). Short-course chemotherapy for tuberculosis in children. *Pediatrics* **72**:801–806.

Acocella, G., Bonollo, L., Garimoldi, M., Mainardi, M., Tenconi, L. T., and Nocolis, F. B. (1972). Kinetics of rifampicin and isoniazid administered alone and in combination to normal subjects and patients with liver disease. *Gut* **13**:47–53.

Addington, W. W. (1979). Patient compliance: the most serious remaining problem in the control of tuberculosis in the United States. *Chest* **76**:741–743.

Alarcon, F., Escalante, L., Perez, Y., Banda, H., Chacon, G., and Duenas, G. (1990). Tuberculous meningitis. Short course of chemotherapy. *Arch. Neurol.* **47**:1313–1317.

American Academy of Pediatrics (1992). Chemotherapy for tuberculosis in infants and children. *Pediatrics* **89**:161–165.

American Thoracic Society (1986). Treatment of tuberculosis and tuberculous infection in adults and children. *Am. Rev. Respir. Dis.* **134**:355–363.

Baciewicz, A. M., Self, T. H., and Bakermeyer, W. B. (1987). Update on rifampin drug interactions. *Arch. Intern. Med.* **147**:565–568.

Blackwell, B. (1973). Patient compliance. *N. Engl. J. Med.* **289**:249–252.

Bowersox, D. W., Winterbauer, R. H., Stewart, G. L., Orme, B., and Barron, E. (1973). Isoniazid dosage in patients with renal failure. *N. Engl. J. Med.* **289**:84–87.

British Thoracic Society (1990). Chemotherapy and management of tuberculosis in the United Kingdom: recommendations of the Joint Tuberculosis Committee of the British Thoracic Society. *Thorax* **45**:403–408.

British Thoracic Society Research Committee (1988). Short course chemotherapy for lymph node tuberculosis: final report at 5 years. *Br. J. Dis. Chest* **82**:282–284.

Centers for Disease Control (1983). Primary resistance to antituberculosis drugs—United States. *MMWR* **32**:521–523.

Centers for Disease Control (1989). Advisory Committee for the Elimination of Tuberculosis: tuberculosis and human immunodeficiency virus infection. *MMWR* **38**:236–238, 243–250.

Centers for Disease Control (1991). Nosocomial transmission of multidrug-resistant tuberculosis among HIV-infected persons—Florida and New York, 1989–1991. *MMWR* **40**:585–591.

Citron, K. M., and Thomas, G. O. (1986). Ocular toxicity from ethambutol. *Thorax* **41**:737–739.

Cohn, D. L., Catlin, B. J., Peterson, K. L., Judson, F. N., and Sbarbaro, J. A. (1990). A 62-dose, 6-month therapy for pulmonary and extrapulmonary tuberculosis. A twice-weekly, directly observed, and cost-effective regimen. *Ann. Intern. Med.* **112**:407–415.

Combs, D. L., O'Brien, R. J., and Geiter, L. J. (1990). USPHS tuberculosis short-course therapy trial 21: effectiveness, toxicity, and acceptability. The report of the final results. *Ann. Intern. Med.* **112**:397–406.

Cross, F. S., Long, M. W., Banner, A. S., and Snider, D. E. (1980). Rifampin-isoniazid therapy of alcoholic and nonalcoholic tuberculosis patients in a U.S. Public Health Service cooperative therapy trial. *Am. Rev. Respir. Dis.* **122**:349–353.

Dautzenberg, B., Grosset, J., Fechner, J., Lucciani, J., Debre, P., Herson, S., Truffot, C., and Sors, C. (1984). The management of thirty immunocompromised patients with tuberculosis. *Am. Rev. Respir. Dis.* **129**:494–496.

Dautzenberg, B., Truffot, C., Legris, S., Meyohas, M-C., Berlie, H. C., Mercat, A., Chevret, S., and Grosset, J. (1991). Activity of clarithromycin against *Mycobacterium avium* infection in patients with the acquired immune deficiency syndrome. A controlled clinical trial. *Am. Rev. Respir. Dis.* **144**:564–569.

D'Esopo, N. D. (1982). Clinical trials in tuberculosis. *Am. Rev. Respir. Dis.* **125**(No. 3, Part 2):85–93.

Dutt, A. K., and Stead, W. W. (1989). Treatment of extrapulmonary tuberculosis. *Semin. Respir. Infect.* **4**:225–231.

Dutt, A. K., Moers, D., and Stead, W. W. (1984). Short-course chemotherapy for tuberculosis with mainly twice-weekly isoniazid and rifampin. Community physicians' seven-year experience with mainly outpatients. *Am. J. Med.* **77**:233–244.

Dutt, A. K., Moers, D., and Stead, W. W. (1986). Short-course chemotherapy for pleural tuberculosis. Nine years' experience in routine treatment service. *Chest* **90**:112–116.

Dutt, A. K., Moers, D., and Stead, W. W. (1989). Smear- and culture-negative pulmonary tuberculosis: four-month short course chemotherapy. *Am. Rev. Respir. Dis.* **139**:867–870.

East and Central African/British Medical Research Council Fifth Collaborative Study (1986). Controlled clinical trial of 4 short-course regimens of chemotherapy (three 6-month and one 8-month) for pulmonary tuberculosis: final report. *Tubercle* **67**:5–15

Ferebee, S. H., Theodore, A., and Mount F. W. (1960). Long-term consequences of isoniazid alone as initial therapy: United States Public Health
Service Tuberculosis Therapy Trials. *Am. Rev. Respir. Dis.* **82**:824–830.

Fox, W. (1979). The current status of short-course chemotherapy. *Tubercle*
60:177–190.

Fox, W. (1990). Drug combinations and the bioavailability of rifampicin. *Tubercle* **71**:241–245.

Geiter, L. J., O'Brien, R. J., Combs, D. L., and Snider, D. E. (1987). United
States Public Health Service Tuberculosis Therapy Trial 21: preliminary
results of an evaluation of a combination tablet of isoniazid, rifampin and
pyrazinamide. *Tubercle* **68**:41–46.

Girgis, N. I., Farid, Z., Kilpatrick, M. E., Sultan, Y., and Mikhail, I. A.
(1991). Dexamethasone as an adjunct to treatment of tuberculous meningitis. *Pediatr. Infect. Dis. J.* **10**:179–183.

Girling, D. J. (1978). The hepatic toxicity of antituberculosis regimens containing isoniazid, rifampicin and pyrazinamide. *Tubercle* **59**:13–32.

Goel, A., Pandya, S. K., and Satoskar, A. R. (1990). Whither short-course chemotherapy for tuberculous meningitis? *Neurosurgery* **27**:418–421.

Gow, J. G., and Barbosa, S. (1984). Genitourinary tuberculosis. A study of 1117
cases over a period of 34 years. *Br. J. Urol.* **56**:449–455.

Grosset, J. (1978). The sterilizing value of rifampicin and pyrazinamide in experimental short-course chemotherapy. *Tubercle* **59**:287–297.

Grosset, J., and Leventis, S. (1983). Adverse effects of rifampin. *Rev. Infect.
Dis.* **5**(Suppl 3):S440–S446.

Hong Kong Chest Service/British Medical Research Council (1987). Five-year
follow-up of a controlled trial of five 6-month regimens of chemotherapy
for pulmonary tuberculosis. *Am. Rev. Respir. Dis.* **136**:1339–1342.

Hong Kong Chest Service/Tuberculosis Research Centre, Madras/British Medical Research Council (1989a). A controlled trial of 3-month, 4-month,
and 6-month regimens of chemotherapy for sputum-smear negative
pulmonary tuberculosis. Results at 5 years. *Am. Rev. Respir. Dis.*
139:871–876.

Hong Kong Chest Service/British Medical Research Council (1989b). Acceptability, compliance, and adverse reactions when isoniazid, rifampin, and
pyrazinamide are given as a combined formulation or separately during
three-times weekly antituberculosis chemotherapy. *Am. Rev. Respir. Dis.*
140:1618–1622.

Hong Kong Chest Service/Tuberculosis Research Centre, Madras/British Medical Research Council (1991). A controlled clinical comparison of 6
and 8 months of antituberculosis chemotherapy in the treatment of patients with silicotuberculosis in Hong Kong. *Am. Rev. Respir. Dis.*
143:262–267.

Hong Kong Tuberculosis Treatment Service/British Medical Research Council (1977). Controlled trial of 6-month and 9-month regimens of daily and intermittent streptomycin plus isoniazid plus pyrazinamide for pulmonary tuberculosis in Hong Kong. The results up to 30 months. *Am. Rev. Respir. Dis.* **115**:727–735.

International Union Against Tuberculosis and Lung Disease (1988). Antituberculosis regimens of chemotherapy. Recommendations from the Committee on Treatment of the IUATLD. *Bull. IUATLD* **63**:60–64.

Iseman, M. D., and Madsen, L. A. (1989). Drug-resistant tuberculosis. *Clin. Chest. Med.* **10**:341–353.

Iseman, M. D., Madsen, L., Goble, M., and Pomerantz, M. (1990). Surgical intervention in the treatment of pulmonary disease caused by drug-resistant *Mycobacterium tuberculosis. Am. Rev. Respir. Dis.* **141**:623–625.

Jacobs, R. F., and Abernathy, R. S. (1985). The treatment of tuberculosis in children. *Pediatr. Infect. Dis. J.* **4**:513–517.

Jawahar, M. S., Sivasubramanian, S., Vijayan, V. K., Ramakrishnan, C. V., Paramasivan, C. N., Selvakumar, V., Paul, S., Tripathy, S. P., and Prabhakar, R. (1990). Short course chemotherapy for tuberculous lymphadenitis in children. *Br. Med. J.* **301**:359–362.

Jindani, A., Aber, V. R., Edwards, E. A., and Mitchison, D. A. (1980). The early bactericidal activity of drugs in patients with pulmonary tuberculosis. *Am. Rev. Respir. Dis.* **121**:939–949.

Jones, F. L. (1982). Rifampin-containing chemotherapy for pulmonary tuberculosis associated with coal workers' pneumoconiosis. *Am. Rev. Respir. Dis.* **125**:681–683.

Judd, K., Miller, R., Luft, H., and Hopewell, P. (1989). Outcomes and costs of tuberculosis treatment strategies in the United States. *Am. Rev. Respir. Dis.* **139**(No. 4, Part 2):A314.

Kim, J. H., Langston, A. A., and Gallis, H. A. (1990). Miliary tuberculosis: epidemiology, clinical manifestations, diagnosis, and outcome. *Rev. Infect. Dis.* **12**:583–590.

Kopanoff, D. E., Snider, D. E., and Caras, G. J. (1978). Isoniazid related hepatitis. *Am. Rev. Respir. Dis.* **117**:991–1001.

Lacroix, C., Guyonnaud, C., Chaou, M., Duwoos, H., and Lafont, O. (1988). Interaction between allopurinol and pyrazinamide. *Eur. Respir. J.* **1**:807–811.

Lacroix, C., Tranvouez, J. L., Phan Hoang, T., Duwoos, H., and Lafont, O. (1990). Pharmacokinetics of pyrazinamide and its metabolites in patients with hepatic cirrhotic insufficiency. *Drug Res.* **40**:76–79.

LeCoeur, H. F., Truffot-Pernot, C., and Grosset, J. H. (1989). Experimental short-course preventive therapy of tuberculosis with rifampin and pyrazinamide. *Am. Rev. Respir. Dis.* **140**:1189–1193.

Lee, C. H., Wang, W. J., Lan, R. S., Tsai, Y. H., and Chiang, Y. C. (1988). Corticosteroids in the treatment of tuberculous pleurisy. A double-blind, placebo-controlled, randomized study. *Chest* **94**:1256–1259.

Lordi, G. M., and Reichman, L. B. (1985). Tuberculosis: when not to order chest roentgenograms. *JAMA* **253**:1780–1781.

Leysen, D. C., Haemers, A., and Pattyn, S. R. (1989). Mycobacteria and the new quinolones. *Antimicrob. Agents Chemother.* **33**:1–5.

Maartens, G., Willcox, P. A., and Benatar, S. R. (1990). Miliary tuberculosis: rapid diagnosis, hematologic abnormalities, and outcome in 109 treated adults. *Am. J. Med.* **89**:291–296.

Malik, S. K., Hehera, D., and Gilhotra, R. (1987). Tuberculous pleural effusion and lymphadenitis treated with rifampin-containing regimen. *Chest* **92**:904–905.

Medical Research Council Working Party on Tuberculosis of the Spine (1986). A controlled trial of six-month and nine-month regimens of chemotherapy in patients undergoing radical surgery for tuberculosis of the spine in Hong Kong. *Tubercle* **67**:243–259.

Miller, R. R., Porter, J., and Greenblatt, D. J. (1979). Clinical importance of the interaction of phenytoin and isoniazid. *Chest* **75**:356–358.

Mitchison, D. A. (1985). The action of antituberculosis drugs in short-course chemotherapy. *Tubercle* **66**:219–226.

Mitchison, D. A., and Nunn, A. J. (1986). Influence of initial drug resistance on the response to short-course chemotherapy of pulmonary tuberculosis. *Am. Rev. Respir. Dis.* **133**:423–430.

Nadler, J. P., Berger, J., Nord, J. A., Cofsky, R., and Saxena, M. (1991). Amoxicillin–clavulanic acid for treating drug-resistant *Mycobacterium tuberculosis*. *Chest* **99**:1025–1026.

O'Brien, R. J., Lyle, M. A., and Snider, D. E. (1987). Rifabutin (ansamycin LM427): a new rifamycin-S derivative for the treatment of mycobacterial diseases. *Rev. Infect. Dis.* **9**:519:530.

Perriens, J. H., Colebunders, R. L., Karahunga, C., Willame, J-C., Jeugmans, J., Kaboto, M., Mukadi, Y., Pauwels, P., Ryder, R. W., Prignot, J., and Piot, P. (1991). Increased mortality and tuberculosis treatment failure rate among human immunodeficiency virus (HIV) seropositive compared with HIV seronegative patients with pulmonary tuberculosis treated with "standard" chemotherapy in Kinshasa, Zaire. *Am. Rev. Respir. Dis.* **144**:750–755.

Pozsik, C. (1989). *Using Incentives and Enablers in the Tuberculosis Control Program*. American Lung Association of South Carolina, Columbia, pp. 1–18.

Ramachandran, P., Duraipandian, M., Nagarajan, M., Prabhakar, R., Ramakrishnan, C. V., and Tripathy, S. P. (1986). Three chemotherapy studies of tuberculous meningitis in children. *Tubercle* **67**:17–29.

Schraufnagel, D. E., Stoner, R., Whiting, E., Snukst-Torbeck, G., and Werhane, M. J. (1990). Testing for isoniazid. An evaluation of the Arkansas method. *Chest* **98**:314–316.

Selwyn, P. A., Hartel, D., Lewis, V. A., Schoenbaum, E. E., Vermund, S. H., Klein, R. S., Walker, A. T., and Friedland, G. H. (1989). A prospective study of the risk of tuberculosis among intravenous drug users with human immunodeficiency virus infection. *N. Engl. J. Med.* **320**:545–550.

Small, P. M., Schecter, G. F., Goodman, P. C., Sande, M. A., Chaisson, R. E., and Hopewell, P. C. (1991). Treatment of tuberculosis in patients with advanced human immunodeficiency virus infection. *N. Engl. J. Med.* **324**:289–294.

Snider, D. E. (1980). Pyridoxine supplementation during isoniazid therapy. *Tubercle* **61**:191–196.

Snider, D. E., and Powell, K. E. (1984). Should women taking antituberculosis drugs breast-feed? *Arch. Intern. Med.* **144**:589–590.

Snider, D. E., and Hutton, M. D. (1989). *Improving Patient Compliance in Tuberculosis Treatment Programs*. Department of Health and Human Services, Public Health Service, Centers for Disease Control, Atlanta, pp. 1–20.

Snider, D. E., Layde, P. M., Hohnson, M. W., and Lyle, M. A. (1980). Treatment of tuberculosis during pregnancy. *Am. Rev. Respir. Dis.* **122**:65–79.

Snider, D. E., Long, M. W., Cross, F. S., and Farer, L. S. (1984). Six-months isoniazid-rifampin therapy for pulmonary tuberculosis. *Am. Rev. Respir. Dis.* **129**:573–579.

Stamatakis, G., Montes, C., Trouvin, J. H., Farinotti, R., Fessi, H., Kenouch, S., and Mery, J. Ph. (1988). Pyrazinamide and pyrazinoic acid pharmacokinetics in patients with chronic renal failure. *Clin. Nephrol.* **30**:230–234.

Starke, J. R. (1990). Multidrug chemotherapy for tuberculosis in children. *Pediatr. Infect. Dis. J.* **19**:785–793.

Steele, M. A., Burk, R. F., and DesPrez, R. M. (1991). Toxic hepatitis with isoniazid and rifampin. A meta-analysis. *Chest* **99**:465–471.

Strang, J. I. G., Kakaza, H. H. S., Gibson, D. G., Girling, D. J., Nunn, P. J., and Fox, W. (1987). Controlled trial of prednisolone as adjunct in treatment of tuberculous constrictive pericarditis in Transkei. *Lancet* **2**:1418–1422.

Styblo, K., and Chum, H. J. (1987). Treatment results of smear-positive tuberculosis in the Tanzania National Tuberculosis and Leprosy Programme: standard and short-course chemotherapy. In *Tuberculosis and Respiratory Diseases*. Professional Postgraduate Services, Tokyo, pp. 122–126.

Sunderam, G., McDonald, R. J., Maniatis, T., Oleske, J., Kapila, R., and Reichman, L. B. (1986). Tuberculosis as a manifestation of the acquired immunodeficiency syndrome (AIDS). *JAMA* **256**:362–366.

Swai, O. B., Aluoch, J. A., Githui, W. A., Thiongo'o, R., Edwards, E. A., Darbyshire, J. H., and Nunn, A. J. (1988). Controlled clinical trial of a regimen of two durations for the treatment of isoniazid resistant pulmonary tuberculosis. *Tubercle* **69**:5–14.

Varughese, A., Brater, D. C., Benet, L. Z., and Lee, C. C. (1986). Ethambutol kinetics in patients with impaired renal function. *Am. Rev. Respir. Dis.* **134**:34–38.

Wilkins, E. G. L., Hnizdo, E., and Cope, A. (1989). Addisonian crisis inducted by treatment with rifampicin. *Tubercle* **70**:69–73.

Working Group on Osteo-articular Tuberculosis in Algeria (1988). Comparison of 3 chemotherapeutic regimens of short duration (6 months) in osteo-articular tuberculosis. Results after 5 years. *Bull. IUATLD* **63**:14–15.

World Health Organization (1991). WHO Model Prescribing Information. *Drugs Used in Myobacterial Diseases*. World Health Organization, Geneva, pp. 14–22.

World Health Organization (1992) Severe hypersensitivity reactions among HIV-positive patients with tuberculosis treated with thioacetazone. *Weekly Epidemiol. Rec.* **67**:1–3.

World Health Organization Tuberculosis Programme (1991). Guidelines for tuberculosis treatment in adults and children in national tuberculosis programmes. Unpublished document, WHO/TUB/91.191.

Wu, J-C., Lee, S-D., Yeh, P-F., Chan, C-Y., Wang, Y-J., Huang, Y-S., Tsai, Y-T., Lee, P-Y., Ting, L-P., and Lo, K-J. (1990). Isoniazid-rifampin-induced hepatitis in hepatitis B carriers. *Gastroenterology* **98**:502–504.

Zierski, M. (1977). Prospects of retreatment of chronic resistant pulmonary tuberculosis patients: a critical review. *Lung* **154**:91–102.

12

Preventive Therapy for Tuberculosis

LAWRENCE J. GEITER

Division of Tuberculosis Elimination
Centers for Disease Control and Prevention
Atlanta, Georgia

I. Introduction

There are three basic strategies for the prevention of tuberculosis. Two means of primary prevention are vaccination and rapid case finding and diagnosis, both of which will prevent new cases from developing. However, both these approaches have their limitations and, even if they operate at 100% efficiency, leave large pools of individuals infected with *Mycobacterium tuberculosis*, who will be the source of cases far into the future. Preventive chemotherapy is a method of secondary prevention that takes advantage of the latent period following infection to prevent the development of clinically recognizable disease, infectiousness, and transmission to others.

II. Clinical Trials of Isoniazid Preventive Therapy

Isoniazid was considered a preventive therapy agent very shortly after its discovery. Edith Lincoln first noted that children receiving isoniazid did not develop complications of a primary tuberculosis infection (Lincoln, 1954). Clinical trials of isoniazid to prevent the development of tuberculosis in previously infected individuals were then undertaken in the late 1950s in Italy (Zorini, 1958), France (Debre et al., 1973), and the United States (Ferebee and Mount, 1962). Since then, placebo-controlled trials of preventive therapy have been conducted in a wide variety of places and situations and are summarized in an excellent review of preventive therapy for tuberculosis (Ferebee, 1969).

In these trials, the average reduction in tuberculosis was about 60%, with a range of 25–92%. These results are based on a comparison of the groups to which the participants were randomized, and the variation in effectiveness in these studies is almost entirely attributable to the degree of adherence of the subjects with the isoniazid regimen. Among study subjects with a high level of adherence, the reduction in the number of tuberculosis cases among those assigned to take isoniazid, compared to a placebo group, was 90% or more. The protection against tuberculosis conferred by isoniazid appears to last at least 19 years and may be lifelong (Comstock et al., 1979).

The most recent large, controlled trial of preventive therapy with isoniazid was a study of individuals with fibrotic lesions but no signs of active tuberculosis and demonstrated that a regimen of three months of isoniazid was not likely to be effective (International Union Against Tuberculosis Committee on Prophylaxis, 1982). Comparing the groups receiving isoniazid to a placebo group, those assigned to a three-month isoniazid regimen had a 21% reduction in the risk of tuberculosis, the six-month regimen a 65% reduction, and the 12-month regimen a 75% reduction. When the results were stratified by adherence with the regimen (adherence defined as taking 80% or more of the assigned medication), the protection conferred on adherent individuals by the 3- and 6-month regimens was similar to that for the groups as a whole, 31% and 69%, but the protection afforded by the 12-month regimen increased to 93%. However, a later analysis showed that the 6-month regimen is actually favored in a cost-benefit analysis (Snider et al., 1986).

III. Recommended Regimens for Preventive Therapy

A. Populations to be Considered for Preventive Therapy

The Advisory Council for the Elimination of Tuberculosis (ACET) has published recommendations for the use of isoniazid preventive therapy (ACET, 1990). All individuals with the following risk factors should be considered for preventive therapy, if they have not already been treated:

1. Tuberculin skin test ≥ 5 mm; human immunodeficiency virus (HIV) infection or risk factors for HIV infection when the HIV infection status is unknown, recent contact with an infectious case of tuberculosis, abnormal chest radiograph with fibrotic lesions indicative of old healed tuberculosis

2. Tuberculin skin test ≥10 mm; intravenous drug users known to be HIV negative, persons with medical risk factors for tuberculosis including silicosis, gastrectomy, jejunoileal bypass, weight 10% or more below ideal body weight, chronic renal failure, diabetes mellitus, prolonged high-dose immunosuppressive therapy, leukemia, lymphoma, and other malignancies.

In addition, preventive therapy should be considered for individuals under 35 years of age:

1. Tuberculin skin test ≥10 mm; if they are in any of the following high-incidence groups; foreign-born persons from high-prevalence countries, medically underserved low-income populations (including high-risk racial and ethnic minorities), residents of correctional facilities, nursing homes, mental institutions, and other long-term care facilities, and other groups defined by the local public health authorities to be at high risk for tuberculosis in that community

2. Tuberculin skin test ≥15 mm; if they are a member of a low-incidence group and lack any of the previously defined risk factors.

Anergy to tuberculin has been identified as a problem when tuberculin skin testing individuals with HIV infection or other immune compromising conditions, and guidelines have been published that suggest testing with purified protein derivative (PPD) tuberculin and two companion delayed-type hypersensitivity (DTH) antigens to assess anergy (CDC, 1991a). Any induration to a DTH antigen ≥3 mm at 48–72 hr is evidence of DTH responsiveness, and a failure to respond to all three antigens is evidence of anergy. These guidelines further suggest that anergic individuals with a personal risk of infection with *M. tuberculosis* of ≥10% should be considered for preventive therapy. One decision analysis, weighing the risks and benefits of preventive therapy, concluded that preventive therapy might be justified for HIV-positive black men and white men and women in the absence of a tuberculin test, even when the risk of infection is a low as 3–8% (Jordan et al., 1991).

B. Dosage Guidelines

The ACET guidelines recommend an isoniazid dosage of 10 mg/kg daily for children and adolescents, and a 5 mg/kg daily dose for adults up to a maximum dose of 300 mg daily. For individuals requiring directly observed therapy to ensure compliance, a twice-weekly dose of 15 mg/kg, to a maximum of 900 mg, should be considered when daily directly observed daily therapy is not possible. Preventive therapy with rifampin, 10 mg/kg up to 600 mg daily, should be considered for infected contacts likely to have been infected by a source case with isoniazid-resistant tuberculosis. All individuals prescribed preventive therapy for tuberculosis should receive a minimum of 6 months and up to 12 months of continuous preventive therapy. Individuals with chest radiographs consistent with past tuberculosis should receive the full 12 months of preventive therapy.

C. Preventive Therapy for HIV-Infected Individuals

HIV infection has been identified as the most potent risk factor for the development of tuberculosis, given infection with *M. tuberculosis*. One estimate places the risk of tuberculosis at over 100 times more likely in the HIV-infected person than in the seronegative individual (Rieder et al., 1989). Selwyn estimated that 7.9% of tuberculin-positive IV drug users, some of whom had previously received preventive therapy, develop tuberculosis each year (Selwyn et al., 1989), but the risk is even higher for HIV-infected individuals recently infected with *M. tuberculosis*. In two tuberculosis outbreaks involving HIV-infected individuals, one reported from Italy (DiPerri et al., 1989) and one from the United States (CDC, 1991b), 40% of HIV-infected persons exposed to patients with active-infectious tuberculosis subsequently developed tuberculosis in the first 2–4 months following infection. This level of risk makes the concept of preventive therapy, or secondary prevention, for those infected with HIV and *M. tuberculosis* all the more important.

Individuals with HIV infection, a tuberculin skin test reaction ≥ 5 mm or tuberculin anergy and an estimated risk of infection with *M. tuberculosis* of $\geq 10\%$, and no signs of active tuberculosis should receive a 12-month course of preventive therapy. However, the optimal length of preventive therapy with isoniazid for individuals infected with both HIV and *M. tuberculosis* has not been established in clinical trials. Preliminary results from one study indicate that a 12-month course of isoniazid may be very effective in preventing tuberculosis, showing an 89% reduction in the development of tuberculosis relative to a placebo group (Wadhawan et al., 1991), but the death rate was nearly equal in the placebo and treatment groups. Additional data from this and other ongoing studies are necessary.

IV. Toxicity Associated with Isoniazid Preventive Therapy

Isoniazid is generally well tolerated and is one of the least toxic of the antituberculosis drugs. Most of the side effects are mild but the occurrence of hepatitis is of concern. Isoniazid-induced hepatitis is rare under the age of 20, but the risk increases with age to a peak of 2–3% in the 50-to-64-year-old age group (Kopanoff et al., 1978). Because of these findings, recommendations limited the use of preventive therapy to reactors at high-risk of developing active tuberculosis and those under 35 years of age and recommended monthly monitoring for adverse reactions. Following these guidelines has been shown to reduce the risk of serious isoniazid hepatitis (Dash et al., 1980).

The risk of isoniazid-associated hepatitis mortality and the decision to recommend isoniazid preventive therapy has been a subject of continued debate. Conflicting decision analysis and cost-benefit analysis have been published supporting (Colice, 1990; Rose et al., 1988) and opposing (Taylor et al., 1981; Tsevat, et al., 1988) the use of isoniazid preventive therapy. However, it is important to bear in mind that the controversy has only concerned low-risk, adult, tuberculin reactors; few question that the benefits of preventive therapy with isoniazid far outweigh the risk of hepatitis for tuberculin reactors at a high risk of tuberculosis, such as those coinfected with HIV, household contacts, and recent skin test converters.

Some of the controversy over the use of preventive therapy has resulted from the estimate of the risk of isoniazid hepatitis mortality. A 57.0/100,000 risk of isoniazid hepatitis mortality was estimated in a United States Public Health Service surveillance study (Kopanoff et al., 1978). While this mortality risk was based on eight cases of fatal hepatitis that occurred during the study and were attributed to isoniazid, seven of the deaths occurred in one study site, Baltimore, Maryland. A subsequent study of deaths in Maryland revealed a significant increase in deaths due to liver disease among persons not receiving isoniazid during the study period. The risk of mortality at the other study sites was estimated as 9.4/100,000. In a recently published paper, the isoniazid hepatitis mortality risk in the United States was estimated to be about 14/100,000 persons starting preventive therapy or 23/100,000 persons completing preventive therapy (Snider and Caras, 1992). These estimates are much lower than the U.S.P.H.S. study–derived figure most often used in the various cost-benefit/ effectiveness and decision analyses published on preventive therapy. Snider and Caras warn that the estimates are very crude and suggest that the truly important question is which groups are actually at highest risk for toxicity and death. Data from their paper and other sources suggest that women, particularly black and Hispanic women in the postpartum period, may be at an increased risk of hepatotoxicity.

V. Adherence with Isoniazid Preventive Therapy

Tuberculosis preventive therapy is a major component of the U.S. effort to control and eliminate tuberculosis. But there is a major problem in its application: namely, the problem of maintaining patient and provider adherence with a preventive regimen that lasts 6–12 months, and preventive therapy with isoniazid is associated with some hepatotoxicity.

State and local health departments are asked to report on the results of tuberculosis program activities to the Division of Tuberculosis Elimination in the Centers for Disease Control. About 90 program areas voluntarily participate in this system each year. According to these program management reports (Centers for Disease Control, unpublished data), approximately nine contacts are identified for each case reported, about 90% are examined, and about 20% of them found to be infected. While program guidelines would call for virtually all the infected contacts to be started on preventive therapy, only 76% were actually started in 1990. Of those started on therapy in 1989, only 67% of this group completed what is considered to be an adequate course of therapy. Therefore, less than half the contacts identified as candidates for preventive therapy received an adequate course. These figures are typical of the experience in the United States each year and indicate the difficulty in delivering preventive therapy.

VI. Alternatives to Isoniazid Preventive Therapy

Because of the limitations placed on preventive therapy by the length of therapy and the concerns about toxicity, short-course regimens of preventive therapy that avoid the use of isoniazid have been investigated. A meeting of experts, convened to discuss alternatives to isoniazid preventive therapy, concluded that the most promising alternatives were a short-course rifampin regimen or a rifampin-pyrazinamide combination (Geiter and O'Brien, 1987). Support for rifampin and rifampin-pyrazinamide regimens later came from the results of studies of preventive therapy in a mouse model (Lecoeur et al., 1989). Four regimens were tested in this animal model, isoniazid alone for 6 months, rifampin alone for 4 months, rifampin and pyrazinamide for 2 months, and isoniazid, rifampin, and pyrazinamide for 2 months. The most effective of the four regimens was the rifampin-pyrazinamide regimen. Interestingly, it was even more effective than the same two drugs in combination with isoniazid. The rifampin-only regimen was also very promising.

Preliminary results have been published from a study of the safety and acceptability of short-course preventive therapy, comparing a 2-month rifampin-pyrazinamide and a 4-month rifampin-only regimen with a control regimen of 6 months of isoniazid preventive therapy. These regimens were tested in tuberculin reactors without special risk factors for reactivation in the United States and Canada (Geiter et al., 1990), Germany (Magdorf et al., 1991), and Poland (Grazcyk et al., 1991). In Germany, the patients were enrolled at a pediatric clinic in Berlin and only children were enrolled. The study population in Poland was mixed, with about equal numbers of children and adults. The study population at the North American centers was limited to adults over 18 years of age.

All three regimens were extremely well tolerated by the children. Adherence with the regimens approached 100% for the children studied in both Germany and Poland. However, in the adult populations, there was much more toxicity and lower rates of adherence than expected. Approximately 10% of the patients on the 2-month rifampin-pyrazinamide regimen had medication withdrawn owing to adverse reactions, many of which were hepatotoxic reactions. However, there was very little evidence of toxicity for the rifampin-only regimen. Adherence with the regimens was best for the group assigned to the 6-month isoniazid regimen, and the adherence rate was significantly lower for the rifampin-only group. Possible explanations for the lower adherence with the therapy was the description of the short-course regimens as experimental, warnings about adverse reactions in the informed consent statement, and a dislike of the orange coloration of body fluids caused by rifampin.

A recently published study of tuberculosis preventive therapy for silicotic patients in Hong Kong confirmed the low toxicity for a rifampin-only regimen and provides an estimate of relative efficacy (Hong Kong Chest Service and Madras/British Medical Research Council, 1992). The study was placebo controlled and regimens of 6 months of isoniazid, 3 months of isoniazid and rifampin, and 3 months of rifampin alone were studied. None of the regimens proved acceptable as preventive therapy for this high-risk population, reducing the risk of disease by only 41–63%. However, all the regimens were more effective than placebo, and although not statistically significantly different from the other two regimens, the 3-month rifampin regimen was the most effective. Examining toxicity, more patients on the isoniazid-containing regimens had significant increases in serum ALT, compared with the rifampin-only regimen, and the mean serum level for the ALT barely changed from baseline for the rifampin-only group.

VII. Preventive Therapy for Contacts of Multidrug-Resistant Cases

Recent outbreaks and an increasing incidence of tuberculosis resistant to both isoniazid and rifampin have made regimens that rely on neither isoniazid nor rifampin a necessity for contacts of these multidrug-resistant tuberculosis (MDR TB) cases. While there are no controlled studies of preventive therapy regimens with other drugs, the Centers for Disease Control has published guidelines for the management contacts of MDR TB (CDC, 1992) recommending that those at the highest risk of infection with MDR TB bacilli and at very high risk of developing tuberculosis following infection with *M. tuberculosis* (e.g., those with HIV infection) be placed on preventive therapy with two drugs to which the presumed source case bacilli are shown to be sensitive. Possible regimens suggested in the document are ethambutol-pyrazinamide and pyrazinamide plus one of the licensed quinolones shown to be active against *M. tuberculosis* (ciprofloxacin or ofloxacin in the United States). A minimum of 6 months of preventive therapy is recommended for immune-competent individuals and 12 months of preventive therapy for HIV-infected and other immune-compromised individuals.

VIII. Conclusion

Preventive therapy with isoniazid has been shown to be an effective strategy for reducing the risk of tuberculosis in those with latent *M. tuberculosis* infection and can be an important component of tuberculosis control and elimination strategies in countries with a low annual risk of infection with *M. tuberculosis*. The high risk of active tuberculosis for HIV-infected individuals increases the importance of preventive therapy programs and may even make preventive therapy a suitable tuberculosis control strategy in countries with a high risk of tuberculosis infection. However, the long treatment course required for isoniazid preventive therapy and the potential for hepatotoxicity have limited the application of preventive therapy. Shorter courses of therapy with drugs other than isoniazid or with combinations of drugs may increase the applicability and effectiveness of preventive therapy programs.

References

Advisory Committee for Elimination of Tuberculosis (1990). The use of preventive therapy for tuberculosis infection in the United States. *MMWR* **39**(RR-8):9–12.

Centers for Disease Control (1991a). Purified protein derivative (PPD)-tuberculin anergy and HIV infection: guidelines for anergy testing and management of anergic persons at risk or tuberculosis. *MMWR* **40**(RR-5):27–33.

Centers for Disease Control (1991b). Tuberculosis outbreak among persons in a residential facility for HIV-infected persons—San Francisco. *MMWR* **40**:649–652.

Centers for Disease Control (1992). Recommendations for the management of persons exposed to multidrug-resistant tuberculosis. *MMWR* 41(RR-11): 59–71.

Colice, G. L. (1990). Decision analysis, public health policy, and isoniazid chemoprophylaxis for young adult tuberculin skin reactors. *Arch. Intern. Med.* **150**:2517–2522.

Comstock, G. W., Baum, C., and Snider, D. E. (1979). Isoniazid prophylaxis among Alaskan eskimos: a final report of the Bethel isoniazid studies. *Am. Rev. Respir. Dis.* **119**(5):827–830.

Dash, L. A., Comstock, G. W., and Flynn J. P. G. (1980). Isoniazid preventive therapy retrospect and prospect. *Am. Rev. Respir. Dis.* 121:1039–1044.

Debre, R., Perdrizet, S., Lotte, A., Naveau, M., and Lert F., (1973). Isoniazid chemoprophylaxis of latent primary tuberculosis: in five trial centres in France from 1959 to 1969. *Int. J. Epidemiol.* 2:153–160.

DiPerri, G., Danzi, M. C., DeChecchi, G., Pizzighella, S., Solbiati, M., Cruciani, M., Luzzati, R., Malena, M., Mazzi, R., Concia, E. and Bassetti, D. (1989). Nosocomial epidemic of active tuberculosis among HIV infected patients. *Lancet*, pp. 1502–1504.

Ferebee, S. H. (1969). Controlled chemoprophylaxis trials in tuberculosis. A general review. *Adv. Tuberc. Res.* 17:28–106.

Ferebee, S. H., and Mount, F. W. (1962). Tuberculosis morbidity in a controlled trial of the prophylactic use of isoniazid among household contacts. *Am. Rev. Respir. Dis.* 85(4):490–521.

Geiter, L. J., and O'Brien, R. J. (1987). Conference on new approaches for tuberculosis preventive therapy. *J. Infect. Dis.* 156(3):536–537.

Geiter, L. J., O'Brien, R. J., and Kopanoff, D. E. (1990). Short-course preventive therapy. *Am. Rev. Respir. Dis.* 141(4, part 2):A437.

Grazcyk, J., O'Brien, R. J., Bek, E., Nimerowska, H., and Geiter, L. J. (1991). Assessment of rifampin containing regimens for tuberculosis preventive therapy: preliminary results of a pilot study in Poland (abstract). *Am. Rev. Respir. Dis.* 143(4, part 2):A119.

Hong Kong Chest Service/Tuberculosis Research Centre, Madras/British Medical Research Council (1992). A double-blind placebo-controlled clinical trial of three antituberculosis chemoprophylaxis regimens in patients with silicosis in Hong Kong. *Am. Rev. Respir. Dis.* 145:36–41.

International Union Against Tuberculosis Committee on Prophylaxis (1982). Efficacy of various durations of isoniazid preventive therapy for tuberculosis: five years of follow-up in the IUAT trial. *Bull. WHO* 60:555–564.

Jordan, T. J., Lewit, E. M., Montgomery, R. L., and Reichman, L. B. (1991). Isoniazid as preventive therapy in HIV-infected intravenous drug abusers. *JAMA* 265(22):2987–2991.

Kopanoff, D. E., Snider, D. E., Jr., and Caras, G. J. (1978). Isoniazid-related hepatitis a U.S. Public Health Service cooperative surveillance study. *Am. Rev. Respir. Dis.* 117(6):991–1001.

Lecoeur, H. F., Truffot-Pernot, C., and Grosset, J. H. (1989). Experimental short-course preventive therapy of tuberculosis with rifampin and pyrazinamide. *Am. Rev. Respir. Dis.* 140:1189–1193.

Lincoln, E. M. (1954). The effect of antimicrobial therapy on the prognosis of primary tuberculosis in children. *Am. Rev. Tuberc.* 69(5):682–689.

Magdorf, K., Arizzi-Rusche, A. F., Geiter, L. J., O'Brien, R. J., and Wahn, U. (1991). Short-course preventive therapy for tuberculosis: a pilot study of rifampin and rifampin-pyrazinamide regimens in children (abstract). *Am. Rev. Respir. Dis.* **143**(4, part 2):A119.

Rieder, H. L., Cauthen, G. M., Comstock, G. W., and Snider, D. E. Jr. (1989). Epidemiology of tuberculosis in the United States. *Epidemiol. Rev.* **11**:79–98.

Rose, D. N., Schecter, C. B., Fahs, M. C., and Silver, A. L. (1988). Tuberculosis prevention: cost-effectiveness analysis of isoniazid chemoprophylaxis. *Am. J. Prev. Med.* **4**:102–109.

Selwyn, P. A., Hartel, D., Lewis, V. A., Schoenbaum, E. E., Vermund, S. H., Klein, R., Walker, A. T., and Friendland, G. H. (1989). A prospective study of the risk of tuberculosis among intravenous drug users with human immunodeficiency virus infection. *N. Engl. J. Med.* **320**:545–550.

Snider, D. E., Jr., and Caras G. J. (1992). Isoniazid-associated hepatitis deaths: a review of available information. *Am. Rev. Respir. Dis.* **145**:494–497.

Snider, D. E., Jr., Caras G. J., and Koplan, J. P. (1986). Preventive therapy with isoniazid: cost-effectiveness of different durations of therapy. *JAMA* **255**:1579–1583.

Taylor, W. C., Aronson, M. D., and Delbanco, T. L. (1981). Should young adults with a positive tuberculin test take isoniazid? *Ann. Intern. Med.* **94**:808–813.

Tsevat, J. Taylor, W. C., Wong, J. B., and Pauker, S. G. (1988). Isoniazid for the tuberculin reactor: take it or leave it. *Am. Rev. Respir. Dis.* **137**:215–220.

Wadhawan, D., Hira, S., Mwansa, N., Tembo, G., and Perine, P. (1991). VII International Conference on AIDS, Florence, Italy, Abstract Book Volume 2, pp. 247, Abstract W.B. 2261.

Zorini, A. O. (1958). Antituberculous chemoprophylaxis with isoniazid: preliminary note. *Dis. Chest*, 32(1):1–17.

13

BCG Vaccination

H. G. TEN DAM

Tuberculosis Unit
Division of Communicable Diseases
World Health Organization
Geneva, Switzerland

I. Introduction

Bacille Calmette-Guérin (BCG) vaccination was introduced over 70 years ago and is currently being used in almost every country, notably in the newborn within the Expanded Programme on Immunization. BCG vaccines and vaccination have been studied extensively, but several aspects, including effectiveness, are still not clear. When, after World War II, mass BCG vaccination campaigns were started by the Scandinavian Red Cross Societies and UNICEF, evidence of the protective effect of BCG vaccination against tuberculosis was scarce, but quite convincing. However, when the World Health Organization (WHO) took over technical responsibility for the mass campaigns, field assessment showed that the quality of the vaccines, and of the vaccinations, was often alarmingly poor. A research and development program was therefore started at a specially created WHO Tuberculosis Research Office. Within a few years the program systematically conducted a series of investigations that solved not only most of the practical problems arising in the field, but also more basic questions of the response of humans to BCG vaccination. A problem that remained, however, was that the strains of BCG commonly used appeared to have widely different characteristics. The original strain of BCG had been distributed to a large number of laboratories, and propagation from culture to culture, through mutation and selection of mutants, mostly accidentally but sometimes deliberately, had given rise to a variety of daughter strains. The issue was complicated because different assay methods produced different results, and a particular assay method often produced different results in different laboratories. Cooperative research was therefore undertaken toward standardizing the assay methods.

By this time the results of a number of controlled field trials became available. Protection from BCG vaccination varied, from trial to trial, between none at all to some 80%. The results have often been described as controversial. This would have been so if an answer had been sought to the simple question of whether BCG vaccination protects against tuberculosis. But clearly this question was never at issue. The trials had not been designed in a systematic way to investigate variables that could possibly influence the protective effect, but rather had been designed as program evaluation in different populations, with different vaccines and different dosages. Collectively, they showed that BCG vaccination protects to a varying degree, but could not show why. Whereas there was circumstantial evidence that extrinsic factors could have forestalled protection being observed in certain trials, it seemed far more obvious at the time that the explanation lay in qualitative differences (strains, viability, dosage) between the vaccines used. Research was therefore directed to improving the quality and identifying the most effective vaccines in experimental models.

Two vaccines that appeared promising in these studies were then tested in a large-scale controlled community trial, in different dosages, in India. They provided no protection at all! A number of hypotheses were suggested to explain this result but most of them could be refuted. Among the remaining factors was the possibility that extrinsic factors played a far greater role than had been assumed in the past.

Mass BCG vaccination campaigns had been superseded by vaccination of the newborn, and such coverage had increased tremendously. The question of whether BCG vaccination of the newborn protects against childhood tuberculosis therefore needed to be answered urgently. An empirical approach was therefore adopted, using relatively simple techniques: case-control and contact studies. These again gave disparate results and no firm indications as to which vaccine would provide the highest level of protection. However, most of the studies showed that protection was highest against hematogenously disseminated forms, especially tuberculosis meningitis and miliary tuberculosis, which are the most serious forms of childhood tuberculosis. Since extrinsic factors are unlikely to play a significant role in young children, the wide variations in protection, observed especially in the case-control studies, pointed again to qualitative differences between the vaccines. Confirmation that qualitative differences can play a role was obtained in a large study where two vaccines could be compared.

II. Vaccines

A. Early History

An account of the early history of BCG has been given by Guérin (1980). BCG is a live attenuated vaccine derived from a culture of a virulent strain of *Mycobacterium bovis* by serial subculturing for 13 years (231 passages) on glycerinated bile-potato medium. During this process the strain gradually lost its virulence for calves and guinea pigs and developed its typical growth characteristics.

The strain, which according to present standards was not really a strain since it had been derived from a culture rather than from a single colony (Frappier et al., 1971), was distributed to many other laboratories. Continuous subculturing in these laboratories has led to a variety of daughter strains that differ widely in their immediate effects in humans and in animals. Thus the characteristics were not as fixed as had been presumed, but the strain never reverted to virulence for guinea pigs or for humans. To the contrary, many strains appear to have become further attenuated. On the other hand, BCG had not lost its virulence for animals altogether: large doses are lethal for hamsters (Bunch-Christensen et al., 1968).

B. Characteristics

BCG vaccination had been observed to induce tuberculin sensitivity, and for a long time it was debated whether tuberculin "conversion" was essential for BCG vaccination to produce protection. This was one of the first issues addressed by the Tuberculosis Research Office (Edwards et al., 1953). It was demonstrated that tuberculin sensitivity induced by BCG was not a qualitative characteristic, i.e. a matter of absence or presence or "positive" or "negative," but a quantitative one. In groups of children vaccinated with the same vaccine, postvaccination tuberculin reactions show a statistically normal distribution, the mean of which depends on the type of vaccine used. For a particular vaccine the response is dose-dependent, in terms of tuberculin sensitivity, vaccination lesion size, as well as risk of suppurative lymphadenitis of the lymph nodes draining the vaccination site. Variations in viability were found to be reflected in the level of tuberculin sensitivity induced, but much less in the size of the vaccination lesion. This provided a basis for the evaluation of vaccines and vaccination programs: a batch of vaccine that induces a relatively low level of tuberculin sensitivity for a usual vaccination lesion size will have had a low viability. Duration of storage and exposure to high temperatures were known to reduce the viability of liquid BCG vaccines, but a surprising finding was that exposure to sunlight for a few minutes reduces the viability by 99%.

It is not known which dose of BCG should be administered to achieve optimal protection, and the policy therefore has been to give the maximum dose that can be reasonably tolerated, considering lesion size and risk of complications. The best results are therefore obtained with a vaccine of high viability. Whether a high viability and the resulting high level of induced tuberculin sensitivity are relevant for protection in humans is not known. In a trial in American Indians, a vaccine batch accidentally produced on a poor medium resulted in a low conversion rate as well as in reduced protection (Aronson and Palmer, 1946), and a tendency for protection to be correlated with viability and tuberculin sensitivity was also seen in a trial in England (D'Arcy Hart et al., 1967).

Freeze drying of BCG vaccine was introduced by 1960, and since then freeze-dried vaccine has replaced liquid vaccine. The advantages of freeze-dried vaccine are that it can be stored much longer than liquid vaccine and that it is less sensitive to higher temperatures, which greatly facilitates transport. Further advantages are that quality control examinations can be terminated before the vaccine is released, which was not possible for liquid vaccine, and that a reference vaccine can be used in the examinations. On the other hand, it is more difficult and costly to prepare a freeze-dried vaccine of good quality. Moreover, the drying process reduces the viability of the vaccine, often by 60–80%. Field assessment has shown, however, that the results obtained with freeze-dried vaccines are comparable to those obtained with carefully stored and transported liquid vaccines.

C. The Seed Lot System

Freeze drying made it possible to replace propagation from culture to culture by simply keeping the BCG strain in dried form and thus to prevent further genetic changes. Production is now based on the seed lot system. A seed lot is a large batch of dried vaccine, generally kept in a deep freezer, from which at frequent intervals an ampule is opened and reconstituted to start a new series of subcultures, which is limited to 12 (or six in case of a secondary seed lot).

D. Quality Control

The first freeze-dried vaccines often showed even larger batch-to-batch variations than the liquid vaccines from which they were prepared. To further uniformity in production, or at least in the products delivered, WHO set up an international quality control system, and requirements for dried BCG vaccine were issued by the WHO Expert Committee on Biological Standardization, first in 1966, with revisions in 1978 and 1985. The tests routinely carried out include physical tests (vacuum of ampule, opacity for bacterial content), microbiological tests (identity, homogeneity, sterility, viability, heat stability), and in vivo control (safety test in guinea pigs, tuberculin sensitivity, and lesion size in children).

Batch-to-batch variations are thus kept under control, and since gross deterioration during transport and storage is almost excluded, routine postvaccination tuberculin testing is no longer required.

E. Differences Between Strains

The availability of the most commonly used strains in the form of seed lots made it interesting to carry out comparisons with a view to identifying those strains that would have the highest immunogenic effect in humans. Evidence that the strains used in the trials that showed disappointing results may have had poor immunogenic properties was produced, *a posteriori*, by Willis and Vandiviere (1961) and Jespersen (1971).

Vallishayee et al. (1974) showed that vaccines produced from 11 different strains differed in terms of tuberculin sensitivity and lesion sizes induced in children. But whereas differences between batches produced from the same strain point to differences in quality, this is not necessarily so for vaccines produced from different strains. It has never been demonstrated conclusively that the immediate effects in humans reflect the immunogenicity of a vaccine, and the level of tuberculin sensitivity observed may depend not only on the BCG but also on the tuberculin used. Ladefoged et al. (1976) demonstrated that 12 strains could be ranked according to the development of tuberculin sensitivity in guinea pigs given the minimum sensitizing dose. Previously a number of strains had been ranked according to the rate of developing immunity in guinea pigs and in bank voles (Ladefoged et al., 1970) and according to the virulence for hamsters (Bunch-Christensen et al., 1968). The rankings obtained in terms of tuberculin reactions in children and in the various animal models were not identical but were concordant in many aspects.

In the absence of firm knowledge of the significance of experimental models for protection in humans, it may well be that a ranking obtained as an "average" is completely irrelevant. It nevertheless seemed wise to select for BCG production a strain that ranks high rather than one that ranks low in the models studied. The vaccines for the large trial in India were selected accordingly.

The strains that ranked high included those that are known to produce a relatively high risk of suppurative lymphadenitis in young children, notably the Paris strain (seed lot 1173 P2) and the Copenhagen strain (seed lot 1331). Lymph node involvement is an integral part of the BCG vaccination process, which aims at producing an artificial primary complex. The occurrence of lymphadenitis therefore may indicate a good "take" of the vaccination, but excessive reactions should of course be avoided. This can be done by reducing the bacterial content of the vaccine: the incidence of suppurative lymphadenitis is linearly related to the dosage (Guld et al., 1955).

III. Protection

A. Early Evidence

The early evidence of a protective effect of BCG vaccination in humans is not just of historical interest, but remains relevant to the potential field of application.

In the early 1920s it was generally held that tuberculosis infection was contracted during early childhood and that disease, also in adults, occurred through reactivation because of some incidental extraneous event. It was therefore considered that the field of application of BCG vaccination was limited to young children.

However, Heimbeck (1949), who was concerned about the high incidence of tuberculosis among student nurses at the Oslo municipal hospital, started tuberculin testing in 1924 and found that less than half the students were positive when they joined the service but that almost all were so at the end of the 3-year training period. Among the students admitted in 1924–1926, 152 were tuberculin positive and 185 negative. Three cases of tuberculosis occurred among the former and as many as 62 cases (with eight deaths) among the latter. From these findings, Heimbeck concluded that tuberculin-positive students were far more resistant than tuberculin-negative students and that rendering the latter tuberculin-positive by artificial means could protect them against tuberculosis. He found that parenteral vaccination with BCG (unlike oral administration) produced a high level of tuberculin sensitivity and offered this to all new students as from 1927. During the following 8 years, 899 students were enrolled. Among these, 436 were tuberculin-positive of whom 27 (6%) developed tuberculosis; 463 were tuberculin-negative of whom 79 developed tuberculosis: 42 (44%) among the 95 who refused vaccination and 37 (10%) among the 368 who accepted it. It thus appeared that BCG vaccination provided significant protection in a situation where the risk of infection was very high.

For similar reasons a controlled trial of BCG vaccination (Aronson et al., 1958) was organized among American Indians in a number of reservations where morbidity and mortality from tuberculosis was very high. The trial started in 1936 and was carried out among subjects aged 1–20 years who were negative to a high-dose tuberculin test. The results after a follow-up of 18–20 years were particularly impressive in view of the observed reduction in mortality:

	BCG vaccinated	Controls
No. of persons	1547	1448
No. of deaths from:		
Violence	45	40
Nontuberculosis diseases	46	42
Tuberculosis	13	68
Total no. of deaths	104	150

In this population BCG vaccination reduced mortality from all causes by 35%, from disease by 50% and from tuberculosis by over 80%.

Hyge (1956) carried out a retrospective study of an epidemic in a state school for girls in the spring of 1943. The girls became exposed to infection at school, 1–3 months after routine tuberculin testing and X-ray examination. One year previously BCG vaccination had been offered at the school, but 46 of the tuberculin-negative girls (12–18 years of age) had refused and another 59 had entered the school afterward. Among the 105 unvaccinated tuberculin-negative girls, 41 developed primary tuberculosis (bacteriologically confirmed in 37) and in 14 progressive disease developed subsequently. Of 105 tuberculin-positive girls, one developed primary tuberculosis and 10 pulmonary disease. Among 133 BCG vaccinated girls, no primary tuberculosis was observed but two developed cavitary pulmonary disease. BCG vaccination apparently protected both against primary tuberculosis and against progressive disease for at least 12 years.

B. Controlled Trials

The trials initiated in the 1950s have been reviewed several times (D'Arcy Hart, 1967; Sutherland, 1971; ten Dam et al., 1976) to find an explanation for the disparity of the results. The main hypotheses put forward were that the vaccines differed in immunogenic potency (strains, viability), that in some trials the method of administration (dosage) was inadequate, and that in some trials the existence of immunity from infection with environmental mycobacteria, as evidenced by the prevalence of low-grade tuberculin sensitivity, forestalled protection being observed, i.e., that BCG did not add to the "natural" immunity.

By using dual tests with tuberculin PPD-S and the new antigens PPD-B, prepared from a nonphotochromogen isolated at the Battey State Hospital (now referred to as *M. intracellulare*), and PPD-Y, prepared from the "yellow" bacillus, a photochromogen isolated in Kansas City (now *M. Kansasii*), Edwards and Palmer (1958) demonstrated that different sensitizing agents occurred in the United States. Evidence that low-grade sensitivity could be associated with immunity against tuberculosis was obtained in longitudinal studies in navy recruits (Edwards and Palmer, 1968): among men with reactions to PPD-S of less than 6 mm the incidence of tuberculosis among those with small reactions to PPD-B was about twice as high as among those with large reactions to PPD-B. Also, in the controlled trial in England, children with low-grade tuberculin sensitivity showed a lower incidence than those with no sensitivity (D'Arcy Hart and Sutherland, 1977). That environmental mycobacteria can induce skin sensitivity, and more so to a homologous product than to a heterologous one, as well as protection against challenge with tubercle bacilli, had been demonstrated by Palmer and Long (1966) in a large experiment in guinea pigs. The degree of protection correlated with the degree of sensitivity to PPD-S. However, the protection was at best not more than 50% of that induced by BCG. Moreover additional BCG vaccination raised protection to the level induced by BCG alone. Thus immunity associated with sensitization by environmental mycobacteria indeed could have reduced the observable protective effect of BCG vaccination in some trials, but alone could not have masked it altogether if a potent BCG product had been used. In the trial in Puerto Rico, where subjects with low-grade sensitivity had been included among the vaccinated and the controls, the protection among them was of the same (low) level as that among the tuberculin-negative (Comstock and Edwards, 1972).

C. The Trial in South India

Since differences in vaccine quality appeared to be the most likely explanation for the disparity of the results obtained in the controlled trials, it was felt that the technological development and the new knowledge acquired from experimental models could make it possible to produce BCG vaccines that would show a high protective effect anywhere. This prompted the start of a new controlled trial.

The trial was organized in South India by the Indian Council of Medical Research in cooperation with the World Health Organization and the Centers for Disease Control, United States Public Health Service. The intake started in 1968 and was completed in 1971; by then about 260,000 participants had been included out of a population of 360,000. The entire population (all ages) was eligible, and in contrast with previous trials, tuberculin reactors were not excluded, though of course the initial tuberculin reactions were carefully recorded so that the results could be analyzed accordingly.

Two vaccines were included, prepared from the Paris strain (seed lot 1173 P2) and the Copenhagen strain (seed lot 1331). To study the effect of dosage, they were used in strengths of 1 mg/ml and 0.1 mg/ml. The seed lots were selected because of their high ranking in experimental models and because the Paris seed lot was being used in 20 and the Copenhagen seed lot in seven national production centers. Moreover, the Copenhagen seed lot had been derived from the strain used to produce the vaccine used in successful trials in England.

The follow-up was both passive and active in 2½ year survey cycles. Case finding aimed at obtaining bacteriological evidence (by microscopy and culture) of pulmonary tuberculosis. The first results, after 7½ years (Tuberculosis Prevention Trial, 1979), showed that there had been no protective effect at all! In fact, regarding those with tuberculin reactions of 0–7 mm at the intake, the incidence in the vaccinated was significantly higher than in the controls. However, this tendency became reversed, and after 10–12½ years there were about equal numbers of cases in all groups (Tripathy, 1983).

The disappointing results seriously challenged the current BCG vaccination policies. A number of more or less obvious explanations, other than that the vaccines had no immunogenic effect, were considered (ICMR/WHO Scientific Group, 1980; WHO Study Group, 1980), and several were studied subsequently:

The methodology was queried by a number of uninformed research workers, but most queries were satisfactorily answered in a comprehensive report (Tuberculosis Prevention Trial, 1980). One weak point, however, was that persons with reactions of 0–7 mm to the initial tuberculin test (3 IU) were considered noninfected. Since the prevalence of infection was high, some infected people may have been included, and since the incidence of disease in the infected was some 20 times higher than among the noninfected, a proportion of the cases observed among those with reaction of 0–7 mm may have stemmed from the infected. This may have masked the effectiveness of BCG to some extent, but certainly not completely.

The quality of the vaccines may have been poor. Quality control by WHO-sponsored laboratories, however, consistently had shown that the various vaccine batches, whether produced in Copenhagen or in Madras, had been of the usual quality in terms of viability and other laboratory tests.

Freeze drying of the seed lots or of the vaccines could have reduced their immunogenicity. This hypothesis was most unlikely in view of the results in experimental models and of the immediate effects in humans. Moreover, a trial in Haiti (Vandiviere et al., 1973) had shown that dried vaccines gave substantial protection.

The South Indian variant of *M. tuberculosis* has low virulence for guinea pigs (Mitchison, 1964). It was suggested that BCG may not protect against infection with this strain. This question was studied by Smith and co-workers. They challenged guinea pigs, vaccinated with a weak or a strong vaccine with strains of low virulence, high virulence, or H37Rv. The weak vaccine protected only against challenge with the low-virulence strain; the strong vaccine against all strains (Hank et al., 1981).

BCG vaccination may be followed by a period of increased susceptibility. This old idea was brought up again in connection with the observed excess incidence in the controls. Smith and co-workers addressed this question by varying the challenge interval in their guinea pig studies. Protection was observed after any interval except 1 week (Edwards et al., 1981). The fact remains that increased initial susceptibility was observed in the trial, probably as the result of something that did not apply in the guinea pig study, and still lacks an explanation.

The host response. Variations in protection may be the result of a possibly genetically determined reduced immunologic response. This hypothesis has been investigated in case-control studies (see below).

The duration of protection from BCG may be very short. If this were so, protection would be observed when most cases occur shortly after vaccination, as in many of the successful studies, or when infection occurs shortly after vaccination and not much later, as in the trial in England. In the latter case, those infected soon after vaccination would continue to have a reduced risk of endogenous reactivation, after immunity had disappeared, simply because they would have fewer residual foci. In the trial in India only very few cases occurred shortly after vaccination, and the risk of infection remained high throughout the follow-up period. Short-lived immunity, therefore, could scarcely have been observed. Circumstantial evidence that immunity may have been of short duration is that BCG-induced tuberculin sensitivity waned rapidly in the first 2 ½ years.

Environmental mycobacteria. In the trial in India lack of protection coincided again (if coincidence there is) with a high prevalence of low-grade sensitivity. Sensitization indeed was massive: by 10 years of age, almost all children were sensitized. If sensitization were associated with the same immunogenic effect as BCG, it is likely that protection would not be observed, at least not in adults. It also could be that previous sensitization with certain environmental bacteria would adversely influence the immunogenic effect of BCG (Rook et al., 1981). These questions were also investigated by Smith and coworkers in their guinea pig model. Infection with mycobacteria of the *avium-intracellulare* complex (isolated in the trial area) provided the same level of protection as BCG, but only against challenge with a low-virulence strain, and the response after BCG vaccination was the same as after subsequent BCG vaccination alone (Edwards et al., 1982). The latter observation confirms that sensitization with environmental mycobacteria does not interfere with the effect of BCG, as had been demonstrated earlier by Palmer and Long (1966). The very fact that the incidence of tuberculosis in the trial area was high indicates that protection associated with sensitization by environmental mycobacteria must have had little impact.

Exogenous reinfection. BCG vaccination cannot be expected to show protection against tuberculosis if disease is the result of exogenous reinfection: the primary infection would determine the level of protection, whether BCG vaccination were given or not. BCG vaccination does not prevent infection with tuberculosis as is clear from animal experiments and was shown in autopsy studies (Sutherland and Lindgren, 1979). From an analysis of the incidence patterns in different protection studies, ten Dam and Pio (1982) found that in studies showing high protection, tuberculosis had been predominantly of the primary and evolutive types. In these studies most cases had been observed early after the intake. The authors therefore proposed that protection was not observed in the trial in India because the type of tuberculosis diagnosed had been the result of exogenous reinfection.

This hypothesis would also explain the initial excess of tuberculosis among the vaccinated. Among the controls a first infection would not lead (according to the hypothesis) to primary or evolutive pulmonary tuberculosis, but among the vaccinated it might resemble reinfection and in some cases lead to the often cavitary "adult" type of tuberculosis, which would have readily been diagnosed in the trial.

The question of whether the "adult" type of tuberculosis is caused by endogenous reactivation or reinfection has been debated for a long time as it was generally impossible to identify the origin of the causative organisms. With the large decreases in the risk of infection in various populations, however, it became apparent that the role of endogenous reactivation had been grossly overestimated. Certain special-risk groups apart (notably the HIV-infected and persons on immunosuppressive treatment), the annual risk of late reactivation is not higher than about 12–15 per 100,000 (Styblo, 1990). During the first 5 years of the trial in England, the average annual incidence among tuberculin reactors was 149 per 100 000. In 1978, among the reactors of the same age group, it was 14.1 per 100 000 (British Thoracic Association, 1980). The large decrease in the risk of reinfection seems the most likely explanation for this more than 10-fold reduction in incidence.

Three observations that, together, are indicative of disease from exogenous reinfection in the study population in India are the low incidence in the uninfected, the high incidence in the infected, and the high risk of infection. The low virulence of the infecting bacilli and the protection associated with low-grade sensitivity could explain the low incidence of primary and evolutive tuberculosis.

D. Studies in Children

The trial in India gave no information on the effect of BCG vaccination on childhood tuberculosis, as childhood tuberculosis was not observed. Some of the hypotheses (infection with environmental mycobacteria, exogenous reinfection) probably would not apply in young children, so that the BCG vaccination policy adopted in most developing countries, i.e., vaccination of the newborn, could still be valid provided the existing vaccines induce protection. A review of vaccination studies in infants (ten Dam and Hitze, 1980) showed that the information was scarce but on the whole favorable. To justify the vaccination policy, however, it was clearly necessary to evaluate the effectiveness of current vaccination programs in an expedient way. The methods proposed were case-control and contact studies. Moreover, a prospective study, which already had started before results of the trial in India were known, had been designed to compare the effects of two vaccines prepared from strains that had ranked quite differently in the experimental models.

E. Case-Control Studies

Case-control studies are relatively simple to perform when the BCG vaccination coverage is not very high or very low and childhood tuberculosis is being diagnosed accurately. The controls must be selected judiciously because they should represent the population that actually produced the cases. The protective effect of BCG vaccination is calculated from the vaccination coverages observed in the cases and in the controls.

Table 1   WHO-Assisted Case-Control Studies on the Efficacy of BCG Vaccination Against Childhood Tuberculosis

Country (vaccine)	Ref.[a]	No. of cases	No. of controls	BCG coverage (%)	Efficacy (%)
Brazil (meningitis) (Rio de Janeiro strain)	1	73	604	91	82–84
Burma (Japan BCG Laboratory)	2	311	1536	64	38
Sri Lanka (various)	3	292	1193	87	20
Argentina (B.A.) (various)	4	175	875	63	73
Argentina (Santa Fe) (various)	3	117	1014	88	2

[a](1) Wünsch Filho et al. (1990); (2) Myint et al. (1987); (3) Smith (1987); (4) Miceli et al. (1988).

The results of WHO-assisted case-control studies are shown in Table 1. The numbers of cases and controls and the BCG vaccination coverage give an indication of the power of the studies. The results again vary widely. This is partly explained by the fact that in some studies the cases included many children with primary tuberculosis against which the protective effect turned out to be relatively low. Protection invariably was highest against disseminated types of disease and when the diagnosis was confirmed by bacteriology. Overdiagnosis may have occurred when the diagnosis was based on clinical evidence only or when (in Santa Fe) a tuberculin test was used. The latter may have introduced bias against the protective effect of BCG.

Table 2 shows the results of some other case-control studies carried out in the 1980s. These studies were carried out in various age groups. It should be noted that when the age group is wide, the observed result is a kind of average of the level of protection at different times after vaccination, since case-control studies show the level of protection at the time of observation, not for the period since vaccination. For most studies protection is considerable.

Of particular interest are the preliminary results of the study in India. It is being carried out in Madras, i.e., near the area of the unsuccessful trial, and is focused on cases of tuberculosis meningitis. The high protective effect observed, if confirmed, indicates that the lack of protection in the trial is not explained by the hypotheses invoking lack of immunogenicity of the strain,

Table 2 Other Case-Control Studies on the Efficacy of BCG Vaccination

Country (vaccine)	Ref.[a]	Age (Years)	No. of cases	No. of controls	Efficacy (%)
Brazil (meningitis) (Rio de Janeiro strain)	1	0–12	45	90	82
Canada (Indians) (Connaught)	2	0–18	71	213	60
Indonesia (Japan BCG Laboratory)	3	0–5	103	412	40
Colombia (various)	3	0–14	178	320	16
Cameroon (Inst. Pasteur)	4	17–26	312	819	63
England (Asians) (Glaxo)	5	0–1	111	555	49
England (Asians) (Glaxo)	6	1–12	108	432	64
Thailand (various)	7	0–14	75	207	83
India (meningitis) (Copenhagen strain)	8	0–12	61	183	85

[a](1) Camargos et al. (1988); (2) Young and Hershfield (1981); (3) Smith (1987); (4) Blin et al. (1986); (5) Rodrigues and Smith (1990); (6) Packe and Innes (1988); (7) Sirinavin et al. (1991); (8) Thilothammal et al. (1992).

dosage, quality of production, freeze drying, or genetic characteristics of the population.

F. Contact Studies

Contact studies are cohort studies, like controlled trials, but differ from these in that there is no random allocation to the vaccinated and unvaccinated groups. In the analysis, this is remedied by stratification for variables that may cause confounding, such as sex and age, degree of exposure, and living conditions. Because all children are contacts of newly diagnosed bacteriologically confirmed cases of tuberculosis, vaccinated and unvaccinated groups are a priori comparable in many respects.

Table 3 WHO-Assisted Contact Studies on the Efficacy of BCG Vaccination Against Childhood Tuberculosis

Country	Ref.[a]	No. of contacts Vacc.	Unvacc.	No. of cases Vacc.	Unvacc.	Efficacy (95% conf. int.)
Thailand (Mérieux)	1	1253	253	218	66	53% (38–64%)
Togo (Glaxo)	2	875	546	62	113	62% (50–70%)
Korea (Paris seed lot)	3	806	417	45	84	74% (62–82%)
Colombia (Paris seed lot)	4	330	88	32	23	64% (36–80%)

[a] (1) Padungchan et al. (1986); (2) Tidjani et al. (1986); (3) Jin et al. (1989); (4) calculated from data supplied by Dr. C. E. Salgado.

The results of the WHO-assisted studies are shown in Table 3. Protection was observed in all studies, but it varied with the type of disease and was highest for the disseminated types such as meningitis and miliary and for cavitary disease and lowest for paratracheal and hilar adenopathy and infiltration without cavity. In these studies disseminated disease was relatively rare since children were given treatment as soon as tuberculosis was suspected. In many cases diagnosis was based on minimal X-ray lesions, and it is likely that overdiagnosis occurred, reducing the observed protective effect.

The studies confirm that BCG can protect against tuberculosis. It should be noted that protection varied according to the types of disease observed and that in this regard the studies varied widely. In the absence of any other hypotheses that would give a satisfactory explanation of the sometimes disappointing results, however, it seems wise to assume that qualitative differences, between the vaccines or in their application, played a major role.

G. A Prospective Comparative Study

A prospective study of the response to BCG vaccination of the newborn was carried out in Hong Kong. Vaccination coverage having reached virtually 100%, it was not possible to carry out a case-control or a contact study to evaluate the protective effect of vaccination and it was not acceptable to undertake a study that would require an unvaccinated control group. However, the Chest Service Central Office, Department of Health, initiated a comparative study, replacing in half of the children the usual Glaxo vaccine by a vaccine prepared from the

Paris seed lot by the Japan BCG Laboratory. Intradermal and percutaneous vaccines were used as these different techniques are routinely employed in Hong Kong. All children born between 1978 and 1982 were included.

The study outline and the first results were presented by Chan at the 26th IUAT World Conference (Chan et al., 1986). As they were not recorded, they are briefly summarized here.

Since vaccines of the Paris seed lot were known to produce suppurative lymphadenitis relatively often, a preliminary calibration study was carried out to find an intradermal dose sufficiently low to avoid too many complaints but high enough to induce a level of tuberculin sensitivity comparable to that induced by the routine Glaxo vaccine. The intradermal dose finally applied was 0.05 ml of a vaccine containing 0.1 mg/ml, which is 1/10 of the usual strength. Percutaneous vaccination was by triangular needle (20 punctures). The concentration of the percutaneous vaccine prepared from the Paris seed lot was 16 mg/ml, which is 1/10 of a concentration found adequate in previous studies of percutaneous vaccination. The Glaxo vaccines were of the usual strengths.

Vaccination was carried out in the six Government hospitals, using the intradermal technique, and in 40 nongovernmental institutes that used percutaneous vaccination. Allocation of the vaccines was by rotation. A random system was prepared by which intradermal vaccination in the six government hospitals was changed every month. In the 40 private institutes the percutaneous vaccine was changed every year, also by a random process. All vaccinations were recorded on individual cards. Cases of tuberculosis were recorded by the tuberculosis service and were sought by monthly visits to all pediatric departments. As the numbers detected appeared low, active follow-up of child contacts was strengthened.

Table 4 shows the study population and the observed incidence of tuberculosis. For both intradermal and percutaneous vaccination, the number of cases after vaccination with the vaccine prepared from the Paris seed lot was smaller than for those given Glaxo vaccine. The summary relative risk is 0.63 with 95%

Table 4 Hong Kong BCG Study 1978/1982–1986: Study Population and Incidence of Tuberculosis

Method	Vaccine	No. vaccinated	No. cases	Cases per 10 000
Intradermal	Glaxo	81,304	37	4.6
	Paris strain	81,649	28	3.4
Percutaneous	Glaxo	70,121	42	5.9
	Paris strain	70,018	22	3.1

Table 5 Hong Kong BCG Study 1978/1982–1986: Disease Incidence by Type

Type	Vaccine	
	Glaxo	Paris strain
Primary TB and effusion	32	29
Glandular	7	8
Pulmonary	16	7
Meningeal alone or combined	11	4
Bone and joint	8	1
Multiple sites	5	1

confidence limits of 0.48 and 0.91. As there was no unvaccinated control group, the absolute levels of any protection cannot be estimated. It may be that the vaccines induced a very high level of protection, so that the absolute difference in effectiveness, in percentage points, is not very high. However, the advantage of the vaccine from the Paris strain was most apparent for the disseminated serious types of tuberculosis, as may be seen from Table 5. The practical significance of the difference observed, therefore, may be greater than suggested by the total figures.

By the end of 1991 another 14 cases had been recorded (S. L. Chan, personal communication): one among those given vaccine from the Paris strain and 13 among those given Glaxo vaccine. The long-term effects may therefore differ substantially, and it will be interesting to continue observations at least well into adolescence, when the risk of tuberculosis is expected to be increased.

The significant difference observed so far clearly indicates that qualitative differences between vaccines can be of practical importance and should be studied further.

IV. Adverse Reactions

A. Local Reactions

Correct intradermal vaccination with a potent vaccine causes a local superficial ulcer, usually seen covered with a crust, which heals in 2–3 months and leaves an often permanent, slightly excavated, round scar 4–8 mm in diameter. With overdosage the tissue destruction will be increased. Occasionally subcutaneous local abscesses are seen that are followed by pronounced, sometimes retracted, scars. They are the result of injecting the vaccine too deeply, with overdosage as a contributing factor (Edwards et al., 1953). In some populations keloid formation can be observed. Its frequency appears to be increased if vaccinations are given too high on the upper arm (over the acromion).

B. Lymphadenitis

Suppurative axillary or cervical lymphadenitis is observed in a small proportion of vaccinated children. Its frequency depends on the age of the subject, the dose, and the strain from which the vaccine has been prepared. Experience has shown that the risk is low for vaccines prepared, for instance, from the London and Tokyo strains and much higher for vaccines from the Paris and Copenhagen strains. In recent years there have been several reports of "outbreaks" of lymphadenitis. They invariably were due to a program switching from a low-reactogenic vaccine to a vaccine of the Paris strain, with poor vaccination techniques probably contributing (Ray et al., 1988). In human immunodeficiency virus (HIV)–infected infants the risk may be somewhat increased, but not alarmingly so (Lallemant-LeCoeur et al., 1991).

Lymphadenitis will heal spontaneously, and it is best not to treat the lesion if it remains unadherent to the skin. An adherent or fistulated lymph gland, however, may be drained and an antituberculosis drug may be instilled locally. Systemic treatment with antituberculosis drugs is ineffective.

C. Disseminated BCG-itis

Disseminated BCG-itis is a rare complication invariably associated with severe immunodeficiency. It has become a matter of concern in view of the rapidly increasing number of infants infected with HIV, particularly in African countries. By 1990, four cases had been reported (ten Dam, 1990). Three of these cases had been treated and improved rapidly upon treatment with isoniazid and rifampicin or ethambutol. Disseminated BCG disease was not observed in two prospective studies, in Congo (Lallemant-LeCoeur et al., 1991) and in Rwanda (Msellati et al., 1991). These observations support the continued practice of vaccinating asymptomatic infants in Africa as early in life as possible. Children born to HIV-infected mothers most often are not infected with HIV and would benefit from the vaccinations, especially since the mothers are at a greatly increased risk of developing tuberculosis. In areas where the risk of tuberculosis is low, however, BCG vaccination may be withheld from individuals known or suspected to be infected with HIV. BCG should be withheld from symptomatic HIV-infected individuals (SPA/EPI, 1987).

Other rare complications include erythema nodosum, iritis, lupus vulgaris, and ostemomyelitis. The latter complication was observed mainly in Sweden and Finland and seemed to be associated with the use of the Gothenburg strain of BCG. These complications should be treated with regimens including isoniazid and rifampicin.

V. Conclusions and Recommendations

Very young contacts are generally infected before the index case is detected, and in a high proportion tuberculosis can be diagnosed by that time. Moreover, young children are prone to developing miliary disease and tuberculous meningitis, which is often fatal or causes permanent brain damage even if treated. BCG should therefore be given as early in life as possible. However, when the risk of infection in the community has become very low, e.g., lower than 0.1% per year, the potential benefit of BCG vaccination may be offset by adverse reactions. Systematic BCG vaccination should then be replaced by selected vaccination of risk groups.

Vaccination or revaccination just before adolescence has been practiced in many European countries and has been demonstrated to be effective. However, the number of vaccinations required to prevent one case of tuberculosis increases as the risk of infection declines. Several countries therefore have abandoned it or are considering doing so. Vaccination at this age has a significant indirect effect. It was shown in England (Sutherland and Springett, 1989) that if vaccination were discontinued now, the incidence in the 15- to 29-year age group would not increase, but it may take some 10–15 years more to reach the same low incidence level as if vaccination were continued. Previous BCG vaccination, by preventing endogenous reactivation, may prevent tuberculosis among people who acquire HIV infection after tuberculosis infection. It may similarly prevent disease from infection with mycobacteria other than *M. tuberculosis* (Källenius et al., 1989). Since BCG should not be given to people known or suspected to have been infected with HIV, the HIV problem should be considered timely when formulating a policy for vaccination of adolescents (or discontinuing an existing program).

BCG vaccination of risk groups, such as medical personnel, used to be practiced widely but in several countries has been abandoned in favor of regular screening by means of the tuberculin test, which makes it possible to give preventive chemotherapy (chemoprophylaxis) when conversion is observed. A point recently raised, however, is that preventive chemotherapy with isoniazid, and perhaps chemotherapy, would not be expected to be effective in a subject infected with multidrug-resistant bacilli.

The results obtained in the more recent studies show that BCG vaccination can provide a substantial level of protection, at least against childhood tuberculosis, but that a varying proportion of the vaccinated children remains unprotected. Program assessment in the contact studies, by measuring the vaccination scars and postvaccination tuberculin sensitivity in the children not suffering from tuberculosis, showed that the quality of the vaccinations may have been far from optimal. In the study in Thailand (Padungchan et al., 1986), over 50% of the children had tuberculin reactions (to 2 TU of RT23 with Tween) of less than

5 mm; in Togo (Tidjani et al., 1986) over 20%, and in Korea (Jin et al., 1989) over 30%. Efforts to increase the effectiveness of vaccination programs, therefore, may be directed in the first place toward qualitative improvements.

The response to BCG vaccination is dose-dependent. Since it has not been possible to determine a threshold dose for any vaccine, the rational procedure is to give the highest dose that is acceptable. Acceptability is determined by the local vaccination reaction (ulcer, scar), but in young children especially by the incidence of suppurative axillary lymphadenitis. Each program should therefore check that the dose of vaccine administered is appropriate for the vaccine used. Special caution is required when a particular vaccine is replaced with another. In practice, switching vaccines is best avoided, because often there are differences in physical characteristics that require special precautions during reconstitution.

Producers of BCG vaccine should assume responsibility in these matters by ensuring that their products are extensively calibrated in the actual target populations, i.e., in the newborn if the vaccine is supplied for use in that group, taking into account that the dose is to be administered in 0.05 ml.

The easiest way to check whether a child has been vaccinated is to see whether it has a lesion or scar. A small percentage of children do not develop a scar, most often because the dose was insufficient. It is therefore practical to verify whether a child has a BCG lesion or scar and to vaccinate if not. BCG vaccination can be given safely at the same time as any other vaccination.

The quality of the administration can be monitored by measuring the scar sizes in groups of some 100 children known to have been vaccinated. The distribution of the sizes, when entered into a histogram, should appear normal (in the statistical sense) and have a small variance and an appropriate mean. If this is observed, it may be assumed that the vaccinations were adequate as far as the injection technique is concerned.

To obtain a measure of the quality of the entire vaccination procedure, groups of some 100 children may be given a tuberculin test 3–5 months after vaccination. If the reaction sizes show a normal distribution and the variance and mean are characteristic for the vaccine and dose used (e.g., are established by an expert team), the entire procedure, from production to injection, has been adequate. The actual effectiveness of the vaccinations may be evaluated by carrying out follow-up studies in child contacts of newly detected cases or case-control studies.

References

Aronson, J. D., and Palmer, C. E. (1946). Experience with BCG vaccine in the control of tuberculosis among north American Indians. *Public Health Rep.* **61**:802–820.

Aronson, J. D., Aronson, D. F., and Taylor, H. C. (1958). A twenty-year appraisal of BCG vaccination in the control of tuberculosis. *AMA Arch. Intern. Med.* **101**:881–891.

Blin, P., Delolme, H. G., Heyraud, J. D., Charpak, Y., and Sentilhes, L. (1986). Evaluation of the protective effect of BCG vaccination by a case-control study in Yaoundé, Cameroon. *Tubercle* **67**:283–288.

British Thoracic Association (1980). Effectiveness of BCG vaccination in Great Britain in 1978. *Br. J. Dis. Chest* **74**:215–227.

Bunch-Christensen, K., Ladefoged, A., and Guld, J. (1968). The virulence of some strains of BCG for golden hamsters. *Bull. WHO* **39**:821–828.

Camargos, P. A. M., Guimareas, M. D. C., and Antunes, C. M. F. (1988). Risk assessment for acquiring meningitis tuberculosis among children not vaccinated with BCG: a case-control study. *Int. J. Epidemiol.* **17**: 193–197.

Chan, S. L., Allen, G., Pio, A., ten Dam, H. G., Sutherland, I., and Kerr, I. (1986). Comparison of the efficacy of two strains of BCG vaccine for the prevention of tuberculosis among newborn children in Hong Kong (abstract). *Bull. Int. Un. Tuberc.* **61**:36–37.

Comstock, G. W., and Edwards, P. Q. (1972). An American view of BCG vaccination, illustrated by results of a controlled trial in Puerto Rico. *Scand. J. Respir. Dis.* **53**:207–217.

Edwards, L. B. and Palmer, C. E. (1958). Epidemiological studies of tuberculin sensitivity. I. Preliminary results with purified protein derivatives prepared from atypical acid fast organisms. *Am. J. Hyg.* **68**: 213–231.

Edwards, L. B., and Palmer, C. E. (1968). Identification of the tuberculous-infected by skin tests. *Ann. NY Acad. Sci.* **154**:140–148.

Edwards, L. B., Palmer, C. E., and Magnus, K. (1953). *BCG Vaccination.* World Health Organization. Monograph Series No. 12, Geneva.

Edwards, M. L., Muller, D., and Smith, D. W. (1981). Influence of vaccination-challenge interval on the protective efficacy of bacille Calmette-Guérin against low-virulence *Mycobacterium tuberculosis*. *J. Infect. Dis.* **143**:739–741.

Edwards, M. L., Goodrich, J. M., Muller, D., Pollack, A., Ziegler, J. E., and Smith, D. W. (1982). Infection with *Mycobacterium avium-intracellulare* and the protective effects of bacille Calmette-Guérin. *J. Infect. Dis.* **145**:733–741.

Frappier, A., Portchance, V., St-Pierre, J., and Panisset, M. (1971). BCG strains: characteristics and relative efficacy. In: *Immunization Against tuberculosis.* Fogarty International Centre Proceedings, No. 14, DHEW publ. No. (NIH) 72–68, pp. 157–178.

Guérin, C. (1980). Early history. In: *BCG Vaccine: Tuberculosis—Cancer*. Edited by S. R. Rosenthal. PSG, Littleton, pp. 35–41.

Guld, J., Magnus, K., Tolderlund, K., Biering-Sörensen, K., and Edwards, P. Q. (1955). Suppurative lymphadenitis following intradermal BCG vaccination of the newborn. *Br. Med. J.* **2**:1048–1054.

Hank, J. A., Chan, J. K., Edwards, M. L., Muller, D., and Smith, D. W. (1981). Influence of the virulence of *Mycobacterium tuberculosis* on protection induced by bacille Calmette-Guérin in guinea-pigs. *J. Infect. Dis.* **143**:734–738.

Hart, P. D'Arcy (1967). Efficiency and applicability of mass BCG vaccination in tuberculosis control. *Br. Med. J.* **1**:587–592.

Hart, P. D'Arcy, and Sutherland, I. (1977). BCG and vole bacillus vaccines in the prevention of tuberculosis in adolescence and early adult life. *Br. Med. J.* **2**:293–295.

Hart, P. D'Arcy, Sutherland, I., and Thomas, J. (1967). The immunity conferred by effective BCG and vole bacillus vaccines, in relation to individual variations in induced tuberculin sensitivity and to technical variations in the vaccines. *Tubercle* **40**:201–210.

Heimbeck, J. (1949). Tuberkoloseschutzmittel BCG, Prinzipien und Resultate. *Schweiz. Ztschr. Tuberk.* **6**:209–224.

Hyge, T. V. (1956). The efficacy of BCG vaccination. *Acta Tuberc. Scand.* **32**:89–107.

ICMR/WHO Scientific Group (1980). *Vaccination Against Tuberculosis*. World Health Organization Tech. Rep. Ser. No. 651.

Jespersen, A. (1971). *The Potency of BCG Determined on Animals*. Statens Seruminstitut, Copenhagen.

Jin, B. W., Hong, Y. P., and Kim, S. J. (1989). A contact study to evaluate the BCG vaccination programme in Seoul. *Tubercle* **70**:241–248.

Källenius, G., Hoffner, S. E., and Svenson, S. B. (1989). Does vaccination with bacille Calmette-Guérin protect against AIDS? *Rev. Infect. Dis.* **11**:349–351.

Ladefoged, A., Bunch-Christensen, K., and Guld, J. (1970). The protective effect in bankvoles of some strains of BCG. *Bull. WHO* **43**:71–90.

Ladefoged, A., Bunch-Christensen, K., and Guld, J.(1976). Tuberculin sensitivity in guinea-pigs after vaccination with varying doses of BCG of 12 different strains. *Bull. WHO* **53**:435–443.

Lallemant-LeCoeur, S., Lallemant, M., Cheynier, D., Nzingoula, S., Drucker, J., and Larouze, B. (1991). Bacillus Calmette-Guérin immunization in infants born to HIV-1-seropositive mothers. *AIDS* **5**:195–199.

Miceli. I., de Kantor, I., Colaiacovo, D., Peluffo, G., Cutillo, I., Gorra, R., Botta, R., Hom, S., and ten Dam, H. G. (1988). Evaluation of the effectiveness of BCG vaccination using the case-control method in Buenos Aires, Argentina. *Int. J. Epidemiol.* **17**:629–634.

Mitchison, D. A. (1964). The virulence of tubercle bacilli from patients with pulmonary tuberculosis in India and other countries. *Bull. Int. Un. Tuberc.* **35**:287–306.

Msellati, P., Dabis, F., Lepage, P., Hitima, D. G., Van Goethem, L., and Vande Perre, P. (1991). BCG vaccination and pediatric HIV infection—Rwanda, 1988–1990. *MMWR* **40**:833–834.

Myint, T. T., Win, H., Aye, H. H., and Kyaw-Mint, T. O. (1987). Case-control study on evaluation of BCG vaccination of newborn in Rangoon, Burma. *Ann. Trop. Paediatr.* **7**:159–166.

Packe, G. E., and Innes, J. A. (1988). Protective effect of BCG vaccination in infant Asians: a case-control study. *Arch. Dis. Childhood* **63**:277–281.

Padungchan, S., Konjanart, S., Kasiratta, S., Daramas, S., and ten Dam, H. G. (1986). The effectiveness of BCG vaccination of the newborn against childhood tuberculosis in Bangkok. *Bull. WHO* **64**:247–258.

Palmer, C. E., and Long, M. W. (1966). Effects of infection with atypical mycobacteria on BCG vaccination and tuberculosis. *Am. Rev. Respir. Dis.* **94**:553–560.

Ray, C. S., Pringle, D., Legg, W., and Mbengeranwa, O. L. (1988). Lymphadenitis associated with BCG vaccination: a report of an outbreak in Harare, Zimbabwe, *Centr. Afr. J. Med.* **34**:281–286.

Rodrigues, L. C., and Smith, P. G. (1990). Tuberculosis in developing countries and methods for its control. *Trans. Roy. Soc. Trop. Med.* **84**:739–744.

Rook, G. A. W., Bahr, G. M., and Stanford, J. L. (1981). The effects of two distinct forms of cell-mediated response to mycobacteria on the protective efficacy of BCG. *Tubercle* **62**:63–68.

Sirinavin, S., Chotpitayasunondh, T., Suwanjutha, S., Sunakorn, P., and Chantarojanasiri, T. (1991). Protective efficacy of neonatal bacillus Calmette-Guérin vaccination against tuberculosis. *Pediatr. Infect. Dis. J.* **10**:359–365.

Smith, P. G. (1987). Case-control studies of the efficacy of BCG against tuberculosis. In: *Tuberculosis and Respiratory Diseases*: Papers presented at the plenary sessions of the 26th World Conference of the IUAT. Tokyo, Professional Postgraduate Services, K. K.

SPA/EPI (1987). Consultation on human immunodeficiency virus (HIV) and routine childhood tuberculosis. *Wkly. Epidemiol. Rec.* **62**:297–304.

Styblo, K. (1990). The elimination of tuberculosis in the Netherlands. *Bull. Int. Un. Tuberc. Lung Dis.* **65**:49–55.

Sutherland, I. (1971). State of the art in immunoprophylaxis in tuberculosis. In: *Immunization in Tuberculosis*. Fogarty International Centre Proceedings, No. 14. DHEW publ. No. (NIH) 72–68, pp. 113–125.

Sutherland, I., and Lindgren, I. (1979). The protective effect of BCG vaccination as indicated by autopsy studies. *Tubercle* **60**:225–231.

Sutherland, I., and Springett, V. H. (1989). The effects of the scheme for BCG vaccination of schoolchildren in England and Wales and the consequences of discontinuing the scheme at various dates. *J. Epidemiol. Commun. Health* **43**:15–24.

ten Dam, H. G. (1990). BCG vaccination and HIV infection. *Bull. Int. Un. Tuberc. Lung Dis.* **65**:38–39.

ten Dam, H. G., and Hitze, K. L. (1980). Does BCG vaccination protect the newborn and young infants? *Bull. WHO* **58**:37–41.

ten Dam, H. G., and Pio, A. (1982). Pathogenesis of tuberculosis and effectiveness of BCG vaccination. *Tubercle* **63**:225–233.

ten Dam, H. G., Toman, K., Hitze, K. L., and Guld, J. (1976). Present knowledge of immunization against tuberculosis. *Bull. WHO* **54**: 255–269.

Thilothammal, N., Prabhakar, R., Krishnamurthy, P. V., and Runyan, D. (1992). Does BCG vaccine prevent tuberculous meningitis in children? Tenth annual meeting of the International Clinical Epidemiology Network, Bali, Indonesia, Abstract 125.

Tidjani, O., Amedome, A., and ten Dam, H. G. (1986). The protective effect of BCG vaccination of the newborn against childhood tuberculosis in an African community. *Tubercle* **67**:269–281.

Tripathy, S. P. (1983). The case for BCG. *Ann. Natl. Acad. Med. Sci. (India)* **19**:12–21.

Tuberculosis Prevention Trial (1979). Trial of BCG vaccines in south India for tuberculosis prevention: first report. *Bull. WHO* **57**:819–827.

Tuberculosis Prevention Trial, Madras (1980). Trial of BCG vaccines in south India for tuberculosis prevention. *Ind. J. Med. Res.* **72**:(Suppl):1–74.

Vallishayee, R. S., Shashidhara, A. N., Bunch-Christensen, K., and Guld, J. (1974). Tuberculin sensitivity and skin lesions in children after vaccination with 11 different BCG strains. *Bull. WHO* **51**:489–494.

Vandiviere, H. M., Dworski, M.; Melvin, I. G., Watson, K. A., and Begley, J. (1973). Efficacy of bacillus Calmette-Guérin and isoniazid-resistant bacillus Calmette-Guérin with and without isoniazid chemoprophylaxis from day of vaccination. *Am. Rev. Respir. Dis.* **108**:301–313.

WHO Expert Committee on Biological Standardization (1987). *Requirements for Dried BCG Vaccine.* World Health Organization. Tech Rep. Ser. No. 745, p. 60.

WHO Study Group (1980). *BCG vaccination policies.* World Health Organization. Tech. Rep. Ser. No. 652.

Willis, S., and Vandiviere, M. (1961). The heterogeneity of BCG. *Am. Rev. Respir. Dis.* **84**:288–290.

Wünsch Filho, V., de Castilho, E. A., Rodrigues, L. C., and Huttly, S. R. A. (1990). Effectiveness of BCG vaccination against tuberculous meningitis: a case-control study in São Paulo, Brazil. *Bull. WHO* **68**:69–74.

Young, T. K., and Hershfield, E. S. (1981). A case-control study to evaluate the effectiveness of mass neonatal BCG vaccination among Canadian Indians. *Am. J. Public Health* **76**:783–786.

14

Contact Tracing in Tuberculosis

SUE C. ETKIND

Division of Tuberculosis Control
Massachusetts Department of Public Health
Boston, Massachusetts

I. Introduction

The Centers for Disease Control estimates that an average investigation of a case of tuberculosis in the United States results in approximately nine contacts identified for each case. Of these, 21% are expected to be infected and another 1% will have already progressed to active disease (Farer, 1986; Moodie and Riley, 1974). Because of the risk for progression to tuberculosis disease, infected contacts have been designated a high-risk group and, as such, are candidates for tuberculosis preventive therapy under current recommendations (CDC, 1990). The examination of contacts or persons exposed to a case of tuberculosis is, therefore, one of the most important methods of case finding for either tuberculosis disease or infection (Capewell and Leitch, 1984). The actual risk of transmission to contacts is related to the characteristics of the source case, the nature of the contact, and the environments they share (American Thoracic Society/CDC, 1983).

Contact tracing is an integral part of any tuberculosis program. This activity encompasses all aspects of tuberculosis control, including surveillance, case containment, and prevention. In many respects, contact tracing corresponds to basic epidemiological methodology, particularly as it relates to surveillance and outbreak control. However, contact tracing is in fact much more. Successful contact tracing requires skills in patient assessment, interviewing, counseling, and evaluation. The quality of contact tracing has been shown to markedly affect the ability to identify potentially infected persons and allow for their integration into the clinical care system (Swallow and Sbarbaro, 1972; Hsu, 1963). Therefore, the ability to perform this investigative process is essential to tuberculosis elimination efforts.

As cases of tuberculosis have retreated into defined pockets of the population (e.g., geographic and risk behavior groups), it has become necessary to modify traditional contact tracing methods in order to address the specific needs of these individuals. Although the basics of epidemiology and follow-up are unchanged, the cultural and/or linguistic barriers, the influence of socioeconomic factors (affecting the homeless population or the injection drug user, for example), the institutional setting, the ramifications of coinfection with HIV, and other factors will affect the type and content of the contact-tracing investigation. This chapter will discuss the purposes of contact tracing as an epidemiological tool and the step-by-step methodology needed to address today's multifaceted tuberculosis problem.

II. Definitions

In discussing contact tracing, a distinction must be made between cases, suspects, and contacts. For the purposes of this chapter, the following definitions will apply:

1. Presenting case—a person with or suspected of having tuberculosis.

2. Index case—the infectious individual who is believed to have transmitted infection to the presenting case.

3. Contact investigation—the process of conducting an epidemiological investigation into a case (or suspected case) of tuberculosis

4. Tuberculosis contacts—those persons who have a risk of acquiring tuberculosis because they have shared air with the presenting case. The degree of risk is dependent on the duration and frequency (times) of exposure and is influenced by the degree of infectiousness of the patient. The risk is also influenced by characteristics of the environment and the new host's (contact) susceptibility to tuberculosis infection or disease.

5. Close contacts—individuals who have shared air with the presenting case for a prolonged period of time (from hours to months, depending on the circumstances).

6. Nonclose (casual) contacts—individuals other than close contacts

III. Need for Contact Tracing

There are several reasons for conducting contact tracing. They include the following:

To identify persons who have been exposed to the presenting case and who, therefore, are at greater risk of developing tuberculosis infection and disease than the general population.

To identify persons who are infected with the tuberculosis bacillus and perform appropriate screening of these individuals.

To ensure access to medical evaluation and preventive therapy as appropriate for these infected individuals in order to prevent disease from occurring.

When possible, to identify the source of tuberculosis disease transmission for the presenting case under investigation. This is particularly important for children with active tuberculosis. When tuberculosis occurs in children, given their age, there is reason to suspect *recent* transmission.

When possible, to identify environmental factors that may be contributing to the transmission of tuberculosis.

To ensure medical evaluation, treatment, and follow-up of any additional cases of active tuberculosis that are identified in the course of the contact tracing.

Contact investigation may also identify a tuberculosis outbreak when more newly infected persons or more tuberculosis cases are discovered during the investigation than were anticipated based on the previous epidemiological data. In this situation, the contact tracing may then lead to expanded outbreak investigation activities.

IV. Methods for Contact Tracing

A. Initiation

Contact investigation is begun once a case/suspect of tuberculosis comes to the attention of the person responsible for infectious disease follow-up (health department, infection control nurse, etc.). Because of the possibility of the existence of other infectious tuberculosis cases related to the reported case, the investigation should begin as soon as possible—ideally, within 3 working days (CDC, 1989).

B. Data Collection

Once a case or suspect of tuberculosis has been reported, the investigator should begin the epidemiological process by collecting all currently available information about the presenting case in a systematic fashion. A case/client record should be opened, and relevant data should be obtained from the medical record review (hospital, clinic, or other health care records), conversations with the health care provider or other reporting source, and laboratory report reviews. Information obtained should include: the tuberculosis disease site, dates/sources and bacteriological results for acid fast bacilli (AFB) and cultures, chest X-ray results including the extent of disease (cavitary/noncavitary), purified protein derivative (PPD) skin test result(s) in millimeters, clinical symptoms, and signs (presence of cough—productive/nonproductive, duration?), and anti-tuberculosis drug regimen including dosages and date initiated.

Armed with this background information, the investigator can then complete the preliminary data collection process by interviewing the presenting case. This patient interview may be conducted in the hospital, at the patient's home, or wherever convenient and conducive to establishing trust and rapport between both parties. The ability to conduct an interview to obtain client and contact information will determine the success or failure of the epidemiological investigation. Good interviewing skills can elicit important information that otherwise might not be forthcoming.

The presenting case interview has many purposes. These include providing opportunities to:

1. establish rapport and trust with the client. Face-to-face contact facilitates building a relationship between the client and the health care provider.

2. obtain information relative to the presenting case's potential level of infectiousness or other needed clinical data (e.g., how long has he/she been symptomatic?).

3. obtain place and time information to establish duration and location of potential exposures.

4. identify potentially exposed contacts.

5. obtain locating/demographic/risk factor and environmental information (living quarters/work/school or leisure activities) for the identified contacts. Environmental factors may include such things as the ventilation, and air volume at the potential exposure sites. For example: Were there complaints about air quality? Was this a "tight" building? Were air quality assessments done in the recent past?

6. provide tuberculosis education on diagnosis, transmission, treatment, and preventive therapy.

7. assess compliance elements as they may relate to the presenting case (that is, are there any factors in the patient's life-style, or daily routines, that could interfere with his/her ability to complete tuberculosis therapy, or is there a previous history of noncompliance with therapy?).

Many factors can interfere with both the case interview and the subsequent contact interviews. These can be attitudinal (on the part of the interviewer or interviewee), social or cultural differences, mistrust of the government or health care system, fear or stigmatization due to tuberculosis, tuberculosis/human immunodeficiency virus (HIV), or other factors. Understanding these potential problems can sensitize the interviewer during the interview process. Furthermore, good communication skills that promote client understanding will enhance the effectiveness of the interview and may potentially result in increasing the number of contacts identified.

C. Tuberculosis Transmission Risk Assessment

The need to set limits and establish priorities for the contact investigation has been well established (Rose et al., 1979; Citron, 1988). Without a systematic approach to the process, the investigative efforts will be diluted and limited resources are likely to be spent on delivering services to persons who are not at demonstrated risk of tuberculosis infection or disease. To focus the contact tracing on those who are most at risk, an assessment of the risk of tuberculosis transmission to the identified contacts can be done prior to the actual field investigation. Transmission risk assessment is best accomplished by organizing the background information into the basic epidemiological categories of person, time, and place. For this chapter, these categories will be defined as:

Person factors: the infectiousness of the presenting case

Time factors: the duration and frequency of exposure

Place factors: the characteristics of the environment

Upon completion of all three aspects of this risk assessment, the investigator will be able to establish the contact tracing priorities.

Person Factors

As one of the purposes of contact tracing is to identify infected individuals who have been exposed to the presenting case, an assessment of the *potential level of infectiousness* of the presenting case must be done. For example, if the presenting

Table 1   Person Assessment Factors

Clinical data	Likelihood of disease transmission	
	High	Low
TB disease location	Laryngeal Pulmonary	Extrapulmonary alone
Smear status	Positive	Negative
Smear source	Spontaneous specimen	Induced or clinical (bronchoscopy, etc.)
Chest X-ray	Cavitary	Noncavitary
PPD result	Large, >15 mm	
Symptoms	Cough	No cough
Anti-TB drugs	No	Yes (2 weeks or more)

case has been shown to have only extrapulmonary disease and no respiratory symptoms, the liklihood of tuberculosis transmission is low and the need for contact tracing would be a lower priority. If however, the presenting case is shown to have cavitary disease, hemoptysis, and a history of coughing productively for several months, the liklihood of disease transmission is much greater and the need for rapid contact tracing is clear. Table 1 lists the person assessment factors to use in assessing the potential infectiousness of the presenting case.

Time Factors

After the investigator has made an assessment of the potential infectiousness of the presenting case, a determination of the *duration of exposure* must be made (that is, how long were the identified contacts potentially exposed to the case while he/she was infectious?). As tuberculosis is an airborne infection, this is normally done by determining the date of the onset of symptoms (particularly coughing) for the presenting case. This date can provide the approximate time frame upon which to focus the investigation. For example, if it is determined during the case interview that the presenting case has had a productive cough for 3 months prior to the diagnosis, then all identified contacts during that 3-month period of exposure may be at increased risk of tuberculosis transmission.

Place Factors

Knowing the level of potential infectiousness of the presenting case and the time frame during which possible exposures may have occurred, the next step in the

Table 2 Place Assessment Factors

	Likelihood of disease transmission	
Factor	High	Low
Volume of air common to the case/contacts	Low	High
Adequacy of ventilation	Poor, <10 CFM/person	Good, >20 CFM/person
Recircularized air	Yes	No
Upper room UV light	Not present	Present

contact tracing process is to establish the *place (or places) where contacts may have been exposed*. In other words, where did the presenting case associate with others during the established time frame? Keeping in mind that the liklihood of transmission is greatest for contacts who have spent the longest number of hours with the presenting case, the closest contacts are usually those persons exposed in the home. However, given the changing risk groups for tuberculosis, the investigation may include other types of domicile such as homeless shelters, correctional facilities, nursing homes, and HIV hospices.

In addition to establishing the exact locations of potential exposures, additional information relative to place assessment is needed to complete the picture. As can be seen in Table 2, environmental factors such as direction of airflow, volume of ventilation, ultraviolet light, crowding, and volume of air space may affect the extent of tuberculosis transmission that occurs at any given identified site. Although this information cannot be precisely obtained until the site visit, background information from the presenting case can assist in further narrowing the limits of the investigation.

For example, the presenting patient states that on most nights during the last 3 months, he slept on the floor in the very crowded lobby of the largest shelter in the city. At 6:00 A.M., all guests were required to leave the shelter and the remainder of the day was spent on the street. Meals were obtained at the local soup kitchen. This information suggests that the contacts who are at greatest risk of transmission are those at the largest shelter and the soup kitchens. Identified ''street'' contacts are assumed to have the least likelihood of transmission, given the dilution of the outside air.

The susceptibility of the host (or contact) to tuberculosis will also affect the liklihood of tuberculosis transmission. Even if all presenting case factors listed above suggest a high probability of tuberculosis disease transmission, an immunocompetent contact who has been previously infected with tuberculosis is rarely reinfected with the organism. However, HIV-infected, immunosuppressed individuals may be reinfected, and although immunocompetent persons with recently acquired tuberculosis infection are at high risk of developing active tuberculosis within 2 years of primary infection (Styblo, 1991), recent information suggests that the risk is increased dramatically for persons infected with HIV (DiPerri et al, 1989; CDC, 1991a; Barnes et al., 1991). Given the higher disease attack rates, shorter incubation periods, and high mortality that has been demonstrated for these individuals, contact tracing assumes as much greater urgency.

In summary, the risk assessment step in contact tracing involves analyzing person, time, and place factors for the presenting case to determine the case's level of infectiousness, the duration and place or places of exposure, and environmental factors that affect the subsequent risk to identified contacts. Once the tuberculosis transmission risk assessment has been completed and potential close and nonclose contacts have been identified, the field investigation may begin.

D. The Contact Field Investigation

The contact field investigation is a mandatory component of the contact tracing process. A personal visit to the identified contacts, whether in the home, shelter, institution, or elsewhere, will assist in establishing rapport and trust between these individuals and the health care provider. The same principles apply to the contact interview as were suggested for the presenting case interview. As prevention of both further disease transmission and further progression to active disease are among the purposes of contact tracing, the timeliness in which the field investigation is conducted is paramount. Current recommendations suggest that high risk contacts be evaluated within 7 days of the presenting case interview and the medical evaluation of these individuals be completed within 1 month (CDC, 1989).

The field visit serves many purposes. It allows the investigator to: (1) interview and skin-test the identified contacts; (2) observe the contacts for any signs or symptoms suggestive of tuberculosis; (3) collect sputum samples from any contact who is symptomatic; (4) identify sources of health care and make appropriate referrals; (5) identify additional potential contacts who may also need follow-up; (6) educate the contacts about the purpose of the investigation and the basics of tuberculosis pathogenesis and transmission; (7) observe the contact's environment for potential transmission factors (crowding, ventilation, etc.); and (8) assess the contact's psycho/social needs and other risk factors that may influence future compliance with medical evaluation recommendations.

The actual skin testing of identified contacts must be done in a logical order. The tuberculosis transmission risk assessment information will allow the investigator to begin with those persons thought to be at greatest risk of tuberculosis infection or disease. However, even with the risk assessment guidelines as outlined thus far, the investigator will still not be able to precisely define the limits of the contact investigation. Although mathematical models exist to analyze potential transmission of tuberculosis (Nardell et al., 1991), the factors affecting both transmission and the acquisition of disease are variable and difficult to calculate. The best measure of actual TB transmission is the actual number of persons who are determined to have been *infected* by the presenting case. The methodology for determining this is described as the concentric circle approach.

The Concentric Circle

The concentric-circle approach (Fig. 1) begins with skin testing the closest contacts to the presenting case (as identified by the risk assessment process). Those persons who are most likely to have been infected by the presenting case make

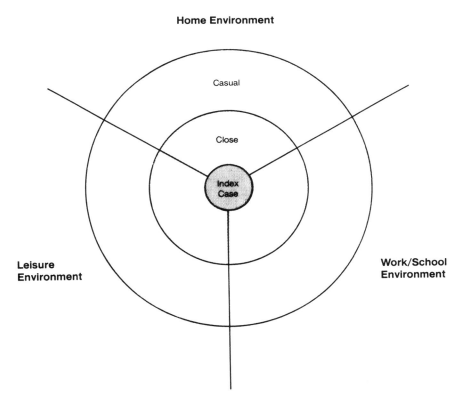

Figure 1 The concentric-circle approach to contact tracing. See text for detailed description.

up the inner circle. If the "inner circle" close contact skin testing reveals that the infection level in this group exceeds that expected for the population, the investigation proceeds to the next circle of contacts—those who frequently share air with the presenting case, but not as often as the close contacts. Examples might be frequent household visitors, close relatives, and close friends. Sometimes infection is found in this group as well, and the investigation is expanded to the third circle of contacts and beyond as necessary. The investigation should stop when a circle of contacts is found to have no more infection than is expected for the general community. If the inner-circle close-contact skin testing reveals that all or most of the contacts have negative skin tests (<5 mm induration), it is usually not necessary to expand the investigation to the next circle of contacts. Exceptions to this might be when the contacts at the next level are determined to potentially pose a greater risk to others (teachers, hospital nursery workers, other health care providers, etc.) or are at greater risk themselves (persons with immunosuppression, etc.).

Inner-circle contacts should receive the highest priority during the investigation and follow-up process. Two groups in particular should be looked upon with a sense of urgency: persons infected with HIV (as described earlier) and children under 5 years of age. Newly infected young children also have a higher disease attack rate and can develop miliary spread, with or without meningitis, within weeks unless given tuberculosis preventive therapy (Comstock et al., 1974). These two high-risk groups should receive a medical evaluation *as soon as possible*.

The advantages of the concentric-circle approach are that when it is used prospectively, groups of contacts can be examined in sequence, beginning with those established to be at greatest risk. This systematizes the investigation by avoiding spending time on low-risk areas initially and allowing for continued contact tracing in areas yielding the greatest tuberculosis infection rates. Retrospectively, this approach documents the degree of infectivity and evaluates the effectiveness of the investigational procedure.

In some settings, such as schools, institutions, or worksites, there may be difficulties in orchestrating the concentric-circle approach. Problems may include: difficulties in narrowing down just who is a part of the inner circle; a reluctance to identify individuals in certain settings; the desire on the part of the employees or administration to overtest individuals to ameliorate the "hysteria" often associated with knowledge of a tuberculosis case; and pressure exerted by various organizations or groups to protect their members through case isolation and/or universal testing. The best method for approaching such situations is to identify and understand the sources of concern. Once this is known, an educational effort can be mounted to alleviate the problem (Kellogg et al., 1987). The Appendix provides a suggested fact sheet that could be used toward that end.

Although the concentric-circle approach allows the investigation to proceed in an orderly fashion, *any* exposed individual who presents himself for examination should be tested regardless of the level of risk.

E. Medical Evaluation of Contacts

Wherever the contact investigation and resultant skin testing are performed (field visit, tuberculosis clinic referral, etc.), arrangements must be made to ensure that the skin test is read in 48–72 hr and that chest X-rays (and sputums as indicated) are obtained for all contacts who need a medical evaluation.

Skin testing of identified contacts should also proceed in an organized fashion. When possible, documentation of previous skin test results should be obtained prior to the actual testing. Contacts who have a documented prior positive PPD, who are not known or likely to be immunosuppressed, need no further evaluation unless they have symptoms suggestive of active tuberculosis. Contacts who have tuberculin skin test reactions >5 mm and who have no history of positive reaction in the past should be considered newly infected with tuberculosis and should be evaluated for preventive therapy, after active tuberculosis has been ruled out (American Thoracic Society/Centers for Disease Control, 1986). (See also Chapter 7.)

All other contacts who are skin-test-negative initially should be retested in approximately 6–12 weeks to allow time for skin test reactivity to occur (unless at the time of the initial skin test, 12 weeks had already elapsed since the last contact with the presenting case).

Although contact tracing relies on skin-testing results to proceed in a stepwise fashion, it must be noted that some high-risk contacts (such as those who are immunosuppressed) may not respond to the standard PPD test, but may well be infected with tuberculosis. For that reason, current recommendations suggest that *any* contact who is known or who is likely to be HIV-infected, or immunosuppressed for other reasons, should be evaluated for anergy at the time of tuberculin skin testing (CDC, 1991b). In addition, contacts who have a history of a prior positive tuberculin skin test, but who are currently known or likely to be immunosuppressed, are at risk for reinfection. These contacts also require a medical evaluation.

The total contact tracing should be completed within 3 months unless concentric-circle testing results require further expansion of the testing process. Contact tracing may need to be reinitiated when a tuberculosis patient becomes a treatment failure or relapses, and the sputum remains smear positive or becomes positive again. In this situation, newly identified contacts must be examined, and exposed, previously uninfected contacts not on preventive therapy should be reexamined. Those with skin test reactions of equal to or greater than 5 mm induration should receive a chest X-ray.

All contacts who are placed on preventive therapy should be followed (preferably with supervised or directly observed therapy) by the health care provider for the duration of their treatment (CDC, 1990).

V. The Contact Investigation Report

The contact-tracing investigation should be well documented and the results analyzed. These findings serve as the basis for decisions regarding future follow-up. The report should include: a summary of the presenting case evaluation including relative infectivity, the environmental investigation, and the collective results of the contact study. Contact study results should include the following: the point when contact with the presenting case was broken for various contacts; the identification, number, and percentage of newly positive, previously positive, documented conversions, negative, and anergic (if known) skin test responses; the identification, number, and percentage of contacts with abnormal chest X-rays, suspects, or new cases; the identification, number, and percentage of contacts placed on preventive therapy or antituberculosis drugs; and recommendations for further contact management or follow-up as needed.

VI. Summary

If tuberculosis elimination efforts are to be successful, prevention activities must be targeted to the groups at highest risk for progression from tuberculosis infection to disease. This chapter has illustrated that contacts to infectious cases of tuberculosis are such a high-risk group and should be priorities for tuberculosis control programs. Although the focus of contact tracing is prevention, other potential benefits of the investigation may include the identification of additional cases of tuberculosis and the opportunity for education about tuberculosis disease, the risk of transmission, the tuberculosis/HIV connection, and so forth.

The actual contact-tracing procedure should be done in a systematic, logical fashion. This chapter has outlined the step-by-step progression of such an investigation beginning with the notification of a case or suspect case of tuberculosis. It has described the collection of needed epidemiological data for planning purposes, the establishment of investigational priorities based on these data, the methodology for contact tracing in the field setting, the utilization of the concentric-circle approach to set the limits of the investigation, and the documentation of the procedures and results of the investigation.

As every case of tuberculosis began as a contact, the ability to rapidly identify tuberculosis cases and to effectively conduct the subsequent contact tracing is the cornerstone of tuberculosis control public health efforts. Without this capacity, transmission of tuberculosis will persist, the tuberculosis case rate will continue to escalate, and tuberculosis elimination will be impossible to achieve.

Appendix: Why, Whom, and When to Skin-Test— A Rational Approach to Tuberculosis Case Finding in the School, Institution, and Workplace for the Administrator and Employer*

1. Why skin-test?
   a. Close contacts of newly diagnosed tuberculosis cases are tested in search of infection transmitted prior to the onset of effective treatment.
   b. Testing of the close contacts sometimes reveals the source case of that infection, as well as others who may have been infected.
2. Who should be tested?
   a. Testing should include those sharing the same breathing space for prolonged periods with a newly diagnosed case of pulmonary tuberculosis. Close contacts are most often in the home, but the workplace, school, and other indoor gathering places are also potential sites for transmission.
   b. Patients with cough, lung cavitation, and smear positivity are most contagious. However, patients without these features have been known to transmit disease, and other patients with these findings may infect no one.
3. How many contacts should be tested?
   a. The number tested in any given case depends on the transmission factors mentioned above, the number of close contacts, and most important, the evidence for or against transmission.
   b. On average, a case of tuberculosis has seven true close contacts, with wide variation.
   c. The concentric-circle concept of stepwise testing suggests that the most intensely exposed contacts be tested first, followed by wider and wider circles if evidence for transmission is found. If there is no transmission to the closest contacts, less intensely exposed individuals may be assumed to be safe.
4. Why not test "everyone" just to be safe?
   Overtesting of contacts may be as bad as undertesting. It has the following undesirable consequences:

---

*From the Bureau of Communicable Disease Control, Division of Tuberculosis Control, Massachusetts Center for Disease Control, Jamaica Plain, Massachusetts.

a. Widespread, unfocused testing reinforces the false fear of epidemic spread of tuberculosis. If everyone is being tested, there must be risk.
b. Widespread testing dilutes the effort aimed at those truly at risk.
c. Widespread testing will detect infection unrelated to the case under investigation. However, it is extremely difficult to convince reactors that their infection is unrelated to the case, even if all the evidence is suggestive. As contacts, reactors may be offered preventive therapy with its attendant risks, who would otherwise not be candidates for treatment because of age.

5.   Why repeat tests on those who test negative?

It takes 1–2 months from the time of infection to the development of a significantly positive PPD. Those who test negative initially may be infected, but not yet positive. Retesting 3 months after the last exposure assures that all those infected will be detected.

6.   Are there false-positive or false-negative tests?

It is safe to assume that anyone testing greater than 10 mm induration (not redness) with 5 TU PPD is infected with *Mycobacterium tuberculosis*. Questionable reactions should be repeated.

Occasionally, those truly infected may test less than 10 mm for technical reasons, or because of an inability to react to skin tests. Control skin tests with common antigens like mumps and yeast can usually help the clinician determine the cause of a negative reaction, if necessary.

In some subjects a tuberculin reaction may have waned. Repetition of a test in a short time (1 week) will reveal those individuals in whom this (boosting) phenomenon has occurred.

References

American Thoracic Society/Centers for Disease Control (1983). Control of tuberculosis. *Am. Rev. Respir. Dis.* **128**:336–342.

American Thoracic Society/Centers for Disease Control (1986). Treatment of tuberculosis and tuberculosis infection in adults and children. *Am. Rev. Respir. Dis.* **134**:355–363.

Barnes, P. F., Bloch, A. B., Davidson, P. T., and Snider, D. E. (1991). Tuberculosis in patients with human immunodeficiency virus infection. *N. Engl. J. Med.* **324**:1644–1650.

Capewell, S., and Leitch, A. G. (1984). The value of contact procedures for tuberculosis in Edinburgh. *Br. J. Dis. Chest* **78**:317–329.

Centers for Disease Control (1989). A strategic plan for the elimination of tuberculosis. *MMWR* **38**(S-3):1–25.

Centers for Disease Control (1990). The use of preventive therapy for tuberculosis infection in the United States: recommendations of the Advisory Committee for the Elimination of Tuberculosis. *MMWR* **39**(RR-8):8–12.

Centers for Disease Control (1991a). Tuberculosis outbreak among persons in a residential facility for HIV-infected persons. *MMWR* **40**:649–652.

Centers for Disease Control (1991b). Purified protein derivative (PPD)—tuberculin anergy and HIV infection: guidelines for anergy testing and management of anergic persons at high risk of tuberculosis. *MMWR* **40**(RR-5):27–33.

Citron, K. M. (1988). Control and prevention of tuberculosis in Britain. *Br. Med. Bull.* **44**:704–716.

Comstock, G. W., Livesay, V. T., and Woolpert, S. F. (1974). The prognosis of a positive tuberculin reaction in childhood and adolescence. *Am. J. Epidemiol.* **99**:131–138.

DiPerri, G., Danzi, M. C., DeChecchi, G., Pizzighella, S., Solbiati, M., Cruciani, M., Luzzati, R., Malena, M., Mazzi, R., Concia, E., and Bassetti, D. (1989). Nosocomial epidemic of active tuberculosis among HIV-infected patients. *Lancet* **23/30**:1502–1504.

Farer, L. S. (1986). *Tuberculosis: What the Physician Should Know*. Centers for Disease Control, Atlanta, GA.

Hsu, K. H. (1963). Contact investigation: a practical approach to tuberculosis eradication. *Am. J. Public Health* **53**:1761.

Kellogg B., Dye, C., Cox, K., and Rosenow, G. (1987). Public health nursing model for contact followup of patients with pulmonary tuberculosis. *Public Health Nurs.* **4**(2):99–104.

Moodie, A. S., and Riley, R. L. (1974). Infectivity of patients with pulmonary tuberculosis in inner city homes. *Am. Rev. Respir. Dis.* **110**:810–812.

Nardell, E., Keegan, J., Cheney, S., and Etkind, S. (1991). Airborne infection: Theoretical limits of protection achievable by building ventilation. *Am. Rev. Respir. Dis.* **144**:302–306.

Rose D. E., Zerbe, G. O., Lantz, S. O., and Bailey, W. C. (1979). Establishing priority during investigation of tuberculosis contacts. *Am. Rev. Respir. Dis.* **119**:603–609.

Styblo, K. (1991). Epidemiology of tuberculosis. In: *Selected Papers, Royal Netherlands Tuberculosis Association*. Vol 24. Edited by J. S. Broekmans. The Hague, The Netherlands, pp. 1–136.

Swallow, J., and Sbarbaro, J. A. (1972). Analysis of tuberculosis case-finding in Denver, Colorado 1965–1970. *Health Serv. Rep.* **87**:135.

Part Three

SPECIAL AND UNIQUE PROBLEMS

15

Drug Resistance in Tuberculosis

PATTISAPU R. J. GANGADHARAM

University of Illinois College of Medicine at Chicago
Chicago, Illinois

I. Introduction

Correct application of the several powerful drugs in the various types of regimens that have evolved from well-planned clinical trials could offer a potentially 100% successful treatment of the disease.* Even though such outcome of chemotherapy could not be seen in developing and undeveloped countries, owing to several factors, many of the developed countries, particularly the United States, have even entertained hopes of eradicating the disease and have established target dates. Unfortunately however, this optimism could not be sustained for long; the downward trend of the disease in the United States, which continued until the mid-1980s, is now taking an upward turn.

Several reasons have been cited for the failure of tuberculosis treatment, chief among them being drug resistance of the tubercle bacilli. Noncompliance, a notoriously persistent worldwide problem, magnifies this because many of the patients who fail to take the drugs for the prescribed period end up with drug-resistant bacilli.

---

*Chemotherapy of tuberculosis is described in detail in Chapter 11.

Table 1 Spontaneous Occurrence of Drug-Resistant Mutants in Wild Strains of *Mycobacterium tuberculosis*

Drug	Probability of resistance
Rifampicin	10^{-8}
Isoniazid, streptomycin ethambutol, kanamycin, PAS	10^{-6}
Ethionamide, capreomycin, viomycin, ethionamide, cycloserine, thiacetazone	10^{-3}

From a microbiological standpoint, resistance and susceptibility are relative terms, since practically all populations of drug-susceptible tubercle bacilli will contain a certain proportion of resistant mutants. These proportions are very small in wild strains that are not exposed to these drugs (Table 1): 1 in 10^6 for standard drugs and 1 in 10^8 for rifampin. From a clinical standpoint, drug resistance can be defined as a temporary or permanent capacity of the organisms and their progeny to remain viable or to multiply in the presence of the concentration of the drug that would normally destroy or inhibit the growth of other cells. According to Mitchison (1961), clinically meaningful drug resistance is indicated by a decrease of susceptibility to a drug of a sufficient degree to be reasonably certain that the strain concerned is different from a sample of wild strains of tubercle bacilli that had never come into contact with the drug.

Epidemiologically, drug resistance in tuberculosis is classified into three types:

1. *Primary drug resistance*, where previously untreated patients are found to have drug-resistant organisms, presumably because they have been infected from an outside source of resistant bacilli.

2. *Acquired drug resistance*, where the patients who initially have drug-susceptible tubercle bacilli later become drug resistant due to inadequate, inappropriate, or irregular treatment or, more important, due to noncompliance in drug taking.

3. *Initial drug resistance* (Mitchison, 1968a) denotes drug resistance in patients who deny history of previous chemotherapy; in reality it consists of true primary resistance and an unknown amount of undisclosed acquired resistance. Since it takes elaborate efforts to check conclusively and determine the possibility of previous but unreported treatment, initial drug resistance has been gaining practical importance. Epidemiological patterns of drug resistance in different communities, discussed later in this chapter, deal mostly with primary or

initial drug resistance. Likewise, in a later section, various factors favoring developing acquired drug resistance are considered.

Historically, the problem of drug resistance was recognized in 1946, almost immediately following the introduction of streptomycin, when Youmans and associates (1946) found that when the drug was given alone, there was at first a striking improvement in the patient's symptoms, together with a rapid decrease in the number of bacilli in the sputum; however, the number of bacilli soon increased and the condition of the patient deteriorated. These investigators found that the bacilli isolated from the patients were drug resistant; i.e., the bacilli, instead of being killed, continued to grow in vitro in the presence of high concentrations of the same drug. This interesting observation was soon followed by a study by Pyle (1947), who showed that during treatment with streptomycin alone, the proportion of drug-resistant bacilli increased progressively from about 1 in 88,750 organisms before the therapy to about 1 in 367 after 15 weeks of treatment. These initial observations were the pioneering studies in the problem of drug resistance in mycobacteria. Subsequent studies have enabled us to recognize that increase in drug resistance following monotherapy was due to the selection of drug-resistant mutants. A significant landmark soon followed with the discovery by Temple and associates (1951), that multiple-drug therapy was able to cure tuberculosis without development of drug resistance. This pioneering work has been confirmed by studies carried out all over the world and has led to the clinical maxim that tuberculosis patients should be treated with multiple-drug chemotherapy only.

The techniques for the detection of drug resistance and the chemotherapeutic and epidemiological importance of the several types of drug resistance had brought forth a vast literature, which was recently summarized by the author (Gangadharam, 1984). Surprisingly, not much progress has occurred over the past several years in the theoretical aspects of drug resistance, although there have been some improvements in technical aspects, particularly in the developed countries where rapid methods have been introduced. No such changes have taken place in developing countries. However, the recent epidemics and upsurge in the incidence of drug resistance in many parts of the world are beginning to reawaken interest in this problem.

II. Theoretical Aspects of Drug Resistance

A. Origin of Drug Resistance

All available evidence shows that drug resistance in *Mycobacterium tuberculosis* occurs only by mutation, the drug acting merely as a selective agent. It has also been shown that resistance of tubercle bacilli to isoniazid and streptomycin develops as a single-step mutation, unlike the gradual multiple-step process observed in penicillin resistance (Rist, 1964). Using fluctuation analysis, David (1970) has calculated the mutation rates and the proportion of resistant mutants for many drugs. The proportion of resistant cells in a given bacillary population is greater than the mutation rate; in addition, some mutants do not survive and some may back-mutate to sensitivity. The mutants resistant to one of several antituberculosis drugs appear once in every 10^7 cells, whereas the proportion of resistant mutants present in the normally susceptible population varies from 1 in 10^5 to 1 in 10^9 cells examined.

B. Mechanisms of Drug Resistance

Among the several theories postulated to explain the mechanisms by which drug resistance develops in microorganisms (Davis, 1957), only three are of relevance to mycobacteria: (1) development of insusceptible metabolic pathways, (2) interference in uptake or penetration of the drug into the bacterial cell, and (3) destruction of the drugs. Among these, the second was considered in great detail by previous investigators. Using the ^{14}C-labeled isoniazid and para-aminosalicylic acid (PAS), Barclay and associates (1954) found that isoniazid-resistant strains take up markedly less radioactive material than the parent strains, though similar findings were not shown with PAS (Barclay, 1955). Youatt (1969) confirmed these findings and suggested that these differences were due to alterations in cell permeability. Similar findings were reported for kanamycin and streptomycin (Nichida, 1959). In contrast to the uptake mechanisms, there was no evidence of the destruction of the drug by resistant tubercle bacilli comparable to that noted in penicillinase-producing, penicillin-resistant organisms. Also, there were no resistant organisms with insusceptible metabolic pathways.

C. Emergence of Drug Resistance

Emergence of drug resistance is due to the selection of preexisting resistant mutants in the original bacterial population. Since the frequency of drug-resistant mutants in the original population is of a low degree (Table 1), large bacterial populations, such as those occurring in big lung cavities, are necessary for the appearance of the drug-resistant mutants in the lesion. In such environments, susceptible organisms will be replaced by the resistant mutants in the presence of the selecting drug. Mutation to resistance thus emerging can be of either high or low degree. Those resistant to ethambutol usually are of low degree while those resistant to rifampin or pyrazinamide will be of high degree (David, 1970). With streptomycin, three types of mutants having different levels of resistance were demonstrated (Mitchison, 1951).

Emergence of different levels of resistance is of clinical significance, since high doses of certain drugs (e.g., isoniazid) can be useful in eliminating the organisms with lower levels of drug resistance (Selkon et al., 1964). In clinical situations, however, a combination of at least two drugs is usually expected to eliminate all mutants except those resistant to both drugs, which are, however, few in number (1 in 10^{10} to 10^{11}) (Cohn et al., 1959). As such, emergence of drug resistance should profitably be discussed separately for single- and double-drug regimens. However, owing to the present widespread use of double- or triple-drug combinations for the treatment of tuberculosis, information on emergence of resistance in patients with single-drug treatments is limited.

Considering the emergence of resistance in patients treated with isoniazid alone, it was found that all patients with unsatisfactory bacteriological response to treatment had strains resistant to the drug (Selkon et al., 1964). Based on the degree of resistance noted in cultures in the first and six months as well as in the rate of inactivation and attainable peak concentration of isoniazid, it was concluded that resistance to isoniazid emerges in two stages. In the first stage, which occurred early in treatment, resistant bacilli grew at any isoniazid dose, but mutants of low resistance were prevented from growing when the peak concentration of isoniazid in the serum was sufficiently high. This probably explains the reduction of the proportion of patients with resistant organisms as the dosage of isoniazid increased since few low-resistance strains developed. In the second stage, organisms with low resistance continued to multiply, though still partly inhibited by isoniazid, and became more resistant, particularly in slow inactivators of isoniazid. It is evident that only the first stage determines the emergence of resistance, since once resistance emerged, its existence was unrelated to the patient's eventual progress.

With streptomycin, early studies showed that resistance appeared readily, and at the end of the first month, as many as 85% of the patients had streptomycin-resistant organisms (Medical Research Council, 1948, 1955). Information on the emergence of resistance to the other antituberculosis drugs, when used alone, is not available, since the use of the single drugs in the initial treatment of tuberculosis is contraindicated. The period during which resistance to individual drugs emerges has been calculated to be 45 days for streptomycin (Medical Research Council, 1948) and 2–5 months for rifampin, ethionamide, and kanamycin (Tsukamura, 1978).

Considering the emergence of resistance under double-drug therapy in patients whose bacilli were originally susceptible to both the drugs, treatment with daily isoniazid and streptomycin showed very little emergence of resistance, since about 95% of the patients would have a bacteriologically favorable response if the treatment was adequately followed (Russell et al., 1959). On the other hand, treatment with daily isoniazid and PAS, or daily streptomycin plus PAS, resulted in emergence of resistance in about 10% of the patients (Daniels and Hill, 1952; Tuberculosis Chemotherapy Center, 1959). The failure to prevent emergence of resistance in the double-drug regimens containing PAS probably is attributable to the inability of PAS to prevent the growth of isoniazid- or streptomycin-resistant mutants. In these regimens, the organisms remained fully susceptible to PAS, thus showing the capacity of the companion drug, mainly isoniazid or streptomycin, to inhibit the growth of the PAS-resistant organisms. The failure of PAS to prevent the emergence of resistance to the companion drug is shown more vividly when it is combined with streptomycin, as was found in the earlier British studies (Daniels and Hill, 1952). In these studies, failure of PAS to inhibit streptomycin-resistant mutants was seen, especially when the bacterial population was large. Thus resistance emerged in 21% of the patients treated with streptomycin and 5–10 g of PAS daily, and in only 4% of the patients treated with streptomycin and 20 g of PAS daily. The smaller dose of PAS was therefore definitely ineffective in inhibiting streptomycin-resistant mutants, though it was much better than streptomycin used alone.

In this connection it is worth pointing out that the role of the companion drug with isoniazid, be it a powerful drug like rifampin or streptomycin or a weak bacteriostatic drug like PAS or thiacetazone, is only to prevent the emergence of resistant mutants to isoniazid (Mitchison, 1979). Synergy was not demonstrated in the treatment of tuberculosis but only with disease caused by *Mycobacterium avium intracellulare* (MAC) complex (Heifets, 1982).

Some information on the emergence of resistance using intermittent and short-course chemotherapy regimens is also available. With the twice-weekly intermittent regimen of streptomycin and isoniazid, the outcome is the same as with daily regimens, but the once-weekly regimens of streptomycin and isoniazid resulted in the emergence of resistance to either streptomycin or isoniazid, even at the end of 1 year of treatment (Tuberculosis Chemotherapy Center, 1970). About 15–20% of the patients still have drug-susceptible organisms at this period, a finding at variance with the experience with daily regimens. Later analysis has shown that in these once-weekly regimens, the level of the companion drug, which is low, either because of the frequency of administration or because of inactivation, is responsible for the failure to prevent the emergence of resistance to the companion drug (Tripathy, 1968).

In the case of the short-course chemotherapy, there is no or minimal emergence of drug resistance because almost all positive cultures isolated from patients at 6 or 9 months of chemotherapy are still drug susceptible and could be re-treated with the same drug combinations (Fox and Mitchison, 1975).

III. Factors Responsible for the Development of Acquired Drug Resistance

Primary drug resistance due to the infection of patients with drug-resistant bacilli generated somewhere else could be a serious epidemiological problem. Increase in such resistance is due to the increase in resistant cases in the

Table 2 Factors that Influence the Chance for Drug Resistance

Increased chance
1. Previous treatment for tuberculosis
   a. Greatest risk if treatment fails or disease relapses while patient is still on drugs
   b. Significant risk if treatment was inadequate (weak drug regimens and/or inappropriate duration)
   c. Treatment received while living in a high-tuberculosis-incidence area [closely related to (b)]
2. Birth and/or recent residence in a high-tuberculosis-incidence area
   a. Particularly Asia, South and Central America, and Africa
   b. Certain localized areas within developed countries (skid row, *barrios*, etc.)
   c. The younger the age, the greater the risk
3. Recent exposure to a known case of drug-resistant disease
4. Infection with mycobacteria other than *M. tuberculosis*

Decreased chance
1. No previous treatment for tuberculosis
2. Birth and/or residence in a low-tuberculosis-incidence area—the longer, the less likely
3. Recent exposure to a known case of drug-susceptible disease

Source: Davidson, 1987.

community and the chances of exogenous infections. Acquired drug resistance, which develops in a patient who had originally drug-susceptible organisms but whose bacilli became resistant can be due to several reasons discussed below. Some of them, most relevant to the United States were recently discussed by Davidson (1987) (Table 2).

1. Biological
   a. Initial bacterial population
   b. Local factors inside the host favorable for the multiplication of drug-resistant bacilli
   c. Presence of drug in insufficient concentrations
   d. Patient's drug inactivation status
2. Clinical
   a. Treatment with single drugs
   b. Inadequate dosage of the drugs

    c. Insufficient duration of treatment
    d. Adding a single drug to a failing regimen
    e. Interference by occult or quack medicine
    f. Interference by other indigenous systems of medicine

3. Pharmaceutical and pharmacological
    a. Insufficient concentration of the pure drug
    b. Inadequate standardization of the bioavailability of the drugs
    c. Improper storage conditions of the preparations
    d. Improper bioavailability of combined tablet preparations
    e. Confusion created by the trade names of the various preparations of combination tablets
    f. Improper or incorrect dispensing of the drugs

4. Administrative
    a. Insufficient supplies of the drugs
    b. Bureaucratic influence in the ordering and supply of the drugs
    c. Substandard drugs purchased because of cost considerations and government regulations
    d. Administrative delays in the release of the drugs from the ports of entry
    e. Administrative controls on the drug dispensing

5. Sociological (patient's cooperation)
    a. Noncompliance
    b. Irregularity in drug intake
    c. Premature discontinuation of drug intake
    d. Avoidance of other exogenous infections with drug-resistant bacilli

Considering the biological reasons, Canetti (1955) showed that cavities that contain liquid necrosis constitute a very favorable medium for the multiplication of drug-resistant tubercle bacilli. Even without cavitation, if bacterial multiplication is allowed for a long time, the proportion of spontaneous resistant mutants may increase, thereby making the entire culture resistant, particularly to the drug used. Drug resistance can also develop even with the use of two drugs, if they are prescribed in insufficient dosages or if sufficient levels are not maintained in vivo, for example, owing to rapid acetylation of isoniazid.

    Single-drug therapy is the most frequent cause for the development of drug resistance. Fortunately, owing to intensive education of tuberculosis treatment practice, most physicians are conscious of the need to use at least two drugs. Unfortunately, however, in some situations, only single-drug treatment is available, the alternative being no treatment at all. Other factors are drug intolerance or the patient's taking one drug selectively instead of all the drugs. Likewise, known or unknown errors in delivering the drugs may occur owing to confusion created by many similar trade names of combined tablets. Since rifampin is active against several infections with gram-positive bacteria, quite frequently it is prescribed for nonmycobacterial infections. While such use has been shown at least in some developed countries such as England (Grunberg et al., 1985; Tofte, 1985), not to result in increased rifampin resistance in tuberculosis, indiscriminate and widespread use in developing countries, where many patients have undisclosed or undiagnosed tuberculosis, may increase the chances of developing drug resistance. These aspects have been recently reviewed (Reichman, 1987).

Another important factor leading to development of drug resistance is adding a single drug to a failing regimen. Such a practice is more common in situations where drug-susceptibility data are not readily available. The organisms develop resistance to the drug added, and this chain reaction will continue until the organisms develop resistance to all the drugs.

Interference in therapy by occult or "quack" medicine may also be important, especially in Africa and Asia. While some of the treatment is administered by authentic and fairly well-developed indigenous systems of medicine, e.g., Ayurveda, Unani in India, classical Chinese medicine, others are simply illegal and unscientific (quack) types. Similarly, an enormous black market for some drugs such as rifampin is noted in many of these countries. These nonscientific forms of treatment may encourage development of drug resistance in a community. Only strict enforcement of legislation regarding clinical practice can rectify this situation.

Pharmacological and pharmaceutical influences on fostering drug resistance have become recognized only recently. While it is assumed that most of the drugs put on the market contain the expected amount of the active ingredients, actually quite often insufficient concentrations are present. Levels of the drugs may also deteriorate due to storage under humid and hot conditions, e.g., in docks before the customs and other formalities are cleared, due to bureaucratic hurdles, or due to a prolonged transportation period (Rao et al., 1968).

An important aspect of bioavailability of the drugs, especially when they are formulated into fixed combination tablets, has been considered by Fox (1990). While many standard original preparations, e.g., Rifater, might be assured of adequate concentrations of the component drugs, many similar types of preparations marketed in developing countries might not be ensured of bioavailability (Fox, 1990). In the absence of regulations, use of such preparations may deliver only substandard amounts of the drugs. This dangerous situation encourages drug resistance.

Another danger is in the confusion that can be created when closely similar trade names are used for single or combination tablets (Gangadharam, 1987). For instance, "Inambutol," which contains isoniazid and ethambutol, could be willfully or erroneously substituted by "Myambutol," which is ethambutol alone.

Similar confusion with rifampin-containing regimens may occur as well: e.g., Rifadin which is only rifampin, instead of Rifanex and Rifinah, which are combinations of rifampin and isoniazid or Rifater, a three-drug combination of isoniazid, rifampin, and pyrazinamide. A pharmacist in a developing country may be unqualified professionally and may readily and indiscriminately substitute a preparation of a single drug for a double-drug preparation with a closely related trade name. In the absence of strict governmental control, and with poor literacy of patients, the risks of getting single-drug therapy are therefore enormous.

Administratively, drug resistance can be fostered quite easily, especially in institutions. Quite frequently in hospitals in developing countries that are controlled by the government, due to administrative, bureaucratic, or budgetary regulations, often bidding favors the lowest-price supplier, which may result in procuring substandard drugs. Similarly, all the drugs may not be purchased at one time, and the hospital pharmacy may have only one drug in stock instead of the two or three drugs, required. The situation might then boil down to giving either one drug or no treatment at all. In many such circumstances, the patients are asked to buy the other companion drugs themselves (Gibson, 1986). These situations can encourage development of drug resistance even in an institutional setting.

By far the most important cause of acquired drug resistance is the failure of the patient to continue treatment for the prescribed period. This shortcoming on the part of the patient occurs most commonly after symptoms disappear, and this may be quite early in the course of therapy. Even if the drugs are supplied free, as is done by several governments, defaults may occur owing to the indolence or preferential attention of the patients to other basic necessities of life, rather than to their disease. Chronic alcoholism and intravenous drug abuse are contributing factors in most developed countries. Supervised intermittent administration of drugs had been a welcome advance (Tuberculosis Chemotherapy Center, 1964; Sbarbaro and Johnson, 1968). More recently, the development of depot-type preparations (Gangadharam et al., 1991), which can deliver sustained drug levels for prolonged periods following single administration in a biodegradable polymer, may solve the problem of noncompliance and thereby avoid the development of acquired drug resistance.

IV. Methods of Avoiding Drug Resistance in Patients

While primary drug resistance cannot be avoided in developing countries where chances of infections with drug-resistant bacilli are enormous, acquired drug resistance, which develops in patients who had drug-susceptible organisms originally, can be avoided by following some basic principles. Some methods can be readily implemented because they are physician or hospital oriented; others depend on the patient's motivation, attitude, and cooperation.

1. At the minimum, double, and preferably triple or more, drug therapy should be given to all patients. Short-course chemotherapy with adequate dosages of the drugs in the well-defined regimens of 6 or 9 months' duration should be followed. Longer therapy may be needed for human immunodeficiency virus (HIV)–infected patients (Centers for Disease Control, 1989). For detailed discussions on the optimal regimens, see Chapter 11.

2. All drugs should be given at the same intervals. A regimen of one drug given intermittently and the other given daily will not be useful (Mitchison, 1954).

3. All drugs to be used should be those to which the patient's organisms are susceptible. If the bacterial population is not susceptible to one drug of a two-drug regimen, it would be similar to giving a single drug, thereby allowing bacilli to develop resistance to the other drug to which they were originally susceptible. If facilities to assess an individual patient's drug resistance do not exist, guidance can be taken from data on the prevalence of drug resistance in the community and from a thorough questionnaire on the history of a patient's previous chemotherapy.

4. The drugs should be dispensed in the proper manner for the prescribed duration. If the drugs are dispensed separately, preferential omission of the less acceptable drug may occur, leading to the development of resistance to the drug taken regularly. Fixed-combination tablets offer great advantage in this respect.

5. Never add a single drug to a failing regimen. This is a common mistake in the absence of susceptibility test results.

6. The most important factor is to see that the patients take the drugs as prescribed for the entire period. *This is the single most important cause for the development of acquired drug resistance.* Depot preparations, if proven satisfactory, may solve this problem.

V. Special Aspects of Drug Resistance

A. Natural Resistance

Natural resistance of tubercle bacilli was found to exist only to two bacteriostatic drugs, PAS and thiacetazone. Both these drugs are becoming obsolescent, although thiacetazone is still used in some developing countries in the initial treatment of tuberculosis. Several years ago it was shown that the Indian strains of tubercle bacilli contain a small proportion (about 0.02%) of organisms that are naturally resistant to PAS (Selkon et al., 1960). However, this low degree of resistance did not seem to influence response of patients to treatment with regimens containing PAS.

Extensive studies were carried out on the natural resistance to thiacetazone, where a geographical distribution was seen (Mitchison, 1968b). Whereas the strains from India, especially those from Madras, have high natural drug resistance to this drug, those from Hong Kong and some European countries have shown remarkable susceptibility, compared to British strains (Mitchison and Lloyd, 1964; Mitchison, 1968b). In India, there was a variation in strains from the north to the south of the country (Gangadharam et al., 1968). The experience with African strains was variable (Mitchison and Lloyd, 1964; Mitchison 1968b). There may be some doubt that some of these African strains could have been *M. africanum*, which shows greater natural resistance to thiacetazone; *M. africanum* was not known at the time of these investigations.

Contrary to the experience with PAS, it was found that the natural resistance to thiacetazone was associated with the likelihood of an unfavorable response of treatment with isoniazid plus thiacetazone. Commenting on this, Mitchison and associates (Mitchison and Lloyd, 1964; Mitchison, 1968b) stated that natural resistance to thiacetazone in countries like India would perhaps be compensated by the low degree of virulence of the organisms.

B. Cross-Resistance

Cross-resistance normally occurs between drugs that have some chemical relationship and has been observed among several antituberculosis drugs. This has great practical clinical importance in that it determines the use and sequence of administration of antituberculosis drugs, especially in re-treatment regimens. With the available knowledge, cross-resistance can be discussed under two broad categories: (1) synthetic antituberculosis drugs (isoniazid, pyrazinamide, ethionamide, and thiacetazone) and (2) aminoglycoside and peptide antibiotics (streptomycin, kanamycin, viomycin, and capreomycin).

Regarding the synthetic antituberculosis drugs, extensive literature is available on ethionamide and thiacetazone. These two drugs appear to be influenced by the manner in which resistance to the individual drugs is developed; for instance, natural resistance to thiacetazone does not involve resistance to ethionamide, and reciprocally, natural resistance to ethionamide does not imply thiacetazone resistance (Rist, 1964). On the other hand, acquired resistance to one drug normally results in resistance to the other drug. A further complication is seen when resistance is developed in combination chemotherapy with isoniazid and thiacetazone (Rist et al., 1959). In this situation, acquired resistance to thiacetazone need not always follow acquired resistance to ethionamide.

With isoniazid and ethionamide (both having the $-NH-NH_2$ group), Canetti et al. (1967) had shown that organisms with low-level isoniazid resistance were often resistant to ethionamide, but those with high resistance to isoniazid were in most cases susceptible to ethionamide. In contrast, no cross-resistance was seen between isoniazid and pyrazinamide although they are structurally similar (Perry and Morse, 1955).

Considerably more information is available on the development of cross-resistance among the aminoglycoside antibiotics. Several investigations have confirmed the existence of one-way cross-resistance between viomycin and capreomycin, viomycin and kanamycin, kanamycin and streptomycin, kanamycin and capreomycin, and kanamycin and amikacin; the last observation on this subject came from our laboratory where we found that strains of *M. tuberculosis* that were resistant to kanamycin were resistant to amikacin in about 50% of cases, whereas strains that were resistant to amikacin were almost always resistant to kanamycin. Since kanamycin is in wide use in initial and re-treatment regimens of tuberculosis and amikacin is rarely used for the treatment of tuberculosis although it is used for the treatment of *M. avium* disease, this observation is helpful in that amikacin may be useful in patients who have kanamycin-resistant organisms.

C. Microbial Persistence

Microbial persistence, which permits tubercle bacilli to exist and not be acted on by the drugs to which they are susceptible, plays an important role in chemotherapy. The proportions of these persisters is very small, about 1 in 10^6 in an actively growing culture, but may be much larger and may even comprise all of the bacterial population in the stationary phase of the culture. Persisters of drug-susceptible tubercle bacilli are also found to exist in great numbers where the bacterial growth is prevented by exposure to anaerobic conditions (Mitchison and Selkon, 1956) or growth in nutritionally deficient media (Schaefer, 1954).

In chemotherapy of tuberculosis, microbial persistence is responsible for the considerable reduction of activity of drugs in lesions of humans compared to their activity in vitro and also for the occurrence of relapses with drug-susceptible organisms even after prolonged courses of chemotherapy (Velu et al., 1960). Most of the persisters reside in macrophages where many drugs either cannot enter or, if they do, may not be able to exercise their activity because of the pH and other intracellular environmental factors (e.g., streptomycin). For this reason, in the chemotherapeutic evaluation, it is essential to test the drugs on intracellularly multiplying or persisting bacilli.

Microbial persistence also has great relevance to drug-parasite interactions. Since powerful drugs such as isoniazid and streptomycin require at least one generation time (e.g., 20–24 hr) to be in contact with the bacilli for effective killing, they will not be active against persistent bacilli which may have only short spurts of growth. On the other hand, rifampin, which has the unique advantage of being able to kill bacteria within a short period of contact (e.g., 15 min), will be able to kill bacteria persisting inside the macrophages. Because of this fact, after the development of rifampin, the duration of chemotherapy could be reduced remarkably from 24 months to 6 or 9 months. These aspects were aptly discussed by Fox and Mitchison (1975).

D. Biological Variations in Mycobacteria Consequent to Drug Resistance

Consequent to the development of drug resistance, tubercle bacilli, particularly those resistant to isoniazid, exhibit some biological variations. These variations include nutritional requirements, enzyme content, and virulence. Among the nutritional requirements, Barry and co-workers (1953) have shown the need for bovine albumin fraction V and hemin; and Cohn and associates (1954) have shown that biotin and carbon dioxide were essential for the growth of isoniazid-resistant tubercle bacilli. Following the observations of Middlebrook (1954) that isoniazid-resistant tubercle bacilli have reduced catalase activity, a finding confirmed by many authors, Knox (1955) demonstrated that catalase possesses a growth-promoting effect on isoniazid-resistant tubercle bacilli that was 100,000 times that of hemin. The catalase from isoniazid-resistant tubercle bacilli was shown to have a normal hemin content and normal complement of cytochromes a, b and c, indicating that the loss in catalase activity in these strains occurred in the genes governing the synthesis of the protein portion of the enzyme molecule (Andrejew et al., 1957).

Concerning changes in virulence, it was observed that isoniazid-resistant strains that were developed in vitro or isolated from patients under treatment with isoniazid have markedly reduced virulence for the guinea pig (Middlebrook and Cohn, 1953). There was a close correlation with the degree of isoniazid resistance, the loss of catalase activity, and reduction of virulence to the guinea pig. On the other hand, isoniazid-resistant, catalase-negative strains do not show diminished virulence for mice. This difference raised questions as to whether or not these organisms would be pathogenic to humans.

Few supporting studies indicate that the infective capacity of isoniazid-resistant organisms in humans will be low. Liebknecht (1964) showed that children exposed for varying periods to isoniazid-resistant tubercle bacilli had different patterns of disease. Of the children who had prolonged contact with individuals with isoniazid-resistant organisms, only 4.5% became infected, in contrast to 11% from sources with susceptible strains. Such differences were not seen after brief contact. Some epidemiological data also support these observations (World Health Organization, 1967). Thus, among 57 contacts exposed to isoniazid-resistant organisms, the infectivity rate was 1.33 for 100 months of exposure, compared to 5.94 for the same period of exposure of 77 contacts of isoniazid susceptible organisms. It should be emphasized, however, that in all these investigations, other factors, besides the attenuated virulence of the isoniazid-resistant strains, may well have had an influence on the low infectivity. For instance, BCG vaccination and differences in the behavior of the patients and the frequency and degree of contact with source case, all may have played important roles.

Such epidemiological studies have excited some workers, who at one time went to the extreme of suggesting that treatment should aim at converting all bacilli into being isoniazid resistant especially in those cases where the bacilli cannot be eliminated completely from the patient's system (Freerksen, 1957). Fortunately, the majority of the experts did not support this, believing that isoniazid-resistant tubercle bacilli are capable of spreading tuberculosis. The current upsurge of drug-resistant tubercle bacilli in the United States and elsewhere confirms the belief that isoniazid-resistant organisms are serious and dangerous pathogens.

VI. Techniques

Soon after the recognition of the problem of drug resistance, which quickly followed the introduction of chemotherapy, bacteriologists all over the world attempted to evolve reliable laboratory methods for identifying and quantitating drug resistance in tubercle bacilli. Since space does not permit a full discussion of this subject, only salient points will be reviewed, and the reader is referred to an earlier monograph (Gangadharam, 1984) and a recent book (Heifets, 1991).

The types of drug susceptibility tests are summarized in Table 3. Among these, the proportion method introduced by Canetti et al. (1969) is now commonly used. In addition, the radiometric method developed by Middlebrook et al. (1977) and Siddiqi et al. (1981) using the BACTEC procedure has also gained great importance in the United States. The Centers for Disease Control (CDC) has adopted a modified version of the proportion method introduced by Canetti. These modifications include (1) slight changes in the critical drug concentrations to be used (Table 4), (2) the critical proportions of drug resistance, and more important, (3) the medium to be used. Some of the changes in drug concentrations are due to the use of 7H10 medium recommended by the CDC instead of the Lowenstein-Jensen (L-J) medium, which is used in European and Asian laboratories. The CDC recommended 7H10 agar medium because its transparency enables growth to be detected earlier, and factors such as heat of inspissation and protein binding, which operate in the L.J. medium, will not influence the results in 7H10 medium. More recently, Heifets (1991) suggested using 7H11 agar medium instead of 7H10 agar medium. Finally, the major deviation from the Canetti report (Canetti et al., 1964, 1969) is in the critical

Table 3 Types of Drug Susceptibility Tests

A. Direct methods
   1. Using 7H10 medium (Middlebrook and Cohn)
   2. Gradient plate method (Bryson and Szybalski)
   3. Using L-J medium (Hobby and Wichelhausen, Mackay, Gangadharam)
B. Indirect methods
   1. Absolute concentration method (Meissner)
   2. Resistance ratio method (Mitchison)
   3. Proportion method (Canetti)
   4. Modified proportion method (Middlebrook, CDC)
C. Simple and rapid method
   1. Slide culture method (Dickinson)
   2. Colony morphology method (Runyon)
   3. Swab method (Gangadharam)
   4. Disk method (Collins, Wayne, Krasnow, and Hawkins)
   5. Radiometric methods (Wagner, Buddemeyer, and Middlebrook)

Table 4 Critical Concentrations of Drugs Recommended for Susceptibility Testing

	Drug concentrations (µg/ml)			
Drug	7H10	7H10 (CDC)	7H11	L-J
Isoniazid	0.2	0.2	0.2	0.2
Rifampin	1.0	1.0	1.0	40.0[a]
Streptomycin	2.0	2.0	2.0	4.0
Ethambutol	2.0	5.0	7.5	2.0
PAS	2.0	2.0	8.0	0.5
Ethionamide	5.0	5.0	10.0	20.0
Kanamycin	5.0	5.0	6.0	20.0
Capreomycin	10.0	10.0	10.0	20.0
Cycloserine	20.0	30.0	30.0	30.0

[a]This is probably due to the considerable loss of the drug in egg-containing media. In some studies, MICs of 5 µg/ml or less have been reported.

proportion for resistance of the various drugs. Canetti recommended 1% for isoniazid, PAS, and rifampin and 10% for the remaining drugs. For strepto-mycin this was changed from 1% in the original report (Canetti et al., 1964) to 10% in a later report (Canetti et al., 1969). In contrast, the CDC manual rec-ommends 1% of proportion for all the drugs. This 1% concept is also adopted in the BACTEC method developed by Middlebrook.

Most American laboratories now follow CDC recommendation and use the modified proportion method in 7H10 agar medium; many have adopted the rapid BACTEC method. In contrast, most laboratories in Europe, Africa, the Far East, and South America, many of which are functioning under cooperation with the World Health Organization and the International Union Against Tuber-culosis and Lung Disease, are using L-J medium and the proportion method of Canetti. These differences should be considered when interpreting the epidemi-ological aspects of drug resistance worldwide.

In addition to the classical drug susceptibility tests, recent attempts in the United States have concentrated on the development of very rapid methods for the diagnosis of tuberculosis. These include DNA probe technology, polymerase chain reaction (PCR), and the more extensively used restriction fragment length polymorphism (RFLP). These sophisticated techniques have been adapted from the rapid developments in bacterial genetics and the original mycobacteriophage techniques and are used to identify the source cases in the spread of drug resis-tance in the "miniepidemics" of drug resistance in the United States.

VII. Clinical Significance of Drug Resistance

The most important feature of drug resistance is its clinical significance. Based on their fundamental properties, this correlation differs considerably among pri-mary and acquired drug resistance. In the case of the former, resistance of the organisms first develops in another individual, and a fresh contact might still have a good chance of controlling his or her disease by developing an in vivo concentration of the concerned drug greater than the minimal inhibitory con-centration for the resistant bacilli. In fact, some clinical studies have corrobo-rated these suggestions (Canetti et al., 1964). With acquired drug resistance, on the other hand, because resistance develops in the same host, its level would normally be determined by the attainable in vivo drug concentration, thus of-fering little chance of achieving any inhibitory effect on the bacilli by further administration of the drug. Further, the widespread use of double- or triple-drug therapy considerably increases the difficulty of assessing the action of single drugs in patients infected by the drug-resistant bacilli. However, the limited ev-idence obtained with the use of a single drug like isoniazid, from a series of controlled clinical trials done in Madras, has shed ample light on this problem

(Ramakrishnan et al., 1962; Tripathy et al., 1969). Thus, only 29% of the patients with primary isoniazid resistance had a favorable response at the end of 1 year compared to 61% of 360 patients with isoniazid-susceptible bacilli. Even with double-drug therapy containing isoniazid plus PAS, only a 29% response was seen in patients with initial primary drug resistance compared to 86% with susceptible organisms (Devadatta et al., 1961).

Similar data were obtained from African studies with isoniazid plus thiacetazone or isoniazid plus PAS regimes (East African/British Medical Research Council, 1963). Thus, while the patients with drug-susceptible organisms had a 77% response, only 36–53% of those having resistant organisms did so. A similar outcome was obtained with a streptomycin-and-isoniazid combination. Thus, the available evidence clearly shows that either monotherapy with isoniazid or combination therapy of isoniazid plus PAS or thiacetazone or streptomycin results only in a poor outcome. Similar poor response with acquired drug resistance also is shown with monotherapy on combination chemotherapy. Thus, of the 57 patients with acquired isoniazid resistance, who were treated with isoniazid alone or with isoniazid and PAS, only 16% had bacteriological conversion compared to 80% of patients with susceptible organisms (Medical Research Council, 1955).

A thorough review of the influence of initial drug resistance on the response of short-course chemotherapy of pulmonary tuberculosis, the now common method of treatment of tuberculosis, has been presented by Mitchison and Nunn (1986). Surveying the results of 12 controlled clinical trials carried out during the past decade in Africa, Hong Kong, and Singapore, among those initially resistant to isoniazid and/or streptomycin, failures during chemotherapy were encountered in 17% of 23 patients given a 6-month regimen of isoniazid and rifampin and 12% of 264 patients given rifampin only in an initial 2-month intensive phase of their regimen. The proportion of failures fell as the number of drugs in the regimen and the duration of treatment with rifampin were increased, to reach 2% of 246 patients receiving four of five drugs including rifampin in the 6-month regimen. The sterilizing activity of the regimen, whether it included rifampin or pyrazinamide, was little influenced by initial resistance; the sputum conversion rate at 2 months was similar to that in patients with initially susceptible or resistant bacilli, and the relapse rates after the chemotherapy were only a little higher. The response in the 11 patients with initial rifampin resistance was, however, much poorer, failure during chemotherapy occurring in five and relapse afterward in an additional three patients. This review demonstrated the value of rifampin in preventing failures caused by the emergence of resistance during treatment and the greater sterilizing activity of rifampin and pyrazinamide, compared with that of isoniazid and streptomycin.

Another detailed analysis of the clinical significance of drug resistance in short-course chemotherapy regimens has been presented by Shimao (1987). Using a monthly scoring system for the intensity of chemotherapeutic regimens for the bactericidal drugs (1.0 for isoniazid, pyrazinamide, and streptomycin; 1.5 for rifampin; and 0 for the resistant drugs), results for the several short-course chemotherapy regimens have been reported for both susceptible and resistant cases for either isoniazid, streptomycin, or both drugs. As can be expected, failure rates of patients with drug-susceptible organisms were minimal, and the score was above 9 in all cases. The failure rates of patients with isoniazid- and streptomycin-resistant organisms were higher, but the rate was low when the score was 9 or above. In cases with organisms resistant to both drugs, the failure rate was high, even in cases with scores of 9–12. The relapse rates of patients with drug-susceptible organisms was low when the score was 17 or above and high when the score was less than 13. Overall, the failure and relapse rates were low with scores greater than 13. In fact, the pretreatment drug susceptibility of the organism seems to have minimal influence if the score is 13 or above.

Based on the goals of the World Health Organization to guide "the choice of the first course of chemotherapy to be given to the patient," there had been several studies (World Health Organization, 1963; International Union Against Tuberculosis, 1964; Poppe De Feguerido, 1969; Hong Kong Tuberculosis Treatment Services/British Medical Research Council Investigation, 1972; Abderrahim et al., 1976) that downplayed the importance of initial drug resistance and expressed the belief that this cause of chemotherapy failure had been greatly exaggerated. The studies, particularly the one from Hong Kong, suggested that drug susceptibility testing for all initial cultures was not important. There have been several discussions by Mitchison (1972) and Fox (1974) in favor of such a decision; however, many others, including Wolinsky (1974), Corpe (1974), and Gangadharam (1980), opposed it. For complete discussion of this controversy, see Gangadharam (1984).

As has been mentioned by the author (Gangadharam, 1984), the Hong Kong studies and the supporting statements by Fox (1974) and Mitchison (1972) have "educated few but confused many." If nothing else, these studies had reduced the interest of many people in continuing drug susceptibility testing. This aspect, along with the overall reduction of interest in tuberculosis worldwide, has perhaps contributed to the tragic upsurge of tuberculosis and, more unfortunately, the increase of drug-resistant strains in the United States and elsewhere. Opinion in the United States, however, has shifted, and it is generally recognized that drug resistance, whether it is primary, initial, or acquired, carries serious therapeutic penalties and should be avoided at all cost.

VIII. Epidemiological Aspects of Drug Resistance

Recognizing its importance, information on the prevalence of drug resistance is being collected from many countries. In developing countries, such information is useful in formulating national programs of chemotherapy. It is suggested that these surveys should be repeated periodically in the same community using the same techniques, so that they will act as an epidemiological tool, or "yard-stick," for measuring the success of chemotherapy programs. In developed countries, even though tuberculosis treatment is individualized, such data will assist in planning proper approaches, especially if the community deals with large numbers of immigrants. In the United States, earlier surveys were made repeatedly by Hobby and associates (1974) in the Veterans Administration population, by the U.S. Public Health Service in the general population (Doster et al., 1976), and more recently by the Centers for Disease Control (Kopanoff et al., 1978).

For reasons advanced by Canetti (1962) and endorsed by other international experts, the problems of drug resistance must be discussed within two broad categories: developed countries on the one hand and the developing countries on the other. In both groups, primary and acquired drug resistances have been studied separately, although in recent years, owing to the difficulty in obtaining accurate histories of previous chemotherapy, most studies are centering on initial drug resistance (Mitchison, 1968a). On the other hand, others (Gangadharam, 1984) have questioned the logic of this kind of dichotomy, especially when it is realized that increases in drug resistance in developed countries have been shown to be due to a large extent to immigrants from developing countries with high prevalence rates (Tables 5–7).

Owing to space constraints, worldwide exhaustive data on primary, initial, and acquired drug resistance prevalence rates will not be presented here. The reader is referred to the earlier monograph (Gangadharam, 1984). Only data accumulated after 1985 are given in this chapter. Data on the developing countries are given for the African, South American, and Asian countries (Tables 8–12). Data on the prevalence in the United States are given with

Table 5 Primary Drug Resistance Rates by Race/Ethnic Group

Race/ethnic group	No. cultures tested	No. cultures with resistant organisms	Resistance rate (%)
White	1170	68	5.8
Black	1135	76	6.7
Asian	111	23	20.7
Hispanic	647	97	15.0
Native American	59	4	6.8
Other	24	3	12.5
Total	3164	271	8.6

Source: Data from Kopanoff et al., 1978.

Table 6 Incidence of Drug-Resistance According to Country of Origin

	USA, Canada	Asia, Africa, Caribbean, Latin America
Isoniazid	7.0	39
Streptomycin	5.0	29
Rifampin	7.0	19

Source: Data from Hershfield, 1987.

Table 7 Primary Drug Resistance Related to Nationality (French Studies)

Nationality	Total no. patients	Percentage resistant cases to:					
		Isoniazid		2 drugs or more		Total resistance	
		No.	%	No.	%	No.	%
French	9,593	357	3.7	255	2.7	881	9.2
North African	1,080	87	8.1	56	5.2	140	13.0
Other	970	55	5.7	38	3.9	125	12.9
Total	11,643	501	4.3	349	3.0	1,146	9.8

Source: Data from Canetti et al., 1972.

Table 8 Drug Resistance in Several African (OCCGE) States

Location	Initial drug resistance to:						Proportion of *M. africanum* in the cultures (%)
	Isoniazid		Streptomycin		Thiacetazone		
	No.	%	No.	%	No.	%	
Bobo-Dioulasso	46	19.5	46	23.9	31	25.8	32
Dori (RHV)	55	8.7	55	6.5	55	47.8	49
Mauritania	71	16.9	90	12.3	71	45.0	57
Benin	125	12.8	125	4.8	125	22.4	62
Ivory Coast	318	5.6	318	6.6	—	—	—
Senegal	?	18.5	?	18.8	?	18.5	25

Source: Data from Rey et al., 1979.

Table 9 Initial Drug Resistance in Selected African Countries (Random Sampling)

Country	Period	No. of subjects	Initial resistance to:							
			H	S	HS	R	HR	E	HE	Total
Africa[a,b]	1988–1989	239	13.0	8.4	12.6	3.3	2.1	3.8	5.4	31.0
Tanzania[b]	1988–1990	921	7.5	2	1.2	0.1	0.2	—	—	11.0
Algeria[b]	1981–1985	1981	1.5	2.0	2.4	—	—	—	—	6.3
Sierra Leone[c]	1978–1984	1754	10.5	—	7.7	1.3	—	0.8	—	6.0
Eastern[d]	1979	453	7.8	0	—	—	—	—	—	11.8
Libya[e]	1986	598	6.1	5.1	—	0	—	5.9	—	13.1

[a]Pooled data from Mali, Mauritania, Rwanda, and Zambia.
[b]Data from WHO (courtesy, Drs. O'Brien and Spinaci).
[c]Adapted from Gibson, 1986.
[d]Adapted from Nielson, 1979.
[e]Adapted from Elghoul et al., 1989.

Table 10 Initial Drug Resistance in Latin American Countries

Country	Location	Initial resistance (%) to:					
		INH	SM	RIF	EMB	TB1	Total
Chile	Santiago	5.9	5.8	0	0	0	14.7
Colombia	Sucra/Boyace	5.0	10.0	0	0	25.0	35.0
	Meta	4.0	12.0	0	0	12.0	20.0
	Cesar	3.8	7.7	0	0	7.7	15.4
	Antioquia	7.7	7.7	7.7	0	0	15.4
Cuba	?	8.8	8.8	0	2.9	8.8	17.6
Haiti	Port-au-Prince	10.0	5.0	5.0	5.0	0	20.0
Mexico	Guanaj/Hidalgo	3.1	9.4	0	0	0	15.6
	Veracruz	8.1	16.2	2.7	2.7	5.4	27.0
	Veracruz	13.5	13.5	0	0	0	16.2
	Oaxaca	2.8	8.3	0	0	0	11.1
Peru	Callao	31.8	54.5	13.6	4.5	4.5	54.5
	Ica	15.0	25.0	5.0	0	10.0	35.0
	Lima	3.0	27.3	6.1	0	6.1	39.4
Total initial resistance		8.5	14.6	2.3	1.0	5.1	22.9

INH, isoniazid; SM, streptomycin; RIF, rifampin; EMB, ethambutol; TB1, thiacetazone.
Source: Data from A. Laszlo, personal communication, 1991.

Table 11   Initial Drug Resistance in Several South American Countries

Country	City	Resistance (%) to: Isoniazid	Resistance (%) to: Streptomycin	Resistance to any drug
Argentina	Chaco	5.9	8.8	11.8
	Jujuy	0	2.7	2.7
Bolivia	La Paz	7.1	9.5	11.9
	Santa Cruz	9.4	12.5	15.6
	Cochabamba	6.3	15.6	21.9
Paraguay	Asuncion	6.1	3.0	12.1
Brazil	Rio G. Sur	2.4	7.1	9.5
	Rio G. Sur	0	13.3	13.3
	Para	5.0	15.0	20.0
	Ceara	3.4	3.4	6.9
	Bahia	25.0	21.4	28.6
	M. Geraes	4.3	8.7	10.9
	Rio de Janeiro	4.2	9.8	9.8
	Rio de Janeiro	2.6	9.0	10.3
	São Paulo	3.2	6.5	9.7

Source: Data from Cepanzo, kindly supplied by Dr. I. N. de Kantor.

respect to the country of origin (Table 13). It should, however, be stressed that unlike the exhaustive study by Kleeberg and Boshoff (1978), in the *World Atlas of Initial Drug Resistance*, on the occurrence of initial drug resistance in developing countries, and the regular surveys done by the Centers for Disease Control, which were discontinued in the mid-1980s, the present summary is rather sporadic. Comparison of data from different countries should not be taken on the face value because of differences in techniques, differences in

Table 12   Initial Drug Resistance in Some Asian Countries (Recent Data)

Country	Period	No. of subjects	H	S	HS	R	HR	E	HE	Total
Korea	1980	108	25.0	4.6	2.8	—	—	5.6	3.8	30.6
	1985	161	13.7	3.7	1.2	2.5	2.5	3.7	3.7	17.4
	1990	115	13.0	6.1	1.8	—	—	0.9	0.9	16.5
India	1990	436	12.2	1.8	3.7	1.8	0.9	0	0.5	21.1

Source: Data from WHO (Drs. R. O'Brien and S. Spinaci, personal communication, 1992).

Table 13   Resistance to Isoniazid, Rifampin, Streptomycin, or
Ethambutol in Tubercle Bacilli Isolated from Patients Without
Prior Treatment

Laboratory	No. of patients	Percentage with resistant organisms
Harlingen, TX	135	14.1
New Mexico	166	13.9
Massachusetts	188	12.2
San Diego, CA	121	11.6
Connecticut	78	11.5
Wisconsin	172	10.6
Miami, FL	58	10.3
Chicago, IL	69	10.1
Maryland	91	9.9
Arizona	136	9.7
New York City	136	9.7
Los Angeles, CA	105	9.5
Minnesota	201	9.5
South Carolina	130	9.2
Cleveland, OH	71	8.5
Mississippi	181	7.7
Philadelphia, PA	58	6.9
Alabama	291	6.5
San Francisco, CA	322	6.5
Tennessee	190	6.3
Louisiana	65	6.2
Washington State	248	5.2
Virginia	48	4.2
Oklahoma	314	4.1
Indiana	50	2.0

Source: Data from CDC, 1991 (kindly supplied by Dr. Cauthen).

intensity of questioning, and other important parameters, which are greatly
relevant to drug resistance. Assuming the same laboratory and questioning
parameters are used, the rates of primary drug resistance do not seem to change
except in some Asian countries, where rifampin resistance seems to increase at
a greater rate than in South American and African countries. This may have
some bearing on the increase of resistance to this drug in some parts of the
United States.

Table 14 Immigrants and Drug Resistance

	Race	Never treated		Previously treated	
		No.	%	No.	%
U.S.-born	White	1452	6.0	125	15.2
	Black	1011	7.4	92	23.9
	American Indian	236	7.2	59	6.8
	Hispanic (any area)	209	11.0	34	15.2
Foreign-born	Europe	53	11.3	—	—
	Central/S. America	342	11.4	53	37.7
	Asia	410	16.1	86	27.9
Overall	U.S.-born	2922	6.9	312	17.0
	Foreign-born	837	13.9	152	32.9

Source: Data from CDC (Dr. Cauthen, personal communication, 1992).

Considering the rates in the United States, the overall percentage seems to be the same or increasing slightly, although some states have shown an upward trend and others, the reverse. The significant aspect is the high occurrence of drug resistance in previously treated patients (Table 14). They contribute the bulk of drug-resistant cases, not only in their home countries, but also in the country of their immigration. Those patients, many of whom might not have been recognized and/or identified as a source of drug resistance at the time of immigration, contribute to the pool of drug-resistant patients in many developed countries.

Two relevant aspects for the increase of drug resistance in the United States should be discussed. First is the high proportion (14.3%) of primary isoniazid resistance in U.S. military beneficiaries in Korea (Berliner and Haupt, 1987). These figures are similar to the 14.8% rate for Asians residing in this country and is much higher than the 6.9% for the general U.S. population. Based on this, chemoprophylaxis with rifampin has been considered. In view of the parallel increase of rifampin resistance identified in many recent outbreaks, this suggestion is debatable (see chapter on preventive therapy).

The other major factor is the increase in drug resistance due to Haitian immigrants. A high incidence of 32% of primary drug resistance to isoniazid in recent Haitian immigrants to Florida, in contrast to 12% of Haitians who have resided for more than 8 months in this country, was reported by Pitchenik and associates (1982). A more recent study (Scalcini et al., 1990) reported lower, but still significantly high, rates of 19% for such patients. The impact of such immigrants on the increase of drug resistance has been stressed repeatedly.

IX. Miniepidemics of Drug Resistance in the United States

Several local epidemics of drug-resistant tuberculosis have occurred in the United States (Centers for Disease Control, 1990; Snider et al., 1991). These have been reported from New York, Florida, Missouri, Michigan, and Mississippi, but we should not delude ourselves into thinking that this is a geographically restricted problem (Dooley, 1991). In these outbreaks, the death rate was very high, ranging from 70 to 90% within a few months and very rapid. Many detailed studies of these outbreaks have compared the progression of the disease in comparison with other HIV-positive patients with drug-susceptible tubercle bacilli or without tuberculosis. Important characteristics such as late diagnosis of tuberculosis, late recognition of drug resistance, ineffective patient isolation, and nosocomial transmission of the disease to health care workers were also studied in detail. Only careful monitoring of drug resistance cases and exhaustive study of the close contacts using sophisticated techniques such as phage typing in earlier studies and, more recently, RFLP studies have enabled investigations to pinpoint source cases. In most instances, they could explain possible modes of infection with such bacilli to patients who were exposed to infected cases and to health care workers. The seriousness of the spread of drug resistance is magnified severalfold when the patients involved are infected with HIV (Pitchenik and Fertel, 1992).

Most of these studies have identified the reasons for the miniepidemics. In all situations, factors such as improper isolation and increased contact with the source case were suggested. The contribution of the immunodeficiency caused by HIV, which accelerated the epidemic, was also highlighted. A distressing observation was that, in most cases, resistance was shown to occur not only to the primary drug, isoniazid, but also to rifampin, the next most powerful drug. In many cases, the organisms were resistant to many other antimycobacterial agents.

Various explanations can be offered for the preferential increase of rifampin resistance in some communities (e.g., Southeast Asia) in contrast to other developing and underdeveloped countries like those from South America and Africa. These may be due to (1) the notoriously common problem of noncompliance, (2) sale of the drugs on the black market, (3) the use of substandard combination tablets, wherein the content or bioavailability of rifampin is reduced (Fox, 1990), and (4) the indiscriminate use of rifampin for nonmycobacterial infections (Discussion Session, 1987).

Highly commendable investigations to identify source cases are only practicable in countries like the United States, which have appropriate laboratory support and the capability for intensive investigations. It would not be an exaggeration to state that such epidemics occur in the thousands in many parts of the world, more so in developing countries. At those sites, it is impossible to do even minimal bacteriological diagnosis of drug resistance, except by clinical judgment or by simple analysis of "fall and rise" of sputum smear positivity for acid-fast bacilli (Toman, 1979). In such situations, it is impossible to trace transmission from source cases to the infection of new contacts.

X. Drug Resistance and HIV Infection

The bad prognostic influence of HIV infection on tuberculosis has been recognized and extensively reviewed (Styblo, 1988; Centers for Disease Control, 1989; Darley et al., 1992; Pitchenik and Fertel, 1992). Likewise, the serious nature of this infection on the influence of drug resistance, often culminating in rapid death, has also been recognized. Although it is not possible to identify the specific reasons for this unfortunate outcome or to determine whether and how the immunodeficiency could foster the spread, the dismal outcome is obvious. The studies performed in the United States during the "miniepidemics" brought this distressing situation to the forefront of concern. The dangers of dual infections (*M. tuberculosis* and HIV) in African countries also are great, and the growing drug resistance is adding further weight to this human tragedy.

XI. A Hypothetical View of Spread of Drug Resistance

In developing countries, *acquired* drug resistance will emerge because of (1) noncompliance, (2) substandard drugs, (3) monotherapy, and (4) indiscriminate use of drugs (especially rifampin) for nonmycobacterial diseases. HIV infection may also have some influence; however, the magnitude of this effect is not clear. All these reasons will contribute to *primary* drug resistance in these countries because of enormous opportunities of exposure to tuberculosis and poor isolation practices (Table 15).

In developed countries, *acquired* drug resistance emerges because of (1) noncompliance and associated factors such as homelessness and frequent dislocation (Pablos et al., 1990), (2) alcohol or drug abuse (which increases noncompliance) (Reichman et al., 1979), and (3) HIV disease. While these factors contribute mostly to the spread of *primary* drug resistance (except in some special cases like some of the miniepidemics, where gross failures of isolation practice were noted), the bulk of primary drug resistance is shown to be due to immigrants from high-prevalence countries. Some of these immigrants who had undiagnosed tuberculosis or drug resistance (a consequence of the enormous delay in laboratory identification of these parameters) would soon develop resistance to rifampin as well. Thus, in the absence of facilities to obtain rapid information on drug resistance, the patient receiving both isoniazid and rifampin

Table 15 Possible Reasons for Acquired and Primary Drug Resistance in the World

Developing countries	Developed countries
Acquired	Acquired
1. Noncompliance	1. Noncompliance
2. Substandard drugs individually or in combination tablets	2. Homelessness and frequent dislocation
3. Monotherapy	3. Alcohol or drug abuse
4. Use for nonmycobacterial disease	4. HIV infection
5. HIV infection	
Primary	Primary
Increased chances for fresh infections with drug-resistant bacilli	Immigrants from high-prevalence countries
Substandard drugs individually or in combination tablets	Failure of containment procedures
HIV infection	HIV infection

(the major drugs in short-course chemotherapy) will, in essence, receive a single drug, rifampin, since he has undiagnosed isoniazid resistance.

To minimize this problem, careful isolation and observation of patients plus the use of rapid methods for the identification of drug resistance are of great importance. Parallel to these approaches, discovery and development of new, powerful bactericidal drugs, with efficacy equal to or greater than that of isoniazid and rifampin, are urgently needed. Since development of resistance is to a large extent due to lack of compliance, new drug development must necessarily include directly observed therapy. (See Chapter 10.) While this is the recommendation for advanced countries like the United States, it is not a practical approach for developing countries, where the bulk of tuberculosis patients with drug resistance live.

Acknowledgments

The author is grateful to Dr. Cauthen and others from the Centers for Disease Control, Dr. Laszlo from Canada, Dr. De Kantor from Brazil, and Dr. O'Brien, Dr. Spinaci, and associates from the World Health Organization for unpublished information of the prevalence rates in the United States, Canada, and several other countries. I am grateful to Ms. Madhavi Paturi, M.S., for excellent secretarial assistance.

References

Abderrahim, K., Chaulet, P., Oussedik, N., Amrane, R., Hansen, C. S., and Mercer, N. (1976). Practical results of standard first line treatment in pulmonary tuberculosis. Influence of primary resistance. *Bull. Int. Union Tuberc.* **51**:359.

Andrejew, A., Gernez-Rieux, C., and Tacquet, A. (1957). Cytochromes et activite cytochrome-oxydasique des mycobacteries sensibles et resistantes a l'1NH, *Ann. Inst. Pasteur*, **93**:281–288.

Barclay, W. R. (1955). In vitro studies with ^{14}C PAS, Trans. Veterans Administration-Armed Forces Conf. Chemotherapy Tuberculosis, pp. 14, 222.

Barclay, W. R., Koch-Weser, D., and Ebert, R. H. (1954). Mode of action of isoniazid. Part II. *Am. Rev. Tuberc.* **70**:784–792.

Barry, V. C., Conalty, M. L., and Gaffney, E. (1953). INH resistant strains of *Mycobacterium tuberculosis*. Preliminary communication. *Mycobacterium tuberculosis. Lancet* **1**:978–979.

Berliner, D. S., and Haupt A. (1987). Implications of emerging isoniazid resistance to *Mycobacterium tuberculosis* in Korea. *Aviat. Space Environ. Med.* 83–85.

Canetti, G. (1955). *The Tubercle Bacillus in the Pulmonary Lesion of Man.* Springer, New York.

Canetti, G. (1962). The eradication of tuberculosis: theoretical problems and practical solutions. *Tubercle* **43**:301–321.

Canetti, G., Rist, N., and Grosset, J. (1964). Primary drug resistance in tuberculosis. *Am. Rev. Respir. Dis.* **90**:792–799.

Canetti, G., Kreis, B., Thibier, R., Gay, P., and LeLirzin, M. (1967). Donnees actualles su la resistance primare deus la tuberculose pulmonaire de "L" adulte en France, deuxieme enquiete In Centre d' estudes sur la resistance orimaine (1) aunees 1965–1966. *Rev. Tuberc. Pneumol.* **31**:433–474.

Canetti, G., Fox, W., Khomenko, A., Mahler, H. T., Menon, N. K., Mitchison, D. A., Rist, N., and Smelev, N. A. (1969). Advances in techniques of testing mycobacterial drug sensitivity and the use of sensitivity tests in tuberculosis control programs. *Bull. WHO* **41**:21–43.

Canetti, G., Gary, P. H., and LeLirzin, M. (1972). Trends in the prevalence of primary drug resistance in pulmonary tuberculosis in France from 1962 to 1970. *Tubercle* **53**:57–83.

Centers for Disease Control (1989). Tuberculosis and human immunodefeciency virus infections, recommendations of the advisory committee for the elimination of tuberculosis. *MMWR* **38**:243–250.

Centers for Disease Control (1990). Outbreak of multi drug-resistant tuberculosis—Texas, California, and Pennsylvania. *MMWR* **39**:369–372.

Cohn, M. L., Kovitz, C., Oda, U., and Middlebrook, G. (1954). Studies on isoniazid and tubercle bacilli. II. The growth requirements, catalase activities and pathogenic properties of isoniazid resistant mutants. *Am. Rev. Tuberc.* **70**:641–664.

Cohn, M. L., Middlebrook, G., and Russell, W. F., Jr. (1959). Combined drug treatment of tuberculosis. I. Prevention of emergence of mutant populations of tubercle bacilli resistant to both streptomycin and isoniazid in vitro. *J. Clin. Invest.* **38**:1349–1355.

Corpe, R. (1974). In discussion on drug sensitivity tests. Annual Conference of the American Thoracic Society, Cincinnati, Ohio.

Daniels, M., and Hill, A. B. (1952). The chemotherapy of pulmonary tuberculosis in young adults. *Br. Med. J.* **1**:1162–1168.

Darley, C. L., Small, P. M., Schecter, G. F., Schoolnik, G. K., McAdam, R. A., Jacobs, W. R., and Hopewell, P. C. (1992). An outbreak of tuberculosis with accelerated progression among persons infected with the human immunodeficiency virus. *N. Engl. J. Med.* **326**:231–235.

David, H. L. (1970). Probability distribution of drug-resistant mutants in unselected populations of *Mycobacterium tuberculosis*. *Appl. Microbiol.* **20**: 810–814.

Davidson, P. T. (1987). Drug resistance and the selection of therapy for tuberculosis. *Am. Rev. Respir. Dis.* **136**: 255–257.

Davis, B. D. (1957). Physiological (phenotypic) mechanisms responsible for drug resistance. In: *Drug Resistance in Microorganisms*. Ciba Fundation Symp. Little, Brown, Boston, p. 165.

Devadatta, S., Bhatia, A. L., Andrews, R. H., Fox, W., Mitchison, D. A., Radhakrishna, S., Ramakrishnan, C. V., Selkon, J. B., and Velu, S. (1961). Response of patients infected with isoniazid-resistant tubercle bacilli to treatment with isoniazid plus PAS or isoniazid alone. *Bull. WHO* **25**:807–829.

Discussion session on tuberculosis control—compliance, resistance and cost. (1987) *Tubercle* **68** (Suppl):47–51.

Dooley, S. (1991). Drug resistance among Tuberculosis cases. In: Conference on Emerging Microbes and Microbial Diseases, sponsored by the National Institute of Allergy and Infectious Diseases and the Forgarty International Center of the National Institutes of Health, Nov 1991. Quoted by Fox, J. L., (1992) Coalition reacts to surge of drug-resistant TB. *ASM News* **58**:135–139.

Doster, B., Caras, G. J., and Snider, D. E., Jr. (1976). A continuing survey of primary drug resistance in tuberculosis. 1961 to 1968. A U.S. Public Health Service Cooperative Study. *Am. Rev. Respir. Dis.* **113**:419–425.

East African/British Medical Research Council pretreatment drug resistant report (1963). Influence of pretreatment bacterial resistance to isoniazid, thiacetazone or PAS on the response to chemotherapy of African patients with pulmonary tuberculosis. *Tubercle* **44**:393–430.

Elghoul, M. T., Joshi, R. M., and Rizghalla, T. (1989). Primary and acquired drug resistance in *Mycobacterium tuberculosis* strains in western region of Libya and Jamahiriya. *Trop. Geogr. Med.* **41**:304–308.

Fox, W. (1974). Drug sensitivity tests. Paper presented at the Annual Conference of the American Thoracic Society, Cincinnati, Ohio.

Fox, W. (1990). Drug combinations and the bioavailability of rafampicin. *Tubercle* **71**:241–245.

Fox, W., and Mitchison, D. A. (1975). Short course chemotherapy for pulmonary tuberculosis. *Am. Rev. Respir. Dis.* **111**:325–328.

Freerksen, E. (1957). The clinical significance of bacterial resistance tests. Symp. Ann. Meet. Int. Union Tuberc., Paris, Sept. 20, 1957, panel discussion. *Bull. Int. Union Tuberc.* **27**:222.

Gangadharam, P. R. J. (1980). Drug resistance and drug susceptibility tests. *Am. Rev. Respir. Dis.* **122**:660–661.

Gangadharam, P. R. J. (1984). *Drug Resistance in Mycobacteria*. CRC Press, Boca Raton, FL.

Gangadharam, P. R. J. (1987). Short course chemotherapy of pulmonary tuberculosis: a new approach to drug dosage in the initial intensive phase. *Am. Rev. Respir. Dis.* **136**:1518.

Gangadharam, P. R. J., Devaki, V., and Mohan, K. (1968). Thiacetazone sensitivity of Indian tubercle bacilli. *Tubercle* **49** (Suppl):48–51.

Gangadharam, P. R. J., Ashtekar, D. R., Farhi, D. C., and Wise, D. L. (1991). Sustained release of isoniazid in vivo from a single implant of a biodegradable polymer. *Tubercle* **72**:115–122.

Gibson, J. (1986). Drug-resistant tuberculosis in Sierra Leone. *Tubercle* **67**: 119–124.

Grunberg, R. N., Emmerson, A. M., and Cremer, A. W. (1985). Rifampicin for non-tuberculosis infections? *Chemotherapy* **31**:324–328.

Heifets, L. B. (1982). Synergistic effect of rifampin, streptomycin ethionamide and ethambutol on *M. intracellulare*. *Am. Rev. Respir. Dis.* **125**:43–48.

Heifets, L. B. (1991). *Drug Susceptibility in the Chemotherapy of Mycobacterial Infections*. CRC Press, Boca Raton, FL.

Hershfield, E. (1987). Drug resistance—response to Dr. Shimao. *Tubercle* **68** (Suppl):17–18.

Hobby, G. L., Johnson, P., and Boytar-Papirnyik, V. (1974). Primary drug resistance: a continuing study of drug resistance in tuberculosis in a veteran population within the United States, X. September 1970–September 1973. *Am. Rev. Respir. Dis.* **110**:95–98.

Hong Kong Tuberculosis Treatment Services/British Medical Research Council Investigation (1972). A study in Hong Kong to evaluate the role of pretreatment susceptibility tests in the selection of regimens of chemotherapy for pulmonary tuberculosis. *Am. Rev. Respir. Dis.* **106**:1–22.

International Union Against Tuberculosis (1964). An international investigation of the efficacy of chemotherapy in previously untreated patients with pulmonary tuberculosis. *Bull. Int. Union Tuberc.* **34**:79.

Kleeberg, H. A., and Boshoff, M. S. (1978). *World Atlas of Initial Drug Resistance*. International Union Against Tuberculosis, Paris.

Knox, R. (1955). Haemin and isoniazid resistance of *Mycobacterium tuberculosis*. *J. Gen. Microbiol.* **12**:191–202.

Kopanoff, D. E., Kilburn, J. O., Glassworth, J. L., Snider, D. E., Farer, L. S., and Good, R. C. (1978). A continuing survey of tuberculosis primary drug resistance in the United States. March 1975 to November 1977. *Am. Rev. Respir. Dis.* **118**:835–842.

Liebknecht, W., personal communication to Dr. Meissner, quoted by Meissner, G. (1964) in The bacteriology of tuberculosis. In *Chemotherapy of Tuberculosis*. Edited by V. C. Barry. Butterworths, London, p. 82.

Medical Research Council (1948). Streptomycin treatment of pulmonary tuberculosis. *Br. Med. J.* **2**:769–782.

Medical Research Council (1955). Tuberculosis Trials Committee. Various Combinations of isoniazid with streptomycin or with PAS in the treatment of pulmonary tuberculosis. *Br. Med. J.* **1**:435–445.

Middlebrook, G. (1954). Isoniazid-resistance and catalase activity of tubercle bacilli. A preliminary report. *Am. Rev. Tuberc.* **69**:471–472.

Middlebrook, G., and Cohn, M. L. (1953). Some observations on the pathogenicity of isoniazid resistant variants of tubercle bacilli. *Science* **118**:297–299.

Middlebrook, G., Reggiardo, Z., and Tigerdt, W. D. (1977). Automatable radiometric detection of growth of *Mycobacterium tuberculosis* in selective media. *Am. Rev. Respir. Dis.* **115**:1066–1069.

Mitchison, D. A. (1951). The segregation of streptomycin-resistant variants of *Mycobacterium tuberculosis* into groups with characteristic levels of resistance. *J. Gen. Microbiol.* **5**:596–604.

Mitchison, D. A. (1954). Problems of drug resistance. *Br. Med. Bull.* **10**:115–124.

Mitchison, D. A. (1961). Primary drug resistance. *Bull. Int. Union Tuberc.* **32**:81.

Mitchison, D. A. (1968a). Sensitivity testing. In *Recent Advances in Respiratory Tuberculosis*. Edited by F. Heaf and N. L. Rusby. J. & A. Churchill, London, p. 160.

Mitchison, D. A. (1968b). Natural sensitivity of *M. tuberculosis* to thiacetazone. *Tubercle* **49** (Suppl):38–46.

Mitchison, D. A. (1972). Implications of the Hong Kong study of policies of sensitivity testing. *Bull. Int. Union Tuberc.* **47**:9.

Mitchison, D. A. (1979). Basic mechanisms of chemotherapy. *Chest* **76** (Suppl):771–781.

Mitchison, D. A., and Lloyd, J. (1964). Comparison of the sensitivity to thiacetazone of tubercle bacilli from patients in Britain, East Africa, South India and Hong Kong. *Tubercle* **45**:360–369.

Mitchison, D. A., and Nunn, A. J. (1986). Influence of initial drug resistance on the response of short-course chemotherapy of pulmonary tuberculosis. *Am. Rev. Respir. Dis.* **133**:423–430.

Mitchison, D. A., and Selkon, J. B. (1956). The bactericidal activities of antituberculous drugs. *Am. Rev. Tuberc.* **74**:109–116.

Nichida, S. (1959). Studies on resistance of microorganisms to various chemicals. 8. Mechanism of acquisition and loss of drug resistance by bacteria. 1. Experiments with anion type of tubercle bacilli. *Ann. Rept. Res. Inst. Tuberc. Kanazawa Univ.* **15**:243; quoted in *Biol. Abstr.* **33**:3847.

Nielsen, N. J. (1979). Primary and secondary resistance of Mycobacterium tuberculosis in Eastern Botswana. *Tubercle* **60**:239–243.

Pablos, M. A., Raigloine, M. C., Ruggero, B., and Ramoux-Zuniga, R. (1990). Drug resistant tuberculosis among the homeless in New York City. *NY State J. Med.* **90**:351–355.

Perry, C. R., and Morse, W. C. (1955). The pyrazinamide susceptibility of isoniazid-resistant mutants of tubercle bacilli. *Am. Rev. Tuberc. Pulm. Dis.* **72**:840–842.

Pitchenik, A. E., and Fertel, D. (1992). Tuberculosis and non-tuberculosis mycobacterial disease. In Medical Management of AIDS patients. *Med. Clin. North. Am.* **76**:121–171.

Pitchenik, A. E., Russell, B. W., Clearly, T., Pejovic, I., Cole, C., and Snider, D. E., Jr. (1982). The prevalence of tuberculosis and drug resistance among Haitians. *N. Engl. J. Med.* **307**:162–165.

Poppe De Figuerido, F. (1969). Treatment of patients with pulmonary tuberculosis classified according to the history of previous chemotherapy and without reference to pretreatment drug sensitivity. *Tubercle* **50**:335–343.

Pyle, M. M. (1947). Relative numbers of resistant tubercle bacilli in sputum of patients before and during treatment with streptomycin. *Proc. Mayo Clin.* **22**:465–473.

Ramakrishnan, C. V., Bhatia, A. L., Devadatta, S., Fox, W., Narayana, A. S. L., Selkon, J. B., and Velu, S. (1962). The course of pulmonary tuberculosis in patients excreting organisms which have acquired resistance to isoniazid. Response to continued treatment for a second year with isoniazid alone or with isoniazid plus PAS. *Bull. WHO* **26**:1–18.

Rao, K. V. N., Eidus, L., Evans, C., Kailasam, S., Radhakrishna, S., Somasundaram, P. R., Stott, M., Subbammal, S., and Tripathy, S. P. (1968). Deterioration of cycloserine in the tropics. *Bull. WHO* **39**:781–789.

Reichman, L. B. (1987). Compliance, resistance and cost: major considerations in tuberculosis control. Proceedings of a symposium held in Singapore, 1986. *Tubercle* **68** (Suppl):1–51.

Reichman, L. B., Felton, C. P., and Edsall, J. R. (1979). Drug dependence: a possible new risk factor for tuberculosis disease. *Arch. Intern. Med.* **139**:337–339.

Rey, J. L., Villon, A., Bichat, B., and Meyran, M. (1979). Les resistances initiales das bacillas tuberculeny don les pays de P[1]) O.C.C.G.E. Consequences practiques. XIX Conference Technique de la O.C.C.G.E. Haute Volta 5–8 Juin 1979. Document No. 7 146/79. Doc Tech O.C.C.G.E. Kindly Supplied by Dr. A. Pio, WHO.

Rist, N. (1964). Nature and development of resistance of tubercle bacilli to chemotherapeutic agents. In *Chemotherapy of Tuberculosis*. Edited by V. C. Barry. Butterworths, London, p. 210.

Rist, N., Grumbach, F., and Libermann, D. (1959). Experiments on the antituberculosis activity of alpha-ethyl-thioisonicotinamide. *Am. Rev. Tuberc.* **79**:1–5.

Russell, W. F., Kass, I., Heaton, A. D., Dressler, S. H., and Middlebrook, G. (1959). Combined drug treatment of tuberculosis. III. Clinical application of the principles of appropriate and adequate chemotherapy to the treatment of pulmonary tuberculosis. *J. Clin. Invest.* **38**:1366–1375.

Sbarbaro, J. A., and Johnson, S. (1968). Tuberculosis chemotherapy for recalcitrant outpatients administered directly twice weekly. *Am. Rev. Respir. Dis.* **97**:895–903.

Scalcini, M., Carre, G. J-B., Hershfield, E., Parker, W. J., Nelz, K., and Long, R. (1990). Antituberculous drug resistance in Central Haiti. *Am. Rev. Respir. Dis.* **142**:508–511.

Schaefer, W. B. (1954). The effect of isoniazid on growing and resting tubercle bacilli. *Am. Rev. Tuberc.* **69**:125–127.

Selkon, J. B., Subbiah, T. V., Bhatia, A. L., Radhakrishna, S., and Mitchison, D. A. (1960). A comparison of the sensitivity to *p*-aminosalicylic acid of tubercle bacilli from South Indian and British patients. *Bull. WHO* **23**: 599–611.

Selkon, J. B., Devadatta, S., Kulkarni, K. G., Mitchison, D. A., Narayana, A. S. L., Nair, C. N., and Ramachandran, K. (1964). The emergence of isoniazid-resistant cultures in patients with pulmonary tuberculosis during treatment with isoniazid alone or isoniazid plus PAS. *Bull. WHO* **31**: 273–294.

Shimao, T. (1987). Drug resistance in tuberculosis control. *Tubercle* **68** (Suppl):5–15.

Siddiqi, S. K., Lebonati, J. P., and Middlebrook, G. (1981). Evaluation of a rapid radiometric method for drug susceptibility testing of *Mycobacterium tuberculosis. J. Clin. Microbiol.* **13**:908–912.

Snider, D. E., Cauthen, G. M., Farer, J. O., Kelly, G. D., Kilburn, J. O., Good, R. C., and Dooley, S. W. (1991). Drug resistant tuberculosis. *Am. Rev. Respir. Dis.* **144**:732.

Styblo, K. (1988). The potential impact of AIDS on the tuberculosis situation in developed and developing countries. *Bull. Int. Union Tuberc. Lung Dis.* **63**:25–28.

Temple, C. W., Hughs, E. J., Mardis, R. E., Towbin, M. N., and Dye, W. E. (1951). Combined intermittent regimens employing streptomycin and para-aminosalicyclic acid in the treatment of pulmonary tuberculosis. *Am. Rev. Tuberc.* **63**:295–311.

Tofte, R. W. (1985). Rifampin no longer just for tuberculosis? *Prostgrad. Med.* **77**:228–230.

Toman, K. (1979). *Tuberculosis Case Finding and Chemotherapy. Questions and Answers.* World Health Organization, pp. 91.

Tripathy, S. P. (1968). Madras study of supervised once-weekly chemotherapy in the treatment of pulmonary tuberculosis: laboratory aspects. *Tubercle* **49** (Suppl):78–80.

Tripathy, S. P., Menon, N. K., Mitchison, D. A., Narayana, A. S. L., Somasundaram, P. A., Stott, H., and Velu, S. (1969). Response to treatment with isoniazid plus PAS of tuberculosis patients with primary isoniazid resistance. *Tubercle* **50**:257–268.

Tsukamura, M. (1978). A comparison of the time of in vivo resistance development of tubercle bacilli to rifampicin, kanamycin, ethionamide, lividomycin an enviomycin (tuberactinomycin-N) in patients with chronic cavitary tuberculosis. *Kekkaku* **53**:495.

Tuberculosis Chemotherapy Center, Madras (1959). A concurrent comparison of home and sanatorium treatment of pulmonary tuberculosis in South India. *Bull. WHO* **21**:51–144.

Tuberculosis Chemotherapy Center, Madras (1964). A controlled comparison of intermittent (twice weekly) isoniazid plus streptomycin and daily isoniazid plus PAS in the domiciliary treatment of pulmonary tuberculosis. *Bull. WHO* **31**:247–271.

Tuberculosis Chemotherapy Center, Madras (1970). A controlled comparison of a twice weekly and three once-weekly regimens in the initial treatment of pulmonary tuberculosis. *Bull WHO* **43**:143–206.

Velu, S., Andrews, R. H., Devadatta, S., Fox, W., Radhakrishna, S., Ramakrishman, C. V., Selkon, J. B., Somosundaram, P. R., and Subbiah, T. V. (1960). Progress in the second year of patients with quiescent pulmonary tuberculosis after a year of chemotherapy at home or in sanatorium and influence of further chemotherapy on the relapse rate. *Bull WHO* **23**:511–533.

Wolinsky, E. (1974). In discussion of the paper by Fox at the Annual Conference of the American Thoracic Society, Cincinnati, Ohio.

World Health Organization (1963). Introduction. *Bull. WHO* **29**:559–563.

World Health Organization Research Project Kenya, (1967). Unpublished observations.

Youatt, J. (1969). A review of the action of isoniazid. *Am. Rev. Respir. Dis.* **99**:729–749.

Youmans, G. P., Williston, E. H., Feldman, W. H., and Hinshaw, C. H. (1946). Increase in resistance of tubercle bacilli to streptomycin. A preliminary report. *Proc. Mayo Clin.* **21**:126.

16

Tuberculosis in Children

JEFFREY R. STARKE

Baylor College of Medicine
Houston, Texas

I. Introduction

A. General Information

Tuberculosis is still a significant cause of both morbidity and mortality for children throughout the world. In many developing countries, tuberculous infection and disease among children have remained commonplace (Murray et al., 1990). In industrialized countries, the incidence of childhood tuberculosis declined substantially between the 1930s and the 1980s, in part owing to improved social conditions, the introduction of antituberculosis drugs and, perhaps, to the use of bacille Calmette-Guerin (BCG) vaccines. Unfortunately, some industrialized countries—especially the United States—have experienced a resurgence of pediatric tuberculosis in the past several years (Starke et al., 1992; Centers for Disease Control [CDC] 1991).

Although tuberculosis can have profound health consequences for the affected child and his or her family, childhood tuberculosis has a limited influence on the *immediate* epidemiology of the disease within a community because children are rarely a source of infection to contacts (International Union Against Tuberculosis and Lung Disease [IUATLD], 1991). However, the occurrence of tuberculosis in children is a marker for ongoing transmission of infection among all age groups in a society (Snider et al., 1988). Infected children also represent a large portion of the pool from which future tuberculosis cases will arise. Programs that target children for treatment of tuberculous infection and disease will have little short-term results on disease rates, but will be critical to effect long-term control of the disease.

B. Limitations on Data

Our knowledge of childhood tuberculosis has been limited substantially by certain characteristics of the disease. The diagnosis of tuberculosis in children rests largely on the results of the clinical history and examination, tuberculin skin testing, radiographic examination, and contact history. Sputum often cannot be obtained from children, and smear and culture results are usually negative when it can be obtained. As a result, the majority of cases of tuberculosis in children in most developing countries are not diagnosed because of the lack of appropriate radiographic and laboratory facilities (IUATLD, 1991). Even in countries with modern clinical and laboratory facilities, the diagnosis of tuberculosis in a child can be confirmed by culture in less than 40% of cases (Lincoln et al., 1958b; Starke and Taylor-Watts, 1989b). The low rate of culture confirmation makes investigations of new diagnostic techniques in children difficult to design and interpret.

The natural history of childhood tuberculosis makes the designing of studies and trials difficult, for several reasons: (1) establishing the diagnosis of tuberculous disease in a child can be imprecise, and it is often not verifiable by culture; (2) definitions of treatment failure and relapse of tuberculosis in a child usually must be on clinical grounds because they are rarely associated with a positive culture; (3) since the natural history of primary pulmonary tuberculosis in a child may be slow, steady improvement, even without drug therapy, studies that measure the effectiveness of interventions must include long-term evaluation; (4) it is difficult to compare results of studies performed in developing countries—where disease tends to be more severe, malnutrition is more common, and supportive care is less available—with those from technically advanced nations; and (5) well-controlled studies in pediatric tuberculosis are rare owing to the fairly small numbers of patients seen at most centers able to perform the studies.

II. Epidemiology

A. Worldwide Disease

It is difficult to assess the worldwide scope of tuberculosis in children because data are scarce and poorly organized. Reported disease rates grossly underestimate the true incidence, and the prevalence of tuberculous infection without disease is completely unknown in most areas of the world. It is estimated that the average annual new tuberculous infection rate for all ages in many areas of Africa and Asia is about 2%, which yields an estimated 218 cases of tuberculosis per 100,000 population per year (Murray et al., 1990). Approximately 15% of these cases occur in children younger than 15 years of age. Between 8 and 20% of deaths caused by tuberculosis in the developing world occur in children. The World Health Organization has recently estimated that, in developing countries, there are 1.3 million cases and 450,000 deaths annually of tuberculosis in children younger than 15 years of age (Kochi, 1991). There is no indication that tuberculosis rates among children in developing nations are declining.

Trends in mortality of pediatric tuberculosis in industrialized nations are well illustrated by data from Europe. The annual mortality from tuberculosis fell from 600:100,000 children in 1860, to 50:100,000 in the late 1930s, and below 0.08:100,000 in 1977 (IUATLD, 1991). The mortality rates for children from newborn to 4 years of age have been and still are about twice that for children ages 5–14 years, mostly because of the higher incidence of tuberculous meningitis in the younger population.

B. Disease in the United States

The most complete recent epidemiological data for pediatric tuberculosis comes from the United States. Reported tuberculosis cases in children younger than 15 years of age declined from 6036 in 1962 to 1261 in 1985, an average annual decline of about 6% (Snider et al., 1988). Case rates declined in a similar fashion, from 10:100,000 children in 1962 to 2.4:100,000 in 1985. However, beginning in 1987, the number of cases began to increase. After a low of 1177 cases in 1987, annual cases in children increased 36% to 1596, by 1990 (CDC, 1991). This increasing incidence means that transmission of infection in the United States is ongoing, and that a new generation of infected individuals will serve as a reservoir of the disease in the future, unless they are treated soon.

Both age and sex are important variables for tuberculosis among children. There is no evidence that the likelihood of infection with *Mycobacterium tuberculosis* is influenced by either; however, both influence the risk of an infected child developing active disease. In 1990, 59% of the pediatric tuberculosis cases in the United States occurred in children younger than 5 years of age, the group traditionally at highest risk for the disease. The interval between ages 5 and 14 years is often called "the favored age," since children in this group consistently have a lower tuberculous disease rate than any other segment of the population. Age also affects the anatomical site of involvement with tuberculosis. Younger children are more likely to develop meningeal, miliary, or lymphatic tuberculosis, whereas adolescents more frequently present with pleural, genitourinary, or peritoneal disease (Table 1). Although tuberculosis in adults

Table 1 Median Age of Tuberculosis by Predominant Site in Persons Younger Than 20 Years of Age: United States, 1986

Site	Percentage of cases	Median age (yr)
Pulmonary	76.1	7
Lymphatic	14.3	5
Pleural	3.3	16
Meningeal	2.4	3
Miliary	1.2	1
Bone–joint	1.0	5
Genitourinary	0.3	12
Peritoneal	0.3	17
Other	1.0	5

Source: Smith (1989).

occurs preponderantly among men, it appears that during the latter part of childhood and during adolescence, girls have a higher incidence of and mortality from tuberculosis than do boys. However, among infants and young children, there is no difference in incidence between the sexes.

At every age—including childhood—in the United States, tuberculosis case rates are strikingly higher in ethnic and racial minority groups than in whites. The difference is most likely a result of environmental factors, such as socioeconomic status, housing conditions, and exposure to high-risk adults. Approximately 80–85% of childhood tuberculosis cases in the United States occur among African–Americans, Hispanics, Asians, and Native Americans (Snider et al., 1988). Although most children with tuberculosis were born in the United States, the proportion of foreign-born children has been increasing. Between 1986 and 1990, the proportion of foreign-born cases rose from 13 to 16% for children younger than 5 years of age, and from 40 to 49% among adolescents aged 15–19 years (Starke et al., 1992). Tuberculosis has become geographically focal; only 11% of counties reported a childhood case in 1990, and the disease is concentrated within cities with populations greater than 250,000.

Transmission of tuberculosis is from person to person, usually by droplets of mucus that become airborne when the ill individual coughs, sneezes, laughs, or sings. Children with primary tuberculosis rarely, if ever, infect other children or adults (Wallgren, 1937). In tuberculous children, tubercle bacilli are sparse in endobronchial secretions, and cough is often lacking in the clinical presentation. When young children do cough, they rarely produce sputum, and they lack the tussive force of adults. Adolescents with reactivation forms of pulmonary tuberculosis, such as cavities or extensive infiltrates, may be infectious to others.

Table 2 Adults at High Risk for Tuberculosis in the United States

Foreign-born persons from high prevalence countries
Persons with HIV coinfection
Residents of correctional institutions
Residents of nursing homes
Homeless persons
Users of intravenous or other street drugs
Poor and medically indigent city dwellers
Persons with certain medical risk factors (e.g., silicosis, diabetes mellitus)
Persons receiving immunosuppressive therapies

Occasionally, transmission of *M. tuberculosis* from a child may occur by direct contact with infected fluids or discharges such as urine or purulent sinus tract drainage. Fomites, such as syringes, gastric lavage tubes, or bronchoscopes, are rare sources of infection (Smith and Marquis, 1987).

Children are usually infected with *M. tuberculosis* by an adult in the immediate household. The current increasing tuberculosis case rates among children in the United States are most likely due to the increasing rates among young adults, especially in urban centers (Bloch et al., 1989). Among adults, tuberculosis has retreated into pockets of high-risk individuals (Table 2). Children cared for or exposed to adults in these groups are most likely to become infected. Casual extrafamilial contact is less frequently the source of infection, but school janitors and teachers, bus drivers, nurses, day care workers, and candy store keepers have been implicated as the source of infection in individual cases and epidemics (Lincoln, 1965; Nolan et al., 1987; Leggiadro et al., 1989). In the Northern Hemisphere, childhood tuberculosis appears to be most common from January to June, perhaps because of increased close indoor contact during winter months and more frequent coughing in adults produced by winter and spring respiratory infections (Smith and Marquis, 1987).

C. Human Immunodeficiency Virus-Related Tuberculosis in Children

The ongoing epidemic of infection with the human immunodeficiency virus (HIV) has had a profound effect on the recent epidemiology of tuberculosis (Bloch et al., 1989). The HIV epidemic can increase the tuberculosis incidence in children by two major mechanisms (Braun et al., 1991; Braun and Cauthen, 1992): (1) HIV-infected adults with tuberculosis may transmit *M. tuberculosis* to children, a portion of whom will develop tuberculous disease; (2) children with HIV infection may be at increased risk of progressing from tuberculous infection to disease.

According to current knowledge, the infectiousness of HIV-seropositive adults with tuberculosis will depend largely on the proportion who have acid-fast smear-positive pulmonary disease. Pulmonary involvement is common among HIV-seropositive adults with tuberculosis, especially when the tuberculosis precedes other opportunistic infections (Chaisson and Slutkin, 1989). In one study from New York City, 45% of HIV-infected adults with pulmonary tuberculosis had a positive sputum smear, compared with 81% of those without HIV infection (Klein et al., 1989). However, studies in Zaire and New York, which involved contact investigations, suggested that HIV-seronegative and HIV-seropositive patients with smear-positive pulmonary tuberculosis infected similar proportions of their contacts with *M. tuberculosis* (Braun and Cauthen, 1992). A retrospective population study in Florida implied that an observed increase in pediatric tuberculosis cases was linked with an increase in cases in HIV-infected adults (Braun and Cauthen, 1992). Although, as a whole, HIV-seropositive adults with tuberculosis may be somewhat less likely than HIV-seronegative adults to transmit tuberculosis, the increased caseload of adult tuberculosis associated with HIV is partly responsible for rising tuberculosis case rates among children.

Information about the risk of tuberculosis in HIV-infected children is surprisingly meager. Up to 1991 in the United States, only seven children with HIV infection and extrapulmonary tuberculosis had been reported (Braun and Cauthen, 1992). Only a handful of case reports of pulmonary tuberculosis in HIV-infected children have been published (Moss et al., 1992; Varteresian-Karanfil et al., 1988). In countries where tuberculous infection rates in children are generally higher than in the United States, such as Zambia (Malek et al., 1989), Brazil (DePaula et al., 1989), and Haiti (Pape et al., 1988), HIV-infected pediatric cohorts have a risk of developing tuberculosis that exceeds background rates. In both developing and technically advanced nations, tuberculosis probably is underdiagnosed in HIV-infected children because of the similarity of its clinical presentation to other opportunistic infections and the difficulty in confirming the diagnosis with positive cultures.

D. Tuberculous Infection

Although there are estimates that about 20% of the world's population is infected with *M. tuberculosis* (Kochi, 1991), it is impossible to determine how many children actually have asymptomatic tuberculous infection. Since all but two countries have used BCG vaccine extensively, population surveys for tuberculous infection using the tuberculin skin test are rarely performed and would be exceedingly difficult to interpret. Even in the United States, the incidence of tuberculous infection is unknown, since a positive skin test is a reported condition in only three states, and national surveys were discontinued in 1971 (Edwards, 1974). At that time, the incidence of tuberculous infection among 5- and 6-year-olds was about 0.2%.

The most efficient method of finding children infected with *M. tuberculosis* is through contact investigations of adults with infectious pulmonary tuberculosis. On average, 30–50% of household contacts will have a reactive tuberculin skin test. Even in countries where BCG is used extensively, a positive tuberculin skin test in a child who has close contact with an adult with infectious tuberculosis probably represents infection with *M. tuberculosis*, and preventive chemotherapy to halt progression of infection to disease should be considered.

In the United States, children in the general population currently have a low risk for infection with the tubercle bacillus. However, several recent studies show that, in some large cities, the risk of infection is high. In Boston public schools, 5.1% of seventh graders and 8.9% of tenth graders are tuberculin skin test-positive (Barry et al., 1990). In Los Angeles and Houston, 2–5% of elementary school children are infected (Davidson et al., 1990; Starke et al., 1988). For some populations, targeted screening and preventive chemotherapy programs will be necessary to diminish the pool of infected children and eliminate future cases of disease.

III. Pathogenesis

A. Primary Tuberculosis in Children

The primary complex of tuberculosis consists of local disease at the portal of entry and the regional lymph nodes that drain the areas of the primary focus. The primary complex may occur anywhere in the body, but it is in the lung in over 95% of cases. While the primary complex is developing, tubercle bacilli usually spread through the bloodstream and lymphatics to many parts of the body. In 1–3% of infections, the dissemination is massive, leading to miliary or meningeal tuberculosis. More commonly, small numbers of bacilli leave tuberculous foci scattered in various tissues, which may or may not develop into clinically significant extrapulmonary tuberculosis later in life. After 4–8 weeks, cell-mediated immunity and delayed hypersensitivity (marked by a positive tuberculin skin test) usually develop. At this time, the primary complex often heals, and further dissemination is arrested. The onset of delayed hypersensitivity may be accompanied by a febrile reaction that lasts 1–3 weeks; at this time, the tissue reaction intensifies, often causing the primary complex to become visible on chest radiographs (Smith and Marquis, 1987).

B. Timetable of Childhood Tuberculosis

There is a fairly predictable timetable of events related to the primary tuberculous infection and its complications (Wallgren, 1948). This timetable is very useful for the clinician, permitting a realistic prognosis, an understanding of what complications to look for and when, and a productive approach to finding the source case for infection (Smith and Marquis, 1987).

When symptomatic lymphohematogenous spread occurs, it does so no later than 3–6 months after the initial infection. Endobronchial tuberculosis, often accompanied by segmental pulmonary changes, usually develops between 4 and 9 months after infection. Clinically significant lesions of bones or joints do not appear until at least 1 year after infection, whereas renal lesions develop 5–25 years later. The interval between the initial infection and reactivation of pulmonary tuberculosis is extremely variable, depending on the age of the child at initial infection; in adolescents, the interval is often months to several years, whereas in infants, it is much longer.

In general, complications of the primary infection in children occur within the first 5 years—and are concentrated in the first year—after initial infection. Complications later in life are often secondary to reactivation of previously dormant bacilli acquired and controlled, but not eliminated, during childhood.

C. Pregnancy and the Newborn

True congenital tuberculosis is very rare, with less than 300 cases being published (Smith and Teele, 1990). There are two major routes for true congenital infection. First, *M. tuberculosis* can pass from the placenta to the fetus through the umbilical vein. The infected infants' mothers frequently suffer from tuberculous pleural effusion, meningitis, or miliary disease during pregnancy or soon after (Grenville-Mathers et al., 1960; Hageman et al., 1980; Nemir and O'Hare, 1985; Stallworth et al., 1980). However, in many cases of congenital tuberculosis, the diagnosis of tuberculosis in the newborn has led to the discovery of the mother's tuberculosis. The intensity of lymphohematogenous spread during pregnancy is one of the factors that determines if congenital infection will occur. Hematogenous dissemination leads to infection of the placenta, with transmission to the fetus (Kaplan et al., 1980). However, even massive involvement of the placenta with tuberculosis does not always give rise to congenital tuberculosis. It is not clear whether the fetus can be infected directly from the mother's bloodstream without a caseous tuberculous lesion forming first in the placenta, although this has been reported in experimental animal models (Smith and Teele, 1990). In either event, bacilli would first reach the fetus' liver, where a primary focus would develop with associated involvement of the periportal lymph nodes. However, the organisms can pass through the liver into the main circulation, leading to a primary focus in the fetal lung. The tubercle bacilli in the lung may remain dormant until after birth, when oxygenation and circulation increase significantly (Smith and Teele, 1990; Hallum and Thomas, 1955).

Congenital tuberculosis also might occur by aspiration or ingestion of infected amniotic fluid. If a caseous lesion in the placenta were to rupture directly into the amniotic cavity, the fetus could inhale or ingest the tubercle bacilli. Inhalation of infected amniotic fluid is the most likely cause of congenital tuberculosis if multiple primary foci are present in the lung or gut and middle ear (Hughesdon, 1946).

In 1935, Beitzke presented criteria for the diagnosis of true congenital tuberculosis: (1) Tuberculosis in the child must be firmly established; (2) there must be a primary complex in the liver; (3) if a primary complex in the liver is lacking or undocumented, the tuberculous lesions must be only a few days old, and extrauterine infection must be excluded with certainty.

Postnatal acquisition of tuberculosis by airborne inoculation is the most common route of infection for the neonate (Jacobs and Abernathy, 1988). It is often impossible to differentiate postnatal infection from true congenital infection on clinical grounds. The distinction is not of major importance for the baby, since the treatment regimens are the same. However, determining the true source of infection is vital for proper evaluation and treatment of the mother and other adults in the baby's environment.

IV. Clinical Forms of Tuberculosis

A. Endothoracic

Asymptomatic Primary Infection

Asymptomatic primary tuberculosis is an infection with *M. tuberculosis* associated with tuberculin skin reactivity, but no clinical or significant radiographic findings. This presentation is more common in school-aged children than in younger infants; 80–95% of infected older children have asymptomatic infections, whereas only 40–50% of infected infants remain free of symptoms or radiographic abnormalities (Miller et al., 1963). Cultures from these children are rarely positive. Children in this category are ideal candidates for so-called preventive chemotherapy, to kill the bacilli before symptomatic disease occurs.

Primary Pulmonary

A primary pulmonary complex includes the parenchymal focus and regional lymphadenitis. Almost 70% of primary foci are subpleural, and localized pleurisy is a common part of the primary complex. The primary complex begins with the deposition of infected droplets into lung alveoli. All lobar segments are at equal risk of being seeded, and, in 25% of cases, there are multiple primary lung foci (Starke and Taylor-Watts, 1989b). The initial parenchymal inflammation usually is not visible on chest radiograph, but a localized, nonspecific infiltrate may be seen. The infection spreads within days to regional lymph nodes. When tuberculin hypersensitivity develops, within 3–10 weeks after infection, the inflammatory reaction in the lung parenchyma and lymph nodes intensifies. The hallmark of primary tuberculosis in the lung is the relatively large size and importance of the hilar, mediastinal, or subcarinal adenitis compared with the relatively small size of the initial parenchymal focus. Because of the patterns of lymphatic drainage, a left-sided parenchymal lesion often leads to bilateral adenopathy, whereas a right-sided focus is associated with right-sided adenopathy only (Smith and Marquis, 1987).

In most children, the parenchymal infiltrate and adenitis resolve early. In some children, especially infants, the lymph nodes continue to enlarge (Fig. 1 and 2). Bronchial obstruction begins as the nodes impinge on the neighboring regional bronchus, compressing it and causing diffuse inflammation of its wall (Daly et al., 1952). The inflammation may intensify, and the lymph nodes erode through the bronchial wall, leading to perforation and formation of thick caseum in the lumen, with partial or complete obstruction of the bronchus (Lincoln et al., 1956; Lorriman and Bentley, 1959; Morrison, 1973). The common radiographic sequence is hilar adenopathy, followed by localized hyperaeration and, eventually, atelectasis (Matsaniotis et al., 1967; Stansberry, 1990). The resulting radiographic shadows have been called "epituberculosis," "collapse-consolidation," or "segmental" lesions. These findings are similar to those caused by aspiration of a foreign body; in primary tuberculosis the lymph node acts as the "foreign body."

Obstructive hyperaeration of a lobar segment may accompany bronchial obstruction (Giammona et al., 1969). This unusual complication occurs most often in children younger than 2 years of age and may be accompanied by wheezing. The obstruction will usually resolve spontaneously, but this may take months to occur. Surgical removal of the lymph nodes may hasten clinical improvement, but is rarely necessary.

The most common complication of the bronchial obstruction is the fan-shaped segmental lesion (see Fig. 1), which results from a combination of the primary pulmonary focus, the caseous material from an eroded bronchus, the host inflammatory response, and the subsequent atelectasis. Up to 43% of children younger than 1 year of age who are infected with *M. tuberculosis* will develop a segmental lesion, compared with 25% for children ages 1–10 years, and 16% for children ages 11–15 years (Miller et al., 1963). Segmental lesions and obstructive hyperaeration can occur together.

Physical signs and symptoms caused by hilar adenopathy and segmental lesions are surprisingly uncommon and are more common in infants. Occasionally, the initiation of the primary infection is marked by fever and cough. As the primary complex progresses, nonspecific symptoms such as fever, cough, night sweats, and weight loss may occur. Most children have no symptoms and are

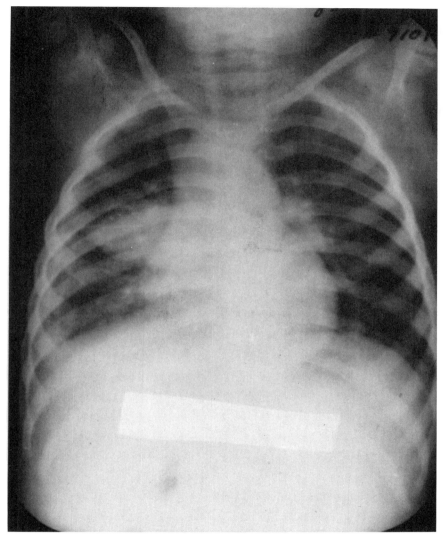

Figure 1 A segmental pulmonary lesion in a child with primary tuberculosis. The complex includes hilar adenopathy, atelectasis, and localized pleural reaction.

discovered only because they are investigated as contacts to an adult case. Pulmonary signs are usually absent. Some children have localized wheezing or diminished breath sounds, which are rarely accompanied by tachypnea or respiratory distress. Nonspecific symptoms and pulmonary signs are sometimes

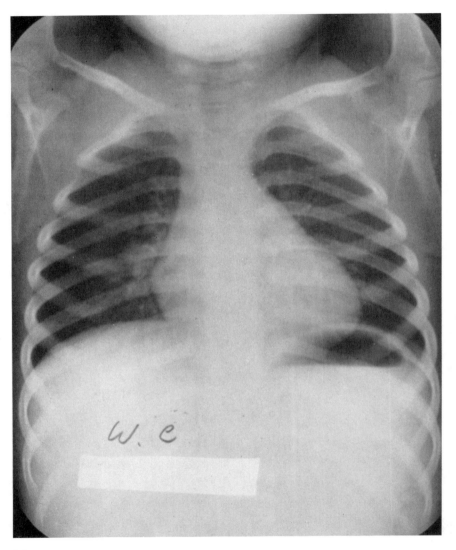

(a)

Figure 2 Chest radiographs of a child with primary complex tuberculosis, showing the importance of obtaining a lateral view. (a) Although the posteo-anterior view appears normal, the (b) lateral view shows hilar adenopathy.

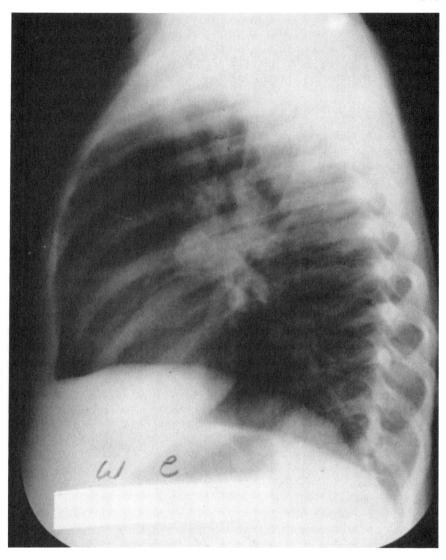

(b)

alleviated by antibiotics, suggesting that bacterial superinfection distal to the bronchial obstruction may be present.

Enlargement of other groups of infected intrathoracic lymph nodes can cause various clinical manifestations. Enlarged subcarinal nodes, which can cause splaying of the large bronchi, may impinge on the esophagus and cause difficulty swallowing or cause a bronchoesophageal fistula. Infected nodes may compress the subclavian vein, producing edema of the hand or arm. Nodes may rupture into the mediastinum and point in the right or left supraclavicular fossa.

Most cases of tuberculous bronchial obstruction in children resolve fully, radiographically, with or without antituberculosis chemotherapy. However, up to 60% of untreated children will have residual anatomical sequelae not apparent on radiographs (Smith and Marquis, 1987). Chemotherapy is given to prevent local progression of disease, dissemination of disease, and future chronic pulmonary tuberculosis. Without therapy, calcification of the caseous lesions is common. Occasionally, healing of the pulmonary segment is complicated by scarring or contraction that may be associated with cylindrical bronchiectasis and bronchial stenosis (Fig. 3). These complications are usually clinically silent when they occur in the upper lobes, and they are quite rare in children who have successfully completed chemotherapy.

Progressive Primary Pulmonary

A rare but serious complication of primary tuberculosis occurs when the primary focus enlarges steadily and develops a large caseous center. The radiograph shows bronchopneumonia or lobar pneumonia. Liquefaction may result in the formation of a thin-walled primary cavity associated with large numbers of tubercle bacilli. A tension cavity develops rarely as a result of a valvelike mechanism, allowing air to enter the cavity but not to escape. The enlarging focus may slough necrotic debris into an adjacent bronchus, leading to further intrapulmonary dissemination. Rupture into the pleural space can lead to bronchopleural fistula or pyopneumothorax.

Unlike with segmental lesions, significant symptoms and signs usually accompany locally progressive disease. High fever, night sweats, weight loss, and severe cough with sputum production are common. Physical signs include diminished breath sounds, rales, dullness, and egophony over the cavity. The clinical picture is similar to that of pyogenic pneumonia caused by *Staphylococcus aureus* or *Klebsiella pneumoniae*. Before the introduction of antituberculosis chemotherapy, prognosis was poor, with a fatality rate of 30–50%. However, with current therapy, the prognosis for complete recovery is excellent.

Chronic Pulmonary

Chronic pulmonary tuberculosis (''adult'' or ''reactivation'' type) represents endogenous reactivation of a site of tuberculous infection established previously. Even before the discovery of antituberculosis drugs, chronic pulmonary tuberculosis occurred in only 6–7% of pediatric patients (Lincoln et al., 1960). Children with a healed primary tuberculous infection acquired before age 2 years

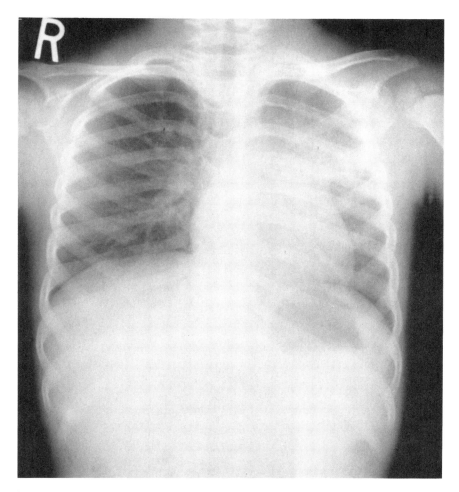

Figure 3 A chronic pulmonary tuberculosis lesion in the left upper lobe of a child who had respiratory symptoms for 8 months before diagnosis.

rarely develop chronic pulmonary disease; it is more common among those who acquire the initial infection after age 7 years, particularly if they become infected close to the onset of puberty (Holm, 1947). The most common pulmonary sites are the original parenchymal focus, the regional lymph nodes, or the apical seedings (Simon foci). This form of disease is identical to pulmonary disease in adults and usually remains localized to the lungs because the presensitization of the tissues to mycobacterial antigens evokes an immune response that prevents further lymphohematogenous spread.

Pericardial

The most common form of cardiac tuberculosis is pericarditis. It is relatively rare, occurring in between 0.4 and 4% of tuberculosis cases in children (Boyd 1953). Tuberculous pericarditis usually arises from direct invasion or lymphatic drainage from subcarinal lymph nodes. Early in the course, the pericardial fluid is serofibrinous or, occasionally, hemorrhagic. Continued fibrosis may lead to obliteration of the pericardial sac, with the development of constrictive pericarditis over months to years. The presenting symptoms are nonspecific, including low-grade fever, malaise, and weight loss. Chest pain is unusual in children with tuberculous pericarditis. As the infection progresses, a pericardial friction rub or distant heart sounds with pulsus paradoxicus may be present. Congestive heart failure is rare. An acid-fast smear of the pericardial fluid rarely reveals the organism, but cultures are positive in 30–70% of cases. Pericardial biopsy may be necessary to confirm the diagnosis. Partial or complete pericardiectomy may be required when constrictive pericarditis is present.

Pleural Effusion

Tuberculous pleural effusions originate in the discharge of bacilli into the pleural space from a subpleural primary pulmonary focus or from subpleural caseous lymph nodes (Smith and Matsaniotis, 1958). The discharge may be small and the pleuritis localized and asymptomatic, or a larger discharge may cause a generalized effusion, usually 3–6 months after infection. The effusion is usually unilateral, but can be bilateral as well (Lincoln et al., 1958a).

Clinically significant pleurisy with effusion occurs in 5–30% of tuberculosis cases in young adults, but is infrequent in children younger than 6 years of age and almost nonexistent in those below age 2 years. It is virtually never associated with a segmental pulmonary lesion and occurs rarely with miliary tuberculosis.

The onset of symptoms and signs is usually abrupt, with fever, chest pain, shortness of breath, dullness to percussion, and diminished breath sounds. Fever can be high and may last for several weeks, even when antituberculosis chemotherapy is given. Diagnosis can be difficult, as the acid-fast stain of the pleural fluid is usually negative, and the culture is positive in only 30–50% of cases. The prognosis of pleural effusion in children is excellent.

B. Lymphohematogenous

It is suspected that tubercle bacilli are disseminated to distant sites from the primary complex in all cases of tuberculous infection. The clinical picture produced by the lymphohematogenous dissemination depends on the quantity of organisms released and the host immune response. The occult dissemination usually produces no symptoms, but it is the event that causes extrapulmonary foci that can become the site of disease months to years after the initial infection. Rarely, children may experience a protracted hematogenous infection caused by the intermittent release of tubercle bacilli when a caseous focus erodes through the wall of a blood vessel. The clinical onset may be acute, with high spiking fevers, but more often, the course is indolent and prolonged. Multiple organ involvement is frequent; the most common findings are hepatosplenomegaly, deep and superficial adenitis, and crops of papulonecrotic tuberculids. Pulmonary findings are common early on, but meningitis is a late complication. Paradoxically, culture confirmation may be difficult and will often require a biopsy of deep tissue such as bone marrow or liver.

Miliary tuberculosis arises when massive numbers of tubercle bacilli are released into the blood stream, resulting in simultaneous disease in two or more organs. This usually is an early complication of the primary infection, occurring within 3–6 months after formation of the primary complex. The disease is most common in infants and young children (Hussey et al., 1991a).

The clinical manifestations of miliary tuberculosis are protean and depend on the numbers of disseminated organisms and the involved organs (Schuitt, 1979). Occasionally, the onset is explosive, the child becoming gravely ill in a matter of days. More often, the onset is insidious, with weight loss, anorexia, malaise, and low-grade fever developing over weeks. Within several weeks, hepatosplenomegaly and generalized lymphadenopathy develop in 50–70% of children. Initially, the chest radiograph may be normal or show evidence of only the primary complex. Within 3–4 weeks, the lung fields become filled with tubercles in over 90% of cases (Hussey et al., 1991a). The child may develop respiratory distress and diffuse rales or wheezing. Meningitis occurs in only 20–30% of cases. Cutaneous lesions are often absent, but the appearance of crops of papulonecrotic tuberculids or nodules may be an important diagnostic clue. Choroid tubercles appear several weeks after onset with variable frequency.

The diagnosis can be difficult, requiring a high index of suspicion by the clinician. Up to 30% of children have a negative tuberculin skin test, especially late in the course. A biopsy of liver or bone marrow may facilitate a more rapid diagnosis. In one recent review, the diagnosis could be confirmed by culture in only 33% of cases (Hussey et al., 1991a). With proper chemotherapy, the prognosis of miliary tuberculosis in children is excellent. However, resolution may be slow, with fever declining in 2–3 weeks, and chest radiograph abnormalities persisting for months.

C. Central Nervous System

Involvement of the central nervous system is the most serious complication of tuberculosis in children. Before the development of chemotherapy, tuberculous meningitis was uniformly fatal. The pathogenesis of central nervous system tuberculosis results from formation of a metastatic caseous lesion in the cerebral cortex or meninges during the occult lymphohematogenous dissemination of the primary infection (Rich and McCordock, 1933). This lesion—the so-called Rich focus—may increase in size and discharge tubercle bacilli into the subarachnoid space. A thick, gelatinous exudate infiltrates the cortical or meningeal blood vessels, producing inflammation, obstruction, or infarction. The brain stem usually is the site of greatest involvement, which accounts for the frequent dysfunction of cranial nerves III, VI, and VII. Eventually, the basilar cisterns become obstructed, leading to a communicating hydrocephalus—the four ventricles are open to the flow of cerebrospinal fluid (CSF), but flow to the spinal column is obstructed.

Tuberculous meningitis complicates about 1 of every 300 primary infections (Jaffe, 1982). This disease is almost unheard of in children younger than 4 months of age because it takes that long for the causative pathological sequence to develop. It is most common in children younger than 4 years of age and usually occurs within 3–6 months of the primary infection.

The clinical onset of tuberculous meningitis in children usually is gradual, but may be abrupt (Waecker and Connors, 1990). The more rapid progression of disease tends to occur in young infants, who may experience symptoms for only several days before the onset of acute hydrocephalus, brain infarct, or seizures (Idriss et al., 1976; Sumaya et al., 1975). More commonly, the onset is gradual over several weeks. The usual course can be divided into three stages. The first stage, which often lasts 1–2 weeks, is characterized by nonspecific symptoms such as fever, irritability, headache, sleepiness, and malaise. There are no focal neurological signs, but infants and young children may experience a loss or stagnation of developmental milestones. The second stage often begins abruptly, with lethargy, convulsions, nuchal rigidity, increased deep-tendon reflexes, hypertonia, vomiting, and cranial nerve palsies. The onset of this stage usually correlates with the development of hydrocephalus, increased intracranial pressure, and meningeal irritation. Some children lack signs of meningeal irritation, but show signs of encephalitis, such as disorientation, abnormal movements, and speech abnormalities (Udani et al., 1971). The third stage is marked by coma, irregular pulse or respiration, hemiplegia, or paraplegia, and eventually, death. Prognosis is directly related to the clinical stage at diagnosis (Ramachandran et al., 1986). The occurrence of the syndrome of inappropriate antidiuretic hormone secretion is common and is also linked to a poor prognosis (Cotton et al., 1991).

The most important clue to the diagnosis of tuberculous meningitis in a child is usually history of a recent contact with an adult with pulmonary tuberculosis. The tuberculin skin test result is negative in up to 40% of cases, and the chest radiograph is normal in up to 50% of cases (Zarabi et al., 1971). The CSF leukocyte cell count ranges from 10 to 500/mm^3; polymorphonuclear cells may be preponderant early, but a lymphocyte preponderance is more typical. The CSF glucose level is typically between 20 mg/dl and 40 mg/dl, whereas the CSF protein concentration is elevated and may be markedly high (>400 mg/dl). The success of microscopic examination of stained CSF and mycobacterial culture is related to the amount of CSF sampled. Computed tomography (CT) may help establish the diagnosis of tuberculous meningitis and can aid in evaluating the success of therapy.

Tuberculoma is manifested clinically as a brain tumor. As many of 30% of brain tumors in a population of children may be tuberculomas, depending on the incidence of tuberculosis in the population. Tuberculomas are most common in children younger than 10 years of age. Whereas most tuberculomas in adults are supratentorial, many in children are infratentorial, most often located at the base of the brain near the cerebellum. Headache, convulsions, fever, and other signs and symptoms of an intracranial space-occupying lesion are common.

D. Other Extrapulmonary Sites

In general, extrapulmonary tuberculosis is more common in children than adults (Reider et al., 1990). Up to 30% of children with tuberculosis will have extrapulmonary manifestations (Starke and Taylor-Watts, 1989b). A complete review of various types is beyond the scope of this chapter, but a few salient points can be emphasized.

The most common form of extrathoracic tuberculosis in children is infection of the superficial lymph nodes, sometimes called scrofula (Margileth et al., 1984). The nodes most commonly involved are in the tonsillar and submandibular regions. Early, the nodes are firm, nontender and discrete, most often unilateral, but can be bilateral. Other than low-grade fever, systemic signs and symptoms are usually absent (Appling and Miller, 1981). Although the nodes generally enlarge slowly, there may be rapid enlargement associated with high fever, tenderness, and fluctuance. If untreated, necrosis of the node usually occurs, accompanied by thinning and erythema of the skin and, eventually, rupture through the skin with formation of a sinus tract.

Skeletal tuberculosis in children is rare in technically advanced countries, but is still common in developing nations. It most commonly affects the vertebrae, resulting in a paravertebral abscess and spondylitis, but also can affect, in order of incidence, the knee, hip, elbow, and smaller joints. Tuberculous peritonitis occurs most often in adolescents and is similar clinically to disease in adults (Chavalittamvong and Talalak, 1982). Extrapulmonary tuberculosis in children affecting the eye, middle ear, kidneys, and skin is fairly rare.

E. Adolescents

Tuberculosis in adolescents falls into two major categories: tuberculosis acquired as an initial infection during adolescence, and tuberculosis acquired in early childhood that is exacerbated during adolescence (Smith 1967). Most commonly, recently infected adolescents develop a classic primary complex, with relatively few signs or symptoms (Nemir, 1986). Occasionally, the primary complex may progress rapidly to chronic pulmonary tuberculosis while the hilar lymph node involvement characteristic of primary tuberculosis is still present.

A primary tuberculous infection in infancy rarely leads to chronic tuberculosis in adolescence. A primary infection acquired between ages 7 and 10 years is more likely to result in reactivation during adolescence. When primary tuberculosis is acquired during adolescence, chronic pulmonary tuberculosis often develops within 1–3 years, a phenomenon that is two to six times more common in girls than in boys (Smith and Marquis, 1987). In both sexes, the adolescent growth spurt is the time of greatest risk. Because of this propensity to progress fairly rapidly to contagious pulmonary tuberculosis, high-risk adolescents are an important target group for tuberculin screening and case finding.

F. Perinatal

The clinical manifestations of tuberculosis in the fetus and newborn vary in relation to the site and size of the caseous lesions (Siegel, 1934). Symptoms may be present at birth, but more commonly begin by the second or third week of life (Cooper et al., 1985). The most common signs and symptoms are respiratory distress syndrome, fever, hepatic or splenic enlargement, poor feeding, lethargy or irritability, lymphadenopathy, abdominal distension, ear discharge, and skin lesions (Hageman et al., 1980; Nemir and O'Hare, 1985). Middle ear abnormalities are especially common when the source of infection is aspiration of infected amniotic fluid (Hertzog et al., 1940). Most neonates have an abnormal chest radiograph, with about 50% having a miliary pattern. Some infants with a normal chest radiograph early in the course will develop profound radiographic abnormalities as the disease progresses.

The clinical presentation of tuberculosis in the newborn can be similar to that caused by bacterial sepsis and other congenital infections, such as syphilis and cytomegalovirus. The major clue to diagnosis is the finding of tuberculosis in the mother, which often is not discovered until after the child becomes ill (Hageman et al., 1980). Diagnosis in the child is often difficult; 50% of cases are discovered at autopsy. The tuberculin skin test is essentially always initially negative. The diagnosis usually is established by finding acid-fast bacilli in gastric aspirates, urine, middle ear fluid, bone marrow aspirate, or a liver biopsy. Fewer than 50% of infected newborns develop meningitis, and the rate of isolation of *M. tuberculosis* from CSF is low.

Numerous studies have shown that infants born to a mother with tuberculosis can be protected from postnatal infection—even when they are not isolated from their mother—by giving them isoniazid (Kendig and Rodgers, 1958; Dormer et al., 1959; Kendig, 1960; Light et al., 1974). If chemotherapy cannot be given to the child, BCG vaccine can be effective if the infant is isolated from the infectious adult while the child develops immunity (Kendig, 1969).

V. Diagnostic Techniques

A. Tuberculin Skin Test

The principles of tuberculin skin testing for children are the same as those for adults (Seibert and Bass, 1990). A positive tuberculin skin test is the hallmark of the primary infection with *M. tuberculosis*. In children, the tuberculin reaction persists for many years, even after successful completion of therapy (Hardy, 1946; Hsu, 1983). However, young infants generally produce less induration in response to tuberculin than do older children and adults. A variety of factors common in children, such as malnutrition, viral infections (especially measles, varicella, and influenza) and, perhaps, administration of live virus vaccines, can lower tuberculin reactivity (American Thoracic Society, 1990). Approximately 10% of immunocompetent children with culture-documented tuberculosis do not initially react to tuberculin, although most become reactive after several months of therapy (Steiner et al., 1980; Starke and Taylor-Watts, 1989b). Parents should not be allowed to interpret their children's skin test results because of unreliable interpretation and reporting (Asnes and Maqbool, 1975; Kenney, 1988).

False-positive reactions to tuberculin in children are most often caused by exposure to environmental nontuberculous mycobacteria (NTM) or previous vaccination with BCG. Skin tests using NTM antigens have been studied recently (Del Beccaro et al., 1989), but standardized products are not currently available. The effect of BCG on the tuberculin test is variable, but is more pronounced in young, recently vaccinated children (Nemir and Teichner, 1983). It appears that the tuberculin reaction can be boosted by repetitive testing in previously vaccinated children (Sepulveda et al., 1988). However, most uninfected, BCG-vaccinated children have no reaction to tuberculin by 3–5 years after vaccination.

B. Smears and Culture

Unfortunately, direct smears and acid-fast stains of body secretions, fluids, and tissues from children with tuberculosis rarely lead to a rapid diagnosis of tuberculosis. The available techniques are too insensitive to detect the relatively small number of mycobacteria that are characteristically present with tuberculosis in children. Sputum is rarely available from children with pulmonary tuberculosis. Acid-fast stains of gastric contents may have a specificity greater than 90%, but the sensitivity is usually below 25% (Klotz and Penn, 1987).

Culture of various fluids and tissues for *M. tuberculosis* is not as helpful for diagnosing tuberculosis in children as it is for adults. Sputum is rarely available. The best available specimen is usually gastric fluid, but tubercle bacilli are isolated from older children in only 30–40% of cases (Lincoln et al., 1958b; Starke and Taylor-Watts, 1989b). For infants with extensive pulmonary disease, the organism may be isolated in up to 80% of cases. If gastric aspirates are obtained correctly, they are more likely to yield the organism than are bronchial washings (de Blic et al., 1991; Toppet et al., 1990; Laff et al., 1956). Aspiration should be performed early in the morning as the child awakens before the stomach empties itself of the overnight accumulation of secretions swallowed from the respiratory tract.

In practice, the difficulty of isolating *M. tuberculosis* from a child with tuberculous disease does not greatly influence the approach to therapy. If the epidemiological, tuberculin skin test, clinical, and radiographic information are compatible with the diagnosis, then the child should be treated for tuberculosis, even if the cultures are negative. If the adult source case culture and susceptibility results are available, they can be used to guide antituberculosis chemotherapy. However, it is important to attempt to isolate *M. tuberculosis* from the child if the diagnosis is in question, no source case information is available, the source case has drug-resistant *M. tuberculosis* infection, or if the child has suspected extrathoracic tuberculosis.

C. Serology and New Techniques

The serodiagnosis of tuberculosis has been envisioned since 1898, when the first agglutination test was developed. In the past 15 years, there have been numerous studies using both whole-cell and specific antigens in various antibody detection systems (Daniel and Debanne, 1987). For adults, most serological tests have a sensitivity and specificity approaching those of a sputum acid-fast smear. Several studies with varying results have used samples from children. One study of a small number of children with pulmonary tuberculosis in Argentina, using a specific mycobacterial antigen in an enzyme-linked immunosorbent assay (ELISA) system, found a sensitivity of 86% and specificity of 100% (Alde et al., 1989). One study of children with tuberculosis, using whole-cell *M. tuberculosis* as the antigen in an ELISA, found a sensitivity of 62% and specificity of 98% (Hussey et al., 1991b). However, a different study that used various whole mycobacterial sonicates had a sensitivity of 26% and specificity of 40% (Rosen, 1990). It is unlikely that serodiagnosis will make a substantial contribution to the diagnosis of pulmonary tuberculosis in children in the near future.

Several new techniques designed to detect the presence of mycobacteria, including using the polymerase chain reaction (PCR) to detect the DNA of *M. tuberculosis* (Brisson-Noel et al., 1989; Eisenach et al., 1991), or detecting the cell wall constituent mycolic acids (French et al., 1987; Brooks et al., 1990) are promising, but have not yet been applied to the diagnosis of pulmonary tuberculosis in children.

VI. Treatment (see also Chapter 11)

A. General Principles

The general principles that have governed the development of antituberculosis chemotherapy regimens in adults also apply to infants and children (Mitchison, 1985). However, there are several special considerations for children with tuberculosis, based on microbiology, natural history of the disease, and product availability (Starke, 1990). First, children usually develop tuberculous disease as an immediate complication of the primary infection. They typically have closed caseous lesions with relatively few mycobacteria (Dutt and Stead, 1982). The large bacterial populations found within cavities or infiltrates that are characteristic of adult pulmonary tuberculosis are absent in children. Since the likelihood of developing resistance to an antimycobacterial drug is proportional to the size of the bacillary population, children are generally less likely than adults to develop drug resistance while receiving therapy, even if compliance is poor. However, secondary drug resistance certainly can occur among children being treated for tuberculosis. When determining the best treatment regimen for a child, it is always safer to overestimate, rather than underestimate, the extent of disease.

Second, children have a higher propensity than adults to develop most extrapulmonary forms of tuberculosis, especially disseminated disease and meningitis. It is important that antituberculosis drugs for children penetrate a variety of tissues and fluids, especially across the meninges. Isoniazid, rifampin, and pyrazinamide cross both inflamed and uninflamed meninges adequately to kill virtually all strains of drug-susceptible *M. tuberculosis* (Donald and Seifart, 1988; Donald et al., 1992).

Third, the pharmacokinetics of antituberculosis drugs differ between children and adults (Reed and Blumer, 1983). In general, children tolerate larger doses per kilogram of body weight and have fewer adverse reactions than adults (Beaudry et al., 1974; Stein and Liang, 1979; O'Brien, et al., 1983). It is unclear whether the higher serum concentrations of drugs achieved in children have any therapeutic advantage (Olson et al., 1981). The lower rates of toxicity in children mean that fewer interruptions in treatment will occur. In general, children with more severe forms of tuberculosis, especially disseminated disease and meningitis, or those with malnutrition, experience more significant hepatotoxic effects than less severely ill children treated with the same doses per kilogram of isoniazid and rifampin, especially if the isoniazid dose exceeds 10 mg/kg per day (Tsagarpoulou-Stinga et al., 1985; Donald et al., 1987). However, many hepatotoxic "reactions" in children taking antituberculosis medications are actually caused by intercurrent infections with hepatitis A and B, or other viruses (Kumar et al., 1991).

Finally, an important difference between children and adults concerns how the medications are administered. Most available dosage forms are designed for use in adults. Giving these preparations to children often involves crushing pills or making up suspensions that are neither standardized nor well studied. Some dosages forms may lead to inadequate absorption of oral medications (Notterman, 1986). Many children experience difficulty taking the several antituberculosis medications required, especially at the beginning of therapy. If these problems are not anticipated and worked out, they may cause significant delays and interruptions of therapy. Currently, fixed-dose combination preparations are not available for children (Acocella, 1990). Technical problems may be difficult; one recent study has demonstrated a marked decline in rifampin concentration over time in suspensions also containing isoniazid or pyrazinamide (Seifart et al., 1991).

B. Antituberculosis Drugs for Children (Table 3)

Isoniazid is familiar to most pediatricians, as it is effective and well tolerated by children. Although it is metabolized by acetylation in the liver, there is no correlation in children between acetylation rate and either efficacy or adverse reactions (Martinez-Roig et al., 1986). The doses of isoniazid in regular use are high enough that drug concentrations are sufficient even in children who acetylate the drug very rapidly. The two major toxic effects of isoniazid in adults are rare in children. Pyridoxine levels are decreased in children taking isoniazid, but peripheral neuritis is exceedingly rare (Pellock et al., 1985). However, in certain children—teenagers with inadequate diets, children from ethnic groups with low milk or meat intake, and breastfeeding babies (who can get pyridoxine-deficiency seizures)—pyridoxine supplementation is recommended (McKenzie et al., 1976; American Academy of Pediatrics, 1992). Hepatotoxicity in children taking isoniazid also is rare. Of children taking isoniazid, 3–10% have transiently elevated liver transaminase levels, but clinically significant hepatitis is exceedingly rare (O'Brien et al., 1973). Adolescents are more likely than younger children to experience hepatotoxicity (Litt et al., 1976). For most children, toxicity can be monitored using only clinical signs and symptoms; routine biochemical monitoring is unnecessary.

Rifampin is well tolerated by children. Hepatotoxicity in children is infrequent, and other adverse reactions, such as leukopenia, thrombocytopenia, and the flulike syndrome, are very rare. Pyrazinamide has been used extensively in children over the past decade. Formal pharmacokinetic studies of pyrazinamide in children have not been reported. A dose of 30–40 mg/kg daily results in adequate CSF levels, is well tolerated, produces little toxicity, and appears to be effective (Donald and Seifart, 1988). Hepatitis and complications of hyperuricemia are exceedingly rare in children. Streptomycin is used less frequently than in the past, but is well tolerated by children. Although safe in infants, it cannot be given to pregnant women because it causes damage to the eighth cranial nerve of the fetus (Snider et al., 1980).

Table 3 Antituberculosis Drugs in Children

Drugs	Dosage forms	Daily dose (mg/kg)	Twice-weekly dose (mg/kg/per dose)	Maximum dose
Isoniazid[a]	Scored tablets: 100 mg 300 mg Syrup: 10mg/ml[b]	10–15	20–40	Daily: 300 mg Twice-weekly: 900 mg
Rifampin[a]	Capsules: 150 mg 300 mg Syrup: formulated in syrup from capsules[c]	10–20	10–20	600 mg
Pyrazinamide	Scored tablets: 500 mg	20–40	50–70	2 gr
Streptomycin	Vials: 1 gr, 4 gr	20–40 (im)	20–40 (im)	1 gr
Ethambutol	Scored tablets: 100 mg 400 mg	15–25	50	2.5 gr
Ethionamide	Tablets: 250 mg	10–20		1 gr
Kanamycin	Vials: 1 gr	15 (im)	15–25 (im)	1 gr
Cycloserine	Capsules: 250 mg	10–20		1 gr

[a]Rifamate is a capsule containing 150 mg of isoniazid and 300 mg of rifampin. Two capsules provide the usual adult (more than 50 kg) daily dose of each drug.
[b]Many experts recommend not using isoniazid syrup, as it is unstable and is associated with frequent gastrointestinal complaints, especially diarrhea.
[c]Marion Merrell Dow issues directions for preparation of this "extemporaneous" syrup.

There is much less experience with the other antituberculosis drugs in children. Ethambutol has not been used widely because of its potential toxicity to the eye and the relatively difficulty monitoring ophthalmological signs and symptoms in young children. However, there is no published evidence of optic toxicity in children, and there is no damage to the fetus when the pregnant woman takes ethambutol (Snider et al., 1980). Ethambutol is not recommended for general use in children, but should be considered strongly for children with suspected drug-resistant tuberculosis. Ethionamide is well tolerated by children, who experience much less gastrointestinal distress than adults. Several aminoglycosides, including capreomycin, kanamycin, and amikacin, have antituberculosis activity and are well tolerated by children.

C. Specific Regimens

Drug-Susceptible Disease

Pulmonary

During the past decade, many treatment trials for tuberculosis in children have been reported. Abernathy et al. (1983) reported successful treatment of 50 children with tuberculosis using isoniazid and rifampin daily for 1 month, then twice weekly for 8 months, a total duration of 9 months. Some patients with only hilar adenopathy were successfully treated with isoniazid and rifampin given for 6 months (Jacobs and Abernathy, 1985). A study from Brazil reported successful treatment of 117 children with pulmonary tuberculosis using isoniazid and rifampin daily for 6 months (Reis et al., 1990). Although these results were impressive, this 6-month regimen for pulmonary tuberculosis in children has not been adopted widely because of limited data and the growing problem of isoniazid or rifampin resistance in many areas of the world. The Brazilian study also demonstrated the difficult problem of noncompliance; even with this fairly simple regimen, 17% of children did not complete treatment.

There have been several studies of 6-month duration of antituberculosis therapy using at least three drugs initially for drug-susceptible tuberculosis in children, presented both in abstracts (Anane et al., 1984; Pelosi et al., 1985; Starke and Taylor-Watts, 1989a; Khubchandani et al., 1990) and articles (Ibanez and Ross, 1980; Varudkar, 1985; Biddulph, 1990; Kumar et al., 1990). Although the regimens used in these trials differed slightly, the most common was a 6-month regimen of isoniazid and rifampin, supplemented during the first 2 months with pyrazinamide. The success of these regimens was the same whether or not streptomycin was also given. Most trials used daily therapy for the first 1–2 months, followed by daily or twice-weekly therapy for the last 4 months. Regimens using twice-weekly therapy under the direct observation of a health care worker were as safe and effective as those using daily therapy. In all trials, the overall success rate was greater than 95% for complete clinical and radiographic cure, and 99% for significant improvement during a 2-year follow-up. The incidence of clinically significant adverse drug reactions—usually gastrointestinal upset or mild skin rash—was less than 2%.

As a result of these clinical trials involving over 1000 children with tuberculosis, the American Academy of Pediatrics (1992) and International Union Against Tuberculosis and Lung Disease (1991) suggest that standard therapy for drug-susceptible intrathoracic tuberculosis in children should be 6 months of isoniazid and rifampin, supplemented during the first 2 months with pyrazinamide. Although daily administration of medications during the first 2 months is preferable, two studies showed that 6 months of twice- or thrice-weekly medications yielded results equivalent to regimens using an initial phase of daily administration (Varudkar, 1985; Kumar et al., 1990). Although a 9-month regimen of isoniazid and rifampin is effective in locales where drug resistance rates are low, the tendency of patients to become more noncompliant as the treatment duration is lengthened makes this regimen less desirable.

Extrapulmonary

Controlled clinical trials comparing treatment regimens for various forms of extrapulmonary tuberculosis are virtually nonexistent. Several 6-month, three-drug regimen trials in children have included cases of lymph node and disseminated tuberculosis; both responded favorably (Anane et al., 1984; Biddulph, 1990; Kumar et al., 1990; Jawahar et al., 1990). Most of the data come from series of extrapulmonary tuberculosis in adults. In general, the 6-month regimen using isoniazid, rifampin, and pyrazinamide initially is recommended for most forms of extrapulmonary tuberculosis. One exception may be bone and joint tuberculosis, which may require a treatment duration of 9–12 months, especially if surgical intervention has not been undertaken (Dutt et al., 1986).

For tuberculous meningitis, treatment with isoniazid and rifampin for 12 months is generally effective (Visudhiphan and Chiemchanya, 1989). A recent study from Thailand showed that both survival and morbidity are improved significantly if pyrazinamide is added to the initial 2 months of treatment, even if the total treatment duration is shortened to 6 months (Jacobs et al., 1992). At least three and usually four drugs should be given initially to guard against unrecognized drug resistance. If the response to therapy is good at the end of 2 months, isoniazid and rifampin alone can be continued to the end of therapy. The duration of therapy should be at least 6 months, but many experts think treatment should be given for 9 to 12 months (IUATLD, 1991).

Human Immunodeficiency Virus-Related

The optimal treatment of tuberculosis in children with HIV infection has not been established. It may be difficult to determine if a pulmonary infiltrate in an HIV-infected child, who has a positive tuberculin skin test or known exposure to an adult with infectious tuberculosis, is due to *M. tuberculosis*. Treatment often must be empiric, based on radiographic and epidemiological information, and should be considered when tuberculosis cannot reasonably be excluded. Most experts think HIV-seropositive children with drug-susceptible tuberculosis should receive the same regimen as HIV-infected adults with tuberculosis: isoniazid, rifampin, and pyrazinamide for 2 months, followed by isoniazid and rifampin to complete a total duration of 9–12 months (Barnes et al., 1991). Preventive therapy for HIV-infected children with drug-susceptible tuberculous infection without disease should be 12 months of isoniazid; rifampin for 12 months is used when the organism is resistant to isoniazid.

Infection Without Disease

The treatment of children with asymptomatic tuberculous infection to prevent the development of tuberculous disease is an established practice. In infected children, the effectiveness of isoniazid preventive therapy has approached 100%, and the effect has lasted for at least 30 years (Hsu, 1984). Tuberculin-positive children with known contact to an infectious adult case are at highest risk of developing disease, and always should be given preventive therapy. Almost all tuberculin-positive children without known contact also should receive therapy, especially adolescents and those younger than 6 years of age. Many BCG-vaccinated children who have contact with an infectious adult also should receive preventive chemotherapy depending on their age and the closeness of the contact (IUATLD, 1991). Children who are tuberculin-negative, including newborn infants, who have contact with an infectious adult should receive isoniazid therapy until 10–12 weeks after contact has been broken by physical separation or chemotherapy. If a repeat tuberculin test at that time is negative, isoniazid can be stopped; if the test is positive, a full course of isoniazid preventive therapy should be given. Rifampin is recommended for preventive therapy for children with asymptomatic infection with isoniazid-resistant *M. tuberculosis*. Although controlled trials are lacking, either isoniazid or rifampin probably will be effective if given twice weekly under direct supervision when compliance with daily therapy cannot be assured. There is no available information concerning the effectiveness of any preventive therapy regimen in children infected with isoniazid- and rifampin-resistant strains of *M. tuberculosis*.

D. Drug Resistance

Patterns of primary drug resistance among children with tuberculosis tend to mirror those found among adults in the same population (Steiner et al., 1983; Steiner et al., 1985). Certain epidemiological factors, such as residence in a country with high rates of drug resistance and history of prior antituberculosis therapy, correlate with drug resistance in adults and their contacts. The development of drug resistance while taking antituberculosis drugs is rare in children, but can occur, especially if the disease is extensive.

The principles of treatment for drug-resistant tuberculosis are the same for children as they are for adults, although few published data are available. When a child has possible isoniazid-resistant tuberculosis, at least three and usually four or five drugs should be given initially until the susceptibility pattern is determined and a more specific regimen can be designed. When isoniazid or rifampin resistance is present, the total duration of therapy is usually extended to 12–18 months.

E. Corticosteroids

Corticosteroids are beneficial in the management of tuberculosis in children when the host inflammatory reaction is contributing significantly to tissue damage or impairment of function. There is convincing evidence that corticosteroids decrease mortality and long-term neurological sequelae in children with tuberculous meningitis by reducing vasculitis, inflammation, and intracranial pressure (Girgis et al., 1991). Children with enlarged hilar, mediastinal, or subcarinal lymph nodes that compromise the tracheobronchial tree—causing respiratory distress, localized emphysema, or segmental lesions—frequently benefit from corticosteroid therapy (Nemir et al., 1967; Toppet et al., 1990). Corticosteroids may also be useful in selected children with miliary disease and alveolar–capillary block, massive pleural effusion, and pericardial effusion. There is no convincing evidence that one form of corticosteroid is more beneficial than the others. Most commonly used are dexamethasone or prednisone for 4–6 weeks.

F. Following the Child on Therapy

Noncompliance with drug therapy is a major problem in tuberculosis control because of the long-term nature of treatment (Sbarbaro, 1979; Anderson and Kirk, 1982). Many children with tuberculosis have few or no symptoms and do not benefit from the dramatic clinical improvement often seen in adults. If the physician suspects any chance of noncompliance with medication administration daily by the family, directly observed therapy given with the aid of the local health authority should be instituted, if possible.

Children taking antituberculosis drugs should be seen frequently to monitor compliance, possible toxic effects of the medications, and success of the treatment. Anticipatory guidance for the family, especially concerning the proper administration of medications, is crucial. The rates of adverse reactions to antituberculosis therapy in children are low enough that routine biochemical monitoring is unnecessary. When blood chemistries are performed, serum liver enzyme elevations of two to four times normal occur rarely and do not necessitate discontinuation of treatment if all other findings are normal.

Radiographic improvement of intrathoracic tuberculosis in children occurs very slowly, and frequent monitoring with chest radiographs is not usually necessary. It often takes 2–3 years for hilar adenopathy to resolve, long after therapy has been discontinued. A normal chest radiograph is not a necessary criterion for stopping therapy; if significant improvement has occurred during treatment, the medications can be discontinued and periodic chest radiographs performed to monitor resolution.

VII. Summary

Tuberculosis continues to occur in children at alarming rates both in developing countries and in the United States. In theory, all cases of childhood tuberculosis could be prevented if tuberculosis in adults could be controlled. In the United States, a sizeable proportion of childhood tuberculosis cases could be prevented if basic principles of tuberculosis control were adhered to more completely (Nolan, 1986; Starke and Taylor-Watts, 1990). Despite the availability of curative therapy for disease and preventive therapy for infection, tuberculosis persists among children. Even in technically advanced nations, the elimination of tuberculosis in children will require an effective vaccine or a greatly shortened length of effective therapy.

References

Abernathy, R. S., Dutt, A. K., Stead, W. W., and Doers, D. L. (1983). Short-course chemotherapy for tuberculosis in children. *Pediatrics* **72**:801–806.

Acocella, G. (1990). The use of fixed-dose combinations in antituberculous chemotherapy. Rationale for their application in daily, intermittent and pediatric regimens. *Bull. Int. Union Tuberc. Lung Dis.* **65**:77–83.

Alde, S. L. M., Pinasco, H. M., Pelosi, F. R., Budani, H. F., Palma-Beltran, O. H., and Gonzalez-Montaner, L. J. (1989). Evaluation of an enzyme-linked immunosorbent assay using an IgG antibody to *Mycobacterium tuberculosis* antigens in the diagnosis of active tuberculosis in children. *Am. Rev. Respir. Dis.* **139**:748–751.

American Thoracic Society (1990). Diagnostic standards and classification of tuberculosis. *Am. Rev. Respir. Dis.* **142**:725–735.

American Academy of Pediatrics Committee on Infectious Diseases (1992). Chemotherapy for tuberculosis in infants and children. *Pediatrics* **89**:161–165.

Anane, T., Cernay, J., and Bensenovci, A. (1984). Resultats compares des regimens et des regimens long dans la chimiotherapie de la tuberculose de l'enfant en Algerie. Presentation at the African Regional Meeting of the International Union Against Tuberculosis, Tunis, Tunisia, October 1984.

Anderson, R. J., and Kirk, L. M. (1982). Methods of improving patient compliance in chronic disease states. *Arch. Intern. Med.* **142**:1673–1675.

Appling, D., and Miller, R. H. (1981). Mycobacterial cervical lymphadenopathy: 1981 update. *Laryngoscope* **91**:1259–1266.

Asnes, R. S., and Maqbool, S. (1975). Parent reading and reporting of children's tuberculin skin test results. *Chest* **68** (Suppl):459–462.

Barnes, P. F., Bloch, A. B., Davidson, P. T., and Snider, D. E., Jr. (1991). Tuberculosis in patients with human immunodeficiency virus infection. *N. Engl. J. Med.* **324**:1644–1650.

Barry, M. A., Shirley, L., Grady, M. T., Etkind, S. W., Almeida, C., Bernardo, J., and Lamb, G. A. (1990). Tuberculosis infection in urban adolescents: Results of a school-based testing program. *Am. J. Public Health* **80**:439–441.

Beaudry, P. H., Brickman, H. F., Wise, M. B., and MacDougall, D. (1974). Liver enzyme disturbances during isoniazid chemoprophylaxis in children. *Am. Rev. Respir. Dis.* **110**:581–584.

Beitzke, H. (1935). Ueber die angeborene tuberkoloese infektion. *Ergeb. Gesamten Tuberkuloseforsch* **7**:1–20.

Biddulph, J. (1990). Short-course chemotherapy for childhood tuberculosis. *Pediatr. Infect. Dis. J.* **9**:794–801.

Bloch, A. B., Reider, H. L., Kelly, G. D., Cauthen, G. M., Hayden, C. H., and Snider, D. E., Jr. (1989). The epidemiology of tuberculosis in the United States. *Clin. Chest Med.* **10**:297–313.

Boyd, G. L. (1953). Tuberculous pericarditis in children. *Am. J. Dis. Child.* **86**:293–300.

Braun, M., Badi, N., Ryder, R., Baende, E., Mukadi, Y., Nsuami, M., Matela, B., Williams, J. C., Kaboto, M., and Heyward, W. (1991). A retrospective cohort study of the risk of tuberculosis among women of childbearing age with HIV infection in Zaire. *Am. Rev. Respir. Dis.* **143**:501–504.

Braun, M. M., and Cauthen, G. (1992). Relationship of the human immunodeficiency virus epidemic to pediatric tuberculosis and bacillus Calmette-Guerin immunization. *Pediatr. Infect. Dis. J.* **11**:220–227.

Brisson-Noel, A., Gicquel, B., Lecossier, D., Levy-Frebault, V., Nassif, X., and Hance, A. J. (1989). Rapid diagnosis of tuberculosis by amplification of mycobacterium DNA in clinical samples. *Lancet* **2**:1069–1071.

Brooks, J. B., Daneshran, M. I., Haberberger, R. L., and Mikhail, I. A. (1990). Rapid diagnosis of tuberculous meningitis by frequency-pulsed electron-capture gas-liquid chromatography detection of carboxylic acids in cerebrospinal fluid. *J. Clin. Microbiol.* **28**:989–997.

Centers for Disease Control (1991). CDC surveillance summaries. Tuberculosis morbidity in the United States: Final data, 1990. *MMWR* **40** (SS-3):23–28.

Chaisson, R. E., and Slutkin, G. (1989). Tuberculosis and human immunodeficiency virus infection. *J. Infect. Dis.* **159**:96–100.

Chavalittamvong, B., and Talalak, P. (1982). Tuberculous peritonitis in children. *Prog. Pediatr. Surg.* **15**:161–167.

Cooper, A. R., Heneghan, W., and Matthew, J. D. (1985). Tuberculosis in a mother and her infant. *Pediatr. Infect. Dis. J.* **4**:181–183.

Cotton, M. F., Donald, P. R., Schoeman, J. F., Aalbers, C., VanZyl, L. E., and Lombard, C. (1991). Plasma arginine vasopressin and the syndrome of inappropriate antidiuretic hormone secretion in tuberculous meningitis. *Pediatr. Infect. Dis. J.* **10**:837–842.

Daly, J. F., Brown, D. S., Lincoln, E. M., and Wilkins, V. N. (1952). Endobronchial tuberculosis in children. *Dis. Chest* **22**:380–398.

Daniel, T. M., and Debanne, S. M. (1987). The serodiagnosis of tuberculosis and other mycobacterial diseases by enzyme-linked immunosorbent assay. *Am. Rev. Respir. Dis.* **135**:1137–1151.

Davidson, P. T., Ashkar, B., and Salem, N. (1990). Tuberculosis testing of children entering school in Los Angeles County, California [Abstract]. *Am. Rev. Respir. Dis.* **141** (Suppl):A336.

de Blic, J., Azevedo, I., Burren, C. P., Le Burgeois, M., Lallemand, D., and Scheinmann, P. (1991). The value of flexible bronchoscopy in childhood pulmonary tuberculosis. *Chest* **100**:688–692.

Del Beccaro, M. A., Mendelman, P. A., and Nolan, C. M. (1989). Diagnostic usefulness of mycobacterial skin test antigens in childhood lymphadenitis. *Pediatr. Infect. Dis. J.* **8**:206–210.

DePaula, M. D. N., Janini, M., and Quieroz, W. (1989). Pulmonary infectious complications in pediatric AIDS patients [Abstract T.B.P. 199]. In *Fifth International Conference on AIDS*, Montreal, 1989. International Development Research Center, Ottawa, Canada, p. 320.

Donald, P. R., Schoeman, J. F., and O'Kennedy, A. (1987). Hepatic toxicity during chemotherapy for severe tuberculous meningitis. *Am. J. Dis. Child.* **141**:741–743.

Donald, P. R., and Seifart, H. (1988). Cerebrospinal fluid pyrazinamide concentrations in children with tuberculous meningitis. *Pediatr. Infect. Dis. J.* **7**:469–471.

Donald, P. R., Gent, W. L., Seifart, H. I., Lamprecht, J. H., and Parkin, D. P. (1992). Cerebrospinal fluid isoniazid concentrations in children with tuberculous meningitis: The influence of dosage and acetylation status. *Pediatrics* **89**:247–250.

Dormer, B. A., Swarit, J. A., and Harrison, I. (1959). Prophylactic isoniazid protection of infants in a tuberculosis hospital. *Lancet* **2**:902–904.

Dutt, A. K., and Stead, W. W. (1982). Present chemotherapy for tuberculosis. *J. Infect. Dis.* **146**:698–704.

Dutt, A. K., Moers, D., and Stead, W. W. (1986). Short-course chemotherapy for extrapulmonary tuberculosis. *Ann. Intern. Med.* **107**:7–12.

Edwards, P. Q. (1974). Tuberculin testing of children. *Pediatrics* **54**:628–630.

Eisenach, K. D., Sifford, M. D., Cave, M. D., Bates, J. H., and Crawford, J. T. (1991). Detection of *Mycobacterium tuberculosis* in sputum samples using a polymerase chain reaction. *Am. Rev. Respir. Dis.* **144**: 1160–1163.

French, G. L., Chan, C. Y., Cheung, S. W., and Oo, K. T. (1987). Diagnosis of pulmonary tuberculosis by detection of tuberculostearic acid in sputum by using gas chromatography–liquid chromatography detection of carboxylic acids in cerebrospinal fluid. *J. Infect. Dis.* **156**:356–362.

Giammona, S. T., Poole, C. A., Zelowitz, P., and Skrovan, C. (1969). Massive lymphadenopathy in primary pulmonary tuberculosis in children. *Am. Rev. Respir. Dis.* **100**:480–489.

Girgis, N. I., Farid, Z., Kilpatrick, M. E., Sultan, Y., and Mikhail, I. A. (1991). Dexamethasone adjunctive treatment for tuberculous meningitis. *Pediatr. Infect. Dis. J.* **10**:179–183.

Grenville-Mathers, R., Harris, W. C., and Trenchard, H. J. (1960). Tuberculous primary infection in pregnancy and its relation to congenital tuberculosis. *Tubercle* **41**:81–87.

Hageman, J., Shulman, S., Schreiben, M., Luck, S., and Yogev, R. (1980). Congenital tuberculosis: Critical reappraisal of clinical findings and diagnostic procedures. *Pediatrics* **66**:980–985.

Hallum, J. L., and Thomas, H. E. (1955). Full term pregnancy after proved endometrial tuberculosis. *J. Obstet. Gynaecol. Br. Emp.* **62**:548–551.

Hardy, J. B. (1946). Persistence of hypersensitivity to old tuberculin following primary tuberculosis in childhood: A long term study. *Am. J. Public Health* **36**:1417–1426.

Hertzog, A. J., Chapman, S., and Herring, J. (1940). Congenital pulmonary aspiration tuberculosis. *Am. J. Clin. Pathol.* **19**:1139–1141.

Holm, S. (1947). *Om der Friske Tuberculose Infection den Klink, Prognose og Behandlung*. Rosenkilde, Copenhagen.

Hsu, K. H. K. (1983). Tuberculin reaction in children treated with isoniazid. *Am. J. Dis. Child.* **137**:1090–1092.

Hsu, K. H. K. (1984). Thirty years after isoniazid. Its impact on tuberculosis in children and adolescents. *JAMA* **251**:1283–1285.

Hughesdon, M. R. (1946). Congenital tuberculosis. *Arch. Dis. Child.* **21**:121–126.

Hussey, G., Chisholm, T., and Kibel, M. (1991a). Miliary tuberculosis in children: A review of 94 cases. *Pediatr. Infect. Dis. J.* **10**:832–836.

Hussey, G., Kibel, M., and Dempster, W. (1991b). The serodiagnosis of tuberculosis in children: An evaluation of an ELISA test using IgG antibodies to *M. tuberculosis*, strain H37RV. *Ann. Trop. Pediatr.* **11**:113–118.

Ibanez, S., and Ross, G. (1980). Quimioterapia abreviada de 6 meses en tuberculosis pulmonar infantil. *Rev. Chil. Pediatr.* **51**:249–252.

Idriss, Z. H., Sinno, A., and Kronfol, N. M. (1976). Tuberculous meningitis in childhood: forty-three cases. *Am. J. Dis. Child.* **130**:364–367.

International Union Against Tuberculosis and Lung Disease (1991). Tuberculosis in children. Guidelines for diagnosis, prevention and treatment. *Bull. Int. Union Tuberc. Lung Dis.* **66**:61–67.

Jacobs, R. F., and Abernathy, R. S. (1985). The treatment of tuberculosis in children. *Pediatr. Infect. Dis. J.* **4**:513–517.

Jacobs, R. F., and Abernathy, R. S. (1988). Management of tuberculosis in pregnancy and the newborn. *Clin. Perinatol.* **15**:305–319.

Jacobs, R. F., Sunakorn, P., Chotpitayasunonah, T., Pope, S., and Kelleher, K. (1992). Intensive short course chemotherapy for tuberculous meningitis. *Pediatr. Infect. Dis. J.* **11**:194–198.

Jaffe, I. P. (1982). Tuberculous meningitis in childhood. *Lancet* **1**:738.

Jawahar, M. S., Sivasubramanian, S., Vijayan, V. K., Ramakrishnan, C. V., Paramasivan, C. N., Selvakumar, V., Paul, S., Tripathy, S. P., and Prabhakar, R. (1990). Short-course chemotherapy for tuberculous lymphadenitis in children. *Br. Med. J.* **301**:359–361.

Kaplan, C., Benirschke, K., and Tarzy, B. (1980). Placental tuberculosis in early and late pregnancy. *Am. J. Obstet. Gynecol.* **137**:858–861.

Kendig, E. L., and Rodgers, W. L. (1958). Tuberculosis in the neonatal period. *Am. Rev. Tuberc.* **77**:418–424.

Kendig, E. L., Jr. (1960). Prognosis of infants born to tuberculous mothers. *Pediatrics* **26**:97–100.

Kendig, E. L., Jr. (1969). The place of BCG vaccine in the management of infants born of tuberculous mothers. *N. Engl. J. Med.* **250**:1969–1972.

Kenney, R. D. (1988). Improving reporting of tuberculin test results in a community hospital pediatric clinic. *J. Pediatr.* **112**:427–429.

Khubchandani, R. P., Kumta, N. B., Bharucha, N. B., and Ramakantan, R. (1990). Short-course chemotherapy in childhood pulmonary tuberculosis [Abstract]. *Am. Rev. Respir. Dis.* **141** (Suppl.):A338.

Klein, N. C., Duncanson, F. P., Lenox, T. H., Pitta, A., Cohen, S. C., and Wormser, G. P. (1989). Use of mycobacterial smears in the diagnosis of pulmonary tuberculosis in AIDS/ARC patients. *Chest* **95**:1190–1192.

Klotz, S. A., and Penn, R. L. (1987). Acid-fast staining of urine and gastric contents is an excellent indicator of mycobacterial disease. *Am. Rev. Respir. Dis.* **136**:1197–1198.

Kochi, A. (1991). The global tuberculosis situation and the new control strategy of the World Health Organization. *Tubercle* **72**:1–6.

Kumar, A., Misra, P. K., Mehotra, R., Gouil, Y. C., and Rana, G. S. (1991). Hepatotoxicity of rifampin and isoniazid. Is it all drug-induced hepatitis? *Am. Rev. Respir. Dis.* **143**:1350–1352.

Kumar, L., Dhand, R., Singhi, P. D., Rao, K. L. N., and Katariya, S. (1990). A randomized trial of fully intermittent and daily followed by intermittent short-course chemotherapy for childhood tuberculosis. *Pediatr. Infect. Dis. J.* **9**:802–806.

Laff, H. I., Golberg, M., and Russell, W. F., Jr. (1956). Bronchoscopy in primary tuberculosis of childhood. *Am. Rev. Tuberc.* **74**:267–289.

Leggiadro, R. J., Callory, B., Dowdy, S., and Larkin, J. (1989). An outbreak of tuberculosis in a family day care home. *Pediatr. Infect. Dis. J.* **8**:52–54.

Light, I. J., Saidleman, M., and Sutherland, J. M. (1974). Management of newborns after nursery exposure to tuberculosis. *Am. Rev. Respir. Dis.* **109**:415–418.

Lincoln, E. M. (1965). Epidemics of tuberculosis. *Adv. Tuberc. Res.* **14**:157–201.

Lincoln, E. M., Harris, L. C., Bovornkitti, S., and Carretero, R. (1956). The course and prognosis of endobronchial tuberculosis in children. *Am. Rev. Tuberc.* **74**:246–256.

Lincoln, E. M., Davies, P. A., and Bovornkitti, S. (1958a). Tuberculous pleurisy with effusion in children. A study of 202 children with particular reference to prognosis. *Am. Rev. Tuberc.* **77**:271–289.

Lincoln, E. M., Harris, L. C., Bovornkitti, S., and Carretero, R. W. (1958b). Endobronchial tuberculosis in children. A study of 156 patients. *Am. Rev. Tuberc.* **77**:39–61.

Lincoln, E. M., Gilbert, L., and Morales, S. M. (1960). Chronic pulmonary tuberculosis in individuals with known previous primary tuberculosis. *Dis. Chest* **38**:473–482.

Litt, I. F., Cohen, M. I., and McNamara, H. (1976). Isoniazid hepatitis in adolescents. *J. Pediatr.* **89**:133–135.

Lorriman, G., and Bentley, F. J. (1959). The incidence of segmental lesions in primary tuberculosis in childhood. *Am. Rev. Tuberc.* **79**:756–763.

Malek, A. N. A., Mukelabai, K., and Luo, N. P. (1989). Pulmonary tuberculosis and HIV disease in infants and children [Abstract M.B.P. 372]. In *Fifth International Conference on AIDS*. Montreal, 1989. International Development Research Center, Ottawa, Canada, p. 284.

Margileth, A. M., Chandra, R., and Altman, R. P. (1984). Chronic lymphadenopathy due to mycobacterial infection. Clinical features, diagnosis, histopathology and management. *Am. J. Dis. Child.* **138**:917–922.

Martinez-Roig, A., Roig, A., Cami, J., Llorens-Terol, J., de la Torre, R., and Perich, F. (1986). Acetylation phenotype and hepatotoxicity in the treatment of tuberculosis in children. *Pediatrics* **77**:912–915.

Matsaniotis, N., Kattamis, C., Economou-Maurou, C., and Kyriazakov, M. (1967). Bullous emphysema in childhood tuberculosis. *J. Pediatr.* **71**:703–707.

McKenzie, S. A., Macnab, A. J., and Katz, G. (1976). Neonatal pyridoxine responsive convulsions due to isoniazid therapy. *Arch. Dis. Child.* **51**:567–569.

Miller, F. J. W., Seale, R. M. E., and Taylor, M. D. (1963). *Tuberculosis in Children*. Little Brown & Co., Boston.

Mitchison, D. A. (1985). The action of anti-tuberculous drugs in short-course chemotherapy. *Tubercle* **66**:219–225.

Morrison, J. B. (1973). Natural history of segmental lesions in primary pulmonary tuberculosis. *Arch. Dis. Child.* **48**:90–98.

Moss, W. J., Dodyo, T., Suarez, M., Nicholas, S. W., and Abrams, E. (1992). Tuberculosis in children infected with human immunodeficiency virus: A report of five cases. *Pediatr. Infect. Dis. J.* **10**:114–116.

Murray, C. J. L., Styblo, K., and Rouillon, A. (1990). Tuberculosis in developing countries: Burden, intervention, and cost. *Bull. Int. Union Tuberc. Lung Dis.* **65**:6–24.

Nemir, R. L. (1986). Perspectives in adolescent tuberculosis: Three decades of experience. *Pediatrics* **78**:399–405.

Nemir, R. L., and O'Hare, D. (1985). Congenital tuberculosis: Review and diagnostic guidelines. *Am. J. Dis. Child.* **139**:284–287.

Nemir, R. L., and Teichner, A. (1983). Management of tuberculin reactions in children and adolescents previously vaccinated with BCG. *Pediatr. Infect. Dis.* **2**:446–451.

Nemir, R. L., Cordova, J., Vaziri, F., and Toledo, F. (1967). Prednisone as an adjunct in the chemotherapy of lymph node–bronchial tuberculosis in childhood: A double-blinded study. II. Further term observation. *Am. Rev. Respir. Dis.* **95**:402–410.

Nolan, C. M., Barr, H., Elarth, A. M., and Boase, J. (1987). Tuberculosis in a day-care home. *Pediatrics* **79**:630–632.

Nolan, R. J., Jr. (1986). Childhood tuberculosis in North Carolina: A study of the opportunities for intervention in the transmission of tuberculosis to children. *Am. J. Public Health* **76**:26–30.

Notterman, D. A., Nardi, M., and Saslow, J. G. (1986). Effect of dose formulation on isoniazid adsorption in two young children. *Pediatrics* **77**:850–852.

O'Brien, R. J., Long, M. W., Cross, F. S., Lyle, M. A., and Snider, D. E., Jr. (1983). Hepatotoxicity from isoniazid and rifampin among children treated for tuberculosis. *Pediatrics* **72**:491–499.

Olson, W. A., Pruitt, A. W., and Dayton, P. G. (1981). Plasma concentrations of isoniazid in children with tuberculous infections. *Pediatrics* **67**:876–878.

Pape, J. W., Verdier, R., and Jean, S. (1988). Transmission and mortality of HIV infection in Haitian children [Abstract 6581]. In *Fourth International Conference on AIDS*. Stockholm, 1988. Swedish Ministry of Health and Social Affairs, Stockholm.

Pellock, J. M., Howell, J., Kendig, E. L., Jr., and Baker, H. (1985). Pyridoxine deficiency in children treated with isoniazid. *Chest* **87**:658–661.

Pelosi, F., Budani, H., Rubenstein, C., Velez, H. D., Bonavena, B., Beltran, O. P., and Gonzalez-Montaner, J. (1985). Isoniazid, rifampin and pyrazinamide in the treatment of childhood tuberculosis with duration adjusted to the clinical status [Abstract]. *Am. Rev. Respir. Dis.* **131** (Suppl.):A229.

Ramachandran, P., Duraipandian, M., Nagarajan, M., Probhakar, R., Ramakrishan, C. V., and Tripathy, S. P. (1986). Three chemotherapy studies of tuberculous meningitis in children. *Tubercle* **67**:17–29.

Reed, M. D., and Blumer, J. L. (1983). Clinical pharmacology of antitubercular drugs. *Pediatr. Clin. North Am.* **30**:177–193.

Reider, H. L., Snider, D. E., Jr., and Cauthen, G. M. (1990). Extrapulmonary tuberculosis in the United States. *Am. Rev. Respir. Dis.* **141**:347–351.

Reis, F. J. C., Bedran, M. R. M., Moura, J. A. R., Assis, I., and Rodrigues, M.E.S.M. (1990). Six-month isoniazid–rifampin treatment for pulmonary tuberculosis in children. *Am. Rev. Respir. Dis.* **142**:996–999.

Rich, A. R., and McCordock, H. A. (1933). The pathogenesis of tuberculous meningitis. *Bull. Johns Hopkins Hosp.* **52**:5–35.

Rosen, E. U. (1990). The diagnostic value of an enzyme-linked immune sorbent assay using adsorbed mycobacterial sonicates in children. *Tubercle* **71**:127–130.

Sbarbaro, J. A. (1979). Compliance: Inducements and enforcements. *Chest* **76** (Suppl.):750–756.

Schuitt, K. E. (1979). Miliary tuberculosis in children. Clinical and laboratory manifestations in 19 patients. *Am. J. Dis. Child.* **133**:583–585.

Seibert, A. F., and Bass, J. B. Jr. (1990). Tuberculin skin testing: Guidelines for the 1990s. *J. Respir. Dis.* **11**:225–234.

Seifart, H. I., Parkin, D. P., and Donald, P. R. (1991). Stability of isoniazid, rifampin and pyrazinamide in suspensions used for the treatment of tuberculosis in children. *Pediatr. Infect. Dis. J.* **10**:827–831.

Sepulveda, R. L., Burr, C., Ferrer, X., and Sorensen, R. U. (1988). Booster effect of tuberculin testing in healthy 6-year-old school children vaccinated with bacille Calmette-Guerin at birth in Santiago, Chile. *Pediatr. Infect. Dis. J.* **7**:578–581.

Siegel, M. (1934). Pathologic findings and pathogenesis of congenital tuberculosis. *Am. Rev. Tuberc.* **29**:297–310.

Smith, M. H. D. (1967). Tuberculosis in adolescents: Characteristics, recognition, management. *Clin. Pediatr.* **6**:9–15.

Smith, M. H. D. (1989). Tuberculosis in children and adolescents. *Clin. Chest Med.* **10**:381–395.

Smith, M. H. D., and Marquis, J. R. (1987). Tuberculosis and other mycobacterial infections. In *Textbook of Pediatric Infectious Diseases*. Edited by R. D. Feigin and J. D. Cherry. W. B. Saunders, Philadelphia, pp. 1342–1387.

Smith, M. H. D., and Matsaniotis, N. (1958). Treatment of tuberculosis pleural effusions with particular reference to adrenal corticosteroids. *Pediatrics* **22**:1074–1087.

Smith, M. H. D., and Teele, D. W. (1990). Tuberculosis. In *Infectious Diseases of the Fetus and Newborn*, 3rd ed. Edited by J. S. Remington and J. O. Klein. W.B. Saunders, Philadelphia, p. 834.

Snider, D. E., Jr., Layde, P. M., and Johnson, M. W. (1980). Treatment of tuberculosis during pregnancy. *Am. Rev. Respir. Dis.* **122**:65–71.

Snider, D. E., Rieder, H. L., Combs, D., Bloch, A. B., Hayden, C. H., and Smith, M. H. D. (1988). Tuberculosis in children. *Pediatr. Infect. Dis. J.* **7**:271–278.

Stallworth, J. R., Brasfield, D. M., and Tiller, R. E. (1980). Congenital miliary tuberculosis proven by open lung biopsy specimen and successfully treated. *Am. J. Dis. Child* **134**:320–323.

Stansberry, S. D. (1990). Tuberculosis in infants and children. *J. Thorac. Imaging* **5**:17–27.

Starke, J. R. (1990). Multidrug therapy for tuberculosis in children. *Pediatr. Infect. Dis. J.* **9**:785–793.

Starke, J. R., and Taylor-Watts, K. T. (1989a). Six-month chemotherapy of intrathoracic tuberculosis in children [Abstract]. *Am. Rev. Respir. Dis.* 139 (Suppl.):A314.

Starke, J. R., and Taylor-Watts, K. T. (1989b). Tuberculosis in the pediatric population of Houston, Texas. *Pediatrics* **84**:28–35.

Starke, J. R., and Taylor-Watts, K. T. (1990). Preventable childhood tuberculosis in Houston, Texas [Abstract]. *Am. Rev. Respir. Dis.* **141**:A336.

Starke, J. R., Taylor, K. T., Martindill, C. A., Pyle, N. D., and Herrin, C. M. (1988). Extremely high rates of tuberculin reactivity among young school children in Houston [Abstract]. *Am. Rev. Respir. Dis.* **137** (Suppl.):22.

Starke, J. R., Jacobs, R. F., and Jereb, J. (1992). Resurgence of tuberculosis in children. *J. Pediatr.* **120**:839–855..

Stein, M. T., and Liang, D. (1979). Clinical hepatotoxicity of isoniazid in children. *Pediatrics* **64**:499–505.

Steiner, P., Rao, M., Victoria, M. S., Jabbar, H., and Steiner, M. (1980). Persistently negative tuberculin reactions: Their presence among children culture positive for *Mycobacterium tuberculosis*. *Am. J. Dis. Child.* **134**:747–750.

Steiner, P., Rao, M., Victoria, M. S., Hunt, J., and Steiner, M. (1983). A continuing study of primary drug-resistant tuberculosis among children observed at the Kings County Hospital Medical Center between the years 1961–1980. *Am. Rev. Respir. Dis.* **128**:425–428.

Steiner, P., Rao, M., Mitchell, M., and Steiner, M. (1985). Primary drug-resistant tuberculosis in children. Correlation of drug-susceptibility patterns of matched patient and source case strains of *Mycobacterium tuberculosis. Am. J. Dis. Child.* **139**:780–782.

Sumaya, C. V., Simek, M., and Smith, M. H. D. (1975). Tuberculous meningitis in children during the isoniazid era. *J. Pediatr.* **87**:43–49.

Toppet, M., Malfroot, A., Derde, M. P., Toppet, V., Spehl, M., and Dab, I. (1990). Corticosteroids in primary tuberculosis with bronchial obstruction. *Arch. Dis. Child.* **65**:1222–1226.

Tsagarpoulou-Stinga, H., Mataki-Emmanouilidou, T., Karida-Kavalioti, S., and Manios, S. (1985). Hepatotoxic reactions in children with severe tuberculosis treated with isoniazid–rifampin. *Pediatr. Infect. Dis.* **4**:270–273.

Udani, P. M., Parekh, U. C., and Dastur, D. K. (1971). Neurologic and related syndromes in CNS tuberculosis: Clinical features and pathogenesis. *J. Neurol. Sci.* **14**:341–357.

Varteresian-Karanfil, L., Josephson, A., Fikrig, S., Kauffman, S., and Steiner, P. (1988). Pulmonary infection and cavity formation caused by *Mycobacterium tuberculosis* in a child with AIDS. *N. Engl. J. Med.* **319**:1018–1019.

Varudkar, B. L. (1985). Short-course chemotherapy for tuberculosis in children. *Indian J. Pediatr.* **52**:593–597.

Visudhiphan, P., and Chiemchanya, S. (1989). Tuberculous meningitis in children: Treatment with isoniazid and rifampin for twelve months. *J. Pediatr.* **114**:875–879.

Waecker, N. J., Jr., and Connors, J. D. (1990). Central nervous system tuberculosis in children: A review of 30 cases. *Pediatr. Infect. Dis. J.* **9**:539–543.

Wallgren, A. (1937). On contagiousness of childhood tuberculosis. *Acta Paediatr. Scand.* **22**:229–234.

Wallgren, A. (1948). The time table of tuberculosis. *Tubercle* **29**:245–256.

Zarabi, M., Sane, S., and Girdany, B. R. (1971). Chest roentgenogram in the early diagnosis of tuberculous meningitis in children. *Am. J. Dis. Child.* **121**:389–392.

17

Tuberculosis and Infection with the Human Immunodeficiency Virus

PHILIP C. HOPEWELL

University of California at San Francisco
and San Francisco General Hospital
San Francisco, California

I. Introduction

For centuries tuberculosis has been recognized to be more common among persons who in some way were in ill health (Keers, 1978). Generally the cause of the underlying condition was unknown, and it was difficult to separate the manifestations of tuberculosis from those of the predisposing disorders. Nevertheless, the connection was widely appreciated.

In more modern times, immunosuppressive diseases have been recognized and immunosuppressive therapies have been developed; as would have been predicted, these seemed to increase the risk of tuberculosis (Table 1) (Root, 1934; Kaplan et al., 1974; Millar and Horne, 1979; Andrew et al., 1980; Wilson, et al., 1985). However, tuberculosis occurring among such immunosuppressed persons contributed very little to the incidence of tuberculosis in the developed world and essentially none (save for the effects of malnutrition) in developing countries.

Quite suddenly, because of the epidemic of infection with the human immunodeficiency virus (HIV), the relative effect of immunosuppression on the incidence of tuberculosis has changed. As a consequence, large proportions of some populations, both in the developed and developing world, are immunocompromised. Moreover, HIV infection is most common among populations in

Table 1 Conditions with Which Tuberculosis May
Occur as an Opportunistic Infection

Malnutrition

Hematological and reticuloendothelial malignancies

Solid tumors

Corticosteroid therapy

Immunosuppression from cytotoxic drug therapy

Diabetes mellitis

End-stage renal disease

Human immunodeficiency virus infection

whom there is a high prevalence of tuberculous infection. As a result of the superimposition of HIV infection and tuberculous infection, rates of tuberculosis have
increased dramatically in many places.

Tuberculosis has emerged as an extremely important disease in HIV-
infected populations for at least three reasons. First is the frequency of tuberculosis as an HIV-associated condition. Second, tuberculosis can be transmitted
from person to person regardless of their HIV status. Third, the disease can be
both prevented and, if diagnosed promptly, treated effectively.

II. Host Defenses Against *Mycobacterium tuberculosis*

Host defenses against *M. tuberculosis* have both nonimmunologic and immunologic components (Bates, 1982; Scordamaglia et al., 1988). These are listed in
Table 2. In persons who have not previously been infected with and sensitized to
M. tuberculosis, only nonimmunologic mechanisms are available to defend
against infection. Because infection with *M. tuberculosis* nearly always occurs

Table 2 Host Defenses Against Tuberculosis

Nonimmunologic
    Filtration in upper airway
    Impaction in large airways and clearance by mucocilliary system
    Nonspecific phagocytosis and killing by alveolar macrophages

Immunologic
    Enhanced phagocytosis and killing by specifically sensitized
        macrophages–monocytes
    Circulating antibodies (? role)

by the airborne route, the initial line of defense consists of the mechanical barriers in the nasal passages and upper airway and the mucociliary clearance system of the lower airways. Larger airborne particles (>5 μm) carrying *M. tuberculosis* cannot penetrate to the alveoli because of these protective mechanisms. Particles that are 5 μm or smaller can reach the alveolar level. Within the alveoli the organisms are engulfed by patrolling alveolar macrophages. Because specific sensitivity to *M. tuberculosis* is lacking, the macrophages have a limited ability to kill the organisms; thus, the organism may proliferate within, and subsequently outside, the cell. In normal hosts, phagocytosis initiates a chain of events that eventually leads to a specific immunologic response to *M. tuberculosis*. Generation of the specific response requires not only phagocytosis of *M. tuberculosis*, but presentation of its antigens to antigen-responsive lymphocytes, particularly T lymphocytes, although B lymphocytes are involved and produce humoral antibodies to several components of *M. tuberculosis*. Sensitized T lymphocytes are then capable of generating lymphokines that activate macrophages, greatly enhancing their killing ability. The time required for this response to become effective is unknown, but probably parallels the development of cutaneous reactivity to tuberculin, approximately 6 weeks.

During the interval between initial implantation of the organism within the alveolus and the subsequent development of specific cell-mediated immunity, there is a (usually) silent tuberculous bacillemia, resulting in seeding of other parts of the lungs as well as other organs. Once the cell-mediated response is mature, infection in all areas is nearly always contained and most organisms are killed. However, killing is not complete, and viable organisms persist in sites that were inoculated during the early bacillemic phase. The factors responsible for the continued containment of *M. tuberculosis* are not well understood, but clearly include maintenance of an intact cell-mediated response.

Soon after infection occurs, before cell-mediated immunity becomes effective, is the time of greatest risk of developing tuberculosis. A variety of studies have shown that the risk of disease is 3–5% in the first year following infection and declines sharply thereafter (Comstock, 1982). The risk for the remainder of the lifetime of the infected person is thought to be in the range of 5%, leading to an overall likelihood of disease of approximately 10%. As was noted previously, conditions that impair cell-mediated immunity may substantially increase this risk, presumably both at the time of new infection and at any later time.

III. Effects of Human Immunodeficiency Virus Infection on Lung Defenses

Although there are still many unknowns concerning the effects of HIV infection on lung defenses, it is well established that HIV directly infects blood monocytes and macrophages (Beck and Shellito, 1989). The effects on macrophage function are not clearly defined; however, it seems likely that the effectiveness of alveolar macrophages in the initial nonspecific response to *M. tuberculosis* may be limited in persons with HIV infection, at least in the later stages of infection. The antigen-presentation function of the macrophage may also be impaired, resulting in a failure to initiate an effective immunologic response.

Because the CD4 receptor-bearing lymphocyte (T-helper cell) is known to be the major target of HIV, it is logical to assume that the responsiveness of these cells when presented with mycobacterial antigens will be limited, both because of reduced numbers and because of functional impairment (Beck and Shellito, 1989). Clonal proliferation in response to antigens and elaboration of soluble factors, such as interferon gamma and interleukin-2 (IL-2), are demonstrably reduced by HIV infection (Clerici et al., 1989). Interferon gamma is necessary for specific activation of macrophages, and IL-2 amplifies T-cell proliferation. Given the presumed essential nature of these responses in the immunologic reaction to *M. tuberculosis*, it is likely that the effects of HIV infection on $CD4^+$ lymphocytes is a major factor in predisposing to tuberculosis. Table 3 summarizes the effects of HIV infection on pulmonary defenses.

IV. Pathogenesis of Tuberculosis in Human Immunodeficiency Virus–Infected Persons

Tuberculosis develops by one of two pathogenetic sequences: (1) direct progression from recently acquired infection to disease and; (2) recrudescence of previously acquired, latent infection. These are shown diagrammatically in Figure 1. It is generally thought that, in areas of low prevalence of tuberculosis, most cases arise from latent infections, because few new infections are occurring. However, because HIV impairs the mechanisms by which new tuberculous infection is contained, the risk of direct progression is much greater in the presence of HIV infection; thus, more cases may be occurring by this sequence.

The mechanisms by which a contained tuberculous infection is kept quiescent are not well understood, but clearly involve cell-mediated immunity. Infection with HIV greatly increases the likelihood of reactivation of this latent tuberculous infection, thereby leading to clinical tuberculosis.

In the normal host, once the cell-mediated immune response to infection with *M. tuberculosis* develops, there is little likelihood of new exogenous infection being acquired. However, because of the HIV-induced immune defect, an HIV-infected person who has been previously infected with *M. tuberculosis* may still be vulnerable to new infection. Preliminary data using restriction fragment length polymorphism (RFLP) analysis suggest that this can occur and may ac-

Table 3 Effects of HIV Infection on Lung Defenses

Monocyte and macrophage function		
Function	Blood monocyte	Alveolar macrophage
Chemotaxis	Decreased or normal	Unknown
Phagocytosis	Normal	Unknown
Intracellular killing	Normal	Normal
Superoxide generation	Normal	Normal
Antibody-dependent cellular cytotoxicity	Decreased normal or increased	Unknown
MHC expression	Decreased or normal	Decreased
Antigen presentation	Decreased	Unknown
IL-1 elaboration		
Resting	Normal or increased	Normal
Stimulated	Decreased or normal	Increased
Tumor necrosis factor elaboration	Decreased or normal	Unknown

Lymphocyte function		
Function	T cells	B cells
Mitogen-induced proliferation	Decreased	Decreased
Interferon gamma elaboration	Decreased	
IL-2 elaboration	Decreased	
Spontaneous immuno-globulin secretion		Increased
Response to new antigen		Decreased

Source: Modified from Beck and Shellito (1989).

count for apparent relapses after successful completion of therapy (Small, P. M., personal communication).

It has been speculated that HIV-infected patients are more likely to acquire tuberculous infection when exposed to *M. tuberculosis* (Daley et al., 1992b). Although this concept is as yet unsubstantiated, it is clear that once an HIV-infected person becomes infected with *M. tuberculosis*, the infection can progress very rapidly to cause clinical disease (DiPerri et al., 1989). In situations during which groups of HIV-infected persons are exposed to a patient with infectious tuberculosis, explosive outbreaks of tuberculosis may occur. For

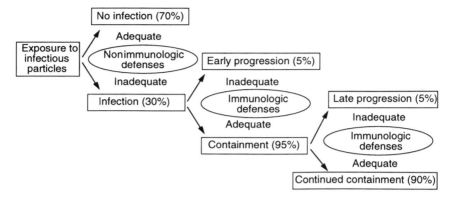

Figure 1 Diagrammatic representation of the consequences of exposure to *M. tuberculosis*. The percentages shown are derived from epidemiological data in persons without recognized immune compromise.

example, in a residential care facility for HIV-infected persons in San Francisco 11 of 30 (37%) residents exposed to a person with infectious tuberculosis developed tuberculosis within 120 days (Daley et al. 1992b). By the use of RFLP analysis it was substantiated that in all 11 of the culture-positive patients tuberculosis was caused by the same strain of organism. This pathogenetic sequence is responsible for the explosive outbreaks of tuberculosis caused by multiple drug resistant organisms that have recently occurred (Centers for Disease Control [CDC], 1991b). Obviously, if the source case in the outbreak reported by Daley and co-workers had been harboring drug-resistant organisms, each of the 11 secondary cases would have had disease caused by organisms with the same resistance pattern.

The development of infectious diseases in persons with HIV infection is a result of the interaction of the specific organism with the defenses of the host. The acquired immunodeficiency syndrome (AIDS)-defining opportunistic infections, such as *Pneumocystis carinii* pneumonia and disseminated *Mycobacterium avium* complex occur late in the course of HIV infection, as indicated by patients with these diseases having markedly reduced CD4 lymphocyte counts (Masur et al., 1989). This probably relates to the virulence of the organism, with lower-virulence organisms not being capable of producing disease until host responsiveness is severely impaired. On the other hand, *M. tuberculosis* is a much more pathogenic organism. Thus, little if any, recognizable impairment of host defenses is required for *M. tuberculosis* to cause disease. Consequently, tuberculosis tends to occur relatively early in the course of HIV infection. This is attested to by the finding of Theuer and associates (Theuer et al., 1990) that HIV-seropositive patients with tuberculosis had a median circulating CD4 lymphocyte count of 354/μl. In this group of 17 patients, tuberculosis was the initial manifestation of HIV infection in all but 2 patients, 1 of whom had limited Kaposi's sarcoma and the other oral candidiasis.

V. Frequency of Tuberculosis in Persons with Human Immunodeficiency Virus Infection

The first report of tuberculosis occurring in patients with AIDS appeared in 1983 and described the illness associated with severe immunosuppression in a group of Haitian patients in South Florida (Pitchenik et al., 1983). Of 20 patients 10 (50%) either had tuberculosis at the time the immune compromise was noted or had previously had the disease. Similarly, in a description of AIDS in Haiti, 11 of 46 patients (24%) had tuberculosis, usually preceding the diagnosis of AIDS (Pape et al., 1983). A second report of Haitian patients with AIDS living in the United States revealed 27 (60%) with tuberculosis (Pitchenik et al., 1984). Subsequently, several reports have described the association between tuberculosis and HIV infection, with and without AIDS (Sunderam et al., 1986; Louie et al., 1986; Chaisson et al., 1987; Handwerger et al., 1987; Pitchenik et al., 1987; Theuer et al., 1990). Common to all of these reports was the occurrence of tuberculosis in individuals and populations that are known to have relatively high rates of tuberculous infection, such as Haitians, intravenous drug users, and minority populations. However, the disease has not been limited to such populations and has occurred in American-born, white, middle-class homosexual or bisexual men as well.

Matching of tuberculosis and AIDS registries in 43 states has revealed that 3.8% of AIDS cases appeared on tuberculosis case registries (CDC, 1989a). However, this percentage is widely variable in different states and areas. In Florida, 10% of AIDS patients have or have had tuberculosis and, in Connecticut and New York, 5% have had the disease. A few states have had no reported cases.

In Africa, although there are no precise data that define the incidence of tuberculosis in HIV-infected populations, it is clear that tuberculosis is the most common HIV-associated lung disease. In Dar Es Salaam, Tanzania, 51% of HIV-infected patients who were evaluated because of lung disease were found to have pulmonary tuberculosis (Daley et al., 1992a). In Bujumbura, Burundi, 49.1% of a similar group of patients were found to have tuberculosis (Kamanfu et al., 1992). These studies confirm numerous anecdotal reports of the frequency of tuberculosis as an HIV-associated diagnosis in Africa.

The frequency with which tuberculosis develops in persons who are infected with both HIV and *M. tuberculosis* is not well established, but appears to be substantially in excess of what would be expected in a non–HIV-infected group. Several early reports suggest that the short-term (2–5 years) risk of tuberculosis is very much in excess of the lifetime risk in a normal host (Rieder and Snider, 1986). Reports of the prevalence of tuberculin reactivity among Haitians arriving in the United States indicated that approximately 75–90% had positive ($\geq$ 10-mm) tuberculin skin test reactions (Pitchenik et al., 1982). Subsequent reports of the frequency of tuberculosis among Haitian patients with AIDS showed that within a 30-month period, 50% had tuberculosis before, at the time of, or after the diagnosis of AIDS (Pitchenik et al., 1983).

More direct data on the frequency of tuberculosis in HIV-infected patients have been provided by Selwyn and co-workers (Selwyn et al., 1989) in a prospective study of tuberculosis among HIV-seropositive and HIV-seronegative intravenous drug users in New York City. Of 49 HIV-seropositive subjects, 7 (14%) drug users, who had been previously known to have positive tuberculin skin test, and 1 anergic patient developed tuberculosis in a 2-year period. This was the equivalent of 7.9 cases per 100 person years of observation. These observations suggest that seven and perhaps all eight patients who developed tuberculosis had preexisting tuberculous infection, indicating that endogenous reactivation was the dominant, if not the only, pathogenetic mechanism for developing tuberculosis. Of additional concern was the observation that 11 and 13% of the seropositive and seronegative subjects, respectively, developed positive tuberculin skin tests during the period of the study. If this is truly indicative of new infections, the rate is very high and suggests that there were numerous infectious cases within the population.

Allen and colleagues (Allen, S., personal communication) have prospectively followed a group of urban women of childbearing age in Kigali, Rwanda and found that the incidence of tuberculosis was approximately 2.5% per year. In comparison with HIV-negative women, the risk ratio for tuberculosis among the HIV-positive women was 22.9. Among the HIV-positive women, having had a positive tuberculin skin test was associated with a significantly increased risk of tuberculosis, but the risk ratio was only 3, and 9 of 17 patients with tuberculosis had negative tuberculin tests, perhaps as a result of anergy.

VI. Prevalence of Human Immunodeficiency Virus Infection Among Patients with Tuberculosis

Several prospective studies in public tuberculosis clinics have described the prevalence of HIV infection among patients with tuberculosis. Pitchenik and co-workers (Pitchenik et al., 1987) reported that 31% of 71 consecutive tuberculosis patients in Miami were HIV-infected. In Seattle, Nolan and associates (Nolan et al., 1988) found 23% of non-Asian adults were HIV-infected. Theuer and colleagues (Theuer et al., 1990) reported that in San Francisco, 28% of non-Asian tuberculosis patients between 15 and 55 years of age were HIV-seropositive.

Beginning in 1988, a systematic nationwide sampling of HIV infection prevalence was undertaken by the Centers for Disease Control (CDC) in 14 urban tuberculosis clinics (Ornorato and McCray, 1992). The median seropositivity rate in the 14 clinics in 4301 persons with, or suspected of having, tuberculosis was 3.4%. The rates varied widely among clinics, ranging from zero to 46%. The highest rate was reported from New York City (46%), followed by Newark (34%), Boston (27%), Miami (24%), and Baltimore (13%).

Data from developing countries are scarce, but indicate a substantial rate of HIV infection among patients with tuberculosis (Mann et al., 1986; Colebunders et al., 1989; Standaert et al., 1989; Gilks et al., 1990). This finding would be expected, given the concomitant high prevalence of both tuberculous infection and infection with HIV in developing countries.

VII. Impact of Human Immunodeficiency Virus Infection on the Incidence of Tuberculosis

The full impact of HIV infection on the epidemiology of tuberculosis has not been defined either in the United States or abroad. Inferential information suggests, however, that the influence may be substantial. Data from the CDC indicate that there have been approximately 28,000 "excess" cases of tuberculosis in the United States between 1984 and 1990 (CDC, 1991a) This was determined by comparing the number of cases actually reported with the estimated cumulative number of cases that would have occurred had the rate of decline in the annual number of cases reported before 1984 continued through 1990. Before 1984 there had been a consistent decrease in the number of newly reported tuberculosis cases, averaging 5–6% per year. However, in 1985 there was no decrease from 1984 and, in 1986, there was a 2.2% increase. In 1987 there were slightly fewer cases than in 1986. In 1988 there was a slight reduction, but in 1989 there was a 4.7% increase compared with 1988, and in 1990 there was a more than 8% increase compared with 1989 (CDC, 1990). Although the excess cases occurring since 1984 are not proved to be attributable to HIV infection, the largest increases have occurred in the areas with the greatest number of AIDS cases and, therefore, the highest prevalence of HIV infection.

Countrywide data tend to underestimate the effects of HIV infection on the incidence of tuberculosis in certain parts of the United States. Perhaps the most profound effects have occurred in New York City. Between 1984 and 1991 the tuberculosis case rate increased from 19.9:100,000 to 36:100,000 population, an 80% rise. The increase in case rates was even more dramatic in Central Harlem, where in 1989, the rate reached 169:100,000 persons, quite similar to case rates in Eastern and Central Africa (Brudney and Dobkin, 1991). These data are illustrated in Figure 2.

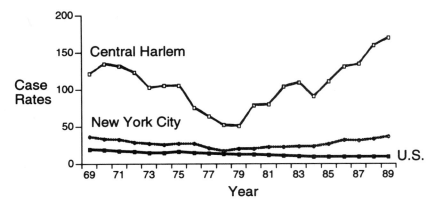

Figure 2 Rates of tuberculosis in the United States, New York City, and Central Harlem. Rates are expressed per 100,000 population. (From Brudney and Dobkin, 1991).

In other areas, although overall rates have not increased so markedly, the demographics of the population with tuberculosis have changed. In San Francisco, for example, although the number of cases has increased only slightly, there has been a decrease in foreign-born and an increase in U.S.-born patients and a shift from older-to younger-aged groups, changes compatible with increasing amounts of tuberculosis associated with HIV infection.

VIII. Diagnosis of Tuberculous Infection and Tuberculosis in Human Immunodeficiency Virus–Infected Patients

A. Tuberculin Skin Testing and Anergy Testing

As would be predicted, the tuberculin skin test commonly shows little or no reaction in persons with advanced HIV infection. However, in earlier stages of the infection, reactivity may be maintained. The ability to respond to tuberculin is an indicator of the status of cell-mediated immunity that, in turn, is an indicator of the stage of HIV infection. Most studies that describe the prevalence of reactive ($\geq$ 10-mm) tuberculin tests indicate that approximately 40% of HIV-infected patients with tuberculosis have positive reactions. However, in the study by Theuer and associates (Theuer et al., 1990), 80% of the HIV-seropositive patients with tuberculosis had positive reactions to tuberculin.

Because of the frequency of blunted skin test responses or anergy, it has been recommended that a reaction of $\geq$ 5-mm induration to 5 tuberculin units (TU) of purified protein derivative (PPD) be regarded as indicative of tuberculous infection (CDC, 1989a). The implications of using 5 mm as the cutting point for defining tuberculous infection have not been determined. In a recent study Graham and associates (Graham et al., 1992) found that a 5-mm cutoff for determining tuberculin positivity underestimated the rates of tuberculous infection and recommended a 2-mm cutoff. However, the practicality of using such a small size would appear to impose significant limitations (Heubner et al., 1992). The effect of boosting the tuberculin response by application of a second skin test soon after a negative initial test has not been examined.

To determine if a negative tuberculin test is the result of immunosuppression or is truly negative, control antigens should be applied. These include antigens made from *Candida* organisms, mumps virus, and tetanus toxoid to which most persons with intact cell-mediated immunity will respond. A negative tuberculin reaction in the presence of positive reactions to one or more of the control antigens can be interpreted as a true-negative. If there is no reaction to any of the antigens, it cannot be determined if the negative tuberculin test is a true- or false-negative result.

B. Clinical Features of Tuberculosis

The clinical manifestations of tuberculosis occurring in patients with HIV infection vary considerably, depending on the severity of the immunosuppression (Pape et al., 1983; Pitchenik et al., 1983, 1984; Louie et al., 1986; Sunderam et al., 1986; Chaisson et al., 1987, Handwerger et al., 1987; Theuer et al., 1990; Batungwanayo et al., 1992) (Table 4). As noted previously, presumably because of the virulence of *M. tuberculosis*, tuberculosis tends to occur earlier in the course of HIV infection. In most series, the majority of tuberculosis diagnoses

Table 4 Clinical Features of Tuberculosis in HIV-Infected Patients

Early in the course of HIV disease
    Typical features
        Predominantly pulmonary
        Upper lobe location
        Cavitation
        Positive tuberculin tests

Late in course of HIV disease
    Atypical features
        Increased proportion of extrapulmonary sites
        Diffuse infiltration

Both early and late
    Infectious
        Good response to therapy

have preceded the identification of an AIDS-defining disease. A substantial number of patients have tuberculosis diagnosed at the time of AIDS diagnosis and, in a smaller number, tuberculosis appears after an AIDS diagnosis. This is partly a semantic distinction, in that the surveillance definition of AIDS, revised in 1987, now includes extrapulmonary tuberculosis in an HIV-seropositive person (CDC, 1987) and is proposed to include pulmory tuberculosis in 1993.

Seemingly, the earlier tuberculosis develops, the more "usual" is its clinical presentation, whereas the later it occurs, the more atypical are its features (see Table 4). This conclusion is somewhat difficult to support from published information, owing largely to the fact that most series in the literature describe the features of tuberculosis in patients who either have or subsequently develop AIDS. Patients identified by crossmatching AIDS and tuberculosis registries clearly are likely to have advanced HIV disease, even if their tuberculosis develops before an AIDS-defining diagnosis appears.

In the earliest report describing tuberculosis in Haitian patients with AIDS, only one of ten patients had pulmonary tuberculosis, whereas one had brain abscesses and the other eight had miliary or disseminated tuberculosis (Pitchenik et al., 1983). There was no immunologic characterization of the patients at the time tuberculosis occurred; thus, the stage of their HIV disease could not be inferred. Nevertheless, tuberculosis occurred 2–15 months before an AIDS-defining diagnosis in seven patients and was concurrent with AIDS in the other three patients.

Subsequent reports focusing on patients who have or develop AIDS have expanded on the atypical presentations contained in the first description (Pitchenik et al., 1984; Louie et al., 1986; Sunderam et al., 1986; Chaisson et al., 1987; Handwerger et al., 1987). These series have emphasized that the disease is frequently disseminated has unusual radiographic manifestations, and nonreactive tuberculin skin tests. Lymph node involvement, including intrathoracic adenopathy, was frequently described. In these series, as well as in individual case reports, a variety of unusual manifestations have been noted. These include central nervous system involvement, with brain abscesses, tuberculomas, and meningitis (Fischl et al., 1985; Bishburg et al., 1986; Sunderam et al., 1986); bone, including vertebral disease (Sunderam et al., 1986; Mallolas et al., 1988); pericarditis (D'Cruz et al., 1986; Sunderam et al., 1986); gastric tuberculosis (Brody et al., 1986); tuberculous peritonitis (Barnes et al., 1986); and scrotal tuberculous (Sunderam et al., 1987). In addition, *M. tuberculosis* has been cultured from the blood as well as bone marrow (Saltzman et al., 1986; Modilevsky et al., 1989; Shafer et al., 1989).

Despite the increased frequency of unusual forms of tuberculosis in persons with HIV infection, several reports have described a preponderance of "standard" pulmonary disease (Pitchenik et al., 1987; Selwyn et al., 1989; Theuer et al., 1990). These reports presented series collected prospectively in which either tuberculosis patients had HIV antibody measured (Pitchenik et al., 1987; Theuer et al., 1990) or HIV-seropositive subjects were followed for the development of tuberculosis (Selwyn et al., 1989). Thus, these patients presumably were less immunocompromised.

C. Radiographic Findings

The atypical findings on chest radiographs of HIV-infected patients who have tuberculosis have received considerable emphasis. In retrospective studies, features that are not regarded as "typical" for pulmonary tuberculosis have been the norm (Pitchenik and Rubinson, 1985; Chaisson et al., 1987). Lower lung zone or diffuse infiltrations commonly have been observed, rather than the usual upper lobe involvement. Cavitation has been unusual, and intrathoracic adenopathy, an unusual finding in nonimmunosuppressed adults with tuberculosis, has been relatively frequent.

In the prospective study by Theuer and colleagues (Theuer et al., 1990), the radiographic finding in patients with HIV infection were indistinguishable from those in patients who were HIV-seronegative. The findings included typical upper lobe infiltration, often with cavitation. A greater prevalence of atypical findings was noted in the prospective study by Pitchenik and colleagues (Pitchenik et al., 1987). These findings included a higher frequency of adenopathy, diffuse or lower lobe infiltration, and a lower frequency of cavitation, compared with HIV-seronegative patients.

D. Bacteriological and Histological Examinations

Most reported series indicate that the prevalence of positive sputum smears and cultures in patients with pulmonary tuberculosis is the same in HIV-infected and HIV-noninfected persons (Chaisson et al., 1987; Pitchenik et al., 1987; Theuer et al., 1990). In some instances, sputum induction or bronchoscopic procedures have been necessary to diagnose pulmonary tuberculosis. Specimens from any site of abnormality in patients with or suspected of having HIV infection should be examined for mycobacteria by smear and culture. Potential high-yield sources include lymph nodes, bone marrow, urine, and blood.

In general, any acid-fast organism identified in any specimen should be regarded as being *M. tuberculosis* until proved otherwise. Such a policy will result in prompt initiation of appropriate therapy for tuberculosis and contact evaluation. With standard techniques, detection of growth and speciation of mycobacteria requires 6–10 weeks. Use of radiometric culture techniques and DNA probes for identification of *M. tuberculosis* and *M. avium* complex can shorten this procedure to 7–10 days, thereby adding greatly to the efficiency of tuberculosis control measures. The use of the polymerase chain reaction should result in a much more rapid diagnoses (Brisson-Noel et al., 1989).

In patients with more advanced HIV infection, mycobacterial infection does not produce classic granulomas (Sunderam et al., 1986). However, because tuberculosis tends to occur earlier in HIV infection, the ability to form granulomas may be intact. Thus, the finding of granulomas either in tissue sections or cytological preparations from needle aspiration should be interpreted as being more consistent with tuberculosis than with nontuberculous mycobacterial disease. It must be remembered, however, that other organisms, including *P. carinii*, may cause granulomas.

IX. Treatment

With a few notable exceptions, reported series of patients with tuberculosis and HIV infection demonstrate a good response to antituberculosis treatment (Pitchenik et al., 1983, 1984, 1987; Louie et al., 1986; Sunderam et al., 1986; Chaisson et al., 1987; Theuer et al., 1990; Small et al., 1991). However, in the series reported by Sunderam and co-workers (Sunderam et al., 1986) there were three patients who did not respond to treatment and had progressive disease. A case report from the same institution described a recurrence of tuberculosis at an extrapulmonary site (scrotal) after apparently successful treatment for pulmonary disease (Sunderam et al., 1987). These reports have led to expressions of concern over the adequacy of current standard 6-month therapy (Iseman, 1987), and subsequently to recommendations that 9 months or 6 months beyond the time of sputum conversion, whichever is longer, be the minimum duration of treatment in HIV-infected patients (CDC, 1989a).

Because in the reported series the regimens used were not uniform in duration or composition, advantages of longer versus shorter durations of treatment cannot be determined. Nearly all patients have been treated with regimens that contained isoniazid and rifampin together with various combinations of pyrazinamide, ethambutol, and streptomycin. Current recommendations indicate that, in adult patients with HIV infection, treatment for tuberculosis should include 300 mg/day isoniazid, 600 mg/day rifampin (450 mg/day for persons weighing less than 50 kg), and 20–30 mg/kg per day pyrazinamide during the first 2 months of therapy; isoniazid and rifampin should be continued for at least another 7 months, making the total duration of therapy at least 9 months (CDC, 1989a). For patients judged to be potentially noncompliant, therapy should be given under direct observation. This can be facilitated by twice-weekly drug administration after an initial phase of daily treatment.

For patients with pulmonary tuberculosis, response to therapy should be determined by bacteriological examination of sputum, as well as by clinical and radiographic examinations. In patients with less accessible sites of disease, generally only clinical and radiographic evaluations can be used to determine the response. It should be kept in mind that worsening clinical and radiographic findings may be caused by other HIV-related diseases.

It appears that the rate of adverse reactions to antituberculosis drugs is greater in persons with HIV infection (Small et al., 1991). Consequently, patients with HIV infection should be followed closely with appropriate laboratory and clinical monitoring. There has been no systematic evaluation of possible interactions of antituberculosis drugs with antiretroviral agents. The potential for increased toxicity should, however, be kept in mind. The antifungal agents ketoconazole and fluconazole both have interactions with isoniazid and rifampin, resulting in reduction in serum concentrations of the antifungal agents (Englehard et al., 1989; Lazar and Wilner, 1990). In addition ketoconazole interferes with the absorption of rifampin (Englehard, et al., 1989).

In view of the generally good response to regimens containing both isoniazid and rifampin reported by all investigators, there appears to be no reason to prolong treatment beyond the recommended period of 9 months, unless bacteriological conversion was delayed, or treatment was interrupted because of noncompliance or adverse reactions. Patients who cannot take isoniazid *and* rifampin together should be treated for a minimum of 18 months, usually with isoniazid *or* rifampin and ethambutol plus pyrazinamide in the initial phase. This recommendation also applies to patients whose disease is caused by organisms that are resistant to isoniazid or rifampin.

Because of the modifications of standard treatment regimens for patients with HIV infection, HIV antibody testing is desirable and should be offered to all patients with new diagnoses of tuberculosis.

X. Tuberculosis Caused By Multiple Drug-Resistant Organisms

Recently, explosive outbreaks of tuberculosis caused by organisms resistant to multiple drugs (usually at least both isoniazid and rifampin) have been reported (CDC, 1991b). These outbreaks have taken place in hospitals and clinics and have preponderantly, although not exclusively, involved HIV-infected patients. Health care workers, both HIV-seropositive and negative, have been infected. Substantial epidemiological and laboratory (RFLP analysis) data indicate that transmission of the resistant *M. tuberculosis* has taken place in the health care facility. Differing patterns of drug resistance have been noted, with some organisms being resistant to all approved antituberculosis agents. These outbreaks have been characterized by very high case fatality rates, ranging from 72 to 89% in median times ranging from 4 to 16 weeks. Also noteworthy are the relatively high rates of tuberculin skin test conversions among exposed health care workers.

There are at least three major factors that have combined to produce these outbreaks. The first is a relatively high prevalence of multiple drug-resistance in the community at large and, particularly, in the groups that in some areas are most likely to be HIV-infected. This prevalence of drug resistance is a predictable outcome of the lack of attention and resources devoted to tuberculosis during at least the last decade (Reichman, 1991).

Second is the effect of HIV on the host response to tuberculous infection. As described in Section IV, recently acquired infection with *M. tuberculosis* in an HIV-infected person may progress very rapidly to cause clinical disease which, in turn, is capable of being transmitted. For example, if tuberculosis in the source case in the outbreak described in San Francisco (Daley et al., 1992b) had been caused by resistant organisms, all 11 secondary cases would have been caused by drug-resistant organisms.

The third factor relates to the fact that tuberculosis in HIV-infected persons may not be so easily recognizable as in persons with a normal immune status. Therefore, the disease may go undiagnosed, perhaps in a hospital or clinic environment, for a relatively prolonged period. During this time, unless adequate infection-control measures are applied presumptively, the patient will be capable of transmitting the infection. Moreover, even if the disease is diagnosed, it may not be appreciated for several weeks that the organisms are multiply-resistant because of the time required for standard techniques to identify drug-resistant organisms.

A fourth factor is the lack of effective means of control of airborne infections in many health care facilities. Even if the disease is recognized, often the isolation measures applied are not effective. Consequently, transmission may occur within the facility (CDC, 1989b). These factors are shown diagrammatically in Figure 3.

Treatment of tuberculosis caused by multiple drug-resistant organisms presents considerable difficulty. First the organism must be recognized to be drug-resistant. With radiometric techniques and direct inoculation of drug-containing media for every specimen, resistance patterns could be known in 7–10 days. However, this is a very inefficient approach and could quickly overload a laboratory. A more efficient approach would be to screen for resistance to one agent, probably rifampin, and infer multiple drug-resistance if there is resistance to rifampin. A more traditional system would be to perform direct susceptibility testing on specimens that are positive for acid-fast organisms on microscopy and to do indirect testing on specimens that are smear-negative, culture-positive. By this last method using radiometric techniques, a result would not be obtained for 14–21 days. If the traditional solid media and indirect testing were done, identification of resistant organisms would require 8–12 weeks.

Given these delays, in areas in which there is a high prevalence of tuberculosis caused by resistant organisms, empiric therapy, based on endemic resistance patterns may be necessary. Such therapy should be based on a knowledge

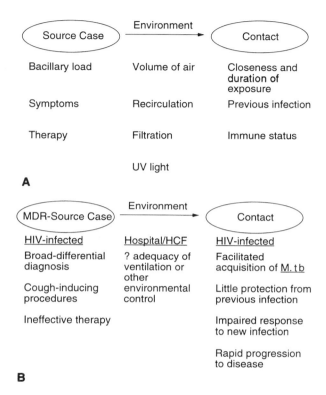

Figure 3 (A) Factors influencing the transmission of *M. tuberculosis* under "usual" circumstances. (B) Factors involved in producing outbreaks of multidrug resistant tuberculosis. MDR, multidrug resistance.

of the prevailing patterns of resistance. Always, at least two agents to which the organisms are thought to be susceptible should be used. In some instances, this may entail use of agents such as the fluorquinolones and amikacin that are not yet approved as antituberculosis drugs.

XI. Prevention

Preventive therapy with isoniazid has been widely effective in preventing tuberculosis among various groups of persons with tuberculous infection (American Thoracic Society and CDC, 1986). Although the effectiveness of isoniazid preventive therapy in persons infected with both HIV and *M. tuberculosis* had not been well documented, there is no reason to assume that it would not work. Moreover, preliminary data from a prospective controlled trial in Zambia

(Wadhawan et al., 1990) indicate substantial protection. Consequently, tuberculin testing should be performed as a routine part of management for patients with HIV infection. Patients with reactions of ≥5 mm to 5 TU of purified protein derivative should be considered as having tuberculous infection and be offered preventive therapy. Although the usual preventive therapy recommendations for persons with normal chest films state that 6 months is sufficient, treatment for 12 months is recommended in the presence of HIV infection (American Thoracic Society and CDC, 1986). There are no data in any group treated with isoniazid preventive therapy that suggest treatment for more than 12 months confers additional protection.

Rifampin should be used as preventive therapy in persons exposed to and presumably infected with isoniazid-resistant organisms, although there are no data to support this recommendation. Recommendations for preventive therapy in persons thought to be infected with organisms resistant to isoniazid and rifampin are difficult to formulate. The use of experimental regimes, such as pyrazinamide and a fluoroquinolone may be the only option.

In HIV-infected persons exposed to a person with infectious tuberculosis, preventive therapy should be given, regardless of the results of tuberculin skin testing. Therefore, it is important to know the HIV status of close contacts of newly discovered cases. Moreover, as opposed to the recommendations that apply in non–HIV-infected close contacts, repeated courses of preventive therapy should be given with subsequent exposures.

Attempts at immunization against tuberculosis with bacille Calmette-Guerin (BCG) should not be undertaken in patients with AIDS because of the possibility of developing disseminated BCG disease. The use of BCG in HIV-infected persons without AIDS, although not shown to be associated with a high rate of adverse reactions, is probably risky, and, at least in areas of low prevalence of tuberculosis such as the United States, should not be done.

XII. Infection Control

As noted in the introduction, tuberculosis is the only common HIV-associated infection that can be transmitted from person to person, including persons who are not HIV-infected. Therefore, it is extremely important that tuberculosis be taken into account in applying infection control measures in persons with HIV infection. In patients who are being evaluated because of respiratory symptoms or findings, respiratory precautions should be applied until tuberculosis is excluded. Sputum induction and bronchoscopy should be performed in areas with adequate ventilation, with the exhausted air not being recirculated to other parts of the building. Similar considerations should apply to areas in which aerosol pentamidine is administered. Transmission of tuberculous infection has occurred in a poorly ventilated clinic where aerosol pentamidine prophylaxis for *P. carinii* pneumonia was being administered to two patients whose sputum contained *M. tuberculosis* (CDC, 1989b). Nosocomial transmission of *M. tuberculosis* has also been described in several other reports.

In general, once a patient is being given effective therapy for tuberculosis, he or she is regarded as being noninfectious. However, because of the potentially severe consequences of new tuberculous infections in immunocompromised patients, it is prudent to be more cautious in persons with tuberculosis who will be in contact with HIV-infected persons. In most patients being treated effectively, because of the decrease in the number of bacilli present in sputum and a decrease in the frequency of coughing, infectivity is reduced by more than 99% within 2 weeks of beginning treatment (Hopewell, 1986). Even with a reduction of this magnitude, sputum smears may still show acid-fact bacilli. To be even more confident that infectiousness is extremely low, precautions may continue to be applied until results of sputum smears are negative. In most instances, however, 2 weeks of therapy is sufficient, assuming the organisms are susceptible to the agents given.

Infection control for HIV is also a major concern. Medical personnel working with tuberculosis patients should use appropriate infection control measures to prevent HIV transmission. In general, universal blood and body substance precautions should be applied. Special care should be taken in blood drawing, administration of tuberculin skin tests, and intramuscular injections. This last consideration is of particular relevance to developing countries where facilities for sterilization are inadequate, but where streptomycin is used commonly.

XIII. Necessary Changes in Tuberculosis Control Policy and Procedures

The basic components of tuberculosis control have been in place with little modification for the past 25–30 years and will continue to be applicable through the dramatic changes we are witnessing in the nature of the disease. Case identification, treatment, case holding, and prevention of disease still provide the basic underpinnings of the public health management of tuberculosis. However, a major change is necessary, not in the elements of tuberculosis control, but in the tempo of their application.

Infection with HIV has caused a telescoping of the natural history of tuberculosis. No longer can it be assumed that only approximately one-third of close contacts of new cases will be infected. As noted previously, there is inferential evidence that HIV-infected persons are more likely to acquire infection with *M. tuberculosis* than is the general population. Perhaps of more importance, it is quite clear that an HIV-infected person who acquires a new infection with *M. tuberculosis* is much more likely to progress rapidly to clinical tuberculosis, as was described by DiPerri and co-workers and Daley and associates. As a consequence of the rapid progression, case fatality rates for tuberculosis are much higher than in nonimmunocompromised patients, with almost all fatalities occurring before treatment is started or in the first month of therapy. Contributing to the higher case fatality rates is the occurrence of tuberculosis caused by multiple drug-resistant organisms. Superimposed on these changes in the nature of the disease is that the HIV-infected patients in whom tuberculosis is of greater likelihood are also more difficult to maintain on a regular treatment regimen. Thus, although because of the immunosuppression, there is less of a "margin of safety" in treating such patients, doing so requires labor-intensive schemes such as directly observed therapy.

The implications of the foregoing are that basic tuberculosis control measures must be applied more quickly and with greater intensity. These concepts work out as follows:

1. At least in hospitals and clinics providing care for HIV-infected persons, rapid radiometric means of detecting growth of mycobacteria should be used, with speciation of organisms by DNA probes or other rapid techniques. If such technology is not available in a given institution, strong consideration should be given to using another laboratory in which they are available.

    Support should be given to developing more rapid diagnostic tests: polymerase chain reaction-based methods, antigen detection, and direct-application DNA probes, for example.

2. Sensitivity testing should likewise be performed as quickly as possible using techniques just described.

3. Contact investigation should be initiated immediately upon identification of a presumed (positive smear) or confirmed case. The contact interview should be performed by a person who has some familiarity with the life-style of the new patient to identify unsuspected settings in which transmission of *M. tuberculosis* may have occurred.

4. All contacts identified should be evaluated promptly. If it is thought that either the case or his or her contacts are at risk of HIV infection, the contact should be asked his or her HIV status or be advised to have the test performed. If the contact is known or thought to be at risk of being HIV-infected, decisions about preventive therapy should not be based on skin test results; rather, preventive therapy should be given to contacts, regardless of the skin test results.

Preventive therapy for persons suspected of having been infected with drug-resistant organisms should be based on prevailing sensitivity patterns.

If it is suspected or known that the contact is HIV-infected, careful questioning concerning possible symptoms of tuberculosis should be undertaken, and the patient should have a thorough physical examination and chest film to exclude current tuberculosis.

5. HIV-infected patients with tuberculosis should be treated initially with isoniazid, rifampin, ethambutol, and pyrazinamide. The last two drugs can be discontinued after 2 months. The duration of therapy (6 or 9 months) is probably less important than the compliance with therapy. Consequently, directly observed therapy is the preferable treatment scheme. As with the contact investigation, supervision of therapy is best done by a health care worker familiar with the patient's life-style.

    If there are problems with compliance or if the response to therapy (judged clinically, radiographically, or bacteriologically) is suboptimal, therapy should be prolonged.

    As noted previously, if drug resistance is known or proved, appropriate regimens based on prevailing patterns or determined sensitivities should be used. In these situations more prolonged therapy should be used.

The changes in the tempo of tuberculous control activities are not only made necessary by HIV infection. Because of the transience of homeless persons and the probability of their being in situations (such as shelters) favoring transmission of *M. tuberculosis*, a rapid-response tuberculosis control program is necessary for this group as well. Likewise rapid response is necessary for other socially marginated groups, such as migrant workers and substance abusers.

References

American Thoracic Society and Centers for Disease Control (1986). Treatment of tuberculosis and tuberculous infection in adults and children. *Am. Rev. Respir. Dis.* **134**:355–363.

Andrew, O. T., Schoenfeld, P. Y., Hopewell, P. C., and Humphreys, M. (1980). Tuberculosis in patients with end-stage renal disease. *Am. J. Med.* **68**:59–65.

Barnes, P., Leedom, J., Radin, D. R., and Chandrasoma, P. (1986). An unusual case of tuberculous peritonitis in a man with AIDS. *West. J. Med.* **144**:467–469.

Bates, J. H. (1982). Tuberculosis: Susceptibility and resistance. *Am. Rev. Respir. Dis.* **125**:20–24.

Batungwanayo, J., Taelman, H., Dhote, R., Bogaerts, J., Allen, S., and Van de Perre, P. (1992). Pulmonary tuberculosis in Kigali, Rwanda: The impact of HIV infection on clinical and radiographic presentation. *Am. Rev. Respir. Dis.* (In press).

Beck, J. M., and Shellito, J. (1989). Effects of human immunodeficiency virus on pulmonary host defenses. *Semin. Respir. Infect.* **4**:75.

Bishburg, E., Sunderam, G., Reichman, L. B., and Kapila, R. (1986). Central nervous system tuberculosis with the acquired immunodeficiency syndrome and its related complex. *Ann. Intern. Med.* **105**:210–213.

Brisson-Noel, A., Lecossier, D., Nassif, X., Gicquel, B., Lévy-Frébault, V., and Hance, A. J. (1989). Rapid diagnosis of tuberculosis by amplification of mycobacterial DNA in clinical samples. *Lancet* **2**:1069–1071.

Brody, J. M., Miller, D. K., Zeman, R. K., Klappenbach, S., Jaffe, M. H., Clark, L. R., Benjamin, S. Z., and Choyke, P. L. (1986). Gastric tuberculosis: A manifestation of acquired immunodeficiency syndrome. *Radiology* **159**:347–348.

Brudney, K., and Dobkin, J. (1991). Resurgent tuberculosis in New York City. *Am. Rev. Respir. Dis.* **144**:745–749.

Centers for Disease Control (1987). Revision of the CDC surveillance case definitions for acquired immunodeficiency syndrome. *MMWR* **36** (Suppl. 1–5): 15–155.

Centers for Disease Control (1989a). Tuberculosis and human immunodeficiency virus infection: Recommendation of the Advisory Committee for Elimination of Tuberculosis. *MMWR* **38**:236–250.

Centers for Disease Control (1989b). *Mycobacterium tuberculosis* transmission in a health clinic—Florida. *MMWR* **38**:256.

Centers for Disease Control (1990). Update: Tuberculosis elimination—United States. *MMWR* **39**:157–169.

Centers for Disease Control (1991a). Cases of specified notifiable diseases—United States. *MMWR* **39**:944.

Centers for Disease Control (1991b). Nosocomial transmission of multidrug resistant tuberculosis among HIV-infected patients. *MMWR* **40**:585–591.

Chaisson, R. E., Schecter, G. F., Theuer, C. P., Rutherford, S. W., Echenberg, D. F., and Hopewell, P. C. (1987). Tuberculosis in patients with the acquired immunodeficiency syndrome. *Am. Rev. Respir. Dis.* **136**:570–574.

Clerici, M., Stocks, M. I., Zajac, R. A., Boswell, N., Lucey, D. R., Via, C. S., and Shearer, G. M. (1989). Detection of three distinct patterns of T-helper cell dysfunction in asymptomatic, human immunodeficiency virus-seropositive patients. *J. Clin. Invest.* **84**:1892–1896.

Colebunders, R. L., Ryder, R. W., Nylambi, N., Nkoko, R., Jeugmanc, J., Kalala, M., Francis, H., Mann, J., Quinn, T., and Piot, P. (1989). HIV infection in patients with tuberculosis in Kinshasa, Zaire. *Am. Rev. Respir. Dis.* **135**:1082–1085.

Comstock, G. W. (1982). Epidemiology of tuberculosis. *Am. Rev. Respir. Dis.* **125**:8–15.

D'Cruz, I. A., Sengupta, E. E., Abrahams, C., Reddy, H. K., and Turlapati, R. V. (1986). Cardiac involvement, including tuberculous pericardial effusion, complicating acquired immune deficiency syndrome. *Am. Heart J.* **112**:1100–1102.

Daley, C. L., Chen, L. L., Small, P. M., Mugusi, F., Aris, E., Cegielski, P., Lalinger, G., Mtoni, I., Mbaga, I. M., and Murray, J. F. (1992a). Pulmonary complications of HIV infection in Tanzania. *Am. Rev. Respir. Dis.* **145**:A821.

Daley, C. L., Small, P. M., Schecter, G. F., Schoolnik, G. K., McAdam, R. A., Jacobs, W. R., and Hopewell, P. C. (1992b). An outbreak of tuberculosis with accelerated progression among persons infected with human immunodeficiency virus: An analysis using restriction-fragment length polymorphisms. *N. Engl. J. Med.* **326**:231–235.

DiPerri, G., Danzi, M. C., DeChecci, G., Pizzighella, S., Solbrati, M., Cruciani, M., Luzzati, R., Molena, M., Mazzi, R., Concia, E., and Bassetti, D. (1989). Nosocomial epidemic of active tuberculosis among HIV-infected patients. *Lancet* **2**:1502–1504.

Englehard, D., Stutman, H. R., and Marko, M. I. (1989). Interaction of ketoconazole with rifampin and isoniazid. *N. Engl. J. Med.* **311**:1681–1683.

Fischl, M. A., Pitchenik, A. E., and Spira, T. J. (1985). Tuberculosis brain abscess and toxoplasma encephalitis in a patients with the acquired immunodeficiency syndrome. *JAMA* **253**:3428–3430.

Gilks, C. F., Brindle, R. J., and Otieno, L. S. (1990). Extrapulmonary and disseminated tuberculosis in HIV seropositive patients presenting to the acute medical services in Nairobi. *AIDS* **4**:981–985.

Graham, N. M. H., Nelson, K. E., Solomon, L., Bonds, M., Rizzo, R. T., Scavotto, J., Astemborski, J., and Vlahov, D. (1992). Prevalence of tuberculin positivity and skin test anergy in HIV-1–seropositive and – seronegative intravenous drug users. *JAMA* **267**:369–373.

Handwerger, S., Mildvan, D., Senie, R., and McKinley, F. W. (1987). Tuberculosis and the acquired immunodeficiency syndrome at a New York City hospital: 1978–1985. *Chest* **91**:176–180.

Hopewell, P. C. (1986). Factors influencing transmission and infectivity of *Mycobacterium tuberculosis*: Implications for clinical and public health management. In *Respiratory Infections*. Edited by M. A. Sande, L. D. Hudson, and R. K. Root. Churchill-Livingstone, New York, pp. 191–216.

Huebner, R. E., Villarino, M. E., and Snider, D. E. (1992). Tuberculin skin testing and the HIV epidemic. *JAMA* **267**:409–410.

Iseman, M. D. (1987). Is standard chemotherapy adequate in tuberculosis patients infected with the HIV? *Am. Rev. Respir. Dis.* **136**:1326.

Kamanfu, G., Mlika-Cabanne, N., Nimubona, S., Mfizi, B., Cishako, A., Roux, P., Girard, P., Couloud, J., Larouze, B., Aubry, P., and Murray, J. F. (1992). The pulmonary complications of human immunodeficiency virus infection in Bujumbura, Burundi. (Submitted).

Kaplan, M. H., Armstrong, D., and Rosen, P. (1974). Tuberculosis complicating neoplastic disease: A review of 201 cases. *Cancer* **33**:850–858.

Keers, R. Y. (1978). *Pulmonary Tuberculosis. Anatomical and Pathological Study*. Bailliere Tindall, London, pp. 20–35.

Lazar, J. D., and Wilner, K. D. (1990). Drug interactions with fluconazole. *Rev. Infect. Dis.* **12**:5327–5333.

Louie, E., Rice, L. B., and Holzman, R. S. (1986). Tuberculosis in non-Haitian patients with acquired immunodeficiency syndrome. *Chest* **90**:542–545.

Mallolas, J., Gatell, J. M., Rovira, M., Conget, J. I., Trilla, A., and Somano, E. (1988). Vertebral arch tuberculosis in two human immunodeficiency virus-seropositive heroin addicts. *Arch. Intern. Med.* **48**:1125–1127.

Mann, J., Snider, D. E., Francis, H., Quinn, T. C., Colebunders, R. L, Piot, P., Curran, J. W., Hzilambi, M., Bosenge, M., Malongam, Kulunga, D., Mzingg, M. M., and Bagala, N. (1986). Association between HTLV-III/LAV infection and tuberculosis in Zaire. *JAMA* **256**:346.

Masur, H., Ognibene, F. P., Yarchoan, R., Shelhamer, J. H., Baird, B. F., Travis, W., Suffredini, A. F., Deyton, L. F., Kovacs, J. A., Falloon, J., Davey, R., Polis, M., Metcalf, J., Baseler, M., Wesley, R., Gill, V. J., Fauci, A. S., and Lane, C. (1989). CD4 counts as predictors of opportunistic pneumonias in human immunodeficiency virus (HIV) infection. *Ann. Intern. Med.* **111**:223–227.

Millar, J. W., and Horne, N. W. (1979). Tuberculosis in immunosuppressed patients. *Lancet* **1**:1176–1178.

Modilevsky, T., Sattler, F. R., and Barnes, P. F. (1989). Mycobacterial disease in patients with human immunodeficiency virus infection. *Arch. Intern. Med.* **149**:2201–2205.

Nolan, C. M., Heckbert, S., and Elarth, A. (1988). Case-control study of the association between human immunodeficiency virus infection and tuberculosis [Abstract]. *Abstracts Fourth International Conference on AIDS*. Abstr. 4620.

Ornorata, I. M., McCray, E., and Field Services Branch (1992). Prevalence of human immunodeficiency virus infection among patients attending tuberculosis clinics in the United States. *J. Infect. Dis.* **165**:87–92.

Pape, J. W., Liautaud, B., Thomas, F., Mathurin, J. R., Stamand, M. M., Boncy, M., Pean, V., Pamphile, M., Larouche, A. C., and Johnson, W. D. (1983). Characteristics of the acquired immunodeficiency syndrome (AIDS) in Haiti. *N. Engl. J. Med.* **309**:945–950.

Pitchenik, A. E., and Rubinson, H. A. (1985). The radiographic appearance of tuberculosis in patients with the acquired immunodeficiency syndrome (AIDS) and pre-AIDS. *Am. Rev. Respir. Dis.* **131**:393–396.

Pitchenik, A. E., Russell, B. W., Cleary, T., Pejovic, I., Cole, C., and Snider, D. E., Jr. (1982). The prevalence of tuberculosis and drug resistance among Haitians. *N. Engl. J. Med.* **307**:162–165.

Pitchenik, A. E., Fischl, M. A., Dickinson, G. M., Becker, D. M., Fouriner, A. M., O'Connell, M. T., Colton, R. M., and Spira, T. J. (1983). Opportunistic infections and Kaposi's sarcoma among Haitians: Evidence of a new acquired immunodeficiency state. *Ann. Intern. Med.* **98**: 277–284.

Pitchenik, A. E., Cole, C., Russell, B. W., Fischl, M. A., Spira, T. J., and Snider, D. E., Jr. (1984). Tuberculosis, atypical mycobacteriosis, and the acquired immunodeficiency syndrome among Haitian and non-Haitian patients in South Florida. *Ann. Intern. Med.* **101**:641–645.

Pitchenik, A. E., Burr, J., Suarez, M., Fertel, D., Gonzalez, G., and Moas, C. (1987). Human T-cell lymphotropic virus-III (HTLV-III) seropositivity and related disease among 71 consecutive patients in whom tuberculosis was diagnosed. *Am. Rev. Respir. Dis.* **135**:875–879.

Reichman, L. B. (1991). The "U"-shaped curve of concern. *Am. Rev. Respir. Dis.* **144**:741–742.

Reider, H. L., and Snider, D. E. (1986). Tuberculosis and the acquired immunodeficiency syndrome. *Chest* **90**:469–470.

Reider, H. L., Cauthen, G. M., Comstock, G. W., and Snider, D. E., Jr. (1989). Epidemiology of tuberculosis in the United States. *Epidemiol. Rev.* **11**:79–98.

Root, H. F. (1934). The association of diabetes and tuberculosis. *N. Engl. J. Med.* **210**:1–13.

Saltzman, B. R., Motyl, M. R., Friedland, G. H., McKitrick, J. C., and Klein, R. S. (1986). *Mycobacterium tuberculosis* bacteremia in the acquired immunodeficiency syndrome. *JAMA* **256**:390–391.

Scordamaglia, A., Bagnasco, M., and Canonica, G. W. (1988). Immune response to mycobacteria: Characterization of immunocompetent cells in tuberculous lesions of humans. In *Mycobacterium tuberculosis: Interactions with the Immune System*. Edited by M. Bendinelli and H. Friedman. Plenum Press, New York, pp. 81–98.

Selwyn, P. A., Hartel, D., Lewis, V. A., Schoenbaum, E. E., Vermund, S. H., Klein, R. S., Walker, A., and Friedland, G. H. (1989). A prospective study of the risk of tuberculosis among intravenous drug users with human immunodeficiency virus infection. *N. Engl. J. Med.* **320**:545–550.

Shafer, R. W., Goldberg, R., Sierra, M., and Glatt, A. E. (1989). Frequency of *Mycobacterium tuberculosis* bacteremia in patients with tuberculosis in an area endemic for AIDS. *Am. Rev. Respir. Dis.* **140**:1611–1613.

Small, P. M., Schecter, G. F., Goodman, P. C., Sande, M. A., Chaisson, R. E., and Hopewell, P. C. (1991). Treatment of tuberculosis in patients with advanced human immunodeficiency virus infection. *N. Engl. J. Med.* **324**:289–294.

Standaert, B., Niragira, F., Kadende, P., and Piot, P. (1989). The association of tuberculosis and HIV infection in Burundi. *AIDS Res. Hum. Retroviruses* **5**:247–251.

Sunderam, G., McDonald, R. J., Maniatis, T., Olecke, Kapila, R., and Reichman, L. B. (1986). Tuberculosis as a manifestation of the acquired immunodeficiency syndrome (AIDS). *JAMA* **256**:362–366.

Sunderam, G., Mangura, B. T., Lombardo, J. M., and Reichman, L. B. (1987). Failure of "optimal" four-drug short-course tuberculosis chemotherapy in a compliant patient with human immunodeficiency virus. *Am. Rev. Respir. Dis.* **136**:1475–1478.

Theuer, C. P., Hopewell, P. C., Elias, D., Schecter, G. F., Rutherford, G. S., and Chaisson, R. E. (1990). Human immunodeficiency virus infection in tuberculosis patients. *J. Infect. Dis.* **162**:8–12.

Wadhawan, D., Mwansa, N., Tembo, G., and Perine, P. L. (1990). Isoniazid prophylaxis among patients with HIV-1 infections. [Abstract] *Sixth International Conference on AIDS.* Abst. ThB 510, 249.

Wilson, W. R., Cockerill, R. F. III, and Rosenow, E. C. III (1985). Pulmonary disease in the immunocompromised host. *Mayo Clin. Proc.* **60**:610–631.

18

Tuberculosis and Human Immunodeficiency Virus Infection in Africa

DONALD A. ENARSON

University of Alberta
Edmonton, Alberta, Canada
and International Union Against Tuberculosis
and Lung Disease
Paris, France

DANIEL S. NYANGULU

Ministry of Health
Lilongwe, Malawi

H. J. CHUM

National Tuberculosis and Leprosy
Programme
Ministry of Health
Dar-es-Salaam, Tanzania

M. ANGÉLICA SALOMÃO

Ministry of Health
Maputo, Republic of Mozambique

M. GNINAFON

National Centre of Pneumophthisiology
Cotonou, Benin

I. Human Immunodeficiency Virus and Acquired Immune Deficiency Syndrome

A. Occurrence of Human Immunodeficiency Virus and Acquired Immune Deficiency Syndrome in Africa

It now seems to be generally accepted that human immunodeficiency virus (HIV) infection initially arose in Africa and spread from there to other parts of the world. In spite of this fact, the numbers of acquired immune deficiency syndrome (AIDS) cases reported from Africa are considerably lower than the numbers reported from the Americas (World Health Organization [WHO], 1990). That this reflects a good deal of underreporting is clear. At present, the Global Programme on AIDS of the World Health Organization estimates that there are 6 million persons infected with HIV in Africa (WHO, 1991). Even from the reported number of AIDS cases each year, it is clear that the difference between numbers of reported cases in Africa compared with the numbers reported from the Americas is rapidly diminishing.

Infection with HIV and AIDS is not evenly distributed throughout the world, throughout each continent, or even within a single country. In calculating rates based on the reported AIDS cases in Africa, it is clear that the highest reported rates are in the countries of central Africa; ranked by descending order of magnitude are Malawi, Uganda, Burundi, Kenya, Congo, Zaire, and Ivory Coast (Styblo and Enarson, 1991). These figures, however, must be viewed with caution, as the extent of reporting may be somewhat limited and may vary from one country to another. Studies of HIV infection within a single country also show wide variation in the prevalence of seropositivity. For example, in Tanzania, the disease was first detected in the Kagera region in 1983, and this area has continued to experience the highest rates in the country; other areas, such as Arusha and Kilimanjaro regions, demonstrate considerably lower levels of seropositivity (Mhalu et al., 1987). Within Kagera region itself, the prevalence of seropositivity varied from 24% in urban areas to nearly 0% in some rural areas (Killewo et al., 1990). In neighboring Rwanda, a national survey of HIV infection in 1986 (Rwandan HIV Seroprevalence Study Group, 1989) revealed a striking difference between urban and rural prevalence (19 vs 4%), with highest rates (30%) in urban residents aged 26–40 years.

Thus, to determine the impact of HIV infection on the tuberculosis situation, it is necessary (and instructive) to compare the situation of one area with that in another, where the levels of the HIV problem differ.

B. Epidemiological Pattern of Human Immunodeficiency Virus in Africa

The mode of spread of HIV infection in Africa is different from that in some other parts of the world, in that it is primarily through heterosexual intercourse, as with other venereal diseases and, to a lesser extent, by means of infected blood, and from mother to infant (Quinn et al., 1986). As a consequence, those with a likelihood of the greatest number of sexual partners are those most affected by the virus: prostitutes, barmaids, truck drivers, armed forces personnel, police, and traveling business persons. The infection has its greatest impact along trucking routes, in large cities, and at work sites where family-living quarters are not available.

II. Relation Between Human Immunodeficiency Virus and Tuberculosis

A. Mechanism of Virus–Tuberculosis Interaction

Sutherland has summarized the mechanisms by which HIV infection will impinge on the tuberculosis situation (Sutherland, 1990); to paraphrase:

1. Through endogenous reactivation of previous tuberculous infection in persons infected with HIV

2. Through exogenous tuberculous infection in persons already infected with HIV

3. Additional cases in the general population caused by infection arising from contact with the increased number of tuberculosis cases among persons infected with HIV in the former two groups

The contribution of the latter group to the tuberculosis situation will depend on the total number of cases arising in the first two groups, the infectivity of such cases, the degree and duration of their contact with HIV-negative persons, and the underlying level and trend of tuberculosis in the community.

The greatest likelihood is that most of the excess new cases at the outset of the HIV epidemic will arise by endogenous reactivation of previous tuberculous infection in those dually infected with both tuberculosis and HIV. It is instructive, therefore, to examine the coincidence of the two infections under various circumstances. Accordingly, we may examine the age-specific prevalence of tuberculous infection at various risk levels of such infection in the community, derived from real data (Grzybowski, 1965; Allen, 1987): rates for the population of native Indians in Ontario, Canada, in 1960 (at a point when chemotherapy was just being introduced), in the nonaboriginal Canadian-born population in 1960 (5 years after the introduction of chemotherapy), and in the nonaboriginal Canadian-born population in British Columbia in 1987 (30 years after the widespread use of chemotherapy) are shown in Figure 1. When the risk of tuberculous infection was high, most of the population had already been infected by the age of 20 years. When the risk of tuberculous infection is very low, almost all infected persons are over the age of 50 years and had been infected many years before.

To determine the expected coincidence of infection with HIV and with tuberculosis in different age groups in Africa, we can superimpose the age-specific prevalence of AIDS cases in Zambia (Fleming, 1990) on the age-specific prevalence of tuberculous infection at various levels in the community (see Fig. 1). The striking difference in potential influence of HIV on tuberculosis between areas with a low, compared with a high, prevalence of tuberculous infection is immediately obvious, in that the overlap of HIV and tuberculous infections is very high in the latter and almost nonexistent in the former. As this is the initiating step in the spiral of exacerbation of the tuberculosis situation, the expected result will be very different under different circumstances. Thus, in Africa, where the annual risk of tuberculous infection is often between 1.0 and 1.5%, the effect of HIV infection would be expected to be rather large.

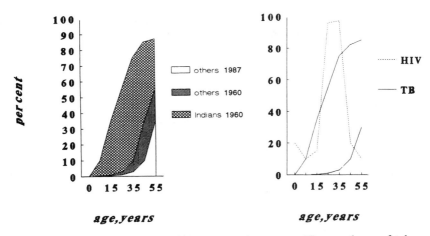

Figure 1 The right-hand figure demonstrates the age-specific prevalence of tuberculous infection at various risk levels of such infection in the community. The left-hand figure shows the superimposition of the age-specific distribution of AIDS patients on these curves.

B. Prevalence of Human Immunodeficiency Virus in Tuberculosis Patients

Because of the uneven distribution of HIV infection, even within one region in Africa, summary figures for the seroprevalence of HIV must be viewed with caution. In particular, it is misleading to take figures from unrepresentative groups of patients or from small areas (particularly the larger cities), as these are heavily biased by the types of patients who receive care in particular institutions or who live in an urban area.

Nevertheless, keeping this caution in mind, some figures are available. Thus, in the far north of Malawi in 1989, of consecutive new cases of tuberculosis, 9 (17%) of 52 men and 5 (10%) of 51 women were seropositive (Ponninghaus et al., 1991). In Abidjan, Ivory Coast in 1989 (De Cock et al., 1991), 40% of 2043 consecutive ambulant tuberculosis patients were positive. In Kampala, Uganda in 1989 (Eriki et al., 1991), 39 (66%) of 59 consecutive cases of pulmonary tuberculosis were seropositive. In 1987 in Kinshasa, Zaire (Perriens et al., 1991), 170 (22%) of 767 consecutive cases of bacillary pulmonary tuberculosis were seropositive. Previous reports from Zaire in 1985 (Colebunders et al., 1988; Mann et al., 1986) had indicated that 40% of 231 cases were seropositive. In Bangui, Central African Republic, in 1987 (Mbolidi et al., 1988), 55% of 55 cases were seropositive. In Zambia in 1988 (Meeran, 1989), 50% of 54 cases were seropositive. In Senegal, of 235 consecutive bacillary pulmonary cases in 1989, 4% were seropositive; in Benin, the figure for 1989 was 6% of 100 cases; in Mozambique, 2% of 1450 cases were seropositive in 1990.

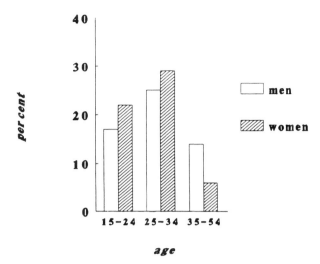

Figure 2 Distribution of HIV seropositivity by age and gender in consecutive patients with tuberculosis, Tanzania, 1989.

Tuberculosis patients are one of the groups in which HIV seroprevalence is high. Figure 2 shows the prevalence by age and sex in consecutive new smear-positive patients with pulmonary tuberculosis in Tanzania in 1989. A similar distribution by age and sex, varying principally in the level, has been observed in other countries. This distribution, with highest levels in young people between the ages of 15 and 34, is to be expected because of the coincidence of the two infections with the resultant endogenous reactivation of latent tuberculous infection. The prevalence of HIV infection in consecutive cases of other forms of tuberculosis (smear-negative pulmonary and extrapulmonary tuberculosis) is even higher, as noted in Zaire in 1985 (where 47% of extrapulmonary, compared with 33% of smear-positive pulmonary cases, were seropositive). Currently, in some areas, a high proportion of all tuberculosis cases are infected with HIV.

III. Effects of Human Immunodeficiency Virus Infection on the Tuberculosis Situation

A. Influence of Human Immunodeficiency Virus on Tuberculosis Rates

Because of the increased rate of development of active tuberculosis from dually infected individuals, it would be expected that the rates of tuberculosis would rise as a result. Indeed, the numbers of cases have risen in Burundi

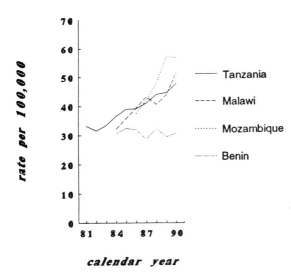

Figure 3 Trend in new smear-positive pulmonary tuberculosis notification rates, Malawi, Mozambique, Benin, and Tanzania.

(Slutkin et al., 1988) and in Tanzania (Murray, 1989) since the first case of AIDS was reported in 1983. Because of the rapid rate of population growth in developing countries, however, it is misleading to look only at the number of cases. Indeed, a comparison of trends in notification rates of bacillary pulmonary cases of tuberculosis in four countries, where reporting has been reasonably complete—Mozambique, Tanzania, Malawi, and Benin—indicates that the rise is not quite as steep as indicated when looking only at the numbers (Fig. 3). Moreover, the notification rates of tuberculosis, even now, although much higher than those at present in North America and Western Europe, are much lower than those in the latter two locations 70 years ago, when the economic situation was more like that in central Africa today. If one compares the level of notifications with those expected based on the estimated average annual risk of infection (Murray et al., 1990), it is possible to compare countries that are more heavily affected by HIV (Malawi and Tanzania) with those less affected (Benin and Mozambique). What is obvious (Fig. 4) is that those countries most heavily affected by HIV do not have strikingly higher notification rates of tuberculosis than those not so much affected. Moreover, in comparing the trend of notification rates observed in Tanzania with those expected (Fig. 5), it is apparent that at least part of the rise in rates is due to extension of the National Tuberculosis and Leprosy Programme throughout the country and the better access to care that this entails. Although there is no doubt that HIV infection will (and already has) worsened the epidemiological situations of tuberculosis, conclusively documenting this effect is not easy.

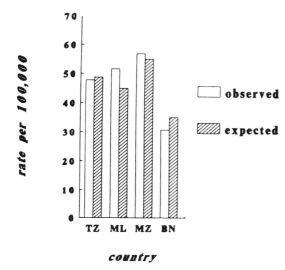

Figure 4 Observed notification rates of smear-positive pulmonary tuberculosis compared with expected rates, Malawi (ML), Mozambique (MZ), Benin (BN), and Tanzania (TZ).

B. Human Immunodeficiency Virus and the Epidemiological Profile of Tuberculosis

The distribution of tuberculosis cases by time, place, and person constitutes the *epidemiological profile* of the disease. We have discussed, in the previous section, the trend in tuberculosis notification rates and the difficulty in definitively

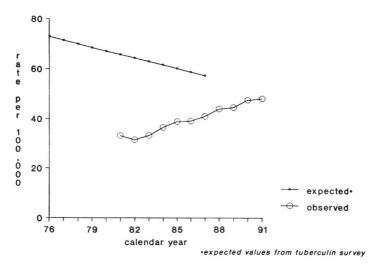

Figure 5 Trend in observed and expected rates of smear-positive pulmonary tuberculosis in Tanzania.

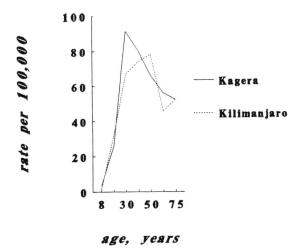

Figure 6 Age-specific notification rates of smear-positive pulmonary tuberculosis in Kagera (with a high prevalence of HIV infection) and Kilimanjaro (with a low prevalence of HIV infection), Tanzania, 1989.

demonstrating the effect of HIV on those rates. We have noted, as well, that the distribution of HIV infection varies markedly by geographic location, both among countries and within countries. The prevalence of tuberculous infection varies similarly. It would be expected that the effect of HIV on tuberculosis would vary accordingly.

The influence of HIV on the age-specific distribution of tuberculosis can be illustrated in Tanzania. A comparison of age-specific notification rates of smear-positive pulmonary tuberculosis between regions with high (Kagera) and low (Kilimanjaro) prevalence of HIV infection in 1989 (Fig. 6). indicates that the effect of HIV infection (the difference between the two curves) is almost totally between the ages of 15 and 44, where it would be most expected owing to the coexistence of the two infections.

The notification rate of new cases of smear-positive pulmonary tuberculosis in 1989 were 30:100,000 population in Kilimanjaro (where HIV is relatively uncommon), compared with 34:100,000 where it is quite common.

C. The Clinical Profile of Tuberculosis in the Presence of Human Immunodeficiency Virus

Several reports indicate a difference in the clinical appearance of tuberculosis in AIDS patients, compared with those not infected with HIV. These differences include a higher proportion of disseminated infections (a number with positive blood cultures); a lower proportion of bacillary infections; the involvement of atypical areas, such as the lower lobes of the lung, on chest radiograph; an increased frequency of hilar lymphadenopathy; and the presence of uncommon forms of extrapulmonary tuberculosis.

A significant change in the clinical appearance of tuberculosis in communities in which HIV infection is common may lead to difficulties in diagnosis of the disease, with a subsequent delay in commencing treatment, resulting in an increased risk of infection in the community and a greater degree of suffering for the patients. In Zaire in 1985 (Colebunders et al., 1988), 13% of cases were extrapulmonary, thought to be an increase from the proportion in previous periods. In Malawi (Reeve, 1989), a series of patients from a large referral hospital contained 38% with pleural effusion, 6% with lymph node tuberculosis, 7% with pericarditis, and 6% with miliary tuberculosis. In Kenya (Gilks et al., 1990), in a series of 506 consecutive cases hospitalized in a referral center, the proportion of extrapulmonary cases was significantly elevated in seropositive, compared with seronegative, patients (nine compared with five cases). The excess was greatest for lymphadenitis and disseminated tuberculosis. These observations should be viewed with great caution as, in most instances, they represent hospital-based series of cases from large referral centers and may represent a biased sample of patients.

To determine whether the clinical picture of the disease in·a community changes when HIV becomes common, we have compared the distribution of cases in communities where HIV is common with that in communities where HIV is uncommon and the trend in the same communities as HIV becomes increasingly common.

Figure 7 shows a distribution comparison of types of cases of tuberculosis in Malawi in 1990 and in Kilimanjaro, Tanzania in 1989. In both locations,

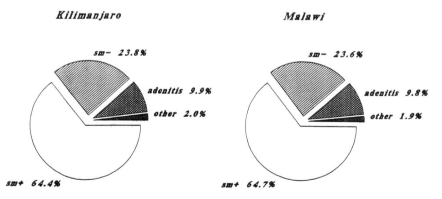

Figure 7 Distribution of types of tuberculosis in Malawi, 1990, compared with Kilimanjaro, Tanzania, 1989. sm⁺; smear-positive pulmonary tuberculosis; sm⁻; smear-negative pulmonary tuberculosis.

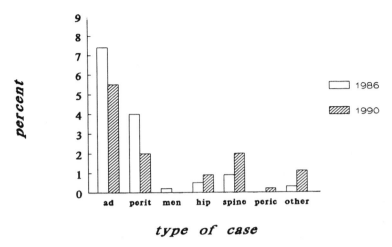

Figure 8 Trend in sites of extrapulmonary tuberculosis in Mangochi Hospital, Malawi, 1986–1990. ad, adenitis; perit, peritonitis; men, meningitis; peric, pericarditis.

infectious smear-positive cases of pulmonary tuberculosis are equally common and account for most of all cases reported.

Figure 8 indicates the distribution of types of extrapulmonary tuberculosis (excluding tuberculous pleurisy) in Mangochi Hospital in Malawi in 1986, compared with 1990. The most common form in both periods was tuberculous lymphadenitis, followed by tuberculous pericarditis and tuberculosis of the spine. It is quite clear, on visiting such a hospital, that unusual cases such as tuberculous pericarditis are seen, but they do not account for the majority of cases and, in general, the appearance of tuberculosis in the community is similar to that in communities with little or no HIV infection, but a similar risk of tuberculous infection.

The influence of HIV infection on the radiographic appearance of tuberculosis is also a matter of interest. We have systematically examined chest radiographs, using a similar method of reading, of consecutive cases of bacillary pulmonary tuberculosis, comparing patients in a setting in which both HIV and tuberculosis are common (Malawi, 1990); in which tuberculosis is common, and HIV is not present (Indians of Canada, 1970); in which tuberculosis is relatively common, but HIV is uncommon (Kilimanjaro region, Tanzania, 1990); and in which neither tuberculosis nor HIV was common (nonaboriginal Canadian-born persons in Alberta, 1989). Whereas the extent of radiographic involvement was related to the amount of tuberculosis in the community (where it was common, the disease was more extensive and vice versa) and unrelated to the presence of HIV (Fig. 9), the presence of cavitation on the chest radiograph was less common in association with a high level of HIV in the community, and unrelated to the level of tuberculosis (Fig. 10).

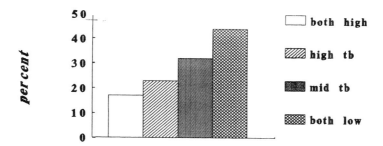

Figure 9 Extent of radiographic involvement (proportion of cases with disease restricted to a single apex) in cases of bacillary tuberculosis, according to the level of tuberculosis and of HIV in the community. both high, high level of tuberculosis and high level of HIV; high tb, high level of tuberculosis and no HIV; mid tb, moderate level of tuberculosis and low level of HIV; both low, low level of tuberculosis and no HIV.

The decline in immunocompetence in AIDS patients might be expected to result in an increasing occurrence of relapse in patients previously cured of tuberculosis. Figure 11 indicates the trend in relapses as a proportion of all cases of smear-positive pulmonary tuberculosis in Malawi. There is no increase in the proportion of relapse cases reported over the period in which HIV infection became well established in the country.

D. Treatment of Tuberculosis Patients Infected with Human Immunodeficiency Virus

The possibility that HIV infection might interfere with the patient's response to chemotherapy raises concerns about the treatment of such cases. The

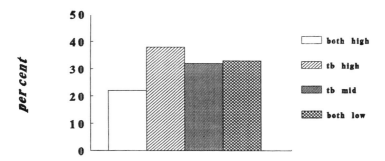

Figure 10 Frequency of cavitation on radiographs of consecutive cases of bacillary pulmonary tuberculosis according to level of tuberculosis and of HIV. For definitions of the groups see legend of Figure 9.

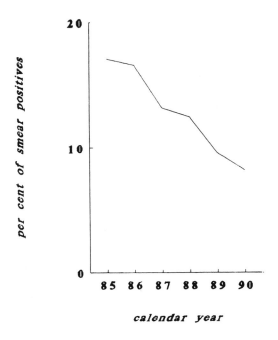

Figure 11 Trend in proportion of relapses among all smear-positive cases of pulmonary tuberculosis, Malawi.

possibility that treatment would not be as effective in the increasing number of cases raises the possibility of a further increase in the risk of transmission of tuberculous infection by leaving a greater number of sources of infection in the community.

It is clear that patients with HIV infection are more likely to die during the course of their treatment than those who are not infected. Thus, 32.5% of HIV seropositive patients, compared with 1.5% of seronegative cases, died while on a 12-month chemotherapy regimen in one report from Zaire (Willarne et al., 1988) and, in another report from Zaire (Perriens et al., 1991), the corresponding figures were 31.3%, compared with 4.4% The difference between the groups in the latter report widened further over the subsequent 12 months of follow-up (57.6% compared with 6.6% of the patients were dead).

Figure 12 indicates the survival of patients with HIV infection compared with those without HIV infection in Tanzania. The HIV-infected patients experience a continuing fatality long after conversion of their sputum smears and after completion of their chemotherapy. At the time of completion of their treatment, approximately one-third had died and by 18 months of follow-up one-half were dead. Most of these patients died of other complications (such as severe diarrhea), and their sputum smears remained negative. This adverse outcome, naturally, makes the overall results of treatment worse. It is unlikely,

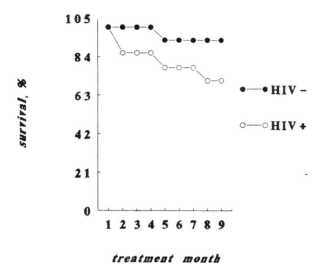

Figure 12 Trend in survival of new cases of smear-positive pulmonary tuberculosis in Tanzania, 1989, according to HIV status.

however, that the problem of relapse after cure in those who are HIV infected at the outset will be common, as the patients are unlikely to survive long enough to be at risk of relapse.

The results of treatment with 12-month chemotherapy (without the use of rifampin) may be worse in tuberculosis patients who are seropositive, compared with those who are seronegative. Thus, in Burundi (Standaert et al., 1989), 11% of cases at a large center were classified as treatment "failures," all of whom were HIV seropositive. In Zaire (Perriens et al., 1991), the relapse rate after 12-month chemotherapy was much higher (18.1%) in seropositive, compared with seronegative, patients (6.0%) in the 12 months after the completion of chemotherapy.

An evaluation of treatment results in National Tuberculosis Programmes that used the "modified" short-course chemotherapy recommended in International Union Against Tuberculosis and Lung Disease (IUATLD)-assisted Programmes shows considerably better results. It is clear that the response to treatment in patients who survive the course of therapy is no different in areas where HIV is common than where it is uncommon, being very good in both situations. For example, in the first half of 1990 in Tanzania, of 179 new cases of smear-positive pulmonary tuberculosis, in the Kagera region, who were still alive at the end of their 8 months of treatment, 170 (95.0%) were cured, compared with 156 (88.6%) of such cases in Kilimanjaro region.

Treatment of tuberculosis in patients with HIV infection is complicated by the danger inherent in giving injections and by the occurrence of adverse reactions to medications. Although the risk for the spread of HIV infection by individual injections given under controlled circumstances is small, the utilization of injections on a large scale throughout a country with meager resources may pose a risk of transmission of the disease. Thus, in a country with 15,000 cases of tuberculosis per year, nearly 1 million injections would be given if streptomycin is used in the initial intensive phase of therapy. If a large proportion of the tuberculosis patients (for example, one-third) are HIV-positive, the risk of transmission of HIV infection through the continued administration of injections is not small, especially because such injections are given at many locations and to an increasing number of patients at each site, stretching the capacity of the staff of the peripheral health institutions to cope. Clearly, the use of streptomycin in the routine treatment of tuberculosis patients where HIV infection is common must be reconsidered.

Of all antituberculosis medications, adverse reactions to thiacetazone (amithiozone) are most serious, with the Stevens–Johnson syndrome associated with a high fatality rate (Nunn et al., 1991). The occurrence of this reaction appears to be greatly increased by the presence of HIV infection. In Malawi, the occurrence of deaths from Stevens–Johnson syndrome increased greatly (to approximately 1% of patients in some centers) by 1990 and appeared to be entirely related to patients who were HIV-positive. This occurrence resulted in efforts to make all clinicians aware of the problem and, when any patient was known to be HIV-positive or at the first sign of any skin reaction, substitution of thiacetazone with ethambutol was advised. Since the institution of this policy, the occurrence rate of the Stevens–Johnson syndrome has been reduced to less than 1 case in 500. The occurrence of these reactions raises serious problems for the treatment of patients in countries with minimal resources and where HIV infection is common, as the substitution of thiacetazone with ethambutol in the continuation phase of treatment greatly increases the cost of treatment.

IV. Mitigating the Effects of Human Immunodeficiency Virus

A. Prevention of Tuberculosis in the Face of Human Immunodeficiency Virus

Although the initial effect of HIV infection is primarily on those who also have tuberculous infection, the more important consequences, as far as the level of tuberculosis in the community is concerned, is the increase in the transmission of tuberculous infection by the excess of infective patients caused by HIV infection. Prevention of tuberculosis is first and foremost primary prevention: the prevention of transmission of tuberculous infection. Primary prevention is achieved by diagnosis, treatment, and cure of as many smear-positive, infectious patients with pulmonary tuberculosis as possible. The control of transmission of tuberculous infection in the community is best achieved in this way (Rouillon et al., 1976). This is as true in the presence of HIV infection as before its entry into the community. As we noted previously, infectious patients continue to be detectable by sputum smear microscopy and curable by the regimens currently employed, even when the level of HIV infection in the community is relatively high. Moreover, the current level of tuberculosis in communities, even in the presence of HIV infection, remains considerably below that experienced in Europe and North America in the early part of this century. With a concerted effort and cooperation of donor-partners, it should be possible to reduce the effect of HIV infection on the transmission of tuberculosis in the community. If action is not taken soon, however, the situation will very likely become unmanageable in some countries.

Secondary prevention of tuberculosis after HIV infection (preventing tuberculous disease in those already infected) should be possible with the use of preventive chemotherapy. The response to chemotherapy of tuberculosis patients with HIV infection gives us some hope that this might be achieved. On the other hand, the disappointing results of "standard" chemotherapy may lend a note of caution. Nevertheless, the evaluation of preventive chemotherapy in this situations is presently being undertaken, although no results are yet available. The widespread application of this measure, however, may be difficult to accomplish in areas where resources are limited and that are not yet even capable of dealing with the active cases.

Secondary prevention of tuberculosis with BCG vaccination is even more difficult to evaluate. It appears that vaccination in those without evidence of immunosuppression is without untoward effects, and its administration even in communities with evident HIV infection is still recommended.

B. Surveillance of Human Immunodeficiency Virus in Tuberculosis Patients

Tuberculosis patients are one of the groups within the community with the highest prevalence of HIV infection. Moreover, the presence and trend of HIV infection among tuberculosis patients has major importance in planning for the future of tuberculosis programs. The increase in the number of cases in several countries in Africa has been noted in the foregoing. The ability to provide regular care for the cases in these countries has depended on the ability to predict the rate of increase in the number of cases so that financial support and material supplies could be planned. Consequently, one of the recommendations of the subregional seminar "Tuberculosis as a Public Health Priority" held in Zimbabwe in mid-1991, was that tuberculosis patients be included among the groups eligible for testing in the routine sentinel surveillance of the National AIDS Programmes in the countries of Africa.

References

Allen, E. A. (1987). Results of tuberculin testing in nonvaccinated members of the general population by age. Division of Tuberculosis Control, Ministry of Health, British Columbia.

Colebunders, R. L., Karahunga, C., Ryder, R., Ririe, D., Nzila, N., and Perriens, G. (1988). Seroprevalence of HIV-1 antibody among tuberculosis patients in Zaire 1985–87. *Int. Congr. Ser.* **810**:222.

De Cock, K. M., Gnaore, E., Adjorlolo, G., Braun, M. M., Lafontaine, M. F., Yesso, G., Bretton, G., Coulibaly, I. M., Gershy-Damet, G. M., Retton, R., and Heyward, W. L. (1991). Risk of tuberculosis in patients with HIV-1 and HIV-2 infections in Abidjan, Ivory Coast. *Br. Med. J.* **302**:496–499.

Eriki, P. P., Okwera, A., Aisu, T., Morrissey, A. B., Ellner, J. J., and Daniel, T. M. (1991). The influence of human immunodeficiency virus infection on tuberculosis in Kampala, Uganda. *Am. Rev. Respir. Dis.* **143**: 185–187.

Fleming, A. F. (1990). Opportunistic infections in AIDS in developed and developing countries. *Trans. Roy. Soc. Trop. Med. Hyg.* **84**(Suppl. 1): 1–6.

Grzybowski, S. (1965). Ontario studies of tuberculin sensitivity. 1. Tuberculin testing of various population groups. *Can. Med. Assoc. J.* **56**:181–192.

Gilks, C. F., Brindle, R. J., Otieno, L. S., Bhatt, S. M., Newnham, R. S., Simani, P. M., Lule, G. N., Okelo, G. B. A., Watkins, W. M., Waiyaki, P. G., Were, J. O. B., and Warrell, D. A. (1990). Extrapulmonary and disseminated tuberculosis in HIV-1 seropositive patients presenting to the acute medical services in Nairobi. *AIDS* **4**:981–985.

Killewo, J., Nyamuryekunge, K., Sandstrom, A., Bredberg-Raden, U., Wall, S., Mhalu, F., and Biberfeld, G. (1990). Prevalence of HIV-1 infection in the Kagera region of Tanzania: A population-based study. *AIDS* **4**:1081–1085.

Mann, J., Snider, D. E., Francis, H., Quinn, T. C., Colebunders, R. L, Piot, P., Curran, J. W., Nzilambi, N., Bosenge, N., Malonga, M., Kalunga, D. Nzingg, M. M., and Bagala, N. (1986). Association between HTLV-III/LAV infection and tuberculosis in Zaire. *JAMA* **256**:346.

Mbolidi, C. D., Cathebras, P., and Vohito, M. D. (1988). Parallel increase in the prevalence of pulmonary tuberculosis and infection with HIV in Bangui. *Presse Med.* **17**:872–873.

Meeran, K. (1989). Prevalence of HIV infection among patients with leprosy and tuberculosis in rural Zambia. *Br. Med. J.* **298**:364–365.

Mhalu, F., Bredberg-Raden, U., and Mbena, E. (1987). Prevalence of HIV-1 infection in healthy subjects and groups of patients in Tanzania. *AIDS* **1**:217–221.

Murray, C. J. L., Styblo, K., and Rouillon, A. (1990). Tuberculosis in developing countries: burden, intervention and cost. *Bull. Int. Union Tuberc. Lung Dis.* **65**:2–20.

Murray, J. (1989). The white plague: Down and out, or up and coming? *Am. Rev. Respir. Dis.* **140**:1788–1795.

Nunn, P., Gathua, S., Brindle, R., Imalingat, N., Gilks, C. F., Omwega, M., Were, J., and Macadam, K. (1991). Cutaneous hypersensitivity reactions due to thiacetazone in HIV-1 seropositive patients treated for tuberculosis. *Lancet* **337**:627–630.

Perriens, J. H., Colebunders, R. L., Karahunga, C., Willame, J. C., Jeugmans, J., Kaboto, M., Mukadi, Y., Pauwels, P., Ryder, R. W., Prignot, J., and Piot, P. (1991). Increased mortality and tuberculosis treatment failure rate among human immunodeficiency virus (HIV) seropositive compared with HIV seronegative patients with pulmonary tuberculosis treated with "standard" chemotherapy in Kinshasa, Zaire. *Am. Rev. Respir. Dis.* **144**:750–755.

Ponninghaus, J. M., Luckson, J., Mwanjasi, J., Fine, P. E. M., Shaw, M. A., Turner, A. C., Oxborrow, S. M., Lucas, S. B., Jenkins, P. A., Sterne, J. A. C., and Bliss, L. (1991). Is HIV infection a risk for leprosy? *Int. J. Lepr.* **59**:221–228.

Quinn, T. C., Mann, J. M., Curran, J. W., and Piot, P. (1986). AIDS in Africa: An epidemiologic paradigm. *Science* **234**:955–963.

Reeve, P. A. (1989). HIV infection in patients admitted to a general hospital in Malawi. *Br. Med. J.* **298**:1567–1568.

Rouillon, A., Perdrizet, S., and Parrot, R. (1976). Transmission of tubercle bacilli: The effects of chemotherapy. *Tubercle* **57**:275–299.

Rwandan HIV Seroprevalence Study Group (1989). Nationwide community-based serological survey of HIV-1 and other human retrovirus infection in a central African country. *Lancet* **1**:941–943.

Slutkin, G., Leowski, J., and Mann. J. (1988). The effects of the AIDS epidemic on the tuberculosis problem and tuberculosis programmes. *Bull. Int. Union Tuberc. Lung Dis.* **63**:21–24.

Standaert, B., Niragira, F., Kadende, P., and Piot, P. (1989). The association of tuberculosis and HIV infection in Burundi. *AIDS Res. Hum. Retrovirus* **5**:247–251.

Styblo, K., and Enarson, D. A. (1991). The impact of infection with human immunodeficiency virus on tuberculosis. In *Recent Advances in Respiratory Medicine*, Vol. 5. Edited by D. M. Mitchell. Edinburgh, Churchill-Livingstone.

Sutherland, I. (1990). The epidemiology of tuberculosis and AIDS. *Commun. Dis. Rep.* **10**:3–4.

Willarne, J. C., Nkoko, B., and Pauwels, P. (1988). Tuberculose et seropositive anti VIH A, Kinshasa, Zaire. *Ann. Soc. Belg. Med. Trop.* **68**:165–167.

World Health Organization (1990). AIDS cases reported as of 1 October 1990. Surveillance, Forecasting and Impact Assessment Unit, Geneva, Switzerland.

World Health Organization (1991). World Health Organization says three-quarters of HIV infections transmitted heterosexually. *WHO Press* WHO/54.

19

Tuberculosis in the Elderly

REYNARD J. McDONALD

University of Medicine and Dentistry of New Jersey–New Jersey Medical School
Newark, New Jersey

I. Epidemiology

Tuberculosis is an important cause of morbidity and death in the world; even though until recently the disease had been in decline in the United States and other industrialized nations. Available estimates indicate that approximately one-third of the world's population has latent tuberculosis infection and that 8 million new cases of tuberculosis and 3 million deaths occur annually worldwide (Styblo and Rouillon, 1981; Centers for Disease Control [CDC], 1989a).

In the United States, an estimated 10 million persons are infected with the tubercle bacillus, and most of the new cases of tuberculosis (approximately 90%) come from this infected pool (CDC, 1991a). Until 1985, the number of cases of tuberculosis reported annually in the United States was in a steady decline. The number of reported cases decreased from 84,304 in 1953, when nationwide reporting began, to 22,255 in 1984 (Fig. 1) (CDC, 1991b). During the same period, tuberculosis case rates decreased from 53:100,000 to 9.4:100,000, respectively (CDC, 1991c). However, since 1985, the number of tuberculosis cases is no longer declining at the expected rate. The downward trend plateaued in 1985 and, subsubsequently, changed to a pattern of modest yearly increases and decreases (Table 1) (CDC, 1991b).

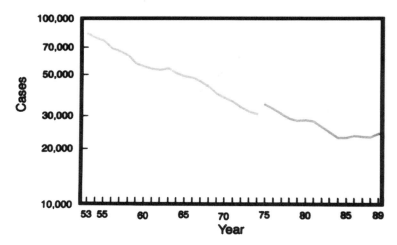

Figure 1 Decline in tuberculosis cases in the United States. (From Tuberculosis Elimination, U.S.A., Division of Tuberculosis Elimination, National Center for Prevention Services, Centers for Disease Control, August, 1991. CDC, 1991b.)

Table 1 Tuberculosis Cases Associated with Leveling of the National Trend

Year	Reported cases	Expected cases	Excess cases	% Associated with change
1985	22,201	21,256	945	4.3
1986	22,768	20,070	2698	11.8
1987	22,517	18,944	3573	15.9
1988	22,436	17,882	4554	20.3
1989	23,495	16,885	6610	28.1
1990	25,701	15,818	9883	38.5

Source: Tuberculosis Elimination, U.S.A., Division of Tuberculosis Elimination, National Center for Preventive Services, Centers for Disease Control, August, 1991. CDC, 1991b.

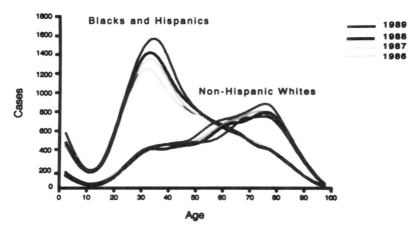

Figure 2 Tuberculosis cases among blacks and Hispanics compared with non-Hispanic whites: United States, 1986–1989. (From Tuberculosis Elimination, U.S.A., Division of Tuberculosis Elimination, National Center for Preventive Services, Centers for Disease Control, August, 1991. CDC, 1991b.)

For 1991, 26,283 verified cases of tuberculosis (10.4:100,000) were reported, a 2.3% increase from the 25,701 cases reported in 1990. These newly reported cases represent approximately 11,000 excess cases for 1991 and increase the estimate of total excess tuberculosis cases to a total of 39,000 for the period from 1985 through 1991.

Although tuberculosis occurs in all segments of the country's population, the increase in morbidity is seen primarily in the younger-aged (25–44 years) groups and is largely because of an increase in tuberculosis cases in persons infected with the human immunodeficiency virus (HIV) (Fig. 2) (CDC, 1989b). Other factors, however, also contribute to the increased tuberculosis morbidity. These include socioeconomic factors, immigration of foreign-born persons with tuberculosis infection, patient noncomliance in following a recommended treatment regimen, and inappropriately prescribed treatment regimens by the physician (CDC, 1990a, 1992).

In the United States, tuberculosis in the non-Hispanic white population is a disease of the elderly ($\geq$ 65 years), but among minorities, it is a disease of the younger-aged groups (Fig. 3). The CDC reported in 1989 that the median age of nonwhite tuberculosis cases was 39 years, compared with 61 years in non-Hispanic whites (Bloch et al., 1989).

For almost a quarter century there has been a progressive decline in tuberculous cases in the geriatric-aged ($\geq$ 65 years) group. In 1965, 9356

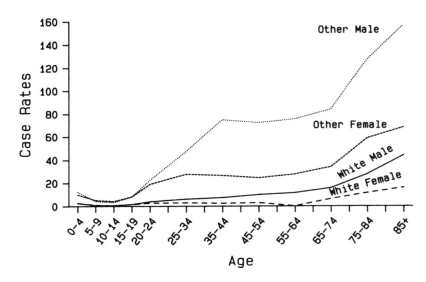

Note: Case rate per 100,000 population.

Figure 3 United States tuberculosis case rates by age and sex, 1989. (From CDC, 1991b.)

tuberculous cases (51.5:100,000) were reported, compared with 6101 cases (19.7:100,000) in 1989 (CDC, 1977, 1991c). Despite this dramatic reduction, a substantial amount of tuberculosis morbidity remains in the elder United States population. Tuberculosis case rates are higher for the over 65-aged group than for any other aged group (CDC, 1990b; Stead and Lofgren, 1983).

In 1989, the United States geriatric population numbered 31 million persons, approximately 90% of whom are white, 8% are black, and 2% are of other races (Native American, Asian/Pacific Islander, and Hispanic) (AARP and AOA, 1990). This elderly cohort represents 12.5% of the United States population, but accounts for 26% of the total number of reported tuberculosis cases (CDC, 1990b).

Among all age groups, regardless of sex, race, or ethnicity, tuberculous case rates are highest in the elderly. Case rates are highest in elderly nonwhite men (100.7:100,000) and are higher in elderly nonwhites than in elderly whites. Rates are also higher in elderly white men (21.3:100,000) than in elderly white women (9.4:100,000) (CDC, 1991c).

The overwhelming majority (95%) of older ($\geq$ 65 years) Americans live in the community, with a much smaller number, 1.5 million persons (5%), residing in nursing homes (Blazer, 1991). Most tuberculosis cases occur among the 95% of the geriatric population who live in the community. However, elderly nursing home residents are at much greater risk of developing disease and, therefore, tuberculous case rates are much higher among the 5% of the geriatric population that reside in nursing homes (CDC, 1989c; Yoshikawa, 1992).

Stead, in a study of tuberculosis in nursing home residents in Arkansas, reported that approximately 80% of new cases of tuberculosis among the elderly occurred in persons living at home and in only 20% in those residing in nursing homes. However, because only 5% of the elderly Arkansas population live in nursing homes, he calculated the tuberculosis case rate to be almost five times greater for nursing home residents than for the elderly living at home (Stead and To, 1987).

A CDC-sponsored study in 1984–1985, reporting several thousand cases of tuberculosis in the elderly from 29 states, found the incidence rate of tuberculosis to be higher (39.2 cases per 100,000) among nursing home residents than among older persons living at home (21.5 cases per 100,000) (CDC, 1990b).

II. Transmission and Pathogenesis

As is true of younger-aged groups, the lungs are the most common site of tuberculosis occurring in the elderly. The lungs are the site of infection in about 83% of cases of tuberculosis in the elderly (CDC, 1991c). This percentage is slightly greater than that reported for those younger than 65 years of age and is partly explained by the increase in extrapulmonary tuberculosis that is occurring in association with HIV infection in the younger-aged groups (Sunderam et al., 1986; Bloch et al., 1989).

In the elderly, tuberculosis arises most commonly as a consequence of endogenous reactivation of previously dormant pulmonary foci that result from exposure to the tubercle bacillus much earlier in life (recrudescent disease) (Riley and O'Grady, 1961; Stead and Dutt, 1989; Bass et al., 1990).

It is thought that with aging many elderly persons lose their tuberculin sensitivity because of complete healing of foci of tuberculous infection that occurred much earlier in life. These immunologically naive individuals are at risk for acquisition of tuberculosis caused by late exogenous reinfection with the tubercle bacillus (Stead and To, 1987; Narain et al., 1985).

The immune response that occurs as a result of infection with *M. tuberculosis* is complicated and is not completely understood. However, recent animal studies suggest that a diminished cell-mediated immune response occurs with increasing age and is probably the major reason for the increased susceptibility of the elderly to tuberculous infection (Yoshikawa, 1992; Orme, 1988). A decline in the ability of aging T lymphocytes to produce interleukin-2 (IL-2) has been reported; however, macrophage function appears to remain intact (Makinodan et al., 1984; Yoshikawa, 1992).

No doubt other confounding influences, including concurrent diseases, malnutrition, and drugs, may all adversely affect the immune system in the elderly.

III. Diagnosis

A. Clinical Manifestations

The clinical manifestations of tuberculosis differ depending on the site of involvement of the disease. In more than 80% of cases of tuberculosis in the elderly, the lung is the site of involvement, and cough is a nonspecific, but common, symptom (American Thoracic Society–CDC; 1990). The cough is usually nonproductive at its onset, but progressive, and may become productive of mucopurulent or blood-streaked sputum. Occasionally, moderate or severe hemoptysis and dull aching chest pain also occur. Chills, fever, night sweats, and myalgia are not infrequent. Pleuritic chest pain is occasionally present and may be associated with the presence of an effusion. Dyspnea is uncommon unless there is widespread parenchymal disease or a large amount of pleural fluid, or unless other concurrent cardiopulmonary disease is present. In most instances, systemic symptoms are not pronounced, but occasionally, an acute toxic febrile course is observed.

Unfortunately, the classic, clinical and roentgenographic features that many physicians have come to recognize as being characteristic of pulmonary tuberculosis may be absent in the elderly (Stead and Dutt, 1989; Morris, 1990). Frequently, symptoms are nonspecific or atypical (Yoshikawa, 1984). Elderly individuals with pulmonary tuberculosis may not manifest the accustomed symptoms of cough, fever, and weight loss and, instead, may present with atypical clinical features or unusual radiographic findings, such as disease involving the lower lung zones (Alvarez et al., 1987; Ip et al., 1986; Chang et al., 1987). The presence of acute or chronic illnesses existing concurrently with tuberculosis may obscure the diagnosis by altering the presentation (MacGee, 1989). Tuberculosis in an elderly person with chronic obstructive pulmonary disease (COPD) or lung cancer may be misdiagnosed, delaying therapy or may be completely missed, only to be found at autopsy (Nagami and Yoshikawa, 1984).

B. Radiographic Features

The usual radiographic features observed in adults, including many elderly adults, with pulmonary tuberculosis are those of recrudescent (reactivation) disease. Roentgenographic findings include parenchymal infiltrates of the apical and posterior segments of the upper lobes and, less commonly, the superior segments of the lower lobes (Bates, 1979; Farman and Speir, 1986). The radiographic pattern of primary tuberculosis that is usually seen in younger-aged groups may occasionally occur in the elderly, such as nursing home residents (Segarra et al., 1963; Parmar, 1967; Berger and Granada, 1974). Recent reports suggest that roentgenographic changes are not restricted to the upper lobes (Morris, 1990). Lymphadenopathy may be unilateral or bilateral and may be present in the absence of parenchymal infiltrates. Diffuse miliary infiltrates also occur.

The lungs are the site of disease in most cases of tuberculosis in the elderly. However, virtually any organ may be involved, and extrapulmonary forms of tuberculosis occur with greater frequency in the elderly (Farer, 1979). These include pleural, skeletal, lymphatic, genitourinary, miliary, central nervous system (CNS), and gastrointestinal forms of tuberculosis. Other sites, including the pericardium, larynx, and middle ear, have also been reported.

Extrapulmonary tuberculosis represents a very difficult diagnostic problem in the elderly, who frequently have concurrent illnesses that obscure the diagnosis of tuberculosis (Slavin et al., 1980).

Chest roentgenography and tuberculin skin test reactivity may be negative in the face of active disease. Diagnosis frequently depends on heightened suspicion, leading to biopsy, with subsequent histological and bacteriological confirmation of tuberculosis. Liver biopsy offers a good diagnostic yield because approximately 97% of cases of extrapulmonary tuberculosis have hepatic involvement (Slavin et al., 1980).

A detailed discussion of extrapulmonary forms of tuberculosis in the elderly is beyond the intended scope of this article, but several publications are available for review (Gertler et al., 1985; Bruckstein, 1988; Yoshikawa, 1992; Dutt and Stead, 1989; Cinman, 1982; Weinburg and Boyd, 1988; Shintani et al., 1990).

C. Smear and Culture

When patients are suspected of having pulmonary tuberculosis because of clinical symptoms, radiographic features, or for other reasons, 10 ml of an early-morning sputum specimen should be collected and submitted for smear and culture for acid-fast bacilli (AFB).

Approximately 50–80% of patients with pulmonary tuberculosis may have a positive sputum smear for AFB. When smears are positive, the collection of three culture specimens on separate days is adequate.

Frequently, the elderly are not able to spontaneously produce sputum. Under these circumstances alternative methods of obtaining sputum specimens become necessary. Sputum induction by inhalation of a saline aerosol is successful in approximately 30–60% of patients (Crawford et al., 1989). Cultures of gastric lavage specimens are positive in 10–34% of patients, but are rarely used in the elderly because of the risk of aspiration and because sputum induction with ultrasonic saline nebulization is equally effective and more accepted by patients. Additionally, gastric lavage specimens are unacceptable for smear because of the presence of saprophytic mycobacteria that are found normally in the gastrointestinal tract, but culture may still be possible. Laryngeal swabbing is effective in approximately 25% of cases. When other lower-risk methods of obtaining sputum are not satisfactory, fiberoptic bronchoscopy with lavage, brushing, and biopsy is a high-yield procedure that may be of benefit to elderly patients in whom sputum cannot be obtained or is negative for AFB on smear.

An unequivocal diagnosis of tuberculosis continues to require culture of *M. tuberculosis* from secretions or tissues of a suspected case. Newer diagnostic methods, using gene probes and immunologic techniques, are increasingly becoming available and allow more rapid and precise identification of *M. tuberculosis* than is possible using traditional culture methods. Although these newer methods will probably eventually replace traditional culture methods, the latter currently remain in widespread use.

D. Tuberculin Skin Test

The tuberculin skin test remains the diagnostic standard for identifying tuberculous infection. It is not a particularly useful tool for diagnosing pulmonary tuberculosis, in which the chest radiograph is usually of much greater diagnostic value; however, the tuberculin skin test may be of particular help when diagnosing extrapulmonary tuberculosis. The reference standard for diagnosing infection with *M. tuberculosis* is the Mantoux test performed by injecting 0.1 ml of Tween-stabilized purified protein derivative (PPD) tuberculin containing 5 TU (tuberculin units) intradermally into the dorsal or volar surface of the forearm. In 48–72 hr the area of induration (not erythema) is measured transversely to the long axis of the arm and recorded in millimeters. If there is a delay in reading a test (e.g., if a patient fails to return for a scheduled reading at the assigned time), positive reactions may be read up to 1 week following placement of the Mantoux test.

A Mantoux test reaction size of 5 mm or more is considered positive in close contacts of infectious tuberculous cases, persons with abnormal chest radiographic findings suggestive of old healed tuberculosis, and persons with known or suspected HIV infection.

A tuberculin skin test reaction of 10 mm or more is considered positive in a second, less high-risk group. This group includes:

1.   Residents of long-term care facilities, such as nursing homes, correctional and mental institutions, and the like

2. Persons with medical conditions that increase the risk of tuberculosis, such as silicosis, gastrectomy, jejunoileal bypass, weight loss (10% or more below ideal body weight), chronic renal failure, diabetes mellitus, hematological disorders (e.g., leukemia and lymphomas), and other malignancies

3. Foreign-born persons from countries in Africa, Asia, and Latin America with high tuberculosis prevalence

4. Medically underserved low-income populations, including high-risk minority populations, especially blacks, Hispanics, and Native Americans

5. HIV-seronegative intravenous drug users

6. Other populations that have been identified in the community as having an increased prevalence of tuberculosis or would potentially pose a hazard to large numbers of susceptible persons

A tuberculin skin test reaction size of 15 mm or more is considered positive in those without known risk (e.g., those having none of the foregoing risk factors) (CDC, 1990c, 1991a; American Thoracic Society–CDC, 1990).

The Mantoux test is especially valuable when repeated periodically in the screening of tuberculin-negative individuals who are at risk of being exposed to tuberculosis, as might occur with residents, employees, and volunteers of a nursing home. A recent Mantoux skin-test conversion is defined as an increase of 10 mm or more within a 2-year period for a person younger than 35 years of age or an increase of 15 mm or more for a person 35 years of age or older (CDC, 1990b). Recent converters are considered newly infected with *M. tuberculosis* and are a high-risk group that should be considered for isoniazid therapy (CDC, 1990c; American Thoracic Society–CDC, 1990).

Once it is acquired, tuberculin sensitivity tends to persist, but may gradually wane over time following the initial sensitization and result in negative reactions in individuals previously known to be positive reactors.

The booster or recall phenomenon refers to enhancement of preexisting, but waning, hypersensitivity to tuberculin induced by the small amount of tuberculin injected in performing a Mantoux test. This results in an increase in the size of the reaction to a subsequent test. This phenomenon can sometimes be misinterpreted as causing an apparent conversion that is indicative of a new infection (Thompson, 1979). Boosting occurs in all age groups, but is most common in those older than 55 years of age. The effect can be seen if a second test is done as soon as a week after the initial tuberculin test. Boosting has been reported as being unusual beyond aged 75 years suggesting that perhaps sensitivity may wane beyond recall (Comstock, 1984).

When tuberculin skin testing is to be repeated periodically, the initial use of a two-step testing procedure is recommended, particularly in the elderly

(Clinical Practice Committee, 1988; Cauthen and Snider, 1986; Gordin et al., 1991). This will reduce the likelihood that a boosted reaction is mistaken as representing a conversion. If the reaction to the first test is negative, a second test is done 1–2 weeks later. If the second test remains negative, the person is classified as not being infected with *M. tuberculosis*. If the second test is positive, however, it would be considered the result of boosting. Conversions that occur to a third tuberculin test within the next 2 years are likely to result from new infection with *M. tuberculosis* during the ensuing interval.

Vaccination with BCG is not usually recommended in the United States. However, many countries continue to use BCG in tuberculosis control programs, particularly in infants. There is no reliable method of differentiating tuberculin reactions caused by BCG as opposed to those occurring naturally, caused by infection with *M. tuberculosis*. Positive tuberculin reactions in persons vaccinated with BCG usually indicate infection with *M. tuberculosis* and should be interpreted as such. These individuals should be considered for isoniazid preventive therapy.

A negative tuberculin test does not exclude the diagnosis of tuberculosis or tuberculous infection. A negative tuberculin reaction may result from severe illness or following therapy with steroids or immunosuppressive drugs. As many as 30% of patients who are HIV-seronegative, and 60% of AIDS patients may have negative tuberculin tests, despite being infected with *M. tuberculosis*. Additionally, recently infected persons may not have had sufficient time to develop a reaction to the tuberculin skin test.

IV. Treatment

A. Preventive Therapy (See Chapter 12)

In 1990, 90% of tuberculosis cases in the United States occurred in persons with remote tuberculous infection and 10% in newly infected persons.

Isoniazid (INH) preventive therapy inhibits infection in those who are exposed to *M. tuberculosis* and tuberculosis in infected persons who have not yet developed disease. Its efficacy, including its use in the elderly, has been convincingly demonstrated (Comstock et al., 1979; International Union Against Tuberculosis, 1982; Stead et al., 1987). Unequivocally, most cases of tuberculosis in this country are potentially preventable through the use of INH preventive therapy.

Shortly after the introduction of INH preventive therapy it became clear that its use is sometimes associated with hepatitis and, in rare instances, death. A U.S. Public Health Service Cooperative Surveillance Study confirmed this fact and also revealed that the association is age-related (Kopanoff et al., 1978). The reason for the cluster of deaths that occurred in 1 of the 21 participating cities (Baltimore) and that increased the case fatality rate has never been fully explained. Comstock has pointed out that, during the year of the study, a peculiar increase in deaths caused by cirrhosis of the liver occurred in Baltimore, but not in the rest of Maryland. If Baltimore had not been included in the study, estimates of the risk of death associated with INH preventive therapy would have been greatly reduced (Comstock, 1981).

The realization that INH caused hepatitis, and occasionally death, led to changes in the recommendations governing its use in preventive therapy. In 1974, INH preventive therapy guidelines were modified to exclude its routine use in positive tuberculin reactors 35 years of age and older who did not have additional risks of developing tuberculosis (American Thoracic Society, 1974, 1986).

However, not everyone agreed with the revised preventive therapy guidelines. Taylor and his co-workers argued that the benefits from INH preventive therapy did not clearly outweigh the risk in young adults whose only risk factor for developing tuberculosis was a positive tuberculin test (Taylor et al., 1981).

To further reduce the risk of hepatitis and death, current recommendations continue to advise restricted use of INH preventive therapy in positive tuberculin reactors 35 years of age and older who do not have other risks. Additionally, they have expanded the number of risk factors and have modified the cutoff point governing the size of what is considered to be a positive tuberculin skin test in certain groups (CDC, 1990c).

Although there was widespread acceptance of the benefits of INH preventive therapy, regardless of age, in treating persons at increased risk of developing tuberculosis, the controversy created by the challenge to its use in young adults may have dimmed enthusiasm for preventive therapy. As stated by Comstock, "Physicians may prefer to accept the improbable risk of being sued for tuberculosis that developed because preventive treatment was not recommended rather than face the more immediate risk of a lawsuit arising from side effects of treatment" (Comstock, 1986). This was particularly unfortunate because it limited the use of INH preventive therapy in a group for whom its use could significantly reduce tuberculosis.

There are several reports that emphasize the efficacy and safety of INH preventive therapy and challenge its restricted use in the elderly.

Cooper, using a decision analysis model, analyzed INH preventive therapy in persons older than 65 years of age with abnormal chest radiographs and concluded that INH preventive therapy would reduce tuberculosis cases without appreciably reducing 5-year survival (Cooper, 1986). Rose, using a similar technique concluded that, although the benefits are smaller for persons aged 65–80 years, low-risk tuberculin reactors of all ages benefit from INH preventive therapy (Rose et al., 1986).

Comstock makes a persuasive argument that the beneficial affect of INH preventive therapy is possibly even greater than Rose concluded because of the prevention of the spread of infection to others, shortened duration of therapy, and reduced INH-related hepatitis case-fatality rate (Comstock, 1986). Stead and his co-workers reported that, in a nursing home setting, INH preventive therapy can dramatically reduce the risk of developing tuberculosis in elderly tuberculin skin test converters. The incidence of hepatic toxicity reported by this group was also quite low (Stead et al., 1987).

Despite these reports favoring the use of INH preventive therapy controversy remains concerning its use in both younger and older groups who have no other risk factors for developing tuberculosis (Tsevat et al., 1988; Snider, 1988; Colice, 1990).

In 1989, Moulding et al. reported 20 INH-associated deaths that had occurred in California and called for a reevaluation of the current indications and precautions used for INH preventive therapy (Moulding et al., 1989).

Snider and Caras, in a limited study of INH-associated hepatitis deaths in persons taking INH preventive therapy in the United States, reported an overall death rate of 14:100,000 and 23.2:100,000 in those who completed therapy. As was true in Moulding's study and the U. S. Public Health Service Surveillance Study, a high proportion of deaths (69%) occurred in women, and an increasing risk of INH-associated hepatitis deaths was noted with increasing age. An unexpected finding was the number of INH-associated hepatitis deaths among persons younger than 20 years of age (Snider and Caras, 1992).

Efforts to carefully select and monitor patients receiving INH preventive therapy should be continued, preventive therapy guidelines for females should be reviewed, better screening for INH-associated hepatitis deaths should be undertaken, and a need for additional research to identify high-risk groups for INH-associated hepatitis death are conclusions reached by Snider and Caras.

Obviously care should be used when selecting and monitoring any elderly patient for INH preventive therapy. However, it should be stated clearly that current evidence favors the use of INH preventive therapy in elderly persons who are at increased risk of developing tuberculosis (CDC, 1990c).

Isoniazid in a single daily dose of 10 mg/kg body weight up to a maximum of 300 mg/day for 6–12 months is the recommended adult dose. An acceptable alternative is to give INH in a dose of 15 mg/kg up to a maximum of 900 mg/day twice a week when directly observed therapy is needed. Twelve months therapy is recommended for tuberculin-positive persons with abnormal chest radiographs compatible with old healed tuberculosis and for tuberculin reactors who have HIV infection.

Preventive therapy using rifampin 600 mg daily for 1 year should be considered in treating close contacts of infectious patients with INH-resistant tuberculosis. Shorter-course preventive therapy regimens using rifampin for 4 months and rifampin and pyrazinamide for 2 months are currently being studied.

Because of a higher risk for hepatotoxicity in the elderly, baseline serum transaminase tests—alanine aminotransferase (ALT) and aspartate aminotransferase (AST)—should be measured before starting INH therapy and periodically during the course of therapy.

Elderly persons should be monitored monthly for signs and symptoms of hepatic toxicity. If symptoms develop, patients should be instructed to discontinue INH therapy immediately and should be seen by a physician and have their liver function evaluated. If serum transaminase levels exceed five times the upper limit of the normal range for that laboratory, discontinuing INH therapy should be strongly considered. Limiting INH to no more than a 1-month supply is important, particularly when treating unreliable patients.

The elderly represent a disproportionately large share of tuberculosis cases in the United States, probably because, as a group, they constitute a majority of the reservoir of persons infected with *M. tuberculosis*. It has even been suggested that the cut point for a positive tuberculin reaction in the elderly should be lowered to 5 mm because of the very high likelihood of their having acquired infection when tuberculosis was common during their youth. As a group, elderly persons (65 years of age and older) have the highest tuberculosis case rates of any group in the United States; the case rate of minority men is highest of all groups (100.7:100,000 population).

Recommendations concerning INH preventive therapy are obviously intended to increase its safe and effective use in the United States. It is the author's bias, however, that under current guidelines, certain elderly persons who should receive the benefit of INH preventive therapy are being excluded. Newly infected elderly tuberculin skin test reactors whose reactions have not increased by more than 15 mm are not considered converters. These individuals, therefore, lacking other risk factors, are not candidates for INH preventive therapy. As an example, under current recommendations, an elderly minority man, residing in a nursing home in a large urban community where there is a high tuberculosis prevalence rate, who is known to have had a negative (0 mm) tuberculin skin test within the previous 2 years, and who presently is found to have a tuberculin skin test reaction of 12 mm, would not be considered a converter and, therefore, would not be a candidate for INH preventive therapy unless he had other risk factors. It is my belief that such individuals should be offered INH preventive therapy and closely monitored.

Guidelines concerning tuberculosis control activities in facilities providing long-term care for the elderly have been published and are a good source of information for administrators and staffs of these facilities, among others (CDC, 1990b).

B. Treatment of Tuberculosis (See Chapter 11)

To treat tuberculosis successfully, therapy must be instituted with at least two drugs to which the mycobacteria are susceptible, and drug ingestion must be continued for a sufficient period with adequate compliance (Reichman and Mc-Donald, 1977). A regimen of 6-months duration consisting of daily INH, rifampin (RIF), and pyrazinamide (PZA) for the initial 2 months, followed by (second phase) daily or twice-weekly INH and RIF for an additional 4 months is the preferred treatment choice (Combs et al., 1990); CDC, 1991a). A regimen of 9-months duration, consisting of daily INH and RIF for the first 1–2 months, followed by (second phase) daily or twice weekly INH and RIF for a total duration of 9 months has been considered an acceptable alternative (American Thoracic Society, 1986).

When INH resistance is suspected or when treating life-threatening tuberculosis, ethambutol (EMB) or streptomycin (SM) should be added to supplement the initial phases of both the 6-month and 9-month regimens. The second phase of treatment would consist of INH and RIF given daily or twice weekly for a total duration of 6 or 9 months, depending on which regimen was initially given.

Because of an alarming increase in rates of multidrug-resistant tuberculosis (MDR–TB) in certain parts of the United States, current recommendations suggest starting patients suspected of having MDR–TB on a five-drug regimen containing INH, RIF, and PZA, plus at least two other drugs that are likely to be effective, while awaiting drug susceptibility test results (CDC, 1991c). A new guideline routinely recommends INH, RIF, PZA, plus either EMB or SM for the initial phase (first 2 months) of treatment for all tuberculosis patients unless INH and RIF resistance is unequivocally shown to be low. The regimen would then be individualized based on the results of drug susceptibility test (CDC, 1993).

In persons with HIV infection, the treatment regimen should include daily INH, RIF, and PZA, along with EMB or SM if there is central nervous system (CNS) involvement or disseminated tuberculosis, or if drug-resistant disease is suspected. the second phase of treatment should always include at least INH and RIF. The duration of treatment should be for a minimum of 9 months and for at least 6 months following documented culture conversion (Fertel and Pitchenik, 1989). If either INH or RIF is not included in the treatment regimen, therapy should continue for a minimum of 18 months and for at least 12 months after culture conversion (CDC, 1989b).

When MDR-TB occurs in HIV-infected persons the addition of a fifth or sixth drug should be considered in the treatment regimen because of the high mortality rate associated with MDR-TB in HIV-infected persons. In general regimens that are effective in the treatment of pulmonary tuberculosis are also effective for the treatment of extrapulmonary disease. Most of the antituberculosis medications that are available for use in the initial treatment of tuberculosis in this country are listed and further discussed in Chapter 11, with their recommended dosages and side affects. Specific side effects related to elderly patients are as follows:

1. Isoniazid enhances the concentration of serum phenytoin levels when they are taken together, requiring monitoring of phenytoin levels when used concomitantly.

2. Rifampin accelerates the hepatic clearance of many medications that are used commonly in treating the elderly. These include warfarin and analogues, steroids, oral hypoglycemic agents, digoxin, and certain anticonvulsants, and may require a dose adjustment.

3. Pyrazinamide causes hyperuricemia, but attacks of gouty arthritis are uncommon.

4. Streptomycin causes renal toxicity and should be used with caution in the elderly. The recommended dose is 10 mg/kg per day up to 750 mg/day.

Other less commonly used antituberculosis drugs are available for treatment; however, because they generally possess greater toxicity, their use is more limited and reserved primarily for treating drug-resistant tuberculosis.

The effectiveness of therapy for pulmonary tuberculosis should be monitored by monthly sputum examinations until culture conversion occurs. More than 90% of patients taking INH and RIF became sputum culture-negative within 3 months of starting therapy. A chest radiograph early during the course of treatment may be helpful (2–3 months) and a chest radiograph should be done at the completion of therapy as a baseline for comparison with any future chest radiographs. For patients who have satisfactory completed therapy, routine follow-up is unnecessary.

Patients whose sputum remains culture-positive beyond 3 months of therapy should be considered treatment failures, either because of drug-resistant organisms or patient noncompliance in taking medications. Drug susceptibility studies should be obtained and while awaiting the results, the original drug regimen may be continued or, in deteriorating patients, at least two drugs not previously given can be added to the regimen. Therapy can then be adjusted in accordance with the susceptibility tests results when they became available. One should never add a single potentially effective new drug to a failing regimen because this may enhance the development of further drug resistance.

V. Summary

Although tuberculosis case rates are disproportionately greater in the elderly than in younger-aged groups in the United States, tuberculosis cases in the elderly have been declining since 1986. Contrary to its occurrence primarily in younger-aged groups in minority populations, tuberculosis in the elderly occurs most commonly in the white population.

Tuberculosis in the elderly occurs from both recrudescent disease, occurring from someone infected in the remote past, and recent infection. The disease may present without accustomed radiographic and clinical features, making diagnosis difficult.

Isoniazid preventive therapy is effective in preventing tuberculosis, and its use should be encouraged in elderly persons who are at high risk for developing disease. Current recommendations favor a 6-month treatment regimen of INH and RIF with PZA for the first 2 months. Four-drug regimens adding either EMB or SM to the initial INH, RIF, and PZA regimen are recommended in treatment of HIV-infected persons and when treating suspected drug-resistant tuberculosis.

References

Alvarez, S., Shell, C., and Berk, S. L. (1987). Pulmonary tuberculosis in elderly men. *Am J. Med.* **82**:602–606.

American Association of Retired Persons (AARP) Administration of Aging (AOA) (1990). A profile of older americans: 1990. Washington, HHS publication No. D 996, pp. 1–14.

American Thoracic Society (1974). Preventive therapy of tuberculosis infection. *Am. Rev. Respir. Dis.* **110**:371–374.

American Thoracic Society (1986). Treatment of tuberculosis and tuberculosis infection in adults and children: Joint statement of the American Thoracic Society and the Centers for Disease Control. *Am. Rev. Respir. Dis.* **134**:355–363.

American Thoracic Society and Centers for Disease Control (1990). Diagnostic standards and classification of tuberculosis. *Am. Rev. Respir. Dis.* **142**:725–735.

Bass, J. B., Farer, L. S., Hopewell, P. C., Jacobs, R. F., and Snider, D. E. (1990). Diagnostic standards and classification of tuberculosis: Joint statement of the American Thoracic Society and the Centers for Disease Control. *Am. Rev. Respir. Dis.* **99**:109–111.

Bates, J. H. (1979). Diagnosis of tuberculosis. *Chest* **76** (Suppl.):757–763.

Berger, H. W., and Granada, M. (1974). Lower lung field tuberculosis. *Chest* **65**:522–526.

Blazer, D. G. (1991). Demography of aging. In *Geriatrics Review Syllabus: A Core Curriculum in Geriatric Medicine*, Vol. 2. Edited by J. C. Beck. American Geriatrics Society, New York, pp. 1–5.

Bloch, A. B., Rieder, H. L., Kelly, G. D., Cauthen, G. M., Hayden, C. H., and Snider, D. E. (1989). The epidemiology of tuberculosis in the United States. *Semin. Respir. Infect.* **4**:157–170.

Bruckstein, A. H. (1988). Abdominal tuberculosis. *N. Y. State J. Med.* **84**:18–21.

Cauthen, G. M., and Snider, D. E. (1986). Delayed tuberculin boosting in the older population. *Am. Rev. Respir. Dis.* **134**:857–858.

Centers for Disease Control (1977). 1975: Tuberculosis in the United States. Atlanta, HEW publication No (CDC)77-8322, pp. 28–29.

Centers for Disease Control (1989a). A strategic plan for the elimination of tuberculosis in the United States. *MMWR* **38**:269–272.

Centers for Disease Control (1989b). Tuberculosis and human immunodeficiency virus infection. recommendations of the Advisory Committee for Elimination of Tuberculosis (ACET). *MMWR* **38**:236–350.

Centers for Disease Control (1989c). A strategic plan for the elimination of tuberculosis in the United States. *MMWR* **38** (Suppl. 5–3):1–25.

Centers for Disease Control (1990a). Screening for tuberculosis and tuberculous infection in high-risk populations. Recommendations of the Advisory Committee for Elimination of Tuberculosis (ACET). *MMWR* **39**:1–7.

Centers for Disease Control (1990b). Prevention and control of tuberculosis in facilities providing long-term care to the elderly: Recommendations of the Advisory Committee for Elimination of Tuberculosis (ACET). *MMWR* **39**:7–20.

Centers for Disease Control (1990c). The use of preventive therapy for tuberculosis infection in the United States: Recommendations of the Advisory Committee for Elimination of Tuberculosis (ACET). *MMWR* **39**:9–12.

Centers for Disease Control (1991a). Core curriculum on tuberculosis. Atlanta, HHS Publication No. (CDC), pp. 7–8.

Centers for Disease Control (1991b). Tuberculosis elimination, U.S.A. (Facsimile of Slides). Atlanta, HHS Publication. (CDC), pp. 1–82.

Centers for Disease Control (1991c). 1989: Tuberculosis statistics in the United States. Atlanta, HHS Publication No. (CDC) 91-8322, pp. 69–79.

Centers for Disease Control (1991d). Nosocomial transmission of multidrug-resistant tuberculosis among HIV-infected persons—Florida and New York, 1988–1991. *MMWR* **40**:585–591.

Centers for Disease Control (1992). Prevention and control of tuberculosis in U. S. communities with at-risk minority populations. Recommendations of the Advisory Council for the Elimination of Tuberculosis. *MMWR* **41**:1–11.

Centers for Diseas Control (1993). Initial therapy of tuberculosis in the era of multiple drug resistance: Recommendations of the Advisory Council for Elimination of Tuberculosis (ACET). *MMWR* (in press).

Chang, S. C., Lee, P. Y., and Perng, R. P. (1987). Lower lung field tuberculosis. Chest **91**:230–232.

Cinman, A. C. (1982). Genitourinary tuberculosis. *Urology* **20**:353–358.

Clinical Practice Committee (1988). The American Geriatrics Society Statement on two-step PPD testing for nursing home patients on admission. *J. Am. Geriatr. Soc.* **36**:77–78.

Colice, G. L. (1990). Decision analysis, public health policy, and isoniazid chemoprophylaxis for young adult tuberculin skin reactors. *Arch. Intern. Med.* **150**:2517–2522.

Combs, D. L., O'Brien, R. J., and Geiter, L. J. (1990). USPHS tuberculosis short-course chemotherapy trial 21: Effectiveness, toxicity, and acceptability: The report of final results. *Ann. Intern. Med.* **112**:397–406.

Comstock, G. W. (1981). Evaluating isoniazid preventive therapy: The need for more data. *Ann. Intern. Med.* **94**:817–819.

Comstock, G. W. (1984). Interpretation of Mantoux test results. In *Guidelines for the Diagnosis of Tuberculous Infection*. Edited by L. B. Reichman. Audio Visual Medical Marketing, New York, pp. 30–38.

Comstock, G. W. (1986). Prevention of tuberculosis among tuberculin reactors: Maximizing benefits, minimizing risks. *JAMA* **256**:2729–2730.

Comstock, G. W., Baum, C., and Snider, D. E. (1979). Isoniazid prophylaxis among Alaskan Eskimos: A final report of the Bethel isoniazid studies. *Am. Rev. Respir. Dis.* **119**:827–830.

Cooper, J. K. (1986). Decision analysis for tuberculosis preventive treatment in nursing homes. *J. Am. Geriatr. Soc.* **34**:814–817.

Crawford, J. J., Eisenach, K. D., and Bates, J. H. (1989). Diagnosis of tuberculosis: Present and future. *Semin. Respir. Infect.* **4**:171–181.

Dutt, A. K., and Stead, W. W. (1989). Treatment of extrapulmonary tuberculosis. *Semin. Respir. Infect.* **4**:225–231.

Farer, L. S., Lowell, A. M., and Meador, M. P. (1979). Extrapulmonary tuberculosis in the United States. *Am J. Epidemiol.* **109**:205–217.

Farman, D. P., and Speir, W. A. (1986). Initial roentgenographic manifestations of bacteriologically proven mycobacterial tuberculosis: Typical or atypical? *Chest* **89**:75–77.

Fertel, D., and Pitchenik, A. E. (1989). Tuberculosis in acquired deficiency syndrome. *Semin. Respir. Infect.* **4**:198–205.

Gertler, R., and Ramages, M. B. (1985). Tuberculous laryngitis—a one year harvest. *J. Laryngol. Otol.* **99**:1119–1125.

Gordin, F. M., Perez-Stable, E. J., Reid, M., Schecter, G., Cosgriff, L., Flahertu, D., and Hopewell, P. C. (1991). Stability of positive tuberculin tests: Are boosted reactions valid? *Am. Rev. Respir. Dis.* **144**:560–563.

International Union Against Tuberculosis Committee on Prophylaxis (1982). Efficacy of various durations of isoniazid preventive therapy for tuberculosis: Five years of follow-up in the IUAT trial. *Bull. WHO* **60**:555–564.

Ip, M. S., So, S. Y., Lam, W. K., and Mok, C. K. (1986). Endobronchial tuberculosis revisited. *Chest* **89**:727–730.

Kopanoff, D. E., Snider, D. E., and Caras, G. J. (1978). Isoniazid-related hepatitis: A U.S. Public Health Service Cooperative Surveillance Study. *Am. Rev. Respir. Dis.* **117**:991–1001.

MacGee, W. (1989). The frequency of unsuspected tuberculosis found postmortem in a geriatric population. *Z. Gerontol.* **22**:311–314.

Makinodan, T., James, S. J., Inamizu, T., and Chang, M. (1984). Immunologic basis for susceptibility to infection in the aged. Gerontology **30**:279–289.

McDonald, R. J., and Sunderam, G. (1989). Tuberculosis in the elderly. *Curr. Pulmonol.* **10**:353–376.

Morris, C. D. W. (1990). Pulmonary tuberculosis in the elderly: A different disease? *Thorax* **45**:912–913.

Moulding, T. S., Redeker, A. G., and Kanel, G. C. (1989). Twenty isoniazid-associated deaths in one state. *Am. Rev. Respir. Dis.* **140**:700–705.

Nagami, P., and Yoshikawa, T. T. (1984). Aging and tuberculosis. Gerontology **30**:308–315.

Narain, J. P., Lofgren, J. P., Warren, E., and Stead, W. W. (1985). Epidemic tuberculosis in a nursing home: A retrospective cohort study. *J. Am. Geriatr. Soc.* **33**:258–263.

Orme, I. M. (1988). A mouse model of the recrudescence of latent tuberculosis in the elderly. *Am. Rev. Respir. Dis.* **137**:716–718.

Parmar, M. S. (1967). Lower lung field tuberculosis. *Am. Rev. Respir. Dis.* **96**:310–313.

Reichman, L. B., and McDonald, R. J.(1977). Practical management and control of tuberculosis. *Med. Clin. North Am.* **61**:1185–1204.

Riley, R. L., and O'Grady, F. (1961). *Airborne Infection: Transmission and Control.* Macmillan, New York, pp. 180.

Rose, D. N., Schecter, C. B., and Silver, A. L. (1986). The age treshold for isoniazid chemoprophylaxis: A decision analysis for low-risk tuberculin reactors. *JAMA* **256**:2709–2713.

Segarra, F., Sherman, D. S., and Rodriguez-Aquero, J. (1963). Lower lung field tuberculosis. *Am Rev. Respir. Dis.* **87**:37–40.

Shintani, S., Kamaki, M., Motohashi, N., Hayashi, M., Toyoda, O., and Wakao, T. (1990). Tuberculous brain infection located in an old cerebral infarct: CT changes with successful conservative therapy. *Neuroradiology* **32**:156–159.

Slavin, R. E., Walsh, T. J., and Pollack, A. D. (1980). Late generalized tuberculosis: A clinical pathologic analysis and comparison of 100 cases in the preantibiotic and antibiotic eras. *Medicine* **59**:352–366.

Snider, D. E. (1988). Decision analysis for isoniazid preventive therapy: Take it or leave it? *Am. Rev. Respir. Dis.* **137**:2–4.

Snider, D. E., and Caras, G. J. (1992). Isoniazid-associated hepatitis deaths: A review of available information. *Am. Rev. Respir. Dis.* **145**:494–497.

Stead, W. W., and Lofgren, J. P. (1983). Does the risk of tuberculosis increase in old age? *J. Infect. Dis.* **147**:951–955.

Stead, W. W., and To, T. (1987). The significance of the tuberculin skin test in elderly persons. *Ann. Intern. Med.* **107**:837–842.

Stead, W. W., To, T., Harrison, R. W., and Abraham, J. H. (1987). Benefit–risk considerations in preventive treatment for tuberculosis in elderly persons. *Ann. Intern. Med.* **107**:843–845.

Stead, W. W. and Dutt, A. K. (1989). Tuberculosis in the elderly. *Semin. Respir. Infect.* **4**:189–197.

Styblo, K., and Rouillon A. (1981). Estimated global incidence of smear-positive pulmonary tuberculosis: Unreliability of officially reported figures on tuberculosis *Bull. Int. Union Tuberc.* **56**:118–126.

Sunderam, G., McDonald, R. J., Maniatis, T., Oleske, J., Kapila, R., and Reichman, L. B. (1986). Tuberculosis as a manifestation of the acquired immunodeficiency syndrome (AIDS). *JAMA* **256**:362–366.

Taylor, W. C., Aronson, M. D., and Delbanco, T. L. (1981). Should young adults with a positive tuberculin test take isoniazid. *Ann. Intern. Med.* **94**:808–813.

Thompson, N. J., Glassroth, J. L., Snider, D. E., and Farer, L. S. (1979). The booster phenomenon in serial tuberculin testing. *Am. Rev. Respir. Dis.* **119**:587–597.

Tsevat, J., Taylor, W. C., Wong, J. B., and Pauker, S. G. (1988). Isoniazid for the tuberculin reactor: Take it or leave it. *Am. Rev. Respir. Dis.* **137**:215–220.

Weinburg, A. C., and Boyd, S. D. (1988). Short-course chemotherapy and role of surgery in adult and pediatric genitourinary tuberculosis. *Urology* **31**:95–102.

Yoshikawa, T. T. (1984). Aging and infectious diseases: State of the art. *Gerontology* **30**:275–278.

Yoshikawa, T. T. (1991). Elimination of tuberculosis from the United States. *J. Am. Geriatr. Soc.* **39**:312–314.

Yoshikawa, T. T. (1992). Tuberculosis in aging adults. *J. Am. Geriatr. Soc.* **40**:178–187.

20

Tuberculosis in Homeless Populations

PHILIP W. BRICKNER

St. Vincent's Hospital and Medical Center
of New York
New York, New York

LAWRENCE L. SCHARER

St. Luke's–Roosevelt Hospital Center
New York, New York

JOHN M. McADAM

St. Vincent's Hospital and Medical Center
of New York
New York, New York

I. Introduction

The medical disorders of homeless human beings are the common illnesses of mankind, magnified by their bizarre living situations and the anxiety of street or shelter life. Psychiatric disease, alcohol and substance abuse, and the sociopathic behavior of themselves and of those around them add to the problem. Routine acute and chronic conditions that we expect to find treatable in their early stages, when neglected, worsen and lead to severe morbidity or death. As a result of these and other factors, the homeless constitute the sickest subgroup of the population in the United States.

Gathered in crowded shelters and flop houses, congregated in food lines and soup kitchens, they transmit with ease common viral respiratory diseases and infestations. Major trauma is commonplace. Chronic leg edema, cellulitis, and leg ulcers routinely result from the need these individuals feel to stand or sit all day, and often all night, for fear of assault. To sleep, even to lie down, is to invite attack. Although the physical consequences of these conditions are uncomfortable and even disabling, the long-term results are controllable if treated and usually do not produce severe danger to life or exposure of others to risk of illness. The development of pulmonary tuberculosis (TB) in the homeless population is more significant.

II. Who Are the Homeless?

To recognize the significance of disease in the homeless of the United States, it is important to attempt a demographic analysis. Which people constitute the mass of humanity we call "the homeless"? How many such persons are there? This is a murky and elusive subject. Estimates of numbers have ranged from about 250,000 to 3 million (Wright, 1990). The variation results from the viewpoint of those doing the counting. The lower figure has been put forth by the federal government; the higher by advocacy groups for the homeless. The correct number, never to be known with accuracy, is somewhere in between and depends on definitions of homelessness.

There is much overlapping of demographic categories (Wright, 1990). The stereotype is a chronic alcoholic man on skid row. Today such individuals make up only about 20% of the whole (Blumberg et al., 1971; Erickson and Wilhelm, 1986; Wright, 1990). Homeless women, essentially unknown in our country two decades ago, now total about 25%. Causative factors include deinstitutionalization from state mental hospitals, the loss of cheap housing, and job discrimination based on sex or age, leading to economic hardship and eviction. Women attempting to survive on the streets or in shelters face problems distinct from those of their male peers. They generally are more easily victimized, assaulted, or raped; chronic mental illness and peripheral vascular disease appear to be more common; and they face pregnancy and child rearing alone (Burroughs et al., 1990).

Children, from newborns to age 18, unknown to our street scene until recent years, form 15%. The youngest are thought of as members of "homeless families," a euphemism for a woman with two to three children, displaced from home by fire, abuse, or inability to pay the rent. Sometimes the children are pregnant as well, but more are prepubertal. And somehow lumped into the category of homeless children are runaway youths. Guesswork suggests that there exist about 2 million such children, often not considered among the homeless, but certainly sharing in their health problems. These estimates include young people who run from their homes, those who are kicked out (also known as "throwaways"), and those whose homes are lost when they became superannuated from foster care.

About one-third of the homeless are chronic substance abusers. Mentally ill persons, some discharged from state mental hospitals through a process known as deinstitutionalization, form a similar proportion (Wright, 1990).

Deinstitutionalization has had a tremendous influence on the numbers of homeless persons. In 1955, an estimated 560,000 people resided in psychiatric institutions; by 1984, this figure had dropped to about 132,000 and has fallen even lower today (Brickner and Scanlan, 1990; Lamb, 1984). The numbers also reflect the blocking of the road back; state judicial and legislative decisions have since made the process of involuntary commitment more arduous.

Shifting the locus of care to the community was prompted by well-documented failures of the state hospital system, but in the process the important function of asylum was lost for those incapable of caring for themselves. Reports from several urban centers suggest that the asylum function has been partly assumed by shelters for the homeless. The aberrant care-seeking behavior and withdrawal of many mentally ill persons, whether a feature of their illness or a product of the institutional experience, pose significant challenges to care providers.

> Irony abounds. Manhattan State Hospital on Ward's Island in New York City discharged many of its chronic patients to the streets during the past twenty years. It became an underutilized facility with empty buildings. At the same time the government of New York City lacked shelter space for a growing number of homeless persons. Logic prevailed, and the state leased the empty space to the city for a nominal sum. Now this city shelter, previously part of the state mental hospital system, houses in substantial number the same people who were previously wards of the state (Baxter and Hopper, 1982).

The only essential distinction is that now they are labeled "homeless" rather than "mentally ill."

Older homeless persons, often unnoticed and rarely considered, if the age of 65 years is the point of definition, make up about 4% of this population. This is a noteworthy figure, recognizing that about 13% of the United States population is that age or older. Why are older homeless persons so underrepresented? In fact, homelessness and the conditions leading to this status accelerate the process of aging. The elderly homeless include a few relics of life on skid row; those with chronic mental illness who lack any form of asylum; economic casualties with no pension, no savings, and no family supports; persons evicted for nonpayment of rent; jail dischargees and demented wanderers. "There is a process of natural selection, and those older individuals who remain on the streets are indeed the 'survivors' who have defied the odds" (O'Connell et al., 1990).

Members of minority groups—blacks and Hispanics, in particular, a considerable number of whom are illegal immigrants—make up a vastly disproportionate number of the homeless in the United States. Overall, about 38% of the homeless are black, 12% Hispanic, and 3% Native American. The corresponding proportions for the United States populace are 11.7%, 6.4, and 0.6, respectively (Wright, 1990; Wright and Weber, 1987).

III.   Tuberculosis and Its Relation to Homelessness

The increase of homelessness in the last two decades and the institution of emergency shelters have resulted in a degree of crowding and lack of access to health care not seen in decades. The association between poverty, crowding, and tuberculosis was made nearly a century ago, and was familiar to physicians in the tuberculosis movement. Studies in England, specifically London and Liverpool, demonstrated decreased tuberculosis death rates with less crowding (Teller, 1988). S. Adolphus Knoph, writing in 1914, believed this to be true in New York City:

> We know that the housing problem is most closely allied to the tuberculosis problem. There is enough statistical evidence to show that tuberculosis is pre-eminently a disease of congestion. This evidence is to be found in the "lung blocks" of our large cities and the congested cheap lodging-houses, in labor camps, prisons, reformatories and schools . . .
>
> Not only in the homes of the poor but also among the homeless, who must be still poorer, bad housing conditions are responsible for much tuberculosis and its concomitant misery (Knopf, 1914).

At the time these comments were written, Manhattan had a population of about 2.3 million and over 17,000 cases of active tuberculosis per year (Knopf, 1914). These figures yield a prevalence rate of over 750:100,000 population. In the United States, tuberculosis case rates have declined dramatically since the rise of public health measures early in the 20th century. Isolating patients who had active, contagious tuberculosis, combined with a general increase in the standard of living, reduced death rates from nearly 200:100,000 to less than 40:100,000 by 1947, when streptomycin became widely available (Centers for Disease Control [CDC], 1978), and tuberculosis became at last a curable disease. In recent decades there had been a steady fall of nearly 7% per year in the annual case rate. This decline stopped in 1985. In 1989, there were 23,495 cases of active tuberculosis in our country, with a case rate of 9.5:100,000 (CDC, 1989a). In 1990, there were 25,701 cases, an increase of 9.4% (CDC, 1990a). Through 1990, an excess of 28,000 cumulative cases had occurred above what would have been expected had the earlier rate of decline continued, according to the CDC (Rieder et al., 1989; Valway, 1991; Snider, 1991).

The situation is exacerbated by the appearance of drug-resistant disease. Early evidence of this problem at homeless shelters was found in Boston during 1983 (Nardell et al., 1986), where a cluster of 49 tuberculous cases was identified at the Pine Street Inn. Of these, 22 were caused by *Mycobacterium tuberculosis* of the same phage type resistant to isoniazid and streptomycin. In New

York City, a retrospective bacteriological study identified drug resistance in 21% of 53 isolates from homeless tuberculous patients diagnosed from 1982 to 1987 (Pablos-Mendez et al., 1990). In New York State, the first recent significant report of fatalities from disease caused by multidrug-resistant bacteria has occurred (Rosenthal, 1991; McFadden, 1991). Thirteen prisoners and one prison guard died during 1991, all immunocompromised. The inmates were human immunodeficiency virus (HIV)-positive and the guard had a malignancy. This is particularly relevant to the homeless shelter experience because of the placement of many ex-offenders in shelter settings. It is inevitable that similar bacteria will be found in major sites housing the homeless, and that deaths from TB will follow.

If we consider the environment at a shelter for homeless persons, it should not be surprising that tuberculosis arises as a problem. Beds in large armory buildings are frequently laid out 1–2 ft apart (Nolan et al., 1991). This situation bears comparison with careful studies of outbreaks among Navy shipboard personnel in which tuberculin conversion rates of 26–80% were found, the variation dependent on where the sailors slept (Ochs, 1962; Houk et al., 1968). An important distinction is that, whereas sailors are examined and found healthy upon joining the armed forces, homeless persons are not required to undergo any sort of initial evaluation on entry into a shelter, yet are found to bear significant amounts of illness (Brickner et al., 1986; Gelberg et al., 1990; Wright, 1990).

Thus tuberculosis continues to be prevalent among the poor, the elderly, the malnourished, those poorly housed in crowded conditions, alcoholics, immigrants from parts of the world where the disease is common, and minorities. These characteristics define the homeless in our country and help partly explain the extraordinary rate of tuberculosis found to exist in these persons through studies in several cities (Knopf, 1914; Rudd, 1985; Stead et al., 1985, 1990; Snider et al., 1989; Nolan and Elarth, 1988; Rieder, 1989; Reichman and O'Day, 1978; Abeles et al., 1970; Braun et al., 1989a, b; Reichman et al., 1979; Friedman et al., 1987; Marsh, 1957; Sherman et al., 1980; Patel, 1985; Capewell et al., 1986; Trachtman and Greenberg, 1978; Barry et al., 1986; Ramsden et al., 1988; Nardell, 1989; New York City Department of Health [NYCDOH], 1989; McAdam et al., 1990a, b).

Prevalence rates of active tuberculosis for homeless persons are estimated to be 150–300 times greater than for the general population (Barry et al., 1986; Slutkin, 1986; Sherman et al., 1980). In October 1991, the U. S. Public Health Service, reporting on data from 109 health care programs for the homeless supported by the Stewart B. McKinney Homeless Assistance Act, noted that tuberculosis had increased fivefold since calendar year 1989 and that children from newborns through age 14 accounted for 17% of the cases (Gaston, 1991).

IV.   Studies in Seven Cities

A.   Centers for Disease Control Recommendations

The CDC published recommendations in 1987 (CDC, 1987a) to improve tuber-culosis control in the homeless population. These focused on the need to assess the magnitude of the problem, case finding and reporting, treatment, and pre-vention. With these parameters we consider here the situation in seven large cities with data provided by staffs of homeless shelters and outreach programs or by the local health department. These cities, with their 1990 national rank-ing for tuberculosis case rates, are New York, New York (5th); San Francisco, California (6th); Los Angeles, California (11th), Chicago, Illinois (15th); Bos-ton, Massachusetts (20th), Seattle, Washington (25th); and Portland, Oregon (28th) (CDC Epidemiology Branch, personal communication, December 1991). Because the data have been gathered variously, precise comparison between cit-ies is not feasible.

Assessment of the Magnitude of the Problem

The definition of homelessness is not uniform from city to city. Persons are usu-ally considered homeless if they give no address or cite a shelter as their resi-dence when interviewed by a health care team (McAdam et al., 1990a). Because many individuals move from one group to another (migrant worker, correctional facility, residential substance abuse facility, shelter), these data have flaws.

The proportion of homeless persons tested in the past 2 years, who were found to have been infected with tubercle bacilli and were reported to us, ranges from 24% in Portland to 47.2% in New York. Homeless persons constituted from 10 to 27% of total cases of tuberculosis in these cities (Tables 1 and 2). The largest total number were in New York City, where approximately 454 of 3520 new cases of active tuberculosis in 1990 were identified as homeless (Adler, 1991). In Los Angeles, the minimum estimated number of homeless patients with TB was 126 in 1989 and 139 in 1990. The latter number represents 49% of the tuberculous patients diagnosed in the city's Central District (Davidson, P., personal communication, November 1991). In San Francisco, the 1990 case rate per 100,000 among the homeless was 420 (San Francisco Department of Health [SFDOPH], 1991). A recent survey (June–August 1991) showed a range of pos-itive reactors of 12–38% at four different locations.

Case Finding

The CDC (CDC, 1987a) advocated both "passive" and "active" approaches to case finding, and all seven cities succeeded in carrying out substantial efforts.

The passive approach implies both screening with tuberculin skin testing of asymptomatic and symptomatic individuals, and educating shelter staffs to

Table 1 Tuberculosis in the Homeless (1988–1989)[a]

City	Boston	Chicago	Los Angeles	New York	Portland	San Francisco	Seattle
Number screened (tuberculin skin tests)	900/yr	227	492	446	1024	403	417
Year	(766 in 1988) including x-ray	(1988)	(1988)	(1988)	(1989)	(1988)	(1986–1987)
Percent returned for reading	55%	74% (estimated)	84%	90%	76%	73%	80%
Percent positive reactions	41%	25%	33%	32%	24%	23%	32% (using ≥5 mm)
Active cases of tuberculosis found by screening	12/3060 (over 3 yr)	0/227	3/492	12/446	4/1024	1/403	5/417

[a]Information provided by:
Boston: Janet Groth, R.N., Public Health Nurse, Boston City Hospital, Healthlink, Boston, Massachusetts.
Chicago: Deborah Benton, N.P., Associate Director of Health Services, Health Care for the Homeless Project, Chicago, Illinois.
Los Angeles: Aaron Strehlow, R.N., UCLA School of Nursing, Health Center at the Union Rescue Mission, Los Angeles, California.
New York: John M. McAdam, M.D., Attending Physician, Department of Community Medicine, St. Vincent's Hospital and Medical Center of New York, New York, New York.
Portland: Dave Houghton, Communicable Disease Division, Multnomah County, Oregon.
San Francisco: Dan Wlodarczyk, M.D., Medical Director, Health Care for the Homeless, San Francisco Department of Health, San Francisco, California.
Seattle: Stacy Kiyasu, R.N., Nursing Coordinator, Downtown Emergency Service Center, Seattle, Washington.

Table 2 Tuberculosis in the Homeless (1990)[a]

City	Boston	Chicago	Los Angeles[b]	New York	Portland[c]	San Francisco	Seattle
Tuberculosis cases (total for city)	150	705	944—city 1936—county	3520	66	334	89—city 113—county
Case rate for city (per 100,000)	20.9	25.3	27.1	48.1	11.3	46.1	17.7
Number of cases in homeless (percent total for city)	27 (18%)	Unknown (10%) estimated	139 (15%)	454 (13%)	20 (30%)	42 (13%)	17 (19%)

[a]Information provided by the CDC and Office of Tuberculosis in the various cities.

		National (from CDC):
Boston:	M. A. Barry, M.D.	
Chicago:	Bapu Arekapudi, M.D.	1990: 25,701 cases
Los Angeles:	Paul Davidson, M.D.	10.3:100,000
New York:	Jack Adler, M.D.	1989: 23,495 cases
Portland:[c]	Dave Houghton	9.5:100,000
San Francisco:	Dan Wlodarczyk, M.D.	
Seattle:	James Nolan, M.D.	

[b]Figures include cases from both the city and county.

[c]Portland defines homeless as living in the Burnside Area, including SROs, shelters, and so forth.

recognize signs and symptoms of tuberculosis, its mode of spread, and the potential hazards of transmission in shelters. Any person with a chronic cough is brought to a location at which health status evaluation can take place, followed by referral for diagnosis and treatment.

The success of this approach varies. In San Francisco, screening of 403 homeless persons without symptoms in 1988 uncovered only 1 case of active tuberculosis (McAdam et al., 1990a). In New York, staff members at a large men's shelter have been screening residents since 1982. They identified 20 active cases of tuberculosis in the 13 months July 1987 through August 1988 (20/446 = 4.5%) (McAdam, J., personal communication, 1991) and 62 between September 1989 and October 1991 (62/1209 = 5.5%) (McAdam, 1991). This shelter study is further discussed below.

On the other hand, the New York City Department of Health screened homeless persons for tuberculosis in several shelters between September 1986 and March 1989 (NYCDOH, 1989). One thousand five hundred fifty persons received skin tests (21% of the estimated shelter population at time of screening) and 3111 chest radiographs were taken (46% of those in shelters). Tuberculin testing led to the finding of three new active cases and radiographs to four new active cases. The health department concluded that the finding of seven new cases over a 3-year period "suggests that a large pool of undiagnosed TB [tuberculosis] cases apparently is not occurring" (NYCDOH, 1989). The health department also noted that the cost of case finding was much lower for purified protein derivative (PPD) screening than for chest radiographs.

The notable distinction between the results of these two passive screening projects in New York probably stems from the fact that the former took place in a shelter clinic where those evaluated included a mixture of persons already sick and those requiring work program physicals, whereas the latter concerned the general shelter population.

The more active approach, perhaps better termed "contact investigation," was used in Boston and Seattle following outbreaks of tuberculosis in shelters. In Boston in 1984 (Barry et al., 1986), 26 new cases of active tuberculosis were diagnosed in the homeless in a short period. Active screening by skin testing, sputum examination, and chest radiographs then took place simultaneously in three shelters during a 4-night period. Of approximately 750 persons in the shelters at that time, 586 were tested and 4 new cases of active tuberculosis identified, all through chest radiographs. Of 362 who accepted skin testing, 187 returned for reading and 42/187 (22%) were positive. There were also 3 documented skin test converters.

Since that time, to enhance communication between shelter staffs and the health department, a computerized listing of all contacts has been developed, incorporating the results of skin testing, radiological studies, sputum smears and cultures, and medications. From 1985 through April 1990, 4500 individuals were screened and 14 new active cases discovered (McAdam et al., 1990a).

The Seattle–King County Health Department reported (Nolan et al., 1991) on tuberculosis identified in clients of a shelter that opened in 1984. Instances were sporadic until late 1986 and early 1987, when seven new cases of tuberculosis were discovered in shelter residents. By tuberculin skin testing, with reactions of 5 mm or greater considered positive, the Seattle health authorities obtained chest radiographs in positive reactors as well as in clients with symptoms. In January 1987, 171 skin tests were applied; 140 (82%) were read and 84/140 (60%) were positive. A similar screening was done in June and September 1987, but these uncovered no further cases. Of interest were conversion rates of 23–30% in clients retested from 1985 to 1988.

Other situations in which vulnerable persons live in close proximity produce similar results. Tuberculosis outbreaks in a residential facility for HIV-infected individuals have been reported in 1991 from Muskegon County, Michigan and San Francisco, California (CDC, 1991a, 1989b). In the first report, there was only one active case, but a documented skin test conversion rate of 22%. In San Francisco, there were 12 cases of active pulmonary tuberculosis (SFDOPH, 1991).

Case Reporting

As the CDC recommends, outpatient clinics and shelters in the seven cities refer tuberculosis suspects for follow-up, and staff often escort individuals to treatment facilities. Despite such efforts, all reported a significant disappearance rate before a diagnosis could be made. Shelter staff have noted that about 25% of homeless persons skin tested in the various programs fail to return for a reading. Following chest radiography in New York City (NYCDOH, 1989), 6% of individuals with abnormal films could not be found for follow-up despite a money incentive for compliance.

Treatment

The CDC recommends that homeless patients with newly diagnosed active tuberculosis be placed in settings that allow full supervision of initial treatment to avoid the possibility of infecting others, such as peers or shelter staff members. If the patient is recalcitrant, treatment should be enforced until the individual is noninfectious, following law, regulation, and due process.

In practical terms, success in treatment over the necessary months depends upon engaging the individual's cooperation. Staff must be sensitive to the patient's concerns, work consistently to establish rapport and show empathy, make the treatment protocol practical by assuring sensible clinic hours, and offer a variety of incentives.

Staff in each of the seven cities, recognizing this point, have developed distinct approaches for seeking compliance, but each is similar in that initial therapy, lasting up to 1 month, is almost invariably started in a hospital, using a standard treatment regimen.

New York City provides various alternatives for treatment following hospitalization. Part of a large shelter on the grounds of Bellevue Hospital has been designated for up to 85 homeless men with active tuberculosis willing to use this facility. Approximately one-third of the city's homeless tuberculosis cases have been treated at this site since it opened in 1988, with a 62% treatment compliance rate as of spring 1990. The remainder are seen in several clinics and shelters with supervised therapy provided, usually 5 of 7 days each week. Detention orders to ensure compliance have been issued by the Health Commissioner, but actual enforcement is left to the hospital, which must provide the supervision.

In San Francisco, homeless persons with active tuberculosis are followed by staff of the Directly Observed Therapy (DOT) program after release from hospital care (Hyman and Wlodarczyk, 1991). Medication is provided 5 days each week at the shelter clinic or, if indicated, brought directly to the patient elsewhere. In 1987, 2 of 22 cases of tuberculosis were lost to follow-up as was 1 of 18 cases in 1988 (McAdam et al., 1990a).

In Boston, homeless persons with tuberculosis have several options for long-term treatment. If compliant, they can receive medications at any of the numerous shelter nurses' clinics. Those who are noncompliant can be forced under Massachusetts law to accept inpatient treatment at a state facility. In Boston, there is a 90% compliance rate, a success attributed to a high nurse/patient ratio.

In Los Angeles County, staff of the Tuberculosis Control Division started a pilot project in 1989 using vouchers for food and hotel accommodations to improve compliance with therapy. Despite an active outreach program, Los Angeles had previously noted only 50% actual compliance among the homeless. With a change to twice-weekly therapy using vouchers valid only from visit to visit and medication taken in a supervised setting, compliance is improved (Davidson, P., personal communication, November 1991). Long-term care facilities are available in Los Angeles county, but are many miles from the downtown skid-row area and are not accessible for the homeless population.

In Portland, the county welfare and health departments arranged that welfare checks of tuberculosis patients who used the Saint Francis Outreach Project were to be distributed by the project director (Good, 1989). This enabled health care workers to monitor clinic visits for twice-weekly therapy in about one-third of homeless cases, assuring very high compliance rates. In time, however, this process overwhelmed the system, and now Portland, as well as Chicago and Seattle, uses DOT with outreach workers and at scattered shelter clinics.

Antituberculous Drug Therapy

All cities follow the CDC guidelines using intensive, multidrug, bactericidal regimens extending at least 6 months. Isoniazid, rifampin, and pyrazinamide are started under daily observation. The next step is a switch to 5 days observed and 2 of unobserved treatment or then to twice-weekly observed therapy using higher drug dosages to complete the 6-month course. Pyrazinamide is usually stopped after the first 2 months.

Staff in all of the cities surveyed felt that previous poor compliance was the usual reason for drug resistance. Other than the outbreak in Boston noted earlier, instances of drug resistance had been isolated until the situation worsened during the fall of 1991 (McFadden, 1991; Rosenthal, 1991). The Seattle outbreak (Nolan et al., 1991) was preponderantly associated with drug-sensitive organisms. Schieffelbein and Snider in 1988 suggested that "if isoniazid-resistant disease is suspected (as it probably should be for most homeless patients), ethambutol hydrochloride should be added." As the frequency of resistance grows, the use of four drugs may be indicated.

Prevention

The CDC recommends application of a broad array of tuberculosis prevention methods. Crowding and poor ventilation enhance the spread of tuberculosis. Therefore, improvement in housing conditions is the best prevention, but also the most complex and least likely to happen. None of the cities has succeeded in making major improvements in housing for homeless persons. All seven have tried to prevent the spread of tuberculosis through early case-finding and treatment. In both Boston and Seattle, following concentrated attention to outbreaks of tuberculosis in the shelters, the number of cases in homeless persons, as a percentage of the total for the city, decreased by 50% (McAdam et al., 1990a; Nardell, 1989).

Programs have attempted, with variable success, to use isoniazid chemo-prophylaxis in this population. Portland reported (Good, 1989) that in 1987, 62 individuals started and 31 completed therapy; in 1988, 69 started and 29 completed therapy, with 17 lost to follow-up. This degree of compliance was ascribed to a particularly effective outreach worker, but includes individuals who received monthly medication, with compliance judged by a pill count. Combining INH prophylaxis with methadone maintenance yielded a compliance rate of 75% (Selwyn et al., 1989).

Following the outbreak of tuberculosis in the shelter in Seattle described in the foregoing, the local health department encouraged 81 individuals to take isoniazid using twice-weekly DOT with 900 mg/dose. Only 28% completed therapy; 30% started, but did not finish, the 6-month course, and 42% never began (Nazar et al., 1990).

Ultraviolet lights are known to decrease the infectiousness of air containing tuberculous droplet nuclei, and have been recommended as an adjunct in control of tuberculosis (Riley, 1982; Riley and Nardell, 1989). The CDC strongly urges the use of ultraviolet lights in the shelters, but the only cities in this report using them are Boston and Seattle. There seems to be a general apathy to this recommendation.

Transmission of tuberculosis in shelters is well documented. Furthermore, the longer individuals stay in the shelter system, the more likely they will be to have a positive skin test (McAdam et al, 1990a, b; Nolan et al., 1991). Early detection of disease in the shelters and prompt therapy has been the most effective way to limit further spread.

V. New York City: A Shelter Analysis, 1982–1991

A. Background

In New York, there were 3520 new cases of active tuberculosis in 1990, an increase of 38.3% over 1989. This case rate, 49.8:100,000, was the highest in over 20 years. The rate in the Central Harlem Health District reached 233.4:100,000 (NYCDOH, 1990). Reliable estimates of the number of homeless persons in New York City do not exist, but an educated guess of 60,000–90,000 persons is generally accepted as realistic. In 1990, there were 454 cases of tuberculosis in homeless persons, or 13% of the total number of cases (Adler, 1991). This would yield a case rate of 504:100,000 to 757:100,000, depending on which homeless population figure is used. This is over twice the rate in the Central Harlem Health District and 10–15 times the overall rate for New York City. In 1991, through the 47th week, the overall number of new cases was 3045, compared with 3121 for the same week in 1990 (CDC, 1991b).

In New York, residents of a men's shelter underwent routine interviews and, where appropriate, tuberculin skin testing, chest x-rays, and sputum collection for smear and culture from July 1982 through August 1988. Care was given on site in the shelter clinic. Significant findings in the 1853 men screened included a 42.8% infection rate (27.0% PPD-positive as tested, 9.8% PPD-positive by history, and 6.0% with active tuberculosis). These data were recorded while staff provided routine primary care at the shelter clinic. Selection was biased toward those presenting for mandatory work program physicals, housing physicals, and also toward those who were ill. Multivariate analysis demonstrated that tuberculous infection was independently associated with increasing age, length of stay in the shelter system, black race, and intravenous drug use. Active tuberculosis was independently associated with age, length of stay in the shelter system, and intravenous drug use. Although not conclusively proved, transmission of tuberculous infection within the shelter environment was strongly suggested, and HIV infection with loss of immunity was thought to be responsible for the higher active tuberculosis rate among intravenous drug users (McAdam et al., 1990b).

An ongoing study at this shelter continues to show the same troubling trend. From September 1989 through October 1991, 1209 men were evaluated. Three-fourths were seen for mandatory work program or housing placement physicals (McAdam and Brickner, 1991).

Compliance rate with skin test readings was 93.6%. Of 1132 men who returned to complete their evaluations, 29.6% were PPD-positive as tested; another 12.1% were PPD-positive by history; and 5.5% (or 62 men) had active tuberculosis. In total, therefore, the infection rate was 47.2%. As previously noted (McAdam et al., 1990b), nonwhite race and increasing age were positively associated with infection. Intravenous drug use versus nonuse was correlated with an increased rate of active tuberculosis (11.2 vs 3.8%), although overall infection rates were similar (49.6 vs 46.4% respectively). Length of stay in the shelter system was positively associated with increased rates of infection and disease. Those in the system 1 day to 3 months had an overall infection rate of 40.8%, including 3.3% with active tuberculosis. Those in the shelter system longer than 24 months had an overall infection rate of 63.2%, including 8.8% with active tuberculosis.

B. Human Immunodeficiency Virus and Tuberculosis

As part of primary medical care services given at this shelter, risk factors for HIV infection are discussed at the time of initial history and physical examinations, or at any clinic visit during which symptoms suggest an infectious etiology. Of the 1209 men evaluated, 383 (or 31.7%) gave histories of high-risk activities for HIV infection. More than one-third (37.1%) of 142 tested were HIV antibody-positive by enzyme-linked immunosorbent assay (ELISA) and Western blot methods. Of the 62 men with active tuberculosis, 32 (51.6%) gave histories of high-risk activities for HIV infection and 24 of the 32 (75.0%) were HIV antibody-positive. Therefore, those men who engaged in high-risk activities who had active tuberculosis were twice as likely to be HIV antibody-positive as those engaging in these same activities, but who did not have active tuberculosis (McAdam and Brickner, 1991).

Today it is unrealistic to consider screening and treatment of tuberculous patients without discussing the impact of HIV on all facets of diagnosis and therapy. Infection with HIV makes both tuberculous infection and disease more difficult to detect by tuberculin skin testing and chest x-ray film, and also may be a factor in the recent increase of multiple drug-resistant tuberculous cases in various populations.

Early in the AIDS epidemic it became apparent that the development of active tuberculosis could be a marker for concurrent HIV infection (Handwerger et al., 1987; Sunderam et al., 1986; Pitchenik et al., 1987). In 1987, the CDC changed its definition of AIDS to include HIV infection plus extrapulmonary tuberculosis (CDC, 1987b). Studies have demonstrated significant rates of HIV infection in homeless persons in Miami (9.8–14.3%), homeless intravenous drug users (IVDUs) in Chicago (33.7%), and homeless men attending a New York City shelter clinic (62%) (Wiebel et al., 1989; Greer et al., 1989; Torres et al., 1990). In New York City, IVDUs have rates of HIV antibody-positivity ranging from 40 to 60% (Robert-Guroff et al., 1986; Des Jarlais et al., 1989; Selwyn et al., 1989). About 20% of the men attending one shelter-based clinic had histories of IVDU, and another 10% were bisexual or homosexual. The overall HIV antibody-positivity rate was 11.7% (McAdam and Brickner, 1991). The combination of a high HIV antibody-positivity rate with 30–50% tuberculous infection rates places the homeless men attending this shelter clinic at high risk for active tuberculosis (McAdam and Brickner, 1991). It is noteworthy that HIV infection has been associated with transmission of tuberculous infection and disease in residential drug treatment centers and group homes for the HIV-infected (CDC, 1991a, c), settings for which residents have medical evaluations before entry. Such evaluations do not generally occur in most shelters for homeless persons. Therefore, HIV infection can threaten the health of all residents and staff within shelters by increasing the risk for development of active tuberculosis in those dually infected. They, in turn, can spread tuberculous infection to others sharing the same facility, regardless of their HIV status.

VI. Compliance and Control Issues

In 1985, tuberculosis patients in New York State in general complied with therapeutic plans at rates of 55.1% (CDC, 1988). With problems of stolen medications, long waiting times in clinics, and more immediate concerns of the daily battle to obtain food, clothing, and shelter, it is expected that compliance will be worse among homeless persons. A recent study in a hospital-based clinic in Central Harlem showed that 89% of a group of over 200 tuberculosis patients were lost to follow-up before completing therapy. Homelessness or unstable housing proved to be significantly related to poor compliance (Brudney and Dobkin, 1991). Two other programs in New York City have yielded better results. The Bellevue Tuberculosis Shelter (see foregoing) has a 62% completion rate of at least 6-months treatment (NYCDOH, 1989). An on-site shelter clinic in an 850-bed men's shelter has a 36% completion rate, with another 13% still receiving therapy at the completion of the study (McAdam et al., 1990b).

VII. Conclusion

Tuberculous infection and disease are relatively common among homeless persons in certain cities. When tuberculosis is known to be a significant problem among the homeless, medical teams placed in shelters should be able to provide care and improve compliance of tuberculosis therapy on-site. Furthermore, such patients can be treated in shelter clinics after hospital discharge, with a reasonable degree of success.

Analyses should be performed periodically to determine the level of tuberculous infection in individual shelters. In this way tuberculosis control efforts can be directed based on results. Cooperation between local shelters and health departments is important in tracking patients receiving therapy and should help prevent repeated rediagnosis of known tuberculous patients. Shelter medical staff should be involved in case finding, and attempt to remove known or suspected active tuberculous patients as early as possible from the shelter environment. Only a few patients with active tuberculosis need to be confined by court order when the usual available measures fail (e.g., incentives, shelter, DOT). Then, involuntary confinement is probably in the best interests of the patient and the community. Of the seven cities we have discussed, only Boston has adequate legal recourse to ensure compliance when a patient with tuberculosis is a genuine threat to the health of others in the environment. Attention to the rights of the individual makes enforcement and treatment difficult, and efforts often fail during a long and expensive legal process or simply from a lack of funds to employ guards in the hospitals. The balance between individual rights to freedom and the good health of the larger public may be awry.

Because of the frequency of combined HIV and tuberculosis among homeless persons, it is important to know the HIV status of patients with tuberculous infection or disease. Most cities have noted a change in the demography of shelter residents, from an older, often alcoholic group, to a younger, illicit drug-oriented population. In New York City an increasing number of the homeless are intravenous drug users, with a high percentage of human immunodeficiency virus (HIV) infection (Selwyn et al., 1989). This same group accounts for many of the newly discovered cases of active tuberculosis. Spread of tuberculosis to HIV-positive individuals in the shelter system is likely to become a major public health problem, as it already is in the New York State prison system. The presence of antibiotic-resistant bacteria has become a serious concern as well.

Chest radiographs are the quickest way to identify new cases of active tuberculosis and should be used whenever mass screening is essential, as in possible shelter outbreaks. With rapid processing and interpretation, radiographs are an effective diagnostic resource and help minimize the disappearance rate of potential patients before proper evaluation. Because of its cost, however, radiography is not justified for routine surveillance, and tuberculin skin testing using 5-mm induration as a positive reaction should be used for standard screening.

Since many shelters are large and populations mobile, evaluating the tuberculous status of every resident and tracking those who are infected often fails.

Therefore, considerable effort should be directed toward minimizing transmission. Ventilation systems should be evaluated and, if necessary, altered to meet the specifications as outlined by the CDC (CDC, 1990b). Ultraviolet lights should be properly installed and maintained (CDC, 1990b).

Providing medications on-site with supervised therapy by staff or health care workers in the shelters where most homeless persons with tuberculosis reside would increase compliance. Conducting a medical clinic in the shelter would help with case-finding as well. Sbarbaro has pointed out that ". . . kindness, understanding, and a committed, loyal, ongoing professional/patient relationship is essential'' to ensure compliance (Sbarbaro, 1979).

Other possible approaches to support effectual tuberculosis treatment include voluntary long-term inpatient therapy (Veager et al., 1986) and the establishment of boarding and living facilities, true hospital beds, and sanatorium-type settings nationally (Sbarbaro and Iseman, 1986). Here, patients could be placed for long-term residential care.

Tuberculosis has emerged among homeless persons in shelters because these sites recreate the worst aspects of pre-20th century urban life. Medical support systems for the poor have deteriorated, whereas homelessness has increased. Infection with HIV serves to make the organism more virulent and active disease more likely. Only if these problems are surmounted can the goal of tuberculosis elimination in the United States become a reality in the 21st century (CDC, 1989b).

References

Abeles, H., Feibes, H., Mandel, E., and Girard, J. A. (1970). The large city prison: A reservoir of tuberculosis. *Am. Rev. Respir. Dis.* **101**:706–709.

Adler, J. (1991). Presentation at the National Health Care for the Homeless Conference, 29 October 1991, Washington, D.C.

Barry, M. A., Wall, C., Shirley, L., Bernardo, J., Schwingl, P., Brigandi, E., and Lamb, G. A. (1986). Tuberculosis screening in Boston's homeless shelters. *Public Health Rep.* **101**:487–494.

Baxter, E., and Hopper, K. (1982). The new mendicancy: Homeless in New York City. *Am. J. Orthopsychiatry* **52**:393–408.

Blumberg, L. U., Shipley, T. E., and Moore, J. D. (1971). The skid row man and the skid row status community. *Q. J. Stud. Alcohol.* **32**:909–941.

Braun, M. M., Truman, B. I., Maguire, B., DiFerdinando, G. T., Wormser, G., Broaddus, R., and Morse, D. L. (1989a). Increasing incidence of tuberculosis in a prison inmate population: Association with HIV infection. *JAMA* **261**:393–397.

Braun, M. M., Truman, B. I., Maguire, B., DiFerdinando, G. T., Wormser, G., Broaddus, R., and Morse, D. L. (1989b). Tuberculosis in correctional institutions [Editorial]. *JAMA* **261**:436–437.

Brickner, P. W., and Scanlan, B. C. (1990). Health care of homeless persons: Creation and implementation of a program. In *Under the Safety Net*. Edited by P. W. Brickner, L. K. Scharer, B. A. Conanan, M. Savarese, and B. C. Scanlan. W. W. Norton & Co., New York, pp. 3–14.

Brickner, P. W., Scanlan, B. C., Conanan, B., Elvy, A., McAdam, J., Scharer, L. K., and Vicic, W. J. (1986). Homeless persons and health care. *Ann. Intern. Med.* **104**:405–409.

Brudney, K., and Dobkin, J. (1991). Resurgent tuberculosis in New York City: Human immunodeficiency virus, homelessness, and the decline of tuberculosis control programs. *Am. Rev. Respir. Dis.* **144**:745–749.

Burroughs, J., Bouma, P., O'Connor, E., and Smith, D. (1990). Health concerns of homeless women. In *Under the Safety Net*. Edited by P. W. Brickner, L. K. Scharer, B. A. Conanan, M. Savarese, and B. C. Scanlan. W. W. Norton & Co., New York, pp. 139–150.

Capewell, S., France, A. J., Anderson, M., and Leitch, A. G. (1986). The diagnosis and management of tuberculosis in common hostel dwellers. *Tubercle* **67**:125–131.

Centers for Disease Control (1978). Tuberculosis case rates and deaths in the United States since 1900. In *Extrapulmonary Tuberculosis in the United States*, Atlanta, DHEW Publication No. (CDC) 78-8322.

Centers for Disease Control (1987a). Tuberculosis control among homeless populations. *MMWR* **36**:257–260.

Centers for Disease Control (1987b). Revision of the CDC surveillance case definition for acquired immunodeficiency syndrome. *MMWR* **36**:3s–15s.

Centers for Disease Control (1988). Tuberculosis in the United States 1985–1986. In *Continuity of Drug Therapy Started in 1985*. Centers for Disease Control. Atlanta, Georgia, Table 64.

Centers for Disease Control (1989a). In *Tuberculosis Statistics in the United States*. HHS Publication No. (CDC) 91-8322, Table 1, p. 5.

Centers for Disease Control (1989b). A strategic plan for the elimination of tuberculosis in the United States. *MMWR* **38**(S-3):1–25.

Centers for Disease Control (1990a). Summaries of notifiable diseases in the United States, 1990. *MMWR* **39**(53):1–12.

Centers for Disease Control (1990b). Guidelines for preventing the transmission of tuberculosis in health-care settings, with special focus on HIV-related issues. *MMWR* **39**(RR-17):7.

Centers for Disease Control (1991a). Transmission of multidrug-resistant tuberculosis from an HIV-positive client in a residential substance-abuse treatment facility—Michigan. *MMWR* **40**:129–131.

Centers for Disease Control (1991b). Table II. *MMWR* **40**:815.

Centers for Disease Control (1991c). Tuberculosis outbreak among persons in a residential facility for HIV-infected persons—San Francisco. *MMWR* **40**:649–652.

Des Jarlais, D. C., Friedman, S. R., Novick, D. M., Sotheran, J. L., Thomas, P., Yancovitz, S. R., Mildvan, D., Weber, J., Kreek, M. J., Maslansky, R., Bartelme, S., Spira, T., and Marmor, M. (1989). HIV-1 infection among intravenous drug users in Manhattan, New York City, from 1977 through 1987. *JAMA* **261**:1008–1012.

Erickson, J., and Wilhelm, C. (1986). Introduction. In *Housing the Homeless*. Edited by J. Erickson and C. Wilhelm. Center for Urban Policy Research, Rutgers University, New Brunswick, N.J., pp. xix–xxxvii.

Friedman, L. N., Sullivan, G. M., Bevilaqua, R. P., and Loscos, R. (1987). Tuberculosis screening in alcoholics and drug addicts. *Am. Rev. Respir. Dis.* **136**:1188–1192.

Gaston, M. (1991). Presentation at the National Health Care for the Homeless Conference, October 1991, Washington, D.C.

Gelberg, L., Linn, L. S., Usatine, R. P., and Smith, M. H. (1990). Health, homelessness, and poverty: A study of clinic users. *Arch. Intern. Med.* **150**:2325–2330.

Good, W. E. (1989). Portland, Oregon Burnside Outreach Project uses KEDS. Department of Human Resources, Portland.

Greer, P., Dickinson, G., Parra, F., Egea, F., Jordahl, L., and Holmes, L. (1989). HIV seropositivity in a clinic for the homeless. Presented at the Fifth International Conference on AIDS; June 5, 1989; Montreal, Quebec.

Handwerger, S., Mildvan, D., Senie, R., and McKinley, F. W. (1987). Tuberculosis and the acquired immunodeficiency syndrome at a New York City hospital: 1978–1985. *Chest* **91**:176–180.

Houk, V. N., Baker, J. H., Sorensen, K., and Kent, D. C. (1968). The epidemiology of tuberculosis infection in a closed environment. *Arch. Environ. Health* **16**:26–35.

Hyman, N., and Wlodarczyk, D. (1991). Tuberculosis among San Francisco's homeless population (draft paper). San Francisco Department of Health, August 1991.

Knopf, S. A. (1914). Tuberculosis as a cause and result of poverty. *JAMA* **63**:1721.

Lamb, H. R. (1984). Deinstitutionalization and the homeless mentally ill. In *The Homeless Mentally Ill*. Edited by H. R. Lamb. American Psychiatric Association, Washington, D.C., pp. 55–74.

Marsh, K. (1957). Tuberculosis among the residents of hostels and lodging-houses in London. *Lancet* **1**:1137–1138.

McAdam, J. M., and Brickner, P. W. (1991). Presentation at the National Health Care for the Homeless Conference, October 28, 1991, Washington, D.C..

McAdam, J. M., Brickner, P. W., Scharer, L. L., Groth, J. L., Benton, D., Kiyasu, S., and Wlodarczyk, D. (1990a). Tuberculosis in the homeless: A national perspective. In *Under the Safety Net.* Edited by P. W. Brickner, L. K. Scharer, B. A. Conanan, M. Savarese, and B. C. Scanlan. W. W. Norton & Co., New York, pp. 234–249.

McAdam, J. M., Brickner, P. W., Scharer, L. L., Crocco, J. A., and Duff, A. E. (1990b). The spectrum of tuberculosis in a New York City men's shelter clinic. *Chest* **97**:798–805.

McFadden, R. D. (1991). Rare TB strain kills 13th inmate in New York prisons. *New York Times,* November 17, p. B1.

Nardell, E. A. (1989). Tuberculosis in homeless, residential care facilities, prisons, nursing homes, and other close communities. *Semin. Respir. Infect.* **4**:206–215.

Nardell, E., McInnis, B., Thomas, B., and Weidhaas, S. (1986). Exogenous reinfection with tuberculosis in a shelter for the homeless. *N. Engl. J. Med.* **315**:1571.

Nazar, V., Oberle, M., and Nolan, C. (1990). Results of a directly-observed, intermittent isoniazid program in a shelter for homeless men. *Am. Rev. Respir. Dis.* **141**:A438.

New York City Department of Health (1989). Tuberculosis among the homeless. *CHI* **8**(7):1–3.

New York City Department of Health (1990). *Tuberculosis in New York City 1990: Information Summary.* Bureau of Tuberculosis Control, pp. 1–10.

Nolan, C. M., and Elarth, A. M. (1988). Tuberculosis in a cohort of Southeast Asian refugees. *Am. Rev. Respir. Dis.* **137**:805–809.

Nolan, C. M., Elarth, A. M., Barr, H., Saeed, A. M., and Risser, D. R. (1991). An outbreak of tuberculosis in a shelter for homeless men. *Am. Rev. Respir. Dis.* **143**:257–261.

Ochs, C. W. (1962). The epidemiology of tuberculosis. *JAMA* **179**:247–252.

O'Connell, J. J., Summerfield, J., and Kellogg, F. R. (1990). The homeless elderly. In *Under the Safety Net.* Edited by P. W. Brickner, L. K. Scharer, B. A. Conanan, M. Savarese, and B. C. Scanlan. W. W. Norton & Co., New York, pp. 151–168.

Pablos-Mendez, A., Raviglione, M. C., Battan, R., and Ramos-Zuniga, R. (1990). Drug resistant tuberculosis among the homeless in New York City. *N.Y. State J. Med.* **90**:351–355.

Patel, K. R. (1985). Pulmonary tuberculosis in residents of lodging houses, night shelters and common hostels in Glasgow: A 5-year prospective study. *Br. J. Dis. Chest* **79**:60–66.

Pitchenik, A. E., Burr, J., Suarez, M., Fertel, D., Gonzalez, G., and Moas, C. (1987). Human T-cell lymphotropic virus-III (HTLV-III) seropositivity and related disease among 71 consecutive patients in whom tuberculosis was diagnosed. *Am. Rev. Respir. Dis.* **135**:875–879.

Ramsden, S. S., Baur, S., and El Kabir, D. J. (1988). Tuberculosis among the central London single homeless: A four-year retrospective study. *J. R. Coll. Physicians Lond.* **22**:16–17.

Reichman, L. B., Felton, C. P., and Edsall, J. R. (1979). Drug dependence, a possible new risk factor for tuberculosis disease. *Arch. Intern. Med.* **139**:337–339.

Reichman, L. B., and O'Day, R. (1978). Tuberculosis infection in a large urban population. *Am. Rev. Respir. Dis.* **117**:705–712.

Rieder, H. L. (1989). Tuberculosis among American Indians of the contiguous United States. *Public Health Rep.* **104**:653–657.

Rieder, H. L., Cauthen, G. M., Kelly, G. D., Bloch, A. B., and Snider, D. E. (1989). Tuberculosis in the United States. *JAMA* **262**:385–388.

Riley, R. L. (1982). Disease transmission and contagion control. *Am. Rev. Respir. Dis.* **125**:16–19.

Riley, R. L., and Nardell E. A. (1989). The theory and application of ultraviolet air disinfection. *Am. Rev. Respir. Dis.* **139**:1286–1294.

Robert-Guroff, M., Weiss, S. H., Giron, J. A., Jennings, A. M., Ginzburg, H. M., Margolis, I. B., Blattner, W. A., and Gallo, R. C. (1986). Prevalence of antibodies to HTLV-I, -II, and -III in intravenous drug abusers from an AIDS endemic region. *JAMA* **255**:3133–3137.

Rosenthal, E. (1991). H.I.V. infection foiling tests that detect deadly TB germ. *New York Times*, December 10, p. A-1.

Rudd, A. (1985). Tuberculosis in a geriatric unit. *J. Am. Geriatr. Soc.* **33**:566–569.

San Francisco Department of Public Health (1991). Outbreak of tuberculosis among residents at an HIV congregate living site. *San Francisco Epidemiol. Bull.* **7**:1.

Sbarbaro, J. A. (1979). Compliance, inducements and enforcements. *Chest* **76**:750–756.

Sbarbaro, J. A., and Iseman, M. D. (1986). Baby needs a new pair of shoes. *Chest* **90**:754–755.

Schieffelbein, C. W., and Snider, D. E. (1988). Tuberculosis control among homeless populations. *Arch. Intern. Med.* **148**:1843–1846.

Selwyn, P. A., Hartel, D., Lewis, V. A., Schoenbaum, E. E., Vermund, S. H., Klein, R. S., Walker, A. T., and Friedland, G. H. (1989). A prospective study of the risk of tuberculosis among intravenous drug users with human immunodeficiency virus infection. *N. Engl. J. Med.* **320**:545–550.

Sherman, M. N., Brickner, P. W., Schwartz, M. S., Viterella, C., Wobido, S. L., Vickery, C., Garippa, J., and Crocco, J. A. (1980). Tuberculosis in single-room-occupancy hotel residents: A persisting focus of disease. *N.Y. Med. Q.* **2**:39–41.

Slutkin, G. (1986). Management of tuberculosis in urban homeless indigents. *Public Health Rep.* **101**:481–485.

Snider, D. (1991). Presentation at the American Epidemiological Society, March 1991, Washington, D.C.

Snider, D. E., Salinas, L., and Kelly, G. D. (1989). Tuberculosis: An increasing problem among minorities in the United States. *Public Health Rep.* **104**:646–652.

Stead, W. W., Lofgren, J. P., Warren, E., and Thomas, C. (1985). Tuberculosis as an endemic and nosocomial infection among the elderly in nursing homes. *N. Engl. J. Med.* **312**:1483–1487.

Stead, W. W., Senner, J. W., Reddick, T. W., and Lofgren, J. P. (1990). Racial differences in susceptibility to infection by *Mycobacterium tuberculosis*. *N. Engl. J. Med.* **322**:422–427.

Sunderam, G., McDonald, R. J., Maniatis, T., Oleske, J., Kapila, R., and Reichman, L. B. (1986). Tuberculosis as a manifestation of the acquired immunodeficiency syndrome (AIDS). *JAMA* **256**:362–366.

Teller, M. E. (1988). *The Tuberculosis Movement*. Greenwood Press, New York, pp. 100–101.

Torres, R. A., Mani, S., Altholz, J., and Brickner, P. W. (1990). Human immunodeficiency virus infection among homeless men in a New York City shelter. *Arch. Intern. Med.* **150**:2030–2036.

Trachtman, L., and Greenberg, H. B. (1978). Surveying 2,020 vagrants for tuberculosis [Letter to the Editor]. *JAMA* **240**:73.

Valway, S. (1991). Workgroup on tuberculosis in congregate housing. Centers for Disease Control, 28 October.

Veager, H. and Medinger, A. E. (1986). Tuberculosis long-term beds. *Chest* **90**:75.

Wiebel, W., Lampinen, T., Chene, D., Jimenez, D., Johnson, W., and Queller, L. Risk of HIV infection among homeless IV drug users (IVDUs) in Chicago. Presented at the Fifth International Conference on AIDs; June 5, 1989; Montreal, Quebec.

Wright, J. D. (1990). The health of homeless people. In *Under the Safety Net*. Edited by P. W. Brickner, L. K. Scharer, B. A. Conanan, M. Savarese, and B. C. Scanlan. W. W. Norton & Co., New York, pp. 15–31.

Wright, J. D., and Weber, E. (1987). *Homelessness and Health*. McGraw-Hill, Washington, D.C.

21

Tuberculosis in Native North Americans

JURE MANFREDA,
EARL S. HERSHFIELD

University of Manitoba, Faculty of Medicine
Winnipeg, Manitoba, Canada

JOSEPH L. BREAULT

Ochsner Clinic
New Orleans, Louisiana

JOHN P. MIDDAUGH,
MICHAEL E. JONES

Section of Epidemiology
Division of Public Health
State of Alaska
Anchorage, Alaska

I. Introduction

Among diseases that have affected the aboriginal–native people of North America after the arrival of Europeans in the 15th century, tuberculosis is the most prominent and long-lasting. Until recently, only a few individuals escaped being infected by the tubercle bacillus at a very young age. The result was an epidemic of the disease that was widespread, with a high case fatality rate. The purpose of this chapter is to review what is known about this epidemic, what actions were undertaken to bring it under control, and to look at the prospects for control and , if possible, elimination of tuberculosis in the aboriginal population of North America in the future. (*Aboriginal* and *native* are used interchangeably in this chapter; aboriginal is preferred in Canada, whereas native is preferred in the United States. The terms *Inuit* and *Eskimo* are used similarly.)

II. Population

North American Indians and Inuit–Eskimos are aboriginal people of Canada and the United States. They settled on the North American continent between

40,000 and 10,000 years ago. In adapting to the varied and sometimes hostile environments, different cultures and tribal groups developed among these people. Until recently, they survived on hunting, fishing, and agriculture. For the purpose of this discussion, four groups are distinguished: Indians and Inuit in Canada, Indians in the contiguous United States, and Alaska natives.

A. Canadian Indians and Inuit

Canadian Indians belong to ten different linguistic families and six different cultures: Woodland Indians in Atlantic and Central Canada, Indians of Southeastern Ontario, Plains Indians on the Prairies, Indians of the Plateau in the interior of the British Columbia, Pacific Coast Indians, and Indians of the Mackenzie and Yukon River Basins. The Inuit belong to the Eskimo–Aleut linguistic family and are divided into several cultural groups. They inhabit the vast area from the Mackenzie river in the West to Labrador in the East (Indian and Northern Affairs Canada, 1990a,b).

In 1981, the total aboriginal population of Canada was approximately 413,000 people, of whom 390,000 were Indians and Metis and 23,000 Inuit. The majority of Indians (335,000 or 86%) were registered with the federal government as Indians according to the terms of the Indian Act. Since statistical data exist for registered, but not for nonregistered Indians and Metis, the discussion of tuberculosis in Canadian Indians will be limited to registered Indians.

Registered Indians form bands; typically one band occupies one reserve (i.e., a tract of land set aside for the use and benefit of a band). In 1980, there were 575 bands in Canada, with the average size of approximately 550 persons. The population of the smallest bands was fewer than 100 persons and the largest approximately 9000. Most of the Indian population lives in bands with fewer than 1000 population.

Approximately 72% of Inuit people live in the Northwest Territories of Canada and the remaining in Northern Quebec (20%) and Labrador. There are 66 Inuit communities scattered over this vast territory, with populations that vary between 100 and 1000.

Canada's aboriginal population is growing rapidly and is expected to almost double between 1981 and 2001 (Hagey et al., 1989). In the 1980s, Indians constituted 1.7% of the total Canadian population, with 37% of them living off reserves, although not necessarily continuously. More females than males live off the reserve. Indian families are larger than the average Canadian families. In comparison with the Canadian average, Indians have less education and lower employment rates. Fishing, trapping, forestry, and related occupations are twice as common among Indians as among the rest of the population. The average income of the Indian population is half that of the general population, and over 40% receive government transfer payments as the major source of income. Living conditions are much poorer than for the non-Indian population: 20% of Indian dwellings have more than one person per room and 24% of dwellings are without a central heating system. Although health indicators have improved over the last 50 years, death rates, particularly before the age of 65 years are still more than twice the national average (Indian and Northern Affairs Canada, 1990a).

B. Indians in the Contiguous United States

Among the Indian population in the contiguous United States, eight major cultural groups (Northeast, Southeast, Great Plains, Southwest, Great Basin, Plateau, California, and Northwest Indians) are further subdivided into numerous tribes. According to the tentative figures from the 1990 Census, there were 1,868,437 American Indians, Eskimos, and Aleuts in the 48 contiguous states, constituting 0.76% of the total population in the United States. This was a 38% increase over the 1980 Census population figures, whereas the total population in the United States increased by 9.8% between the 1980 and 1990 Census. The states with the largest number of American Indians in the 1990 Census were Oklahoma (252,420), California (242,164), Arizona (203,527), New Mexico (134,355), and Washington (81,483). Approximately 49% of the Indian population lives in these five states. The states with the largest percentage of their total population who are Indians are New Mexico (8.9%), Oklahoma (8.0%), South Dakota (7.3%), Montana (6.0%), and Arizona (5.6%). In 34 of the 48 states, Indians represent less than 1% of the population (Bureau of the Census, U. S. Department of Commerce News, CB91-100, March 11, 1991). Approximately 53% of the Indians in the contiguous 48 states live in metropolitan areas. The metropolitan areas with the largest numbers of Indians were Los Angeles (83,258) and San Francisco, California (34,357), Tulsa (34,126) and Oklahoma City, Oklahoma (25,085), and New York (22,930) (Bureau of the Census, US Department of Commerce News, CB91-229, July 5, 1991).

Approximately one-quarter (436,222) of all Indians in the contiguous 48 states were living on 309 reservations or trust lands (Bureau of the Census, American Indian and Alaskan Native Areas: 1990, June 1991). In 1990, the total land held in trust by the federal government of the United States for Indians was 54.4 million acres. This land is administered by the Bureau of Indian Affairs, an agency of the Interior Department that is 87% staffed by American Indians. The ten most populous Indian reservations (some of which include trust lands) in 1990 were Navajo, Arizona–New Mexico–Utah (143,400); Pine Ridge, Nebraska–South Dakota (11,200); Fort Apache (9,800), Gila River (9,100), and Papago, Arizona (8,500); Rosebud, South Dakota (8,000); San Carlos, Arizona (7,100), Zuni Pueblo, Arizona–New Mexico (7,100); Hopi, Arizona (7,100); and Blackfeet, Montana (7,000) (Bureau of the Census, 1990 Census Profile, No.2, June 1991).

The American Indian population tends to be younger than the total population in the United States. Poverty is a serious problem for many Indian tribes and this has a notable effect on health, nutrition, and housing. On reservations, about half of the students do not graduate from high school, unemployment is at least 40%, birth and death rates are high, life expectancy is shorter, and suicides occur at twice the national average.

C. Alaska Natives

Alaska is about one-fifth the size of the contiguous United States. In 1990, 86,000, or 16%, of the Alaska population were Alaska natives, which include Eskimos, American Indians, and Aleuts. Eskimos comprise two major groups: the Inupiat, who inhabit the northern and coastal areas of Alaska; and the Yupik Eskimos, who live in the southwest of Alaska. Among Indians, the Athapaskans occupy the vast areas of the interior Alaska, while the Tlingit, Haida, and Tsimshian live on the coast of the panhandle. Aleuts include the residents of the Aleutian Chain of Alaska and the Pribilof Islands (Fitzbugh and Crowell, 1988; Morgan, 1979).

Approximately 70% of the Alaska natives live in 171 villages, with populations ranging from 30 to 3500 (Alaska Department of Labor, 1990). Although the health status of Alaska natives has been significantly improved in the past 40 years, both infant and total mortality remain more than twice the rate in non-native ethnic groups (Alaska Department of Labor, 1990)

III. Epidemic of Tuberculosis

The question of whether or not tuberculous infection was brought to the Americas by Europeans has not been resolved (Buikstra, 1981; Paulsen, 1987). However, the real rise in tuberculosis undoubtedly began after the settling of North America by Europeans. Because Europeans were heavily infected by the tubercle bacillus, they greatly increased the number of sources of tuberculous infection and, thereby, increased the opportunity for the native population to become infected. The native populations are believed to have been very susceptible to tuberculous infection because they had little previously acquired resistance. In addition, the arrival of Europeans profoundly affected the biological basis of the native populations, their social organization, and culture. This resulted in periods of starvation, chronic malnutrition, and epidemics of other communicable diseases, which further increased susceptibility to tuberculosis. Conditions for epidemic outbreaks of tuberculosis in the aboriginal population of the Americas were thus met.

Regions that first came in contact with the Europeans were the first to be affected by the tuberculosis epidemic. Among Indians in the contiguous United

States and in Canada, the epidemic was widespread in the second half of the 19th century, whereas, in Alaska and in the Canadian Arctic, the epidemic peaked in the 20th century.

When the epidemic reached its zenith in Saskatchewan, Canada, in 1890, the incidence of the disease was 9000:100,000 population (Ferguson, 1934). One-third of the population was affected by tuberculosis of lymph nodes. In one school in Saskatchewan in 1906, approximately 20% of children had excision of tuberculous glands (Ferguson, 1934). The dominant type of disease was the acute form, and the affected individuals frequently died within 1 year of diagnosis. The highest mortality was in the age group 1–5 years (Ferguson, 1934). Following the peak of the epidemic in 1890, the incidence of the disease declined to 800:100,000 population by 1926. The course of the disease became less acute, and the glandular form of the disease almost disappeared; it affected 1% of children in 1932 in comparison with 20% in 1890. The highest mortality shifted to the age group 15–19 years during 1927–1932 (Ferguson, 1934).

James Walker came as the physician to the Pine Ridge Reservation in South Dakota in 1896. In 1908, he reported 600 cases of tuberculosis among approximately 7000 Indians (i.e., 8839 cases per 100,000 persons (Walker, et al. 1980). Dr. Walker implemented sanitary measures and the safe disposal of waste and sputum. Between 1897 and 1903 he noted that the annual incidence of tuberculosis declined by 49% and mortality from tuberculosis by 44%.

Between 1926 and 1930, 982 (35.5%) of the 2767 deaths among Alaska natives were attributed to tuberculosis, in comparison with 80 (4.7%) of 1704 deaths among white Alaskans. The average annual mortality rate per 100,000 was 655 among Alaska natives and 56 per 100,000 in Alaskan whites (Fellows, 1934). In 1946, tuberculosis was still listed as the cause of death on 43% of all death certificates for that year. In 1953, a chest x-ray survey of 200 Alaska National Guardsmen—all of whom were Alaska native men between the ages of 18 and 43 years—showed evidence of tuberculosis in 40%, with 10% in an apparently active state (Alaska's Health, 1954).

It appears that the Canadian Inuit were the last aboriginal population in North America to be exposed to tuberculosis. Although some Inuit communities were exposed to tuberculosis as early as the 1820s, there were others who, because of their isolation, were not exposed to tuberculous bacilli until the 1920s (Rabinowitch, 1936; Grzybowski et al., 1976b). Wherrett (1969) estimated that between 1937 and 1941, the mortality from tuberculosis in the Northwest Territories was 3150:100,000 population. In 1950, the mortality from tuberculosis in Inuit in the Northwest Territories was 718:100,000 population, one of the highest in the world at that time (Grzybowski et al., 1976b).

At the height of the epidemic of tuberculosis, the rates of infection, incidence of active disease, and mortality caused by tuberculosis, were extremely high, particularly among the younger-aged groups. During the decline of the epidemic, the probability of infection was reduced, and the infection occurred later in life. The incidence of active disease declined faster in younger- compared with older-aged groups. The mortality was also drastically reduced. The interval between infection and the onset of disease was short during the peak of the epidemic. During the decline of the epidemic, the proportion of the disease from remote infection increased and the proportion of primary tuberculosis decreased. In addition, during the epidemic peak, it was impossible to distinguish population groups with different risks for tuberculosis. This became possible when the epidemic declined. Among the Canadian Inuit people, individuals at the highest risk of developing active disease were those with inactive tuberculosis. They relapsed at a rate of 85:10,000 per year. Next were those with a positive tuberculin test, no bacille Calmette-Guérin (BCG) vaccination, and a normal x-ray film, who developed the disease at a rate of 62:10,000 per year. In comparison, the risk of the BCG-vaccinated population, with normal x-ray films, was 19:10,000 per year (Grzybowski et al., 1976b).

During the decline of the epidemic, relapses were frequent. In the Inuit, the greatest risk of relapse occurred approximately 12 years after becoming inactive. This is contrary to observations in nonaboriginals for whom the highest risk of relapse is shortly after completion of therapy. The long interval between the completion of therapy and relapse in the Inuit people may be due to a lower natural resistance to tuberculosis that cannot prevent multiplication of a small number of bacilli remaining in the body at the end of treatment (Chan-Yeung et al., 1971).

IV. Program Implementation

The awareness of the extent of the epidemic of tuberculosis and its effect on the North American aboriginal population developed slowly. Although some information was available at the end of the 19th century, the situation among Indians in the contiguous United States and in Canada became well documented only about 1930. Similarly, the devastating effect of tuberculosis among Alaska natives was documented for the first time in the 1930s (Fellows, 1934), but the government's and the public's concern focused on the problem about 1950, when the full extent of the problem was documented. A special health survey team reviewed the health status of Alaskans in 1954 and found that the most pressing health problems fell disproportionately on Alaska natives, and that their main finding was the epidemic of tuberculosis (Alaska's Health, 1954). As a result of the devastating conditions documented by the health survey team, emergency programs were initiated in 1953 and 1954 by the territorial government of Alaska and by the United States government to address the most pressing and urgent problem of public health in Alaska.

The Indian Health Services of the Canadian Department of National Health and Welfare became involved in the control of tuberculosis in 1946, but a comprehensive treatment program was not developed and implemented until the beginning of the 1950s (Grzybowski et al., 1976b).

V. Hospitalization

The earliest tuberculosis control program for the aboriginal population was based on hospitalization of persons with active disease. In the late 1800s and early 1900s the sanatorium movement tried to isolate persons with active disease away from population centers. Many Indian patients resisted being taken out of their communities. In 1926, the Miriam Commission, impaneled by the United States Congress to investigate conditions among Indians, reported that "No sanatorium in the Indian Health Service meets the minimum requirements of the American Sanatorium Association." Sanatoria were often located in "abandoned forts and other discarded buildings" that were grossly inadequate and often unsafe (Aberdeen Area Indian Health Service, 1985). The situation improved somewhat later. As recently as the early 1960s, hospitalization was still the essential component of treatment of tuberculosis in Canadian Inuit, who were evacuated to sanatoria in southern Ontario for 18 months (Grzybowski et al., 1976b). All tuberculosis hospital beds were closed by the United States Indian Health Service in the mid 1970s. Similarly, in Canada, the average hospital stay was reduced to 2.9 months (Grzybowski et al., 1976b) in early 1979.

VI. General Preventive Measures

In the 1930s, in Saskatchewan, Canada, it was recognized that boarding schools were important for both the transmission and control of the disease. The following preventive measures were introduced: a selective x-ray and physical examination survey of the Indian schoolchildren; exclusion and segregation of sick children; elimination of bovine tuberculosis; education about sanitation; and application of general health principles in school (Ferguson, 1934).

A. Radiography

The availability of chest radiography, and especially mass miniature radiographs in the 1940s, made it possible to search for unknown sources of infection. In the case of the Canadian Inuit, the total population was periodically screened. At the present time, x-ray examinations are used to identify tuberculosis cases among contacts when a case or an outbreak occurs.

B. Tuberculin Testing

Tuberculin testing was, and still is used to estimate the proportion of the aboriginal population infected with *Mycobacterium tuberculosis*; to estimate changes in the infection rate over time; and to identify contacts (i.e., those who may have become infected when exposed to a known case). Tuberculin testing was of little value in the Canadian aboriginal population because the majority had been BCG-vaccinated.

C. Chemotherapy

In the 1950s chemotherapy was introduced for treatment of tuberculosis in the North American aboriginal population. Streptomycin, *p*-aminosalicylic acid (PAS), isoniazid, and other drugs were used. Efficacious chemotherapy had a profound effect on the tuberculosis program in American Indians and Inuit. It was possible to shorten hospitalization, which was particularly disliked because patients were frequently moved far away from their communities. Ambulatory chemotherapy was instituted. Potent new drugs made it possible to shorten the duration of treatment and to administer it on an intermittent (two to three times a week) basis. Experience in controlling tuberculosis in Alaska led to innovative strategies for implementing programs. The development, in the 1950s, of ambulatory treatment under supervision by selected individuals was critical in remote villages. The benefit of this program was not only improved compliance with treatment, but the evolution of the Alaska community health aide program that has become an integral component of Alaska's medical and public health delivery system over a 20-year period.

D. BCG Vaccination

Although the documentation is unclear, administration of BCG seems to have been fairly standard throughout the United States Indian Health Service until the mid-1950s, when isoniazid came into use (Aberdeen Area IHS Office, 1985). BCG vaccination was used in Alaska for only a short period before being abandoned in the mid-1950s. Vaccination of Indian and Inuit children at birth was introduced in Canada in the 1940s and became the official policy in the 1960s. Currently, between 50 and 80% (Young and Hershfield, 1986; Houston et al., 1990) of children are vaccinated at birth. The most important difference between the tuberculosis control programs for the aboriginal people in the United States and in Canada is that those in the United States are not BCG-vaccinated, whereas those in Canada are.

There were several trials of BCG vaccine among Indian children. In 1935–1938 2046 Indians aged 1–10 years from Pima, Arizona; Wind River, Wyoming; Turtle Mountain, North Dakota; and Rosebud, South Dakota, along with 961

Alaska natives were divided between BCG and control groups. In terms of cases per 1000 person-years, the rates were 24.3 for controls and 4.7 for the vaccinated (Aronson and Palmer, 1946). In 1936, in a study of 3008 BCG-vaccinated Indian children in the western United States, followed for about a decade, a 75% reduction in cases of tuberculosis was estimated (Comstock, G., personal communication). In 1938, a study of 262 Indian newborns in the north central United States, followed-up for 6–8 years, demonstrated a 59% reduction in cases (Comstock, G., personal communication). In 1949, 27,000 children attending federal and mission schools were studied: 11,500 were BCG-vaccinated, 3500 were controls, and 12,000 were tuberculin reactors. There were no deaths reported in the vaccinated group, 1 in the control group, and 13 in the reactor group (Palmer and Shaw, 1953).

A randomized clinical trial to determine the efficacy of BCG vaccination was conducted in Saskatchewan between 1933 and 1947 (Ferguson and Simes, 1949). They vaccinated 306 children and 303 served as controls; 6 cases occurred in the vaccinated (2.9:1000 person-years of observation) and 29 (15.7:1000 person-years) in controls. The rate of active disease in the vaccinated was 0.19 of the rate in controls, suggesting an approximate 80% protection by the vaccine in this highly infectious environment.

It was regularly observed that tuberculosis also develops in children who had been vaccinated. In Frobisher Bay, the clinical picture and the course of tuberculosis did not differ between the BCG-vaccinated and nonvaccinated patients. In both groups, approximately 80% of tuberculosis was primary. This was unexpected for the vaccinated children (Wilson et al., 1973).

Because of doubts about the efficacy of BCG vaccination, especially when the infection rate and the disease incidence rate have decreased, two case-control studies were carried out in which a case of tuberculosis was matched with two or more controls without tuberculosis (Young and Hershfield, 1986; Houston et al., 1990). A history of BCG vaccination was compared between cases and controls. Both studies found a similar degree of protection [i.e., 60% (Young and Hershfield, 1986) and 57% (Houston et al., 1990)]. However, because of the case-control design used in these two studies, it was not possible to distinguish between the efficacy of the vaccine and the effectiveness of vaccinating a population at high risk of developing tuberculosis. It is possible that children with a lower risk of developing disease were vaccinated, whereas those with a higher risk were not.

E. Chemoprophylaxis

Chemoprophylaxis with isoniazid was introduced in the late 1950s and early 1960s as the last component of the tuberculosis control program. Because this approach was perceived as very effective, BCG vaccination was abandoned by the Alaska tuberculosis program.

In 1957, a controlled study was initiated in the Bethel area of Alaska (Hanson et al., 1967). Alaska natives with untreated nonactive tuberculosis were given either isoniazid or placebo for 1 year. During the 6-year follow-up, 12% of the placebo group, in comparison with 4% of the isoniazid treated group, developed active tuberculosis, in spite of the fact that only one-third of the treatment group took 80% or more of the prescribed annual dose, and one-sixth took less than 40%. On the basis of these results, chemoprophylaxis with isoniazid was introduced in Alaska in 1963, initially as a demonstration project (Comstock and Woolpert, 1972).

In Frobisher Bay, Canada, between 1971 and 1974, 587 high-risk Inuits (i.e., those with inadequately treated tuberculosis and those with large positive tuberculin reactions with or without BCG vaccination) were enrolled in a randomized clinical trial. A randomly selected group was given isoniazid and ethambutol three times a week over a period of 18 months in a supervised manner. More than 90% of subjects completed the treatment. Over a follow-up period of 10 years, 3 cases occurred among the vaccinated (0.1%) and 13 (1.0%) among the controls. During the first 36 months, there were no cases among the vaccinated and 9 cases in the controls. Results of the study suggested that prophylactic treatment in high-risk individuals was highly protective and that this protection may last at least 10 years, although it tends to weaken somewhat with time lapsed since treatment (Grzybowski et al., 1976a; Dorken et al., 1984).

VII. Decline in Mortality, Incidence of Active Disease, and Rate of Infection

Application of case-finding, isolation, and treatment brought about a dramatic reduction in the rates of mortality, the rate of active cases, and the rate of infection between 1940s and the present (Comstock and Philip, 1961; Kaplan et al., 1972; Johnson, 1973). Key to these efforts were innovative programs using portable chest x-ray surveys in rural villages, institution of ambulatory chemotherapy using isoniazid and PAS with supervised home care, and initiation of chemoprophylaxis of household contacts (Comstock et al., 1979).

A. Mortality

Canadian Indians

Between 1950 and 1960, the annual mortality rate from tuberculosis declined from 290:100,000 to 23:100,000 population—13 times less (Statistics Canada, personal communication).

Canadian Inuit

The annual tuberculosis mortality rate per 100,000 population in Inuit in Northwest Territories declined from 718:100,000, in 1950, to 3:100,000 in

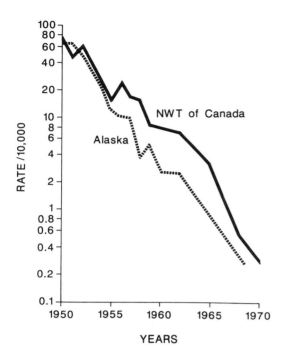

Figure 1 Tuberculosis death rates among the Eskimos of the Arctic, Alaska, U.S.A., the Northwest Territories of Canada (1950–1972). (Modified from Grzybowski et al., 1976b.)

1972—approximately 40% annual reduction depicted in Figure 1 (Grzybowski et al., 1976b).

United States Indians

Tuberculosis death rates among American Indians on reservations were reported for 13 states in 1887 and ranged from 95:1000 deaths in Nevada to 625:1000 deaths in New York. Between 1901 and 1903, more than 36% of 255 deaths in a Southwest reservation of 3000 American Indians were caused by tuberculosis (Rieder, 1989a). Age-adjusted tuberculosis death rates dropped from 57.9:100,000, in 1955, to 3.3:100,000, in 1983 (Rhoades et al., 1987).

Alaska Natives

In 1950, the mortality rate was 653:100,000 and declined to fewer than 4:100,000 in 1967 (see Fig. 1). This decline was similar to that observed in the Canadian Inuit. Although rates for Alaska natives were slightly lower than for the Canadian Inuit throughout the period, the difference was greater between 1955 and 1965 than in the beginning of the 1970s (Johnson, 1973; Grzybowski et al., 1976b).

B. Incidence of Active Disease

Canadian Indians

Enarson and Grzybowski (1986) estimated that the incidence of active tuberculosis in Canadian Indians between 1970 (approximately 150:100,000) and 1980 (approximately 83:100,000 population) declined annually by 4%. In the following decade, the rate of the decline was smaller. The rate was 72:100,000 population in 1990 (Statistics Canada, personal communication). Figure 2 compares the rate of active disease for the Canadian registered Indians and for the Indians in the United States. It is important to point out that the annual rates of tuberculosis among the Canadian Indians are two to three times higher than for Indians in the United States. The reasons for this are not clear from our review, nor has this been recognized or speculated on in the literature. One possibility is the definition of the Indian population; in Canada it consists only of registered In-

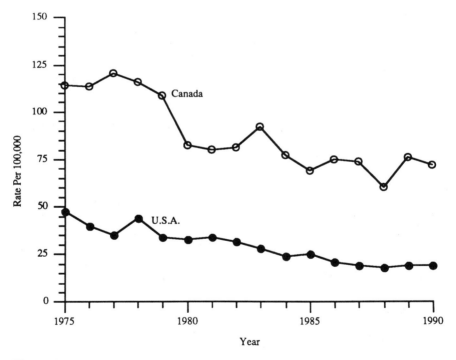

Figure 2   Incidence of active tuberculosis (per 100,000 population) between 1975 and 1990 in Canadian registered Indians (Canadian Center for Health Information, Statistics Canada) and in Indians in the United States (Courtesy of the CDC) (see text).

dians, whereas in the United States it is the total native population. This discrepancy requires further review and analysis.

Canadian Inuit

Data for Inuit in the Northwest Territories were not available until 1960, when the annual incidence was approximately 1095:100,000; it declined to 549:100,000 in 1970 and 18:100,000 in 1974. Since 1970, the decline has accelerated. Until the early 1970s, the rates in Alaska natives were two to three times higher than those in Canadian Inuit (Grzybowski et al., 1976b). Enarson and Grzybowski (1986) estimated that the incidence of active tuberculosis in the Inuit between 1970 and 1980 declined annually by 16%. The average rate of 129:100,000 population between 1979 and 1983 declined to 77:100,000 between 1984 and 1989 (Brancker, 1990).

United States Indians

Incidence of active tuberculosis is available for the period 1975–1990 (see Fig. 2). It declined from 48:100,000 in 1975 to 19:100,000 in 1990, representing an annual 4% reduction. The decline in incidence rate observed over several decades slowed down at the end of the 1980s (Sugarman et al., 1991).

Alaska Natives

In 1952, the annual rate was 1854:100,000; it declined to 442:100,000 in 1960 and to 162:100,000 in 1970 (Johnson, 1973; Grzybowski et al., 1976). The succeeding two decades, 1970s and 1980s, were marked by a continuous, slow decline in annual tuberculosis morbidity to 60.7:100,000 population in 1990.

C. Rate of Infection

Canadian Indians

Between 1933 and 1947, 54% of Indian children became tuberculin-positive by the age 10 years, giving a 5.9% annual average infection rate (Ferguson and Simes, 1949). Because of BCG vaccination of the Canadian aboriginal population at birth since the 1950s, more recent estimates of the rate of infection cannot be easily obtained.

Canadian Inuit

In 1971, a study of 377, 9-year-old Inuit children in Frobisher Bay, most of whom were BCG vaccinated, showed that 29% of them had a tuberculin reaction greater than 9-mm induration. This would approximate a 4.2% annual risk of infection (Grzybowski et al., 1976b). The risk of infection in Frobisher Bay may have underestimated the risk in many other Canadian Inuit communities, particularly in the Western Arctic. On the other hand, it is higher than in Alaska natives, probably because the tuberculosis program was started earlier in Alaska than in the Canadian Arctic (Grzybowski et al., 1976b).

United States Indians

In 1959, 50–60% of 6- to 10-year-old Navajo children were estimated to be tuberculin-positive. In 1972, a tuberculin skin test survey among 5- to 9-year-old Navajo children showed 3.7% were tuberculin-positive (Rieder, 1989b). In 1990, a tuberculin skin testing survey among 388 Oglala Sioux children in elementary and high schools showed 0.5% were tuberculin-positive. In 1991, a chart review of tuberculin status among 650 Oglala Sioux adult diabetic patients showed 70.3% were tuberculin-positive (Breault, J., unpublished data).

Alaska Natives

Kaplan et al. (1972) summarized results of five tuberculin surveys carried out in Eskimo children in Alaska (Fig. 3). These surveys were carried out with similar, although not identical, methods. Among 7- and 8-year-old children, 92% were reactors in 1949–1951, 83% in 1957, 69% in 1960, 9% in 1963–1964, and 2% in 1969–1970. The risk of infection was decreasing throughout the time interval, although the reduction seems to have been accelerating between 1960 and 1970.

In 1952, results of a tuberculin test survey of rural Alaskan children through age 14 carried out from 1948 to 1951 were reviewed. The proportion of children in the 5- to 8-year aged group with positive purified protein derivative (PPD) skin test results ranged from 89% for Yupik Eskimos to 22% for Southeast Indians, suggesting variability between different subgroups (Weiss, 1953).

VIII. Tuberculosis in the 1980s

The North American aboriginal population still bears a burden of tuberculous infection and disease that is disproportionate to their number. The persistently higher rates of tuberculosis among North American Indians and Eskimos have been, in part, a legacy of the remarkably intense transmission of *M. tuberculosis* during the first half of this century.

In the 1980s, Canadian aboriginals represented 1.7% of the total Canadian population, but experienced 15% of all active tuberculous cases. Between 1984 and 1989, the rate of active tuberculosis was approximately 70:100,000 population in both Indians and Inuit people, whereas the rate for the total Canadian population was approximately 10:100,000. Very few aboriginals died of tuberculosis, and mortality was essentially no different from that for other segments of the Canadian population.

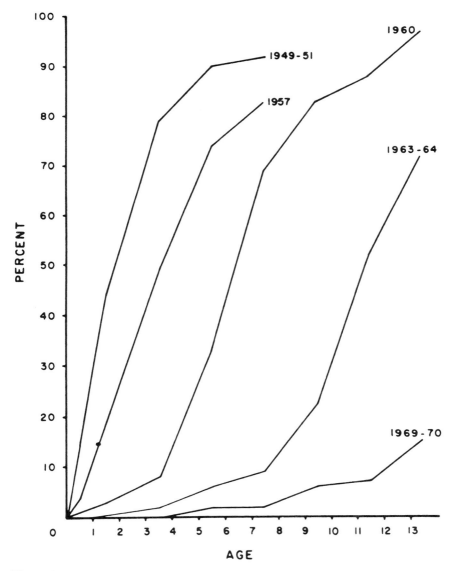

Figure 3 Prevalence of tuberculin sensitivity among Eskimo children 0–14 years of age from the Yukon–Kuskokwim Delta of Alaska in five successive surveys. (From Kaplan et al., 1972.)

Although Alaska natives compose 16% of the population, they have accounted for 50–90% of all tuberculosis cases reported in Alaska in the 1980s. Between 1988 and 1990, Alaska natives accounted for 43 (90%) of the 48 cases younger than 20 years. In this group the presence of tuberculosis implies active transmission to children and adolescents (Middaugh and Jones, 1989). For the period 1986–1990, the mean age adjusted incidence rate of active tuberculosis for Alaska natives was 61.8:100,000, in comparison with 14.7 for all Alaska residents and 9.1 for the entire United States.

For American Indians in the 48 contiguous states in 1990, there were 319 cases of tuberculosis among a population of 1,868,437 (17.1:100,000 population). This is 4.1 times higher than the rate for the non-Hispanic whites in the United States (4.2:100,000 population). Case rates for Indians are declining nearly as fast as those for the total population in the United States. Rates in Indians continued to fall through the end of 1990, in contrast with the leveling of rates seen in other races, believed to be due to the spread of human immunodeficiency virus (HIV) among tuberculous-infected Americans. American Indians have a larger proportion of child and young adult cases, indicating lack of control of infection (CDC, personal communication).

In the United States, most of the tuberculous cases among Indians occur in a few states. The CDC's databank for the 6 years from 1985 to 1990 shows a total of 1803 tuberculosis cases in the 48 states. Most these cases (51.7%) occurred in four states: Arizona (344 cases), Oklahoma (264), New Mexico (164), and California (160). Almost three-quarters (74.2%) of all the tuberculous cases in Indians in the 48 states occurred in eight states: the previous four plus South Dakota (120 cases), Washington (114), Montana (91), and Minnesota (80).

Most cases of tuberculosis in the 1980s were pulmonary. Among Alaska natives, pulmonary tuberculosis was the only, or the major form of the disease in 119 (86%) of the 138 cases reported during 1988–1990. The CDC 1990 data show 80% pulmonary tuberculosis in Indians in the contiguous United States. In Canadian aboriginals, in the 1980s, respiratory tuberculosis accounted for 85–87% of cases. This proportion is similar to that for Canadian-born non-aboriginals (Brancker, 1990). Between 1971 and 1981, the proportion of primary tuberculosis was higher in Indians (20%) than in Inuit (8%) (Enarson and Grzybowski, 1986), suggesting a greater transmission of infection to the non-infected persons in Indian than in Inuit communities. In Canada, over 90% of reported tuberculous cases are bacteriologically examined (Enarson and Grzybowski, 1986). More than 80% of pulmonary tuberculosis is culture-positive, and more than 55% is smear-positive (Enarson and Grzybowski, 1986). In 1990, 82% of the tuberculous cases occurring in the native Americans in the 48 contiguous states were bacteriologically confirmed (262 of 319 cases) (Breault, J., personal communication).

In Canada, nonrespiratory tuberculosis accounts for 13–16% of tuberculous cases in the aboriginal population. Of these, 3–5% is genitourinary tuberculosis and 5–7% tuberculosis of lymph nodes (Brancker, 1990). In Saskatchewan (Canada), tuberculous lymphadenitis has become the most common form of extrapulmonary tuberculosis and is much more common in Indians (38:100,000 population) than in the nonnative Canadian-born population (0.2:100,000 population; Martin et al., 1988). In British Columbia and in Manitoba, tuberculous peritonitis is more common in Indians than in other ethnic groups in the province (Jakubowski et al., 1988; Marrie and Hershfield, 1978).

In the United States, approximately 25% of tuberculosis is extrapulmonary in Indians, in comparison with 16% for the white non-Hispanic group (Rieder et al., 1990a). In Alaska natives, the frequency of exclusively extrapulmonary tuberculosis cases during 1988–1990 was as follows: pleural: 7 (5%), lymphatic 2 (1.5%), genitourinary 4 (3%), and other 3 (2%). Meningeal tuberculosis is rare in Alaska: six cases were reported in the state during the 11-year period from 1980 through 1990; two of the three Alaska native patients were young children.

Relapses are common in the aboriginal population. Of the 138 cases reported among Alaska natives during 1988–1990, 22 (16%) had histories of prior tuberculous disease and had either failed to complete recommended therapy or had been treated with now obsolete antibiotic regimens. Registered Indians in Manitoba, Canada, were at higher risk of relapse than other segments of the population, particularly if the disease was extensive (Johnson et al., 1985).

Resistance to drugs is becoming an increasing problem. In Alaska natives, antibiotic-resistant strains were cultured from 5 (3.6%) out of 138 individuals between 1988 and 1990. Five of these patients had strains that were resistant to isoniazid alone. An isoniazid-resistant strain of *M. tuberculosis* caused an outbreak of tuberculosis in the village of Chevak in 1989. It occurred in a school and affected primarily schoolchildren. The index case, a 14-year-old boy, with a cavitary pulmonary infiltrate, was initially overlooked because his respiratory problems were not prominent and because investigators expected to find an adult index case. Of 150 previously tuberculin-nagative students in the school, 50 (33%) were infected during the outbreak; 4 developed isoniazid-resistant tuberculous disease.

In the 1980s, tuberculosis manifested itself through small outbreaks in various communities. Sources of infection were usually adults who relapsed. Epidemics occurred because there were many susceptible children and adolescents in these communities. In these small outbreaks, young susceptible children were most affected (Mah and Fanning, 1991). From 1987 through late 1991, 13 villages in Alaska had clusters of three or more tuberculosis cases. Occurrence of tuberculosis is becoming more common in Indians living off reserves in urban centers, and is brought back on the reserves. It seems, however, that small outbreaks on reserves, under present conditions of tuberculosis control, do not seem to slow down the declining trend of incidence of active tuberculosis (Poffenroth, personal communication). Persons affected in these outbreaks are usually young. The outbreaks are usually detected by tuberculin skin-testing surveys of schoolchildren or through investigation of contacts of an identified case.

IX. Risk Factors

Tuberculosis is both a socioeconomic and a medical problem. The cause of the disease, the tubercle bacillus, is known, effective treatment is available, and methods of prevention and control are well understood. Once infected, however, certain population groups have a higher risk of developing active disease (Grzybowski et al., 1972). Persons with the highest risk for developing disease are those who have had tuberculosis in the past and have received no, or inappropriate, antituberculous chemotherapy. Included in this group are persons who are presumed to have had tuberculosis in the past and who present with a positive tuberculin test and upper lobe scarring. The risk of active disease for this latter group has been calculated for the Inuit population and is between 74:10,000 and 85:10,000 population per year. The risk for Inuits with a positive tuberculin reaction and a normal chest x-ray film varies from 57:10,000 to 62:10,000 persons in comparison with the risk of 14:10,000 to 19:10,000 population per year for BCG-vaccinated population with a normal x-ray film (Grzybowski et al., 1976b).

The North American native population was believed to have a lower natural resistance against the tubercle bacillus than those of European origin. There is no evidence that this difference might be due to genetic factors. The exception might be the observation that over 95% of Inuit are rapid inactivators of isoniazid, in comparison with 63% of Indians and a smaller proportion of whites (Armstrong and Peart, 1960; Jeanes et al., 1972). This might increase the probability of treatment failure, including preventive therapy with isoniazid alone, particularly if irregular (Jeanes et al., 1972).

The risk of relapse of tuberculosis and of progression from infection (indicated by a positive tuberculin test) to active disease is caused by a lowering of the resistance of a person to the tubercle bacillus. The most important known conditions that are associated with lowering of the resistance against tubercle bacillus in the North American aboriginal population are age, malnutrition, diabetes, and substance abuse, including alcohol.

Because of the lowering of resistance with age, the risk of relapse increases with age. Diabetes is a growing problem among North American Indians. Diabetics are 2–3.5 times more likely to progress from a positive tuberculin status to active tuberculosis (Boucot et al., 1952; Warwick, 1957; Oscarrson and Silwer, 1958; Opsahl et al., 1961; Henri and Bennett, 1985). A recent study in Pine Ridge Reservation shows that the odds ratios of developing active tuberculosis among tuberculin-positive diabetics was 5.2 in comparison with nondiabetic tuberculin-positive controls (Mori et al., 1992).

Social, economic, and cultural factors play a critical role in making tuberculosis an important public health problem of the North American aboriginal population. Poverty is common, both on and off reserves, and is a major factor among American Indians (Coetzee et al., 1988). Poverty results in malnutrition and lowered natural resistance against the disease. Overcrowding, poor housing, and inadequate sanitation facilitate the spread of the infection among susceptible persons, usually children. In a Canadian urban area (Vancouver), the incidence of tuberculosis was higher in poorer than in more affluent census tracts (Enarson et al., 1989). Urban Indians (including those temporarily off-reserves) are more likely to live in these areas. One-quarter of the North American Indian cases occur in persons living in cities of 100,000 or more, so urban Indians contribute significantly to the tuberculosis problem. Alcoholism is closely associated with tuberculosis (Friedman et al., 1987). It is also closely associated with poor social and economic conditions. It contributes to the lowering of resistance against tuberculosis and is a major reason for poor compliance with treatment and chemoprophylaxis.

Cultural factors are important because the aboriginal population may be less likely to seek medical treatment early or at all, or to comply with prescribed therapy or chemoprophylaxis (Jenkins, 1977). Although poor socioeconomic conditions increase the probability of active disease in those infected with the tubercle bacillus, on one hand, and facilitate the spread of infection to noninfected susceptible individuals in native communities, on the other hand, cultural characteristics of the native population may impede the effectiveness of the tuberculosis control measures, such as early diagnosis, compliance with chemotherapy, and chemoprophylaxis.

Current literature suggests that no significant effect of acquired immune deficiency syndrome (AIDS) on tuberculosis has yet been noted in the American aboriginal population up to and including 1990.

X. Health Services and Programs

Health Services for American Indians in the United States are based in Indian Health Service (IHS) facilities on or near reservations or near large groups of native Americans. The IHS was transferred from the Department of the Interior to the Public Health Service in 1955. The IHS divides its services into independent service units. The Navajo Reservation, which is massive, is divided into eight service units. For other reservations, the service unit is the reservation and enrolled members in the immediately surrounding counties. In Oklahoma and areas that do not have reservations, a service unit consists of enrolled members within a geographic area.

In recent years, several tribes have used Public Law 638 (PL 638) to transfer funds for health care from the IHS to the tribe to manage their own health care facilities. In some areas, for example North and South Dakota, Arizona, and New Mexico, PL 638 programs are the exception. In other areas, for example, California, almost all health care for American Indians is delivered under PL 638 programs. The IHS contributes technical and support staff to PL 638 programs on an individual basis, and these can vary widely.

Indian Health Service facilities are understaffed and preventive services are often postponed to deal with the crisis on hand. This increases the susceptibility of the American Indian population to tuberculosis.

In Alaska, health care facilities for the native population are located in the larger population centers throughout the state. IHS maintains a tertiary care hospital in Anchorage and supports 11 small hospitals in rural towns. The IHS provides medical care for Alaska natives and other U. S. Public Health Service (USPHS) beneficiaries, as well as some nonnatives in rural areas. There are four major referral hospitals in Alaska: the Alaska Native Medical Center (IHS) in Anchorage, two private hospitals in Anchorage, and one private hospital in Fairbanks. Fourteen community hospitals provide care for persons living in smaller towns.

In Canada, the role of Medical Services Branch (Department of National Health and Welfare of the federal government) in relation to tuberculosis control in Indian health is all-encompassing. It ensures that health care providers recognize aboriginal people as a high-risk group for tuberculosis and that they keep a high index of suspicion in their assessment of disease. A diagnosis of tuberculosis requires that patients are provided with appropriate treatment, that contacts are assessed and provided with preventive chemotherapy as necessary, and that follow-up for both groups is continued within established guidelines. Routine chest x-ray screening surveys, once an important part of active case-finding, are no longer done.

The Indian Health Service in the United States adopted and implemented recommendations of the United States Centers for Disease Control (CDC), "Strategy for Elimination of Tuberculosis in the United States" (CDC, 1988, 1990a,b; Beller and Middaugh, 1989; Welty and Follas, 1989). Key components are

1. Rapid diagnosis and meticulous treatment under direct-observed therapy of all culture-confirmed cases of pulmonary tuberculosis

2. Identification, through epidemiological investigation of all cases of pulmonary tuberculosis, and of individuals who have been infected and need appropriate chemotherapy to prevent future tuberculosis disease

3. Effective surveillance to detect new transmission of tuberculosis through routine, periodic, annual skin testing of schoolchildren, and vigorous application of epidemiological investigation to identify cases actively transmitting tuberculosis whenever a skin test converter is identified

4. Directly observed therapy of all individuals to ensure meticulous compliance with drug treatment recommendations

5. Vigorous use of prophylactic isoniazid to prevent tuberculosis among those recently infected

The tuberculosis control program of the Medical Services Branch, Health and Welfare Canada is integrated with the provincial programs. The program consists of

1. Extensive case-finding with clinical examinations, chest x-ray examination, sputum or gastric mycobacterial examination in symptomatic individuals

2. Case-holding, with registration of each case and recording of treatment and compliance

3. Treatment—usually 2 months with isoniazid, rifampin, and pyrazinamide or ethambutol and a fourth drug where indicated, daily, followed by 4 months of isoniazid and rifampin, usually directly observed, twice a week

4. Contact follow-up, including tuberculin testing, x-ray follow-up, and institution of preventive treatment where indicated

5. BCG at birth (as recommended by Medical Services Branch, Health and Welfare Canada)

Because of vast distances in Alaska, remote villages, limited transportation, and high cost, reliance on village-based supervision of treatment is a key component of successful tuberculosis control. Community health aides are paid to provide directly observed treatment to all individuals with active disease and to those receiving isoniazid preventive treatment.

Use of routine chest x-ray surveys was discontinued in Alaska in 1986 when a review determined the lack of efficacy and high cost (Beller and Middaugh, 1989). Essential is the availability of portable radiography to enable chest x-rays films to be done in villages during investigations of infectious cases.

A critical component of Alaska's tuberculosis program is routine annual tuberculin skin testing of schoolchildren. Because BCG vaccination was used in Alaska for only a short period before being abandoned in the mid-1950s, routine tuberculin skin testing provides a reliable and inexpensive surveillance system for detection of disease transmission. Trained nurses and physicians conduct an epidemiological investigation on all cases of tuberculin skin test conversion to find the index case and establish treatment regimens.

A 1991 survey of 9 of the 11 largest service areas of the Indian Health Service in the 48 states suggests that, on average, 2.5 persons per 1000 started isoniazid for prophylactic purposes (infection, no disease) (Breault, J., unpublished data).

Directly observed chemoprophylaxis in these service areas was done in 61% of cases (Breault, J., unpublished data). A high dropout rate is a common problem in any tuberculosis control program when 6–12 months of isoniazid is prescribed on a daily unsupervised basis. To help minimize dropouts at the Pine Ridge Reservation, personnel meet weekly to review charts and records of those who have not picked up their isoniazid from the pharmacy and home delivery is arranged. People who do not complete an adequate (at least 6-month) course of isoniazid because of noncompliance, allergy or aminotransferase (SGOT) levels that are five times the upper limit of normal or more, are placed on the high-risk list.

XI. The Future

Among North American aboriginals, tuberculosis remains a serious health problem. It will continue to be a formidable problem in the last decade of this century and into the 21st century. Cases of infectious pulmonary tuberculosis continue to occur, primarily in two groups: younger adults aged 29–35 who have severe substance abuse, including dependency on alcohol; and in the elderly, who have long-standing tuberculous infection and who may have received inadequate or inappropriate drug regimens in the past. In addition, compliance in this latter group may also have been a problem.

Alaska native children now have an extremely low prevalence of tuberculin skin test reactivity. Recent experience with several village outbreaks had demonstrated the potential for infectious cases to infect large numbers of susceptible individuals. Village outbreaks have been discovered through routine, periodic tuberculin testing of schoolchildren, with epidemiological investigation of convertors, or through epidemiological investigation of reported infectious cases. Because sporadic infectious cases continue to occur, cases of primary tuberculosis are still being reported. These newly infected individuals run the risk of severe disease, including meningeal and miliary tuberculosis. Those who do not develop disease early and who are undetected through contact follow-up have a lifetime risk of developing active disease and becoming infectious, thereby continuing the cycle of spread.

Tuberculosis has gone from a major killer of native Americans to one of the many causes of their morbidity. Alcoholism, substance abuse, diabetes, and poverty are disproportionate problems for native Americans and account in part for the fact that tuberculosis rates among native North Americans are almost twice those of the nonnative locally born citizens of the United States and Canada. For reasons that are not clear, native Americans are 11 times more likely to have peritoneal tuberculosis that non-Hispanic whites. Strategies have been developed to reduce the rates of active tuberculosis and the risks of infection for the uninfected and must now be fully implemented. Since tuberculosis is more a socioeconomic than a medical disease, attention must be directed at improving the living standards of this group. Better housing, better nutrition, and improved access to health care are a must if this disease is to be eliminated. Individuals with active tuberculosis must be placed on appropriate regimens that are carried to completion to ensure cure. Since patients' compliance is a major problem, the institution of directly observed therapy for all potentially infectious cases of tuberculosis must be the core of any tuberculosis program. An infrastructure to deliver medications and to ensure patients' compliance must be developed. In addition, this infrastructure can at times be used in the diagnosis of suspect cases by collecting sputum from symptomatic individuals and having the specimens sent for examination. Thus health care personnel in the field can, with the proper instruction, be employed in many aspects of tuberculosis control.

As more potent drugs are developed and better regimens designed, the disease can be brought under control. Drug combinations of the various drugs into one capsule with demonstrated bioavailability will make supervision easier. Government programs must ensure that appropriate antibiotic therapy is available to all who suffer from tuberculosis.

In developing these strategies, adequate attention must be given to the social and cultural characteristics of the aboriginal population. Incorporation of native healing practices may be an important catalyst in gaining the confidence of the target population. With each new step, proper involvement of tribal–band councils in decision-making is essential. The provision of educational materials and the transfer of technology to the tribal–band councils and through them to the population will be a linchpin for this successful endeavor.

Long-term goals need to be assessed and confirmed by the participating groups. A feeling of control over their own destiny is extremely important. Case-finding, including contact follow-up, case-holding, preventive treatment, and appropriate regimens and follow-up must be designed with the local conditions in mind. This transfer, however, should not isolate the health care of the Indian and Eskimo populations from the local provincial or state health authorities, who should ensure that facilities for diagnosis and appropriate supplies of testing materials and drugs are readily available. Responsibility of the local authorities is to quality-control the efforts for diagnosis, prevention, and treatment. It is also important that record-keeping be emphasized and that cases are reported promptly and accurately to provincial or state authorities so that individual cases and groups of cases can be detected early to prevent small outbreaks from occurring. Innovative treatment and control modalities taking into account local characteristics are extremely important.

There are two potential problems for tuberculosis control on the horizon. The first is the occurrence of multidrug-resistant strains of *Mycobacterium tuberculosis.* Recent studies have indicated that this is on the increase, and the consequences of being infected by a multidrug-resistant tubercle bacillus carries with it great potential risks. To prevent this from happening, patient compliance (''taking the treatment to cure'') is essential. Without this attention to detail, multidrug-resistance will become widespread and cause a more complicated clinical picture, prolonged treatment, and increased mortality.

The second major problem is the presence of infection with the human immunodeficiency virus (HIV). Because of the alteration of the cellular immune system in persons infected with HIV. the response to infection by the tubercle bacillus is altered. Thus, in dually infected individuals, the incidence of active tuberculosis is higher than in the general population, the time from infection to disease is shorter, and the risk of infecting other persons is increased.

Tuberculosis in native North Americans can be controlled by the judicious effort of local, provincial, and state public health authorities, and the tribal–band councils of the native groups in the areas involved. The essential ingredient for the elimination of tuberculosis in this group is the appropriate transfer of knowledge to those who have a desire to control their own destinies and to understand the necessity for proper and long-term public health measures.

References

Aberdeen Area Indian Service (1985). *Tuberculosis Manual.* Aberdeen Area Indian Health Service, pp.4–5, 28–29.

Alaska Department of Labor (1990). *Alaska Population Overview.* State of Alaska, Juneau.

Alaska's Health (1954). A survey report to the United States Department of the Interior by the Alaska Health Survey Team, Thomas Parran, Chief. Max Q. Elder, Editor. The Graduate School of Public Health, University of Pittsburgh.

Armstrong, A. R., and Peart, H. E. (1960). A comparison between behaviour of Eskimos and non-Eskimos to administration of isoniazid. *Am. Rev. Respir. Dis.* **81**:588–594.

Aronson, J. D., and Palmer, C. E. (1946). Experience with BCG vaccine in the control of tuberculosis among North American Indians. *Public Health Rep.* **61**:802–819.

Beller, M., and Middaugh, J. P. (1989). Surveillance for tuberculosis in Alaska, 1986. *Alaska Med.* **31**:4–8.

Boucot, K. R., Dillon, E. S., Cooper, D. A., and Meier, P. (1952). Tuberculosis among diabetics: The Philadelphia survey. *Am. Rev. Tuberc.* **65**(Suppl.):1–50.

Brancker, A. (1990). Recent patterns and trends in tuberculosis incidence in Canada. Presented at the "Workshop on Tuberculosis in Aboriginal People." Winnipeg.

Buikstra, J. E. (ed.). (1981). *Prehistoric Tuberculosis in the Americas.* Northwestern University Archeological Program. Chicago.

Centers for Disease Control. (1988). A strategic plan for the elimination of tuberculosis in the United States. *MMWR* **38**(S-3):1–25.

Centers for Disease Control. (1990a). Case definitions for public health surveillance. *MMWR* **39**(RR-13):39–40.

Centers for Disease Control. (1990b). Screening for tuberculosis and tuberculous infection in high risk populations: and the use of preventive therapy for tuberculosis infection in the United States: Recommendations of the Advisory Committee for the Elimination of Tuberculosis. *MMWR* **39**:1–12.

Chan-Yeung, M., Galbraith, J. D., Sculson, N., Brown, A., and Grzybowski, S. (1971). Reactivation of inactive tuberculosis in Northern Canada. *Am. Rev. Respir. Dis.* **104**:861–865.

Coetzee, N., Yach, D., and Joubert, G. (1988). Crowding and alcohol abuse as risk factors for tuberculosis in the Mamre population: Results of a case-control study. *S. Afr. Med. J.* **74**:352–354.

Comstock, G. W., and Philip, R. N. (1961). Decline of the tuberculosis epidemic in Alaska. *Public Health Rep.* **76**:19–24.

Comstock, G. W., and Woolpert, S. F. (1972). Preventive treatment of untreated, nonactive tuberculosis in an Eskimo population. *Arch. Environ. Health* **25**:333–337.

Comstock, G. W., Baum, C., and Snider, D. E., Jr. (1979). Isoniazid prophylaxis among Alaskan Eskimos: A final report of the Bethel isoniazid studies. *Am. Rev. Respir. Dis.* **119**:827–830.

Comstock, G. W., Ferebee, S. H., and Hammes, L. M. (1967). A controled trial of community-wide isoniazid prophylaxis in Alaska. *Am. Rev. Respir. Dis.* **95**:935–943.

Dorken, E., Grzybowski, S., and Enarson, D. A. (1984). Ten year evaluation of a trial of chemoprophylaxis against tuberculosis in Frobisher Bay, Canada. *Tubercle* **65**:93–99.

Enarson, D. A., and Grzybowski, S. (1986). Incidence of active tuberculosis in the native population of Canada. *Can. Med. Assoc. J.* **134**:1149–1152.

Enarson, D. A., Wang, J. S., and Dirks, J. M. (1989). The incidence of active tuberculosis in a large urban area. *Am. J. Epidemiol.* **129**:1268–1276.

Fellows, F. S. (1934). Mortality in the native races of the Territory of Alaska, with special reference to tuberculosis. *Public Health Rep.* **49**:289–298.

Ferguson, R. G. (1934). The Indian tuberculosis problem and some preventive measures. *Can. Med. Assoc. J.* **30**:544–547.

Ferguson, R. G., and Simes, A. (1949). BCG vaccination of Indian infants in Saskatchewan. *Tubercle* **30**:5–11.

Fitzbugh, W. W., and Crowell, A. (1988). *Crossroads of Continents. Cultures of Siberia and Alaska.* Smithsonian Institution Press. Washington D.C.

Friedman, L. N., Sullivan, G. M., Rocco, P. B., and Loscos, R. (1987). Tuberculosis screening in alcoholics and drug addicts. *Am. Rev. Respir. Dis.* **136**:1188–1192.

Grzybowski, S., Galbraith, J. D., and Styblo, K., (1972). Tuberculosis in Canadian Eskimos. *Arch Environ Health* **25**:329–332.

Grzybowski, S., Galbraith, J. D., and Dorken, E. (1976a). Chemoprophylaxis trial in Canadian Eskimos. *Tubercle* **57**:263.

Grzybowski, S., Styblo, K., and Dorken, E. (1976b) Tuberculosis in Eskimos. *Tubercle* **57** (Suppl.):S1–S42.

Hagey, N. J., Larocque, G., and McBride, C. (1989). Highlights of aboriginal conditions 1981–2001. Part I. Demographic trends. Indian and Northern Affairs Canada, Ottawa.

Hanson, M., Comstock, G. W., Haley, C. E. (1967). Community isoniazid prophylaxis program in an underdeveloped area of Alaska. *Public Health Rep.* **82**:1045–1056.

Henri, J., and Bennett, O. H. (1985). Tuberculosis and NIDDM: New dimensions to an old problem. *Abstracts from the 12th Congress of the IDF.* Sept. 23–28, Madrid, Spain. Elsevier Science Publishers, Amsterdam, p. S234.

Houston, S., Fanning, A., Soskolne, C. L., and Fraser, N. (1990). The effectiveness of the bacillus Calmette-Guérin (BCG) vaccination against tuberculosis. A case-control study in Treaty Indians, Alberta, Canada. *Am. J. Epidemiol.* **131**:340–348.

Indian and Northern Affairs Canada (1980). Indian conditions. A survey. Ottawa.

Indian and Northern Affairs Canada (1990a). *The Canadian Indian.* Minister of Supply and Services Canada, Ottawa.

Indian and Northern Affairs Canada (1990b). *The Inuit.* Minister of Supply and Services Canada. Ottawa.

Jakubowski, A., Elwood, R. K., and Enarson, D. A. (1989). Clinical features of abdominal tuberculosis. *J. Infect. Dis.* **158**:687–692.

Jeanes, C. W. L., Schaefer, O., and Eidus, L. (1972). Inactivation of isoniazid by Canadian Eskimos and Indians. *Can. Med. Assoc. J.* **106**:331.

Jenkins, D. (1977). Tuberculosis: The native Indian viewpoint on its prevention, diagnosis, and treatment. *Prev. Med.* **6**:545–555.

Johnson, I. L., Thomson, M., Manfreda, J., and Hershfield, E. S. (1985). Risk factors for reactivation of tuberculosis in Manitoba. *Can. Med. Assoc. J.* **133**:1221–1224.

Johnson, M. W. (1973). Results of 20 years of tuberculosis control in Alaska. *Health Serv. Rep.* **88**:247–254.

Kaplan, G. J., Fraser, R. I., and Comstock, G. W. (1972). Tuberculosis in Alaska, 1970: The continued decline of the tuberculosis epidemic. *Am. Rev. Respir. Dis.* **105**:920–926.

Mah, M. W., and Fanning, E. A. (1991). An epidemic of primary tuberculosis in a Canadian aboriginal community. *Can. J. Infect. Dis.* **2**:133–141.

Marrie, T. J., and Hershfield, E. S. (1978). Tuberculosis peritonitis in Manitoba. *Can. J. Surg.* **21**:533–536.

Martin, T., Hoeppner, V. H., and Ring, E. D. (1988). Superficial mycobacterial lymphadenitis in Saskatchewan. *Can. Med. Assoc. J.* **138**:431–434.

Middaugh, J. P., and Jones, M. E. (1989). The epidemiology of tuberculosis in Alaska, 1987. *Alaska Med.* **31**:9–16.

Morgan, L. (ed.). (1979). *Alaska's Native People* Vol. 6, No. 3. Alaska Geographic.

Mori, M. A., Leonardson, G., and Welty, T. K. (1992). The benefits of isoniazid chemoprophylaxis and risk factors for tuberculosis among Oglala Sioux Indians. *Ann. Intern. Med.* **152**:547–550.

Opsahl, R. Riddervold, H. O., and Aas, T. W. (1961). Pulmonary tuberculosis in mitral stenosis and dsiabetes mellitus. *Acta Tuberc. Scand.* **40**:290–296.

Oscarrson, P. N., and Silwer, H. (1958). Incidence of pulmonary tuberculosis among diabetics. *Acta Med. Scand.* **161** (Suppl.):23–48.

Palmer, C. E., Shaw, L. W. (1953). Present status of BCG studies. *Am. Rev. Tuberc.* **68**:462–466.

Paulsen, H. J. (1987). Tuberculosis in the Native American: Indigenous or introduced? *Rev. Infect. Dis.* **9**:1180–1186.

Rabinowitch, I. M. (1936). Clinical and other observations on the Canadian Eskimos in the Eastern Arctic. *Can. Med. Assoc. J.* **34**:487–490.

Rhoades, E. R., D'Angelo, A. J., and Hurlburt, W. B. (1987). The Indian Health Service record of achievement. *Public Health Rep.* **102**:356–360.

Rieder, H. L. (1989a) Tuberculosis among American Indians of the contiguous United States. *Public Health Rep.* **104**:653–657.

Rieder, H. L. (1989b) Notes on the history of an epidemic: Tuberculosis among North American Indians. *IHS Primary Care Provider* **14**(5):45–50.

Rieder, H. L., Snider, D. E., and Cauthen, G. M. (1990). Extrapulmonary tuberculosis in the United States. *Am. Rev. Respir. Dis.* **141**:347–351.

Sugarman, J., Chase, E., Johannes, P., and Helgerson, S. D. (1991). Tuberculosis among American Indians and Alaskan Natives 1985–1990. *IHS Primary Care Provider* **16**:186–190.

Walker, J. R., DeMallie, R. J., and Jahner, E. A. (1980). *Lakota Belief and Ritual.* University of Nebraska Press, Lincoln, pp. 8 and 12.

Warwick, M. T. (1957) Pulmonary tuberculosis and diabetes mellitus. *Q. J. Med.* **26**:30–34.

Weiss, E. S. (1953). Tuberculin sensitivity in Alaska. *Public Health Rep.* **68**:23–27.

Welty, T. K., and Follas, R. (1989). IHS standards of care for tuberculosis. *IHS Primary Provider* **14**:54–58.

Wherrett, G. J. (1969). A study of tuberculosis in Eastern Arctic. *Can. J. Public Health* **60**:7–14.

Wilson, J. M., Galbraith, J. D., and Grzybowski, S. (1973). Tuberculosis in Eskimo children: A comparison of disease in children vacinated with BCG and non-vaccinated children. *Am. Rev. Respir. Dis.* **108**:559–564.

Young, T. K., and Hershfield, E. S. (1986). A case-control study to evaluate the effectiveness of mass neonatal BCG vaccination among Canadian Indians. *Am. J. Public Health* **76**:783–786.

22

Tuberculosis in the Inner City

CHARLES P. FELTON and JEAN G. FORD

Columbia University College of Physicians and Surgeons
and Harlem Hospital Center
New York, New York

I. Introduction

Following years of steady decline, tuberculosis (TB) has resurfaced as a menacing public health problem (Snider and Roper, 1992). In 1990, 25,701 cases of tuberculosis were reported in the United States. Of these, 9883 or 38.5% were in excess of the expected number of cases, based on previous trends (Centers for Disease Control [CDC], 1992). This new tuberculosis epidemic is closely related to the human immunodeficiency virus–acquired immunodeficiency syndrome (HIV/AIDS) epidemic, and it has most severely affected certain urban areas, especially "inner-city" communities (Reider et al., 1989a,b; CDC, 1992; Barnes et al., 1991). We recognize the nonhomogeneity of urban populations and that, strictly speaking, the term *inner city* could describe the residential area for communities rich or poor, and of diverse ethnic backgrounds. However, for the purposes of this discussion, *urban* will refer to cities or towns with a population of more than 250,000 and *inner city* will refer to urban areas of concentrated poverty.

Throughout the 1990s, minority groups in the United States will continue to suffer disproportionate morbidity and mortality (McCord and Freeman, 1990; Schwartz et al., 1990) from this disease, which is entirely preventable and curable. If the 1980s is the decade in which the AIDS epidemic came into full bloom, the current decade is already indelibly marked by the worsening tuberculosis epidemic, most ominously, the increasingly prevalent multidrug-resistant *Mycobacterium tuberculosis* (MDR-TB) (Snider and Roper, 1992).

Circumstances that promote the spread of tuberculosis include (1) the existence of a reservoir consisting of infected individuals, (2) susceptible hosts, and (3) the absence of adequate treatment and control programs. All these factors exist in certain inner-city communities in the United States today, because a reservoir exists that has never been brought under control in these communities (Bloch et al., 1989). Other factors that contributed to this reservoir are the increased prevalence of substance abuse and homelessness, as well as the influx of foreign-born persons from countries with a high prevalence of tuberculous infection (Reider et al., 1989a,b; CDC, 1990). With the rising incidence and prevalence of HIV infection in these communities, the risk for tuberculous disease increased dramatically, especially for HIV-positive hosts (Sunderam et al., 1986; Barnes et al., 1991). Finally, the deterioration of tuberculosis control programs in inner-city communities in the United States provided the ideal environment for a public health nightmare to materialize (Brudney and Dobkin, 1991 a,b).

In this chapter, we review some special issues in the control of tuberculosis in inner-city populations. Since New York City is most severely affected by the current epidemic (CDC, 1992), the experience of this city will be particularly emphasized.

II. Historical Perspective

At the turn of the century, tuberculosis was the most frequent cause of death in those countries for which reliable statistics were collected (Comstock, 1986). However, in the United States, in the late 1800s the tuberculosis case rate had begun to drop significantly as a result of general improvements in public health measures, nutrition, sanitation, and living standards (Comstock, 1986). Effective drugs began to be used in public health programs in the late 1940s, and the first nationwide reporting system for active tuberculosis cases became operational in 1953. From that point, a steady nationwide annual decline was noted over three decades in the number of active tuberculosis cases (Rieder et al., 1989a). Important factors promoting this decline were the development of new drugs, widespread implementation of effective drug regimens, and programs for prevention and cure of tuberculosis, including prolonged hospitalization. Aggressive public health programs focused on early detection, isolation, and management of clinical disease; screening programs aimed at identifying infected contacts; directly observed therapy was administered by public health nurses and community outreach workers; and research efforts focused on development of new chemotherapeutic agents. With realization of effective chemotherapy, lengthy isolation in hospitals and sanatoria became unnecessarily expensive, and ambulatory, home treatment of shortened duration became possible (Sbarbaro and Iseman, 1986; Yeager et al., 1986). As confidence grew in available drug regimens, an increasing number of tuberculous patients were cared for by generalists, rather than physicians especially trained in the care of such patients.

However, troubling disparities in the epidemiology and demography of the affected population persisted (Bloch et al., 1989; Rieder et al., 1989a,b). The decline in incidence and prevalence was steeper among whites than among other racial groups, and in suburban areas, rather than in inner-city areas (Bloch et al., 1989; Rieder et al., 1989a,b). In the context of the fiscal constraints of the 1970s and 1980s, support for governmental programs was curtailed sharply (Brudney and Dobkin, 1991a,b; Leff and Leff, 1989). During the 1970s, poverty became more spatially concentrated in American cities, with increasing prevalence of poverty in minority communities and an increase in the number of poverty areas (Wilson, 1987). Although incomes of whites increased in the 1970s, despite the recession and inflation, the concentration of poverty during the same period affected principally blacks outside the western United States, and Latinos in the Northeast (Massey and Eggers, 1990). Cities such as New York, Newark, and Washington D.C. saw significant increases in poverty, particularly in black and Latino communities (Massey and Eggers, 1990). Within these communities the deterioration of the housing stock left many homeless or unstably housed (Wallace, 1988).

This situation was further aggravated by U. S. governmental policies in the 1980s, which resulted in a redistribution of income favoring the more affluent (Phillips, 1990).

With diminished revenues from federal sources, cities struggled to cope with a lower tax base and a higher demand for services and, consequently, cut back on health care allocations. A subsequent survey of major metropolitan tuberculosis control programs found wide variation among the programs in screening, drug toxicity monitoring, and posttreatment follow-up (Leff and Leff, 1989). Meanwhile, the prevalence of joblessness, homelessness, and substance abuse increased. Foreign immigrants took up residence in urban areas, especially inner-city communities, and the proportion of the tuberculosis caseload in the foreign-born rose steadily (CDC, 1991c). With the convergence of these factors, it is not surprising that, following decades of decline, an increase in tuberculosis incidence could be demonstrated in certain inner-city communities several years ahead of national statistics, and well before the advent of the HIV/AIDS epidemic (Reichman et al., 1979; Council of Lung Association of New York, 1981; Brudney and Dobkin, 1991a). Finally, with the AIDS epidemic, the incidence of tuberculosis increased dramatically (Barnes et al., 1991). Yet, even as certain urban communities saw increases in their caseloads, support for tuberculosis control programs continued to diminish (Brudney and Dobkin, 1991a).

III. The Urban Environment

The relation of urban living conditions to morbidity and mortality from tuberculosis has long been recognized. Among Navy recruits who had lived all their lives in a metropolitan area, 4.1% were tuberculin reactors, compared with 2.7% among lifetime residents on farms (Lowell et al., 1969). In 1987, the 177 U.S. towns and cities with more than 100,000 inhabitants accounted for 25.4% of the U.S. population, but 47.1% of tuberculous cases. Within these municipalities, the risk of tuberculosis increased with population size, and cities with a population greater than 250,000 had an incidence rate three times higher than towns of fewer than 100,000 population, where 74.7% of the U.S. population lived (Bloch et al.,1989). In the 1980s, the gap in case rates between urban and rural areas widened, and this trend still continues. Between 1979 and 1987, the tuberculous case rate decreased from 9.6:100,000 to 6.6:100,000, or by 31%, in communities of fewer than 100,000 (Bloch et al., 1989; CDC, 1992). During the same period, it increased from 14.8 to 17.2 cases per 100,000 population, or 16.3% in towns of 100,000–250,000 (Bloch et al., 1989).

The observed increase in tuberculosis incidence with population size is not uniform. Of 64 cities with a 1990 Census population greater than 250,000, New York, Los Angeles, Chicago, and Houston accounted for 52.6% of the cases, but 34.1% of the population (CDC, 1991, unpublished data). However, Newark, one of the least populated of these cities, had the highest incidence rate (Table 1). Although Milwaukee counted more than twice the population of Newark, it

Table 1   U.S. Cities with Highest Tuberculosis Incidence Rates, 1990

City	Incidence rate[a]	Population
Newark, New Jersey	68.3	275,221
Miami, Florida	66.1	358,548
Atlanta, Georgia	51.5	394,017
Oakland, California	49.2	372,242
New York City, New York	48.1	7,322,564
San Francisco, California	46.1	723,959

[a]Per 100,000 population
Source: CDC, unpublished data (1991).

Table 2 U.S. Cities[a] with Highest Tuberculosis Incidence Rates in Blacks or Hispanics, 1990

Blacks		Hispanics	
City	Rate[b]	City	Rate[b]
Miami, Florida	158.5	New York, New York	50.6
New York, New York	111.4	San Francisco, California	39.7
Newark, New Jersey	100.8	Los Angeles, California	32.4
Tampa, Florida	85.0	Oakland, California	30.9
Austin, Texas	75.2	Miami, Florida	29.9

[a]Only those cities with more than 50,000 blacks or Hispanics are considered.
[b]Per 100,000 population.
Source: CDC, unpublished data (1991).

had one of the lowest incidence rates. Table 2 lists the cities with more than 50,000 blacks or Hispanics and the highest incidence of tuberculosis in these racial and ethnic groups. At the other extreme, in 1990, blacks in Norfolk, Virginia and Hispanics in Tucson, Arizona had incidence rates of 5.0:100,000 and 5.1:100,000, respectively (i.e., one-half that of the U.S. population in general) (CDC, 1991, unpublished data). We suspect that a difference in the concentration of poverty between cities is the main factor determining these extreme differences in incidence rates.

The preponderance of tuberculous cases in certain urban areas is partly attributable to greater efficiency of transmission of *Mycobacterium tuberculosis* (Mtb) in overcrowded living quarters. Overcrowding increases the probability that previously unexposed individuals will inhale infected droplet nuclei and thus become infected with Mtb (Houk et al., 1968). Thus, in high school students in Maryland, a better quality of housing and lack of overcrowding correlated with lower rates of positive tuberculin reactions (Kummerer and Comstock, 1967). Overcrowded housing facilities are more likely to exist with increasing poverty, and they are more common in inner-city communities. This situation has worsened as a result of the deterioration of housing in the 1970s and 1980s in urban ghettos in the United States (Wallace, 1988). Homeless shelters, prisons, and jails, institutions in which inner-city residents, particularly blacks and Latinos, are disproportionately represented (CDC, 1987a–d; Stead, 1989), are known to be frequently overcrowded. They have a high incidence and prevalence of both tuberculous and HIV infection, and their populations can be highly mobile between and within facilities. Special problems of tuberculosis control in these settings are discussed in Chapters 20, 22, and 25.

As of 1986, the prevalence of positive tuberculin skin tests was 28.4% in close contacts of tuberculous patients, and 14.4% in other-than-close contacts (CDC, 1989a). One investigator had estimated that to become infected a hospital worker would have to breathe air contaminated by patients with untreated tuberculosis for 600–800 h (Riley, 1957). However, in a recent outbreak in a housing facility for HIV-infected persons in San Francisco, active tuberculosis developed in 11 of 30 persons, or 37% of those exposed to possible infection, and 4 others converted their tuberculin skin tests (Daley et al., 1992). Of 28 staff members with possible exposure, 6 had tuberculin skin test conversions, and 3 were tuberculin-positive without previous skin testing (Daley et al., 1992). These results, as well as data from recent outbreaks of drug-resistant disease (Pitchenik et al., 1990; CDC, 1991a,b; Monno et al., 1991), serve as a reminder of the efficiency with which certain individuals aerosolize mycobacteria and transmit infection, especially HIV-positive individuals. Under these circumstances, overcrowding is likely to favor the spread of tuberculosis with increased frequency.

IV. Socioeconomic Status

Within urban areas, case rates vary widely, being greatest in areas where poor people live (Rieder, 1989a,b). Indeed, an inverse relation has been noted between the incidence of tuberculosis and household income (Fig. 1). In the National Health Examination Survey, a negative tuberculin skin test correlated with higher educational level, increasing income, skilled occupation, and a larger number of rooms in the home (Engel and Roberts, 1977). In large cities, for persons under aged 35 years, tuberculosis mortality in both sexes is three times higher in the lowest than in the highest economic group. This difference increases for men over 35, in whom the ratio may reach 6:1 (Rieder, 1989a,b). There is a linear relation between the unemployment rate by zip code and the incidence of tuberculosis, particularly in communities for which the unemployment rate is greater than 20% (Fig. 2).

Within municipalities, extreme variations are known to occur in the incidence of tuberculosis according to socioeconomic status. For instance, in 1990, the incidence of tuberculosis in Central Harlem was the highest in New York City and was 32 times that of the more affluent, neighboring Kips Bay–Yorkville sections of Manhattan. In fact, during that year, the incidence rate in Kips Bay–Yorkville was 7.4:100,000 population, compared with 10.3:100,000 for the U.S. population in general (N.Y. City Tuberculosis Bureau, 1991; CDC, 1992).

This strongly suggests that city-living alone does not explain the spread of tuberculosis. In poor urban communities, the high incidence of tuberculosis is

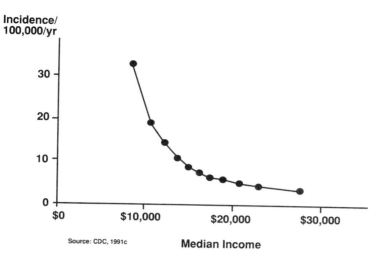

Figure 1 Tuberculosis incidence by income level in zip code of residence. (From CDC, 1991c.)

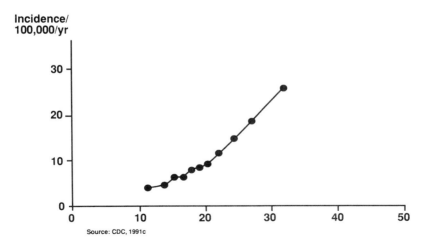

Figure 2 Tuberculosis incidence by unemployment level in zip code of residence. (From CDC, 1991c.)

better explained by poverty in its diverse manifestations, rather than urban life itself. Since African–Americans and Latinos are more likely than whites to be poor, to live in inner-city neighborhoods, and to be foreign-born, it is not surprising that tuberculous case rates are highest among nonwhites.

V. Access to Care

Restricted access to primary care is an important barrier to adequate tuberculosis control in inner-city populations. Minorities, the groups at increased risk for tuberculosis, are disproportionately represented among the nearly 40 million U.S. residents without adequate access to health care services (American College of Physicians, 1990). Consequently, they are more likely to encounter delays or be denied access to needed medical care (Tallon et al., 1989; Schwartz et al., 1900). Twenty-two percent of African–Americans do not have health insurance, and 20% do not have a regular source of health care; but for whites, the comparable numbers are 16 and 14%, respectively (Robert Wood Johnson Foundation, 1987; U.S. Census Bureau, 1987).

Lower-income individuals, irrespective of race, postpone seeking primary care until their need for treatment becomes urgent, and they tend to rely on emergency rooms and hospital clinics for health services (National Center for Health Statistics, 1985). Although this is often assumed to represent risk-taking behavior, the institutional barriers that discourage poor urban residents from seeking medical care are not sufficiently emphasized and are frequently overlooked.

Moreover, poor patients generally receive less intensive medical services than more affluent ones, and nonwhites less than whites (Yergan et al., 1987). In one study, nonwhites were observed to receive fewer consultations, fewer surgical procedures, and less intensive care than expected, and at lower levels than whites (Yergan et al., 1987). Even though the overall rate of treatment completion for tuberculosis in 1988 at Harlem Hospital was dismal at 10%, multivariate analysis showed significantly better compliance for patients with AIDS (Brudney and Dobkin, 1991a). This difference is best explained by enrollment in an AIDS treatment program, which establishes a source of comprehensive primary care. In New York City, about half of the tuberculous patients are cared for at municipal hospitals and related clinics (Brudney and Dobkin, 1991b). There, laboratory facilities too often lag far behind available technologies, and sometimes standard tests such as drug-sensitivity studies are unavailable, simply for lack of reagents. This severely impairs the ability of clinicians to provide state-of-the-art care. Many of these patients are homeless, and in most municipal hospitals and departments of health, adequate mechanisms are not in place for reaching out to this population. Long waiting periods for appointments are common, clinic hours are too often inconvenient, and clinic sites are commonly unattractive. In addition, although alcohol and drug abuse are highly prevalent in the population afflicted with tuberculosis, progressive cutbacks in funding have curtailed treatment programs and social support services.

VI. Racial Factors

Racial susceptibility to tuberculous infection has been hypothesized to contribute to the higher incidence rate observed in races of darker pigmentation. However, serious methodological questions arise as we examine the relation of race to tuberculosis (Hahn, 1992). A National Center for Health Statistics study found that 5.8% of persons reporting themselves as black were classified as white by interviewers, and 32.3% of self-reported Asians and 70% of self-reported Indians were classified as "white" or "black" (Massey, 1980). According to the Census Bureau, in 27 states, among those who specified a race, 93% of blacks and 33% of whites who reported being Mexican–American did so incorrectly, and 33% of the Mexican–American population estimated for those states was misclassified (U.S. Bureau of Census, 1982). Given the extent of miscegenation in the United States, race correlates more closely with socioeconomic status than with genetic makeup (Osborne and Feit, 1992).

Available data suggest that racial differences in incidence of active tuberculosis are mostly attributable to differences in risk of tuberculous infection, and the latter is strongly related to socioeconomic status. These differences increase with increasing age, but the decline in race- and sex-specific incidence rates has been uniform among children across racial groups (Rieder, 1989a,b), an observation that does not support racial predisposition to infection during childhood. In the bacille Calmette-Guerin (BCG) vaccination trial in Puerto Rico, no significant differences in incidence of tuberculosis were observed between black and white tuberculin reactors after follow-up of numerous participants (Comstock et al., 1974b). This suggests that, once infected, blacks are equally likely as whites to develop active tuberculosis, but because of disparities in the rate of decline in prevalent infection, blacks constitute a more concentrated reservoir for reactivation of disease (Rieder, 1989a,b).

Results of several studies have been interpreted as suggestive of racial differences in genetic susceptibility to tuberculosis (Comstock et al., 1974a; Rook, 1988; Ferebee, 1970). Among Filipinos in the U.S. Navy, the rate of disease caused by *M. tuberculosis* was observed to increase with duration of enlistment (Comstock, 1974a). The opposite was true in blacks and whites. In Great Britain, Asians have a 30 times greater risk of tuberculosis than do whites, and this difference has been hypothesized to relate to both genetic and environmental factors (Rook, 1988); namely, genetically determined dark skin, which results in reduced photosynthesis (Webb and Holick, 1988), and insufficient exposure to sunlight and ingested vitamin D. However, there is significant overlap between and within racial groups in the range of circulating vitamin D, and the minor differences in serum level could not explain the magnitude of the observed disparities. Tuberculous case rates among infected persons living in Denmark in the 1950s were only 28:100,000 (Horwitz et al., 1969), in striking contrast with annual rates of 1500:100,000 to 1800:100,000 in Eskimo populations in Alaska and Greenland (Ferebee, 1970). However, the wide disparities in standard of living and available public resources between these two populations make such a conclusion subject to serious question.

A recent study found a higher tuberculous infection rate in black compared with white nursing home residents. Of 25,398 initially tuberculin-negative residents, evidence of new infection was present for 7.2% of whites, compared with 13.8% of blacks (Stead et al., 1990). However, interpretation of these results is difficult because (1) 30% of the residents did not undergo tuberculin testing 60 or more days after initial testing (Felton et al., 1990), and (2) the authors did not control for use of immunosuppressive agents, diabetes, end-stage renal disease, or other chronic conditions (Rosenman, 1990).

Minorities in the United States and the foreign-born appear to be at increased risk for extrapulmonary tuberculosis (Rieder et al., 1990). In 1986, although 63% of tuberculous cases occurred in racial or ethinic minorities and the foreign-born, the association of extrapulmonary tuberculosis with minority status or birth in a foreign country was even stronger. In the same year, 17.5% of all tuberculous cases in the United States were extrapulmonary, and 71.2% of these cases occurred among racial or ethnic minorities (Rieder, 1990). However, these data do not facilitate differentiation between genetic and environmental determinants of disease.

A recent study in Denver found that tubercle bacilli grew faster in successfully infected macrophages from six black than from those of eight white donors, especially in the presence of black donor serum (Crowle and Elkins, 1990). Although the experimental design allowed for control of exposure to mycobacteria and vitamin D levels, the few participants and the uncertain relation between race and genetic makeup make the result of this study difficult to interpret. Various histocompatibility antigen (HLA) phenotypes have been shown to be associated with tuberculosis in different ethnic groups (Papiha et al., 1985; Hwang et al., 1985; Cox et al., 1988). At this point, interpretation of these associations is complicated by the nonspecificity of these haplotypes across ethnic groups. Consequently, race-related risk cannot be assigned on this basis. Clearly, more research is needed.

Although racial differences in susceptibility to tuberculous infection may exist, a genetic, rather than socioeconomic, basis for them remains to be convincingly demonstrated. Since drugs are available that are effective against tuberculosis in all races, regardless of HIV status, differences in susceptibility are unlikely to explain racial differences in the burden of suffering from this disease. Rather, failure to identify and appropriately manage those infected with the disease seems to be the principal problem.

Future studies should further clarify the contribution of host factors to the pathogenesis of tuberculosis. Because of genetic heterogeneity within racial groups, models need to be developed to assess individual susceptibility to tuberculosis on the basis of immunogenetic makeup. These studies must control for socioeconomic status, as it is likely to be an important confounding variable.

VII. Tuberculosis and Human Immunodeficiency Virus Infection

The relation of tuberculosis to HIV infection is covered in detail in Chapter 17, but will be discussed briefly here. In AIDS patients, the incidence of tuberculosis is 500 times that of the general population (Pitchenik et al., 1988). States and cities with the largest number of cases of AIDS also have the highest number of tuberculous cases and, as the number of AIDS cases have increased, so have the number of tuberculous cases (Barnes et al., 1991). The demographic groups with the highest prevalence of AIDS (i.e., blacks and Latinos 25–44 years of age) also have the highest incidence of tuberculosis (CDC, 1992). Finally, HIV infection is the strongest risk factor for reactivation of latent tuberculous infection (i.e., HIV-positive persons who are tuberculin-positive have an 8% risk per year of developing active tuberculosis if left untreated (Selwyn et al., 1989).

The rate of HIV infection is increasing fastest in poor urban populations and, with the passage of time, HIV infection will be preponderant in blacks and Latinos (Barnes et al., 1991). Compared with patients with AIDS only, patients with both AIDS and tuberculosis were also more likely to be Haitians, U.S.-born blacks, or Hispanic. That is, tuberculous infection among AIDS patients was reported in 2% of non-Hispanic whites, 7% of Hispanics, 15% of U.S.-born blacks, and 29% of Haitians (Bloch et al., 1989).

Perhaps most ominous of all is the rapid rise in cases of multidrug-resistant tuberculosis (MDR-TB), a subject that is discussed in detail in Chapter 15. In the United States, the impact of this epidemic has been felt most severely in New York and Miami, with outbreaks reported in hospitals and prisons (CDC, 1991a; Monno et al., 1991; Pitchenik et al., 1990). Thus far, most of the cases have been reported in persons with AIDS, and case fatality rates have been very high, up to 90% (CDC, 1991a). Inner-city populations and health care workers will be at greatest risk for this evolving epidemic.

VIII.   The Foreign-Born (See Chapter 24)

The proportion of tuberculous cases nationwide in the foreign-born has risen steadily over recent years (Bloch et al., 1989). Extrapulmonary tuberculosis is more common in minorities and the foreign-born than in the U.S. population in general (Rieder et al., 1990). Not only are disease rates high among foreign-born individuals, but the infecting organisms are frequently resistant to commonly used antituberculosis drugs, especially isoniazid and streptomycin (Bloch et al., 1989). If not recognized and managed appropriately, drug-resistant disease and infection may lead to treatment failure. Eighty percent of foreign-born tuberculous patients in the United States were reported from eight states, including California, New York, Florida, Massachusetts, and New Jersey (Bloch et al., 1989). In 1989, in certain states, namely, California, Rhode Island, and Hawaii, the foreign-born accounted for more than 55% of the tuberculous caseload (CDC, 1991c). During the same year, in Oregon, Minnesota, Idaho, Colorado, and Washington, between 32 and 47% of tuberculous patients were foreign-born (CDC, 1991c). Many of them live in poor urban neighborhoods, and most developed active disease within 5 years of arrival in the United States (Bloch et al., 1989). Eight countries account for nearly two-thirds of tuberculous cases in the foreign-born. These include Mexico (22%); the Indochinese countries of Kampuchea, Laos, and Vietnam (13%); the Philippines (12%); Haiti (6%); South Korea (6%); and China (4%) (Bloch et al., 1989). In 1987, 48.5% were younger than 35 years of age at the time the case was reported, and another 18.1% who were older than 35 years at the time of case report, were younger than 35 years at the time of arrival in the United States. Disease rates among the foreign-born are highest in the first few years after arrival. As many as 67% of foreign-born cases were potentially preventable, had they been identified on arrival in the United States as infected and given preventive therapy (Bloch et al., 1989).

IX.   Issues in Tuberculosis Control in Urban Communities

Control and containment of tuberculosis in the community are dependent on three basic public health approaches: (1) Early identification, isolation, and treatment of persons with clinically active tuberculous disease; (2) identification and preventive treatment for individuals who have tuberculous infection, but not active disease; (3) prevention of conditions that facilitate transmission of disease, such as HIV infection, chemical substance abuse, and overcrowding in households, shelters, and correctional facilities.

Curative treatment of active cases is the priority in urban populations today, because it removes sources of new infection from the community. The high frequency of nonadherence to therapy among tuberculous patients in poor urban communities is the most important obstacle to control of this disease. Nothing, including age, sex, race, socioeconomic status, income level, and occupation, predicts adherence to therapy (Sbarbaro, 1990). Therefore, directly observed therapy, especially in combination with positive incentives, is the best method for ensuring that patients are taking prescribed medications (McDonald et al., 1982; Sbarbaro, 1985). Completion rates higher than 90% can be achieved using this modality, even in severely nonadherent patients (Brudney and Dobkin, 1991a).

For hospitalized patients, a careful discharge plan must be elaborated by the tuberculosis management team and discussed with each individual patient. The patient's social needs should be identified, and responsive action should be taken. Supportive social services should be a key ingredient in management of tuberculous patients. Adequate numbers of well-trained community public health workers are needed to follow all patients through their course of treatment. Tools need to be developed for patient education, their effectiveness evaluated, and the results rapidly disseminated. In addition, potential barriers such as clinic or pharmacy waiting time, and lack of availability of evening clinic, should be identified and eliminated (Cuneo and Snider, 1989). Approaches to optimizing adherence to therapy are discussed in more detail in Chapter 10.

Alternative approaches to outpatient treatment for the homeless need to be developed. For some, this might entail voluntary participation in treatment programs involving the use of incentives, one of which is housing itself. In addition, community and culturally based directly observed therapy programs should be tested as a means of improving the rate of completion of therapy.

The importance of coordinated efforts between local providers and departments of health is self-evident. Too often a patient presents in a local hospital with active tuberculosis, and no database can be efficiently consulted on recent hospitalization for tuberculosis, culture results, drug susceptibility patterns, or adherence to therapy. Computerized data-bases are needed to connect providers to their local Department of Health. This need is most acute in homeless shelters and jails, for which turnover of active cases can be rapid. Prompt reporting of cases and culture results through these data-bases could make current information available to clinicians.

Special emphasis must be placed on identification and treatment of contacts of active cases and all patients dually infected with *M. tuberculosis* and HIV. The tuberculin skin test result is a poor marker of infection in patients who are HIV-seropositive (Huebner et al., 1992). In a recent nested case-control study, changing the definition of a positive tuberculin skin test from the current CDC recommendation of 5 mm (CDC, 1991b) to 2 mm significantly improved identification of those infected with *M. tuberculosis* (Graham et al., 1992) and, therefore, eligible for preventive therapy. A decision analysis found that in HIV-seropositive intravenous drug users, except tuberculin-negative black women, isoniazid (INH) preventive therapy was beneficial and resulted in an average increase in life expectancy of as much as 285 days (Jordan et al., 1991). Therefore, anergy testing should be performed on all patients who are HIV-positive (CDC, 1991b), and guidelines need to be developed for preventive treatment of anergic, HIV-seropositive patients.

On the other hand, although INH chemoprophylaxis was shown to prevent tuberculosis in dually infected patients (Selwyn et al., 1989), the rising incidence of drug-resistant disease in certain areas, particularly in New York and Miami, raises questions about which agent(s) to use for chemoprophylaxis. Guidelines are currently being prepared, and more research is needed in this area.

Finally, provider education efforts should aim to raise the index of suspicion for tuberculosis and guide decisions on when to consult professionals especially trained in the management of the disease, namely, pulmonary and infectious disease specialists. Indeed, given the rising incidence of drug-resistant disease, the time may be here for management of all tuberculous cases by a specialized multidisciplinary team, including these subspecialists, social workers, infection control nurses, and community outreach workers.

X. Sociolegal Issues in Tuberculosis Management

Never before have our technological capabilities been so advanced, yet they are dwarfed by the magnitude of the social issues underlying the spread of this disease. The medical and public health community today is called upon to respond to this epidemic, which is yet another symptom of urban decay, increasing poverty, and a disintegrated public health infrastructure. Technological improvements and new drugs are needed to reduce the time to diagnosis, to determine the sensitivity patterns of *M. tuberculosis*, and to shorten the duration of therapy. Nevertheless, success in control of urban tuberculosis will depend principally on our ability to convince disenfranchised individuals, preponderantly blacks and Latinos, to take medication with significant toxicities for several months in *the* "public interest," usually defined by individuals who are preponderantly white and socioeconomically stable.

Consequently, important ethical and legal issues arise. The responsibility of the health authorities is to prevent the public at large from becoming infected with *M. tuberculosis*. At what point does the public interest take precedence over individual rights? Who is to determine that, and on what basis? This dilemma sets the tone for the current debate on how to deal with this potentially devastating crisis.

We have come full circle. At the turn of the century, changes in the quality of life were the most important determinant for the decline in incidence of tuberculosis. Today, available tools, particularly molecular biology, are being applied in the fight against this disease. Already, the polymerase chain reaction makes it possible to diagnose *M. tuberculosis* in sputum with high sensitivity and specificity within hours (Eisenbach et al., 1991), and analysis of restriction fragment length polymorphisms has proved an important tool in outbreak investigations (Daley et al., 1992). However, technological solutions alone are unlikely to prevail in this crisis, which is rooted in poverty and complicated by the AIDS epidemic. Moreover, the degree of alienation and demographic instability of the population at greatest risk for tuberculosis is greater today than it was at any other time during this century.

Whereas overwhelming emphasis has been placed on delivering chemotherapy to tuberculous patients, the role of community education in the response to this epidemic has received little attention. This may result in failure to mobilize an important resource in the fight against tuberculosis in inner-city communities.

Although certain patient demographic characteristics, particularly homelessness, are often invoked to explain treatment failures and poor results of tuberculosis control programs, institutional and provider responsibility are too often overlooked. Although the reduction in available resources has been identified as an important factor in the current epidemic, mismanagement of existing resources may be a complicating issue (Brudney and Dobkin, 1991b). For instance, patients who are drug- and alcohol-dependent should be routinely offered appropriate treatment before adherence to therapy is to be expected. However, too often these and other psychosocial support services for tuberculous patients are inadequate. Until such basic measures are systematically implemented, institutional noncompliance to minimal standards of care will contribute to patient nonadherence to prescribed therapy.

However, even with consistently appropriate institutional care, a few patients will show a clear pattern of nonadherence. In this small minority of tuberculous patients, involuntary treatment may be necessary. Demographic characteristics of 33 patients detained for therapy in New York City between January 1988 and April 1991 are 79% black, 12% Latino, 61% male, 52% homeless, median age 34 years; 61% were IVDU or crack users, and 46% were alcohol-dependent. The mean number of hospitalizations for this population was 4.73, and 73% of their isolates were resistant to at least one antituberculous medication. Only one of these patients took drugs long enough to be cured (New York City Department of Health, 1991, unpublished data).

The law in New York City currently allows detention only until the patient is no longer infectious, and efforts are underway to provide for detention to cure. However, this will be no substitute for rebuilding our public health infrastructure. The potential for institutional abuse of statutes providing for involuntary treatment is enormous. Since the overwhelming majority of these patients are poor and nonwhite, the requirement for cultural competence cannot be overemphasized. Clear criteria will need to be established for involuntary treatment of these patients, including participation of multiple disciplines and community, as well as credibly enforced minimum standards of care and institutional accountability.

The outcome of detention for treatment must be critically evaluated, both for individual recruits and for its effect on the epidemic. However, even if the necessary resources are expended to support detention to cure where appropriate, the likelihood of success of this approach remains open to serious question. For, as long as individuals are being released to conditions of homelessness, unemployment, and widespread drug abuse, tuberculosis in our inner cities is here to stay.

References

American College of Physicians (1990). Position paper: Access to health care. *Ann Intern. Med.* **112**:641–661.

Barnes, P. F., Bloch, A. B., Davidson, P. T., and Snider, D. I. (1991). Tuberculosis in patients with human immunodeficiency virus infection. *N. Engl. J. Med.* **324**:1644–1650.

Bloch, A. B., Rieder, H. L., Kelly, G. D., Cauthen, G. M., Hayden, C. H., and Snider, D. E., Jr. (1989). The epidemiology of tuberculosis in the United States. Implications for diagnosis and treatment. *Clin. Chest Med.* **10**:297–313.

Brudney, K., and Dobkin, J. (1991a). Resurgent tuberculosis in New York City. *Am. Rev. Respir. Dis.* **144**:745–749.

Brudney, K., and Dobkin, J. (1991b). A tale of two cities: Tuberculosis control in Nicaragua and New York City. *Semin. Respir. Infect.* **6**:261–272.

Centers for Disease Control (1987a). Tuberculosis among Hispanics—United States, 1985. *MMWR* **36**:568–569.

Centers for Disease Control (1987b). Tuberculosis control among homeless populations. *MMWR* **36**:257–260.

Centers for Disease Control (1987c). Tuberculosis in blacks—United States. *MMWR* **36**:212–220.

Centers for Disease Control (1987d). Tuberculosis in minorities—United States. *MMWR* **36**:77–80.

Centers for Disease Control (1989a). A strategic plan for the elimination of tuberculosis in the United States. *MMWR* **38**(Suppl.):1–25.

Centers for Disease Control (1989b). *Tuberculosis in the United States 1965–1985.* U.S. Government Printing Office, Washington, D.C., HHS publication (CDC)89-8322.

Centers for Disease Control (1990). Update: Tuberculosis elimination—United States. *MMWR* **39**:153–156.

Centers for Disease Control (1991a). Nosocomial transmission of multidrug-resistant tuberculosis among HIV-infected persons—Florida and New York, 1988–91. *MMWR* **40**:585–591.

Centers for Disease Control (1991b). Purified protein derivative (PPD)-tuberculin anergy and HIV infection: Guidelines for anergy testing and management of anergic persons at risk of tuberculosis. *MMWR* **40**(Suppl. RR-5):27–33.

Centers for Disease Control (1991c) *Tuberculosis Elimination, U.S.A.* Atlanta, Georgia.

Centers for Disease Control (1992). Tuberculosis morbidity in the United States: 1990. Final data. *MMWR* **40**:23–28.

Comstock, G. W. (1986). Tuberculosis. In *Public Health and Preventive Medicine*. Edited by J. M. Last. Appleton and Lange, Norwalk, Connecticut, pp. 222–233.

Comstock, G. W., Edwards, L. B., and Livesay, V. T. (1974a). Tuberculous morbidity in the U.S. Navy: Its distribution and decline. *Am. Rev. Respir. Dis.* **110**:572–580.

Comstock, G. W., Livesay, V. T., and Woolpert, S. F. (1974b). The prognosis of a positive tuberculin reaction in childhood and adolescence. *Am. J. Epidemiol.* **99**:131–138.

Council of Lung Associations of New York (1981). *New Approach to a Resurging Crisis. Report of the Task Force on Tuberculosis in New York, 1980.* New York Lung Association, New York.

Cox, R. A., Downs, M., Neimes, R. E., Ognibene, A. J., Yamashita, T. S., and Ellner, J. J. (1988). Immunogenetic analysis of human tuberculosis. *J. Infect. Dis.* **158**:1302–1308.

Crowle, A. J., and Elkins, N. (1990). Relative permissiveness of macrophages from black and white people for virulent tubercle bacili. *Infect. Immun.* **58**:632–638.

Cuneo, W. D., and Snider, D. E. (1989). Enhancing patient compliance with tuberculosis therapy. *Clin. Chest Med.* **10**:375–380.

Daley, C. L., Small, P. M., Schecter, G. F., Schoolnik, G. K., McAdam, R. A., Jacobs, W. R., Jr., and Hopewell, P. C. (1992). An outbreak of tuberculosis with accelerated progression among persons infected with the human immunodeficiency virus. *N. Engl. J. Med.* **326**:231–235.

Eisenach, K. D., Sifford, M. D., Cave, M. D., Bates, J. A., and Crawford, J. T. (1991). Detection of *Mycobacterium tuberculosis* in sputum samples using a polymerase chain reaction. *Am. Rev. Respir. Dis.* **144**:1160–1163.

Engel, A., and Roberts, J. (1977). Tuberculin skin test reaction among adults 25–74 years. United States, 1971–72. *Vital and Health Statistics: Series 11, no. 204.* U.S. Government Printing Office, Washington, D.C., DHEW Publication no. (HRA)77-1649, pp. 1–31.

Felton, C. P., Smith, J. A., and Ehrlich, M. H. (1990). Racial differences and *Mycobacterium tuberculosis* infection. *N. Engl. J. Med.* **322**:1670–1671.

Ferebee, S. H. (1970). Controlled chemoprophylaxis trials in tuberculosis: A general review. *Adv. Tuberc. Res.* **17**:28–106.

Graham, N. M. H., Newson, K. E., Solomon, L., Bonds, M., Rizzo, R. T., Scavotto, J., Astemborski, J., and Vlahov, D. (1992). Prevalence of tuberculin positivity and skin test anergy in HIV-1-seropositive and -seronegative intravenous drug users. *JAMA* **267**:369–373.

Hahn, R. A. (1992). The state of federal health statistics on racial and ethnic groups. *JAMA* **267**:268–271.

Horwitz, O., Wilbeck, E., and Erickson, P. A. (1969). Epidemiologic basis of tuberculosis eradication. 10. Longitudinal studies on the risk of tuberculosis in the general population of a low-prevalence area. *Bull. WHO* **41**:95–113.

Houk, V. N., Baker, J. H., Sorensen, K., and Kent, D. C. (1968). The epidemiology of tuberculosis infection in a closed environment. *Arch. Environ. Health* **16**:26–50.

Huebner, R. E., Villarino, M. E., and Snider, D. E., Jr. (1992). Tuberculin skin testing and the HIV epidemic. *JAMA* **267**:409–410.

Hwang, C. H., Khan, S., Ende, N., Mangura, B. T., Reichman, L. B., and Chou, J. (1985). The HLA-A, -B, and -DR phenotypes and tuberculosis. *Am. Rev. Respir. Dis.* **132**:382–385.

Iseman, M. D., and Sbarbaro, J. A. (1990). Short course chemotherapy of tuberculosis. Hail Britannia (and friends)! *Am. Rev. Respir. Dis.* **143**:697–698.

Jordan, T. J., Lewit, E. M., Montgomery, R. L., and Reichman, L. B. (1991). Isoniazid as preventive therapy in HIV-infected intravenous drug abusers. *JAMA* **265**:2987–2991.

Kuemmerer, J. M., and Comstock, G. W. (1967). Sociologic concomitants of tuberculin sensitivity. *Am. Rev. Respir. Dis.* **96**:885–892.

Leff, D., and Leff, A. R. (1989). Tuberculosis control policies in major metropolitan health departments in the United States. IV. Standards in 1988. *Am. Rev. Respir. Dis.* **139**:1350–1355.

Lowell, A. M., Edwards, L. B., and Palmer, C. E. (1969). *Tuberculosis.* Harvard University Press, Cambridge, Mass., pp. 137–138.

Massey, D. S., and Eggers, M. L. (1990). The ecology of inequality: Minorities and the concentration of poverty, 1970–1980. *Am. J. Sociol.* **95**:1153–1188.

Massey, J., (1980). Using interviewer observed race and respondent reported race in the Health Interview Survey. In *Proceedings of American Statistical Association Meetings: Social Statistics Section.* American Statistical Association, Alexandria, Va., pp. 425–428.

McCord, C., and Freeman, H. P. (1990). Excess mortality in Harlem. *N. Engl. J. Med.* **322**:173–177.

McDonald, R. J., Memon, A. M., and Reichman, L. B. (1982). Successful supervised ambulatory management of tuberculosis treatment failures. *Ann. Intern. Med.* **96**:297–302.

McFadden, R. D. (1991). A drug-resistant TB results in 13 deaths in New York prisons. *New York Times*, Nov. 16, p. A1.

Monno, L., Carbonara, S., Costa, D., Angarano, G., Coppola, S., Quarto, M., and Pastore, G. (1991). Emergence of drug-resistant *Mycobacterium tuberculosis* in HIV-infected patients. *Lancet* **337**:852.

National Center for Health Statistics (1985). *Persons With and Without a Regular Source of Medical Care. United States.* Series 10, no. 151. Washington, D.C.

New York City Tuberculosis Bureau (1991). *Tuberculosis in New York City, 1990.* New York City Department of Health, New York.

Papiha, S. S., Wentzel, J., Behjati, F., and Argawal, S. S. (1985). Human leukocyte antigens and circulating immunoglobulin levels in Indian patients with pulmonary tuberculosis. *Tubercle* **66**:25–33.

Phillips, K. P. (1990). *Politics of Rich and Poor. Wealth and the American Electorate in the Reagan Aftermath.* Random House, New York.

Pitchenik, A. E., Burr, J., Laufer, M., Miller, G., Cacciatore, R., Bigler, W. J., Witte, J. J., and Cleary, T. (1990). Outbreaks of drug-resistant tuberculosis at an AIDS centre. *Lancet* **336**:440–441.

Pitchenik, A. E., Fertel, D., and Bloch, A. B. (1988). Mycobacterial disease: Epidemiology, diagnosis, treatment and prevention. *Clin. Chest Med.* **9**:425–441.

Reichman, L. B., Felton, C. P., and Edsall, J. R. (1979). Drug dependence, a possible risk factor for tuberculous disease. *Arch. Intern. Med.* **139**:337–339.

Rieder, H. L., Cauthen, G. M., Comstock, G. W., and Snider, D. E., Jr. (1989a). Epidemiology of tuberculosis in the United States. *Epidemiol. Rev.* **11**:79–98.

Rieder, H. L., Cauthen, G. M., Kelly, G. D., Bloch, A. B., and Snider, D. E., Jr. (1989b). Tuberculosis in the United States. *JAMA* **262**:385–389.

Rieder, H. L., Cauthen, G. M., Kelly, G. D., Bloch, A. B., and Snider, D. E., Jr. (1989b). Tuberculosis in the United States. *JAMA* **262**:385–389.

Riley, R. L. 81957). The J. Burns Amberson Lecture: Aerial dissemination of pulmonary tuberculosis. *Am. Rev. Tuberc.* **76**:931–941.

Robert Wood Johnson Foundation (1987). *Access to Health Care in the United States: Results of a 1986 Survey.* Robert Wood Johnson Foundation, Princeton, N.J.

Rook, G. A. W. (1988). The role of vitamin D in tuberculosis. *Am. Rev. Respir. Dis.* **138**:768–770.

Rosenmann, K. D. (1990). Racial differences in *Mycobacterium tuberculosis* infection. *N. Engl. J. Med.* **322**:1670.

Sbarbaro, J. A. (1979). Compliance: inducements and enforcements. *Chest* **76**:750–756.

Sbarbaro, J. A. (1985). Strategies to improve compliance with therapy. *Am. J. Med.* **79**:34–37.

Sbarbaro, J. A. (1990). The patient–physician relationship: Compliance revisited. *Ann. Allergy* **64**:325–331.

Sbarbaro, J. A., and Iseman, M. D. (1986). Baby needs a new pair of shoes. *Chest* **90**:754–755.

Schwartz, E., Kofie, V. Y., Rivo, M., and Tuckson, R. V. (1990). Black/white comparisons of deaths preventable by medical intervention: United States and the District of Columbia 1980–1986. *Int. J. Epidemiol.* **19**:591–598.

Selwyn, P. A., Hartel, D., Lewis, V. A., Schoenbaum, E. E., Vermund, S. H., Klein, R. S., Walker, A. T., and Friedland, G. H. (1989). A prospective study of the risk of tuberculosis among intravenous drug users with human immunodeficiency virus infection. *N. Engl. J. Med.* **320**:545–550.

Snider, D. E., and Roper, W. L. (1992). The new tuberculosis. *N. Engl. J. Med.* **326**:703–705.

Stead, W. W. (1989). Special problems in tuberculosis. *Clin. Chest Med.* **10**:397–405.

Stead, W. W., Senner, J. W., Reddick, W. T., and Lofgren, J. P. (1990). Racial differences in susceptibility to infection by *Mycobacterium tuberculosis*. *N. Engl. J. Med.* **322**:422–427.

Sunderam, G., McDonald, R. J., Maniatis, T., Oleske, J., Kapila, R., and Reichman, L. B. (1986). Tuberculosis as a manifestation of the acquired immunodeficiency syndrome (AIDS). *JAMA* **256**:362–366.

Tallon, J. R., Jr. (1989). A health policy agenda proposal for including the poor. *JAMA* **261**:1044.

United States Bureau of the Census (1982). *Persons of Spanish Origin by State: 1980*. U.S. Government Printing Office, Washington, D.C., U.S. Dept. of Commerce Publication PC80-S1-7.

United States Bureau of the Census (1987). *Current Population Survey*. U.S. Government Printing Office, Washington, D.C., U.S. Department of Commerce.

Wallace, R. (1988). A synergism of plagues: "Planned shrinkage," contagious housing destruction, and AIDS in the Bronx. *Environ. Res.* **47**:1–33.

Webb, A. R., and Holick, M. F. (1988). The role of sunlight in the cutaneous production of vitamin D_3. *Annu. Rev. Nutr.* **8**:375–469.

Wilson, W. J. (1987). *The Truly Disadvantaged: The Inner City, the Underclass, and Public Policy.* University of Chicago Press, Chicago.

Yeager, H., and Medinger, A. E. (1986). Tuberculosis long-term beds: Have we thrown out the baby with the bathwater? *Chest* **90**:752–753.

Yergan, J., Flood, A. B., LoGerfo, J. P., and Diehr, P. (1987). Relationship between patient race and the intensity of hospital services. *Med. Care* **25**:592–603.

23

M. avium Complex, *M. kansasii*, *M. fortuitum*, and Other Mycobacteria Causing Human Disease

PAUL T. DAVIDSON

County of Los Angeles
Department of Health Services
Public Health Programs
and University of Southern California School of Medicine
Los Angeles, California

I. Introduction

Mycobacteria other than those belonging to the "tuberculosis complex group" were, until recently, uncommon causes of human disease. Their importance has increased in recent years because of their association with patients with the acquired immunodeficiency syndrome (AIDS). Criteria for the diagnosis of disease caused by these organisms, primarily *Mycobacterium avium–M. intracellulare* complex (MAC), when they should be treated, with what regimens, and for how long remain controversial. Despite the number of cases reported, there are no data on long-term controlled clinical trials evaluating the efficacy of any treatment regimen. Research into the pathogenesis, virulence, and treatment is sorely needed. Most of the recent interest has been directed at the MAC and, in particular, the disseminated form that occurs in AIDS patients. Far less attention has been given to the chronic pulmonary form of MAC disease and disease caused by other nontuberculous mycobacteria (Wolinsky, 1979; Wallace et al., 1990; Davidson, 1985, 1989a,b). There are several recent publications summarizing information and proposed guidelines concerning these organisms (American Thoracic Society, 1987; Wallace et al., 1990; Ellner et al., 1991; Young et al., 1986).

II. Epidemiology

Most species of mycobacteria do not depend on a mammalian host for survival and are nonpathogenic for humans or animals.

Exposure to multiple species of environmental mycobacteria is the norm. Under certain poorly understood conditions, some of the species may become pathogenic in humans. They should be considered opportunists in these circumstances, but they can cause progressive and potentially destructive disease. The epidemiology, pathogenesis, and management of disease with these mycobacteria is not well understood or documented. Many species have never been reported as causing disease. Rare reports of disease with some species can be found in the medical literature; for example, *M. terrae* (Cianciulli, 1974; Edwards et al., 1975), *M. gordonae* (Kurnik et al., 1983), or *M. triviale* (Dechairo et al., 1973). These unusual generally saprophytic mycobacteria may be increasing in prevalence as causes of disease in humans, particularly with the advent of AIDS (Collins et al., 1986).

MAC and *M. kansasii* frequently cause human disease. Other species infrequently cause disease, but clearly are pathogenic under certain circumstances. These include *M. marinum*, *M. szulgai*, *M. xenopi*, *M. fortuitum* complex, and *M. simiae*. This chapter will emphasize MAC and to a lesser extent *M. kansasii*, since they are more common causes of disease.

A discussion of the taxonomy of mycobacteria is beyond the scope of this chapter. Considerable headway has been made in characterizing the genus in recent years by applying new technological procedures (Laszlo and Siddiqi, 1984; Butler et al., 1986; Wallace et al., 1990). There remains some debate over terminology to apply for clinical convenience. *Tuberculosis* is frequently defined as a communicable disease caused by *M. tuberculosis*. What to call disease cause by other mycobacteria is less certain, as is the best term for these species as a group. "Nontuberculous mycobacteria" or "nontuberculosis-causing mycobacteria," both abbreviated to NTM, seem the most popular designations in recent years, particularly among lung specialists. "Atypical mycobacteria" and "mycobacteria other than tuberculosis" (MOTT) still remain in use. When the specific species is known, it should be used in association with the disease process (i.e., "lung infection with MAC"). What to call or how to describe the disease in general also has several options including "mycobacteriosis," or "tuberculosis caused by (specific species name)." A detailed proposal for clinical terminology has been published elsewhere (Davidson, 1981).

MAC and other species are often found in water and soil (Wolinsky and Rynearson, 1968; Collins et al., 1984). Studies have documented significant contamination of certain natural waters with virulent MAC strains and have demonstrated methods by which such strains can be aerosolized and carried inland, where presumably they can be inhaled by humans and animals (Gruft et al., 1981; Meissner and Falkinham, 1986). If certain, as yet poorly defined, host factors exist, disease may thus occur, or a predisposition in the host may be established. With the advent of AIDS in humans and as a result of epidemiological studies done in domesticated animals, it appears that ingestion of MAC is an important route of infection as well, with dissemination occurring from the gastrointestinal tract (Damsker and Battone, 1985). The MAC is subdivided into several serotypes, some classified as *M. avium* and others as *M. intracellulare* or *M. scrofulaceum*. The MAC isolates from patients with AIDS are almost always *M. avium* serotypes. Three serotypes predominate, types 4 (40%), 8 (17%), and 1 (9%) (Yakrus and Goad, 1990). Isolates from AIDS patients are more likely to contain plasmids and are more virulent in the beige mouse model than isolates from other sources (Gangadharam et al., 1988). Plasmid studies have also indicated similarities between isolates from the environment and those from patients, supporting the hypothesis that the environment is the source of human MAC infection (Jucker and Falkinham, 1990).

Direct environmental inoculation, either accidently or with an injury, is also a documented method of disease transmission. This is the usual circumstance with *M. marinum*, a frequent inhabitant of water (Mollahan and Romer, 1961; Collins et al., 1985), and *M. fortuitum* complex disease (Gremillion et al., 1983).

Inapparent infection with mycobacteria, such as MAC, without any evidence of disease exists in humans, as evidenced by the high percentage of individuals in some areas of the United States who react to a purified protein derivative (PPD) skin test made from MAC to a greater extent than to PPD made from *M. tuberculosis* (Edwards and Palmer, 1955). Whether this "infection" is in any way analogous to infection with *M. tuberculosis* is highly uncertain. There is no current evidence that a "positive" reaction denotes the presence of dormant organisms or a potential risk of "reactivation," as with *M. tuberculosis*.

Colonization of the human body by environmental mycobacteria is very common. The upper airways, the skin, and the gastrointestinal tract commonly harbor mycobacteria. Even though these areas may not be regularly colonized by mycobacteria, there may be repeated episodes of contamination by mycobacteria from the environment. In addition, specimens obtained from patients are commonly contaminated by mycobacteria.

The histopathology and pathogenesis of disease is variable. In the normal host, the response to disease will be similar to that seen with *M. tuberculosis* and cannot be differentiated on histological criteria alone. Occasionally the response may present as an acute or chronic bacterial infection. In AIDS or other immunosuppressed patients, many of the histological characteristics of chronic mycobacterial diseases are absent (Pitchenik et al., 1988).

III. Clinical Presentation

MAC and *M. kansasii* most commonly cause lung disease in humans. Disseminated disease, particularly with MAC, is emerging as a common manifestation of disease in patients with AIDS (Fauci, 1984; Armstrong et al., 1985; Young et al., 1986; Horsburgh and Selik, 1989), but is rare in immunocompetent hosts.

The symptoms of pulmonary disease are similar to those caused by *M. tuberculosis*, but are often less severe and more chronic. Fever, chills, and rapid weight loss are less common. Underlying lung diseases, such as chronic obstructive lung disease, bronchiectasis, pulmonary fibrosis, or other conditions, are common. These underlying conditions frequently cause symptoms that may be difficult or impossible to differentiate from those caused by the mycobacterial disease. Progression of symptoms or disease may also be largely related to the underlying condition, rather than to the mycobacterial disease.

Pulmonary disease occurs more often in older immunocompetent individuals (average age older than 50). Patients with *M. kansasii* are, on the average, somewhat younger than those with MAC. Disease is probably equally distributed between men and women. In the past, there was a preponderance in men (Davidson et al., 1981). It is unclear why a shift has occurred. The radiologic appearance of disease in the lung is often no different from that of *M. tuberculosis* disease. Cavitary changes are common. A more diffuse, nodular interstitial process without cavitation is also found and appears to be more common in women and in patients without recognized predisposing lung conditions. Disease may be localized to one lobe of the lung, but frequently involves multiple lobes and both lungs. Mediastinal lymph node involvement and pleural effusions are uncommon.

Pulmonary disease caused by *M. fortuitum* complex, *M. simiae*, *M. xenopi*, and other species is rare and generally without specific clinical characteristics. Achalasia of the esophagus may be a predisposing condition for *M. fortuitum* complex disease of the lung, presumably related to chronic aspiration.

Extrapulmonary sites of disease occur in a variety of circumstances. Localized lymph node disease caused by MAC and *M. kansasii*, particularly in the cervical and submandibular chains, is relatively common in otherwise healthy children 5 years of age or younger. The node may increase in size relatively rapidly, but this is usually not associated with fever, pain, or much tenderness. Spontaneous drainage may occur. Disease is probably self-limiting in many children and may, in fact, often go unrecognized. Involvement of other lymph node groups has been observed (inguinal, epitrochlear, popliteal), but multiple node involvement is rare. Older children and adults rarely develop this condition.

Mycobacterium fortuitum complex and *M. marinum* cause skin disease and localized abscesses, usually associated with trauma. A localized granuloma on the skin of an extremity is characteristic of *M. marinum* and is acquired through abrasion or injury to the skin while exposed to contaminated water. Abscesses and infections have been caused by *M. fortuitum* complex through puncture wounds or in association with injection or surgical procedures (Borghous and Stanford, 1973; Fox et al., 1978; Gremillion et al., 1983; Petrini et al., 1980), including breast augmentation (Centers for Disease Control [CDC] 1978; Clegg et al., 1983), cardiac valve replacement (Repath et al., 1976; Narasimhan and Austin, 1978), the sternal split approach to coronary bypass (Robicsek et al., 1978; Hoffman et al., 1981; Sethi et al., 1985), and total hip replacement (Horadam et al., 1982).

Localized lesions in bone, kidneys, and other organs have been caused by MAC and *M. kansasii*. Disseminated disease with multiple organ involvement is rare except in patients with AIDS. In the absence of AIDS, other serious underlying conditions are often present. The prognosis is poor if the disease is not successfully treated. Organisms may be found in bone marrow, liver, lungs, and other tissues. It has become common to isolate MAC from the stool and blood of patients with AIDS in association with dissemination (CDC, 1987). Fever, sweats, anorexia, weight loss, and weakness commonly occur in patients with disseminated mycobacterial disease, particularly that associated with AIDS (Ellner et al., 1991).

IV. Diagnosis

Isolation of environmental mycobacteria from specimens such as sputum is common. Because of the possibility of colonization and contamination, care must be taken to assess the clinical significance of a particular mycobacterial isolate. The first laboratory test done is usually an acid-fast stain. If acid-fast baccilli (AFB) are found on smear, they are present in relatively large numbers. Currently, it is not possible to definitely identify the species on the basis of the staining alone. Consequently, a positive smear result should be considered as indicative of *M. tuberculosis* until proved otherwise. Therapy for *M. tuberculosis* should be started immediately, since it is a communicable disease (particularly if smear-positive), a potentially serious condition for the patient, and a hazard to the patient's contacts. When culture results or other definitive tests indicate a different species, further consideration must be given to the diagnosis. The smear is frequently not positive, and the culture report is the first to indicate a mycobacterial isolate. A systematic and careful evaluation must be undertaken to establish a correct diagnosis, since finding atypical mycobacteria in sputum does not necessarily establish a cause-and-effect relation for a pulmonary condition under investigation. Every effort should be made to assure the correct diagnosis. This is particularly important if the patient will be subjected to potentially toxic or dangerous treatments that are of limited or uncertain benefit. This problem most commonly arises with the isolation of MAC.

As a general rule, the more often and the larger the number of MAC isolated from sputum over time in a patient with an otherwise undiagnosed pulmonary condition, the more likely that that condition is caused by MAC. It is often possible and safe to follow a patient with suspected pulmonary MAC disease for several months as part of the clinical evaluation to establish a diagnosis.

A definitive diagnosis of disease is established when MAC or other mycobacteria are isolated from a normally sterile site such as blood, cerebral spinal fluid, bone marrow, or lymph node tissue. The nature of the disease may not be clearly established with this finding, but a disease process caused by or related to the organism must be accepted. Likewise, the isolation of only one species of *Mycobacterium* from biopsy material with the histological changes of tuberculosis must be considered diagnostic.

Disseminated disease in AIDS patients is best diagnosed by blood culture, using radiometric methods (Hawkins et al., 1986; Wallace and Hannah, 1988). Bone marrow smear and culture are probably the best indicators for early dissemination (Poropatich et al., 1987). Positive acid-fast smears of bone marrow and positive cultures from bone marrow or liver have the same significance as positive cultures of blood (Young, 1988).

Beyond the preceding definitive circumstances, there will be, by necessity, a collection of factors that, in the aggregate, support the evidence for disease to a greater or lesser degree in a given patient. The stronger the factors, the more likely the diagnosis. The presence of one or two stronger factors may suffice in a given clinical situation to establish a diagnosis, whereas several weaker factors are necessary to increase the likelihood of a correct diagnosis. This weighing of factors is more critical in the non-AIDS patient, since isolation of an atypical *Mycobacterium* may be less important in this setting. In all instances, all other reasonable causes for the disease process must be excluded.

The following are strong factors supporting the diagnosis of disease: (1) The patient has a clinical syndrome compatible with disease caused by a mycobacterial species other than *M. tuberculosis* (this will most often be MAC). Mycobacteria have been isolated repeatedly in large numbers from a nonsterile source, and no other pathogen has been found. The larger the number of positive cultures, the more organisms present on each culture, the longer the period of observation, the more likely the diagnosis. (2) A patient with a positive AFB smear has clinical worsening during appropriate antituberculosis chemotherapy. This may include increased symptoms or radiological progression. The evidence becomes stronger if MAC or another mycobacterial species other than *M. tuberculosis* is found on culture.

The following conditions are supportive factors in establishing a diagnosis: (1) A single species of *Mycobacterium* (usually MAC) is identified from a sputum specimen that was AFB smear-positive. (2) A mycobacterial species, such as MAC, that is associated with colonization is not eliminated or significantly reduced in numbers in the sputum of a patient following 1–3 months of vigorous daily bronchial hygiene (Ahn et al., 1979, 1982). (3) A mycobacterial species is consistently isolated from the sputum of a patient with a known predisposing lung condition. (4) The same mycobacterial species is always isolated from the sputum of a patient, but only in small numbers. (5) A patient has cavitary changes in the lung as well as a known predisposing lung condition, but no evidence of a risk for *M. tuberculosis* disease. The tuberculin skin test reaction is negative or small and there has been no *M. tuberculosis* exposure. (6) A patient with AIDS has a positive AFB smear, but the culture is negative for mycobacteria. (7) A patient with AIDS has MAC identified on stool culture. The diagnosis is more likely with multiple positive smears and cultures and may indicate dissemination.

The following are weaker factors supporting the diagnosis of disease: (1) A patient suspected of a mycobacterial disease has a negative tuberculin skin test. (2) A single isolate of a mycobacterial species other than *M. tuberculosis* is obtained on a sputum culture. (3) The patient has a known underlying lung condition that predisposes to mycobacterial disease. (4) A patient with AIDS has a positive AFB smear. This should be considered strong evidence for *M. tuberculosis* infection until proved otherwise because of the serious public health implications. Consequently, this finding, in and of itself, must be considered weak support for infection with other mycobacteria even though, in the past, MAC has been more commonly isolated in AIDS patients. (5) The patient is known to have human immunodeficiency virus (HIV) infection.

Patients with no symptoms and no clinical findings have no disease, even if a mycobacterium such as MAC is found on sputum culture.

The application of the preceding suggested factors to help establish a diagnosis is intended only to support the clinical judgment and experience of the clinician. A single strong factor is frequently sufficient to make the diagnosis until proved otherwise. The more supportive and weaker factors present, the more likely the diagnosis. As a guideline, at least three such factors should be present. One or more of these should be in the supportive group. A diagnosis based only on weak factors is highly suspect and potentially detrimental to the patient.

The recommended diagnostic criteria for pulmonary disease caused by nontuberculous mycobacteria suggested by the American Thoracic Society (Wallace et al., 1990) differentiates between patients with cavitary or noncavitary disease and includes a quantitation guideline that may be helpful to some clinicians.

Isolation of more than one species of mycobacteria from a specimen may occur. If one of the species is *M. tuberculosis*, it should always be considered a pathogen and treated accordingly. Often the other species such as MAC or *M. fortuitum* complex is present in small numbers and may disappear along with the *M. tuberculosis* following treatment of the latter condition. Even if it persists in the sputum specimum, it is usually only as a colonizer and requires no further therapy. In rare circumstances both the *M. tuberculosis* and the other mycobacterial species are causing disease. More aggressive therapy than that for *M. tuberculosis* alone may be necessary, depending on the species.

V. Treatment

Treatment of *M. tuberculosis* infection and disease is based on years of experience, supported by numerous controlled clinical trials. Similar information is not available for managing disease with other mycobacteria, largely because of the relatively infrequent occurrence of disease and the few patients available for study to any one investigator or institution. There is also a lack of good supportive data in laboratory and animal models. Recent efforts to develop an animal model, using the beige mouse for MAC disease, have met with some success (Gangadharam et al., 1983; Bertram et al., 1986). Extensive studies of in vivo antimicrobial sensitivity and synergy have been done using this model (Klemens and Cynamon, 1991). A variety of drugs and combinations have shown an effect by producing a significant reduction in the number of MAC organisms in the lungs and spleens of infected beige mice. These results have not established any clear-cut treatment guidelines and have not as yet been correlated with results in humans. The beige mouse model, infected intravenously, may be appropriate to study disseminated mycobacterial disease in an immunodeficient host, and in a recent report, beige mice, orally infected with MAC, developed disseminated MAC that more closely resembled infection in humans (Bermudez et al., 1992). However, conclusions drawn in such studies may not apply to the human counterpart (i.e., AIDS patients) and are certainly questionable in application to the immunocompetent human.

The penetration of drugs into tissue or cells is a likely controlling factor for efficacy against mycobacteria. Therefore, infected macrophage models are of interest, since MAC survives well intracellularly. This model is important in evaluating drugs targeted against MAC (Yajko et al., 1989; Ellner et al., 1991).

Any in vivo or in vitro model results will have to be substantiated in humans. No prospective controlled clinical trials for treating MAC disease have yet been reported, but clearly are needed (Wallace et al., 1991).

Combinations of drugs used against *M. tuberculosis* have been used against diseases caused by other mycobacteria, with variable success. In many cases, successful response has occurred, despite that some degree of in vitro drug resistance to one or more of the standard antituberculosis drugs is invariably present. Unfortunately, consistent and agreed-upon standards for conducting drug susceptibility studies for these organisms have yet to be established. The laboratory results also frequently fail to have any predictive value concerning outcome, although one study suggested a correlation (Horsburgh et al., 1987). Many types of antibiotics, in addition to the antituberculosis drugs, have been tested or used against the various species of mycobacteria, also with highly variable results. In conclusion, drug susceptibility studies have a limited role in the management of atypical mycobacterial diseases. The guidelines suggested by the American Thoracic Society are appropriate at present (Wallace et al., 1990).

The clinician is left with an array of incomplete or anecdotal data on which to base a decision concerning the treatment of disease in a given patient. The decision may be relatively easy under certain conditions. *Mycobacterium kansasii* is susceptible to rifampin and, to a lesser degree, other antituberculosis drugs. Response to a well-tolerated drug regimen including rifampin is to be expected. Cervical lymphadenopathy in children is cured by surgical excision. (Altman and Margileth, 1975; MacKellar, 1976; Schaad et al., 1979; Taha et al., 1985). Surgical drainage or removal of a foreign body is often curative for *M. fortuitum* complex disease. When the best therapy appears to be an experimental or potentially toxic regimen with unpredictable results, the choice becomes more difficult. This is often the situation with MAC. A cautious approach is indicated. The certainty of the diagnosis and its role in the patient's clinical course must be established. This may require a longer period of observation or additional laboratory testing. Certain factors may indicate no current need for treatment, such as stable or absent symptoms or no evidence of clinical progression. If the patient is known to be allergic or to have toxic reactions to the drugs, treatment should be avoided. Surgical excision may be risky in some patients. Elderly patients often do not tolerate multiple drug regimens. Patients with AIDS often are taking many other medications and can be expected to have more drug intolerance.

Fortunately, disease is often self-limiting or slowly progressive in many patients. The value of toxic, unpredictable treatment is then questionable. This is particularly true for patients with the combination of pulmonary disease and underlying chronic obstructive lung disease. Treatment may not prolong life or improve symptoms to an extent that warrants the risks. Even a child with adenopathy in the neck can be observed and go without surgical treatment if such an approach has a significant risk of permanent damage. Despite the persistent drainage, it will eventually heal without specific therapy.

Patients with AIDS and disseminated MAC infection are seriously ill. Multiple drug regimens are often not well tolerated. Response to therapy is unpredictable. Treatment may have little effect on survival time (Hawkins et al., 1986; ATS/CDC, 1987). However, studies indicate that AIDS patients with disseminated MAC have a significantly shorter survival than AIDS patients without disseminated MAC when a sterile body site was cultured within 3 months of their first AIDS-defining episode of *Pneumocystis carinii* pneumonia (Jacobson et al., 1991). Patients with significant symptoms should always be given the benefit of a treatment trial, since symptoms will often improve. Treatment should be continued if there is a response. The use of experimental drugs may improve the clinical outcomes in some patients. When disseminated MAC is diagnosed, it now appears clear that treatment is indicated (Ellner et al., 1991).

There may be circumstances for which treatment is indicated even when the disease appears stable or asymptomatic. A younger patient with localized pulmonary disease caused by MAC has more to gain by a surgical excision. The surgery is more likely to be tolerated at a younger age, and removal may prevent progression of disease at some future time when drug treatment would be less well tolerated. This may also apply to a younger patient who is not a surgical candidate, but otherwise has stable disease. They may better tolerate medications at this stage than when they become older. The treatment might also prevent disease from progressing in the future when treatment may be less well tolerated or effective.

Chemotherapy is frequently the only treatment choice available to those patients with symptomatic and progressive disease. The guidelines included in this chapter are largely based on my own personal experience as well as information in the medical literature. Because of the relative degree of resistance of certain strains of mycobacteria to the drugs, the highest tolerated dose is usually suggested. Table 1 lists most of the drugs and dosages that are discussed in the following sections.

A. *Mycobacterium avium* Complex

The experience in treating MAC in the past was primarily with pulmonary forms of the disease. Antituberculosis agents in various combinations were generally used. During the past decade, MAC has been diagnosed with increasing frequency in patients with AIDS, usually in a disseminated form. Today the number of cases of MAC in patients with AIDS markedly exceeds that of those with lung disease without AIDS. These AIDS patients have received therapy with a broadened spectrum of agents, many of which are not generally used for treating *M. tuberculosis*. This probably partly reflects the experience of the clinicians involved. Those taking care of AIDS patients are generally familiar with treating a wide spectrum of infections with a wide array of antimicrobial agents. They

Table 1 Drugs and Dosage for Difficult to Treat Mycobacterial Infections

Drug	Dosage
Ciprofloxacin	500–750 mg twice daily
Clofazimine	100–300 mg/day in a single dose
Cycloserine	500–1000 mg/day usually in divided doses
Doxycycline	100 mg twice daily
Ethambutol	25 mg/kg daily in a single dose until culture-negative for 6 months, then 15 mg/kg daily thereafter
Ethionamide	500–1000 mg/day usually in divided doses
Isoniazid	300–600 mg/day in a single dose
Macrolid (azithromycin, clarithromycin)	500–2000 mg/day in divided doses
Pyrazinamide	20–40 mg/kg per day in a single dose not to exceed 3 g
Rifabutin	150–300 mg/day in a single dose
Rifampin	600–900 mg/day in a single dose
Injectables	
Streptomycin Capreomycin Kanamycin	15 mg/kg up to 1 g once daily 5 times a week. When culture-negative or significant toxicity occurs, dosage can be reduced or the drug given less frequently.
Amikacin	7.5–15.0 mg/kg per day intravenously or intramuscularly in divided doses

are less familiar with treating tuberculosis, particularly drug-resistant tuberculosis, and with the antituberculosis drugs for this situation, such as ethionomide, cycloserine, kanamycin, and capreomycin. Those treating MAC pulmonary disease in the past are more familiar with drugs for treating drug-resistant *M. tuberculosis*. It may be that the two approaches are both valid, but, as stated earlier, no drug treatment regimen has been adequately studied in humans. It seems likely that as more information is accumulated about better and less toxic treatment regimens, a more effective regimen for all forms of MAC disease, whether in AIDS patients or not, will emerge. This would be similar to the situation for treating *M. tuberculosis*. In the meantime, it should be remembered that the expected response and prognosis is significantly different between the AIDS and non-AIDS patient with MAC.

Once it is established that treatment of MAC in a non-AIDS patient is necessary, two options exist: chemotherapy or surgery. Most patients have been treated with chemotherapy consisting of two or more antituberculosis drugs. Results with this approach have been variable, but in general disappointing (Corpe, 1964; Carruthers and Edwards, 1965; Fischer et al., 1968; Lester et al., 1969; Dutt and Stead, 1973; Yeager and Raliegh, 1973; Rosenzweig, 1979; Davidson et al., 1981; Iseman et al., 1985; Etzkorn et al., 1986; Hornick et al., 1988; Reich and Johnson, 1991). Better results are usually obtained with combinations of four or more drugs. Numerous agents, in addition to the antituberculosis drugs, have been tested or tried in patients with MAC. Among the more notable are rifabutin (Sanfilippo et al., 1980), clofazimine (Heyworth, 1967; Schonell et al., 1968; Watson and Smyth, 1968; Damle et al., 1978; Davidson, 1979; Gangadharam et al., 1981), amikacin (Armstrong et al., 1985; Hawkins et al., 1986), clarithromycin (Dautzenberg et al., 1990), ciprofloxacin and imipenim–cilastatin (Young et al., 1986). Newer rifamycins, macrolids, and quinolones may prove effective. A clearly superior regimen among all those reported has not yet been established.

Surgical excision is possible in some patients with localized disease and may be the way that a diagnosis is first established when a solitary pulmonary lesion is removed and is found to contain a granuloma caused by MAC. The patient may have an established diagnosis of pulmonary MAC that has not responded to treatment or has become symptomatic. Surgery may be quite effective in eradicating MAC disease if it is localized. Chemotheraphy may not be necessary, and long-term results are good (Corpe and Laing, 1960; Lewis et al., 1960; Law et al., 1963; Law, 1965; Corpe, 1981; Moran et al., 1983).

The best results occur with lobectomy or pneumonectomy. Segmental or subsegmental resections have a high rate of failure and complications. It is essential that the patient have the ability to tolerate the procedure as well as have localized disease only. Without this, relapse and failure are more likely to occur (Davidson et al., 1981).

Chemotherapy is the only alternative for most patients with MAC pulmonary disease. Because multiple drugs are necessary, toxicity is a frequent problem. Response to treatment is also unpredictable. This requires individualized management of the available alternatives to best serve the patient. The following is a suggested management strategy for the various types of patients encountered with MAC.

The first type of patient has an abnormal chest x-ray film suggestive of *M. tuberculosis*. They may or may not be symptomatic. They may be sputum AFB smear-positive or negative. This patient should be started on a standard antituberculosis regimen and be managed as a tuberculous suspect. Once the organism has been identified as MAC, the patient is handled as described in the following for the second type of patient if asymptomatic, or like the third type of patient if symptomatic.

The second type of patient is asymptomatic, but has proved disease. If the disease is localized, surgical excision should be considered. An alternative in the patient who is not suitable for surgery is to clinically observe the patient or treat with isoniazid (INH), rifampin (RIF), and ethambutol (EMB). This regimen is continued until the patient is culture-negative for 18–24 months. If the patient remains sputum culture-positive, but is clinically stable, the regimen may be discontinued after 6–12 months. If symptoms return or disease progresses, the same regimen can be reinstituted and continued indefinitely if the patient remains clinically stable or improving. If there is progression, it may be necessary to manage the patient as described for the fourth type of patient.

The third type of patient presents initially with moderate to severe clinical disease, usually with symptoms and evidence of progression. Surgery should be considered for localized disease. This might include removing an entire lung. Treatment with RIF, INH, and EMB should be given. Treatment is continued until sputum cultures are negative for 18–24 months. In patients who remain culture-positive but stabilize clinically, chemotheraphy is discontinued after 24 months. Should symptoms return or the disease progress, the same regimen can be reinstated and continued indefinitely if the patient improves. When progression or symptoms persist for 3–6 months despite therapy, the patient should be managed as indicated for the fourth type of patient.

The fourth type of patient has progressive disease that has not responded to drugs as described in the foregoing. Surgery may still be possible for patients with localized disease. Otherwise, RIF, INH, and EMB should be continued and other drugs added, usually streptomycin (SM) or capreomycin (CM), ethionamide (ETA), and/or cycloserine (CS). This regimen should be continued until the patient is culture-negative for 18–24 months. It may be necessary to discontinue some of the drugs earlier because of toxicity. As with the other types of patients, those who remain culture-positive, but stabilized clinically, should have chemotherapy discontinued after 24 months. Should symptoms or progression of disease continue or return, the same regimen can be continued or reinstituted and be given indefinitely if the patient stabilizes clinically. If progression or symptoms continue or recur for 3–6 months while receiving treatment, the patient should be managed as indicated for the fifth type of patient.

The fifth type of patient has progressive pulmonary disease that is not responding to multiple drugs. Experimental or unproved drugs should be considered. Ciprofloxacin, clarithromycin, and clofazimine should be given, in addition to as many drugs as can be tolerated from the approach described for the fourth type of patient. Amikacin (AK) should be substituted for SM or for CM if they were used previously. Treatment is continued until the patient is sputum culture-negative for 18–24 months. Some drugs may have to be discontinued earlier because of toxicity. Those patients remaining culture-positive, but clinically stable, for many months may have the drugs stopped after 24 months. If symptoms return or progression occurs after discontinuation, the same regimen may be reinstated and all or some of the drugs continued indefinitely when stability or improvement occurs. A period of at least 6 months of treatment should be tried before concluding that no benefit will result. Little can be done if progression continues despite therapy. Different combinations of drugs can be tried again in the hope of finding something that will stabilize the condition. Drugs should be stopped if they clearly are not working and, in particular, if they may be causing significant side effects or risks to the patient.

A sixth type of patient, with disseminated MAC, but without AIDS, should be managed initially as the fifth type of patient just described. The drug regimen should include INH, RIF, EMB, SM or CM, ETA or CS, and ciprofloxacin and clarithromycin. Very few such patients exist, but there are reports of successful multiple drug treatment and long-term survival (Davidson et al., 1981; Horsburgh et al., 1985). Whether these patients should now be treated the same as those with AIDS is problematic. No long-term results have been reported in AIDS patients with disseminated MAC.

Patients with AIDS and disseminated MAC are a seventh type of patient and should be treated particularly to control symptoms. A three- or four-drug regimen should be tried: RIF, EMB, ciprofloxacin, and clofazimine and AK are commonly used and are under investigation (Ellner et al., 1991). The role of AK is uncertain, but it probably should be used, despite potential toxicity. Clarithromycin and azithromycin will probably emerge as important agents in combination with the other drugs. The length of therapy remains uncertain. In general, most patients continue to receive therapy until they die of AIDS-related complications. Some clinical studies suggest that most patients have significant clinical and microbiological responses by 4–6 weeks, suggesting that an initial period of intensive multiple drug therapy can be followed by a maintenance phase of fewer drugs. (Agins et al., 1989; Chiu et al., 1990). In all patients, care should be taken to treat with a regimen that will also kill *M. tuberculosis*. Some clinicians include INH until *M. tuberculosis* has been ruled out.

There is also emerging interest in the possibility of prophylaxis in AIDS patients to prevent disseminated disease with MAC. Which drug or drugs would have this effect is uncertain. However, rifabutin is currently under study and shows promise. Recent treatment reports suggest that results of treating disseminated MAC in AIDS patients are improving over earlier results, even with oral drug regimens alone. (Hoy et al., 1990; Kemper et al., 1990). This may partly reflect earlier diagnosis and treatment, better management of AIDS in general, and better compliance in taking medication.

The eighth and last type of patient has lymphadenopathy or a solitary pulmonary nodule and is immunocompetent. Surgical excision is the treatment of choice. Chemotherapy may be indicated in some patients, particularly if they are initially a *M. tuberculosis* suspect, in which case, they are managed as the first type of patient. If the disease is caused by MAC and is removed surgically, chemotherapy is stopped.

B. *Mycobacterium kansasii*

Rifampin-containing regimens are highly effective in treating disease with this species of mycobacteria. Even before rifampin was available, *M. kansasii* disease responded well to standard antituberculosis regimens (Davidson et al., 1972; Harris et al., 1975; Ahn et al., 1981). Surgery for localized disease is not necessary. A three-drug regimen, consisting of daily RIF, INH, and EMB for 18 months is effective. Because of a relative degree of resistance to INH, the dosage should be increased up to 600 mg daily. Success with treatment for 12 months, including intermittent streptomycin therapy, has been reported (Ahn et al., 1983). Acquired or increased resistance of *M. kansasii* to RIF, INH, and SM has been reported (Davidson and Waggoner, 1976). Treatment with other drugs may be necessary in such patients. Three drug regimens containing ethionamide, cycloserine, SM, capreomycin, or kanamycin have given good results in drug-resistant patients (Davidson, 1976b). Pyrazinamide is not a useful drug for treating *M. kansasii* because all isolates are resistant. *Mycobacterium kansasii* is the second most common cause of atypical mycobacterial disease in patients with AIDS (Horsburgh and Selik, 1989). Although response to therapy should be good with rifampin-containing regimens in AIDS patients, results thus far have been disappointing (Sherer et al., 1986; Jost and Hodges, 1991).

C. *Mycobacterium marinum*

Skin lesions caused by this organism usually heal spontaneously, and specific chemotherapy is unnecessary. Occasionally, deeper infection occurs or the superficial lesions progress. Various forms of chemotherapy have been used with success, including antituberculosis drugs (Wolinsky et al., 1972), co-trimoxazole (trimethoprim–sulfamethoxazole) (Black and Eykyn, 1986), tetracycline (Kim, 1974; Izumi et al., 1977), minocycline (Loria, 1976), and trimethoprim–sulfamethoxazole (TM/S) (Barrow and Hewitt, 1971; Kelly, 1976). A combination of RIF and EMB or RIF alone are probably the most useful (Donta et al., 1986), with tetracycline or TM/S as a substitute. Treatment should be continued until the lesions have completely subsided.

D. *Mycobacterium fortuitum* Complex

The *M. fortuitum* complex consists of *M. fortuitum* and *M. chelonae*, with its two subspecies, *M. chelonae chelonae* and *M. chelonae abscessus*. They are generally very resistant to antituberculosis drugs. Surgical excision, debridement, or drainage is often the treatment of choice, with chemotherapy playing no or only a minimal role. In those circumstances for which surgery is impossible or ineffective, drug therapy should be tried. Several antibiotics, singly or in combination, have been used clinically, with sporadic reports of success including doxycycline and amikacin (Dalovisio et al., 1981), sulfonamides (Graybill et al., 1974; Wallace et al., 1981), antituberculosis drugs (Dreisen et al., 1976), and cefoxitin (Casal and Rodriguez, 1982; Kuritsky et al., 1983). Wolinsky (1979) has suggested a combination of AK, ETA, and erythromycin. The American Thoracic Society suggests AK and cefoxitin (Wallace et al., 1990). Because of unpredictable results and uncertain efficacy of drugs, it may be worthwhile to perform drug susceptibility studies with several antibiotics to determine the most effective regimen for a given patient. In general, the *M. chelonae* subspecies are more resistant than *M. fortuitum*; unfortunately, they may also be more virulent. Therapy should be continued for 3 months or more after cultures have become negative or successful surgical intervention has occurred.

E. Other Species

Sporadic cases of disease caused by a variety of species that are ordinarily saprophytic have been reported (Dechairo et al., 1973; Cianciulli, 1974; Edwards et al., 1975; Casimir et al., 1982; Kurnik et al., 1983; Collins et al., 1986). There are no treatment guidelines, since they are so rare. Drug susceptibility studies may be of some help in selecting drugs. Multiple drug regimens are presumed to be more effective than single-drug therapy in most cases.

Several species are more commonly associated with disease in humans. *Mycobacterium ulcerans* is a tropical disease, rarely seen in the United States, causing extensive skin ulceration. Wide excision and skin grafting appear to be the best therapy, although RIF and SM are effective in vitro, and clofazimine has been used in humans (Lunn and Rees, 1964; Revill et al., 1973). Pulmonary disease and colonization occur with *M. simiae*, a highly drug-resistant organism, that is photochromogenic and niacin-positive in the laboratory. A very limited experience in treatment exists (Valdivia-Alvarez, 1973; Krasnow and Gross, 1975; Rose et al., 1982; Bell et al., 1983). Results have not been good thus far. Patients with disease from *M. szulgai* respond well to regimens containing RIF, INH, and EMB (Marks et al., 1972; Schaefer et al., 1973; Davidson, 1976a). Pulmonary disease caused by *M. xenopi* is reported to respond to two- or three-drug regimens, presumably because it is generally susceptible to INH, RIF, SM, and cycloserine in the laboratory (D'Esopo et al., 1979; Bogaerts et al., 1982; Dornetzhuber et al., 1982). Banks et al. (1984) have questioned these results and conclude that both drug susceptibility and response to therapy are unpredictable. *Mycobacterium malmoense* has been increasingly reported as a cause of disease since it was first described (Schroder and Jaklin, 1977; Portaels et al.,

1991). In the laboratory it may be confused with MAC or *M. terrae*. It is, however, more likely to show drug susceptibility than MAC and should arouse suspicion (Jenkins, 1985). The treatment approach is unclear, but a combination of RIF, INH, and EMB for 18 months or longer appears to give the best results (Banks et al., 1985).

Other species of mycobacteria are reported as causes of disease in humans. Because of their rarity, details about *M. shimoidei* (Tortoli and Simonetti, 1991), *M. haemophilum* (Holton et al., 1991), and others are not included here.

Acknowledgment

The author wishes to acknowledge the fine technical help of Bonnie Cooley in the preparation of the manuscript.

References

Agins, B. D., Berman, D. S., Spicehandler, D., El-Sadr, W., Simberkoff, M. S., and Rabol, J. J. (1989). Effect of combined therapy with ansamycin, clofazimine, ethambutol, and isoniazid for *Mycobacterium avium* infection in patients with AIDS. *J. Infect. Dis.* **159**:784–787.

Ahn, C. H., Lowell, J. R., Onstad, G. D., Ahn, S. S., and Hurst, G. A. (1979). Elimination of *Mycobacterium intracellulare* from sputum after bronchial hygiene. *Chest* **76**:480–482.

Ahn, C. H., Lowell, J. R., Ahn, S. A., Ahn, S., and Hurst, G. A. (1981). Chemotherapy for pulmonary disease due to *Mycobacterium kansasii*: Efficacies of some individual drugs. *Rev. Infect. Dis.* **3**:1028–1034.

Ahn, C. H., McLarty, J. W., Ahn, S. S., Ahn, S. I., and Hurst, G. A. (1982). Diagnostic criteria for pulmonary disease caused by *Mycobacterium kansasii* and *Mycobacterium intracellulare*. *Am. Rev. Respir. Dis.* **125**:388–391.

Ahn, C. H., Lowell, J. R., Ahn, S. S., Ahn, S. I., and Hurst, G. A. (1983). Short-course chemotherapy for pulmonary disease caused by *Mycobacterium kansasii*. *Am. Rev. Respir. Dis.* **128**:1048–1050.

Altman, R. P., and Margileth, A. M. (1975). Cervical lymphadenopathy from atypical mycobacteria: Diagnosis and surgical treatment. *J. Pediatr. Surg.* **103**:419–422.

American Thoracic Society–Centers for Disease Control (1987). Mycobacterioses and the acquired immunodeficiency syndrome. *Am. Rev. Respir. Dis.* **136**:492–496.

Armstrong, D., Gold, J. W. M., Dryjanski, J., Whimbey, E., Polsky, B., Hawkins, C., Brown, A. E., Bernard, E., and Kiehn, T. E. (1985).

Treatment of infections in patients with the acquired immunodeficiency syndrome. *Ann. Intern. Med.* **103**:738–743.

Banks, J., Hunter, A. M., Campbell, I. A., and Jenkins, P. A. (1984). Pulmonary infection with *Mycobacterium xenopi*: Review of treatment and response. *Thorax* **39**:376–382.

Banks, J., Jenkins, P. A., and Smith, A. P. (1985). Pulmonary infection with *Mycobacterium malmoense*—review of treatment and response. *Tubercle* **66**:197–203.

Barrow, G. I., and Hewitt, M. (1971). Skin infection with *Mycobacterium marinum* from a tropical fish tank. *Br. Med. J.* **2**:505–506.

Bell, R. C., Higuchi, J. H., Donovan, W. N., Drasnow, I., and Johanson, W. G. (1983). *Mycobacterium simiae*. Clinical features and follow-up of twenty-four patients. *Am. Rev. Resp. Dis.* **127**:35–38.

Bermudez, L. E., Petrofsky, M., Kolanoski, P., and Young, L. S. (1992). An animal model of *Mycobacterium avium* complex disseminated infection after colonization of the intestinal tract. *J. Infect. Dis.* **165**:75–79.

Bertram, M. A., Inderlied, C. B., Yadegar, S., Kolanoski, P., Yamada, J. K., and Young, L. S. (1986). Confirmation of the beige mouse model for study of disseminated infection with *Mycobacterium avium* complex. *J. Infect. Dis.* **154**:194–195.

Black, M. M., and Eykyn, S. (1986). The successful treatment of tropical fish tank granuloma (*Mycobacterium marinum* infections). *Arch. Intern. Med.* **146**:902–904.

Boguerts, Y., Elinck, W., Van Penterghem, D., Pauwels, R., and Van Der Straeten, M. (1982). Pulmonary disease due to *Mycobacterium xenopi*. Reports of two cases. *Eur. J. Respir. Dis.* **63**:298–304.

Borghous, J. G. A., and Stanford, J. L. (1973). *Mycobacterium chelonei* in abscesses after injection of diphtheria–pertussus–tetanus–polio vaccine. *Am. Rev. Respir. Dis.* **107**:1–8.

Butler, W. R., Ahearn, D. G., and Kilburn, J. O. (1986). High performance liquid chromotography of mycolic acids as a tool in the identification of *Corynebacterium*, *Nocardia*, *Rhodococcus*, and *Mycobacterium* species. *J. Clin. Microbiol.* **23**:182–185.

Carruthers, K. J., and Edwards, F. G. (1965). Atypical mycobacteria in Western Australia. *Am. Rev. Respir. Dis.* **91**:887–895.

Casal, M., and Rodriguez, F. (1982). In vitro susceptibility of *Mycobacterium fortuitum* and *Mycobacterium chelonei* to cefoxitin. *Tubercle* **63**:125–127.

Casimir, M. T., Fainstein, V., and Papadapolous, N. (1982). Cavitary lung infection caused by *Mycobacterium flavescens*. *South. Med. J.* **75**:253–254.

Centers for Disease Control (1987). Diagnosis and management of mycobacterial infection and disease in persons with human immunodeficiency virus infection. *Ann. Intern. Med.* **106**:254–256.

Centers for Disease Control (1978). Mycobacterial infections associated with augmentation mammoplasty, Florida, North Carolina, Texas. *MMWR* **27**:513.

Chiu, J., Nussbaum, J., Bozzette, S., Tilles, J. G., Young, L. S., Leedom, J., Heseltine, P. N. R., McCutchan, A., and California Collaborative Treatment Group (1990). Treatment of disseminated *Mycobacterium avium* complex infection in AIDS with amikacin, ethambutol, rifampin, and ciprofloxacin. *Ann. Intern. Med.* **113**:358–361.

Cianciulli, F. D. (1974). The radish bacillus (*Mycobacterium terrae*): Saprophyte or pathogen? *Am. Rev. Respir. Dis.* **109**:138–141.

Clegg, H. W., Foster, M. T., Sanders, W. E., and Baine, W. B. (1983). Infection due to organisms of the *Mycobacterium fortuitum* complex after augmentation mammoplasty: Clinical and epidemiological features. *J. Infect. Dis.* **147**:427–433.

Collins, C. H., Grange, J. M., and Yates, M. D. (1984). Mycobacteria in water. *J. Appl. Bacteriol.* **57**:193–211.

Collins, C. H., Grange, J. M., Noble, W. C., and Yates, M. D. (1985). *Mycobacterium marinum* infections in man. *J. Hyg. (Camb).* **94**:135–149.

Collins, C. H., Grange, J. M., and Yates, M. D. (1986). Unusual opportunist mycobacteria. *Med. Lab. Sci.* **43**:262–268.

Corpe, R. F., and Laing, J. (1960). Surgical resection in pulmonary tuberculosis due to atypical *Mycobacterium tuberculosis. J. Thorac. Cardiovasc. Surg.* **40**:93–97.

Corpe, R. F. (1964). Clinical aspects, medical and surgical, in the management of Battey-type pulmonary disease. *Dis. Chest* **45**:380–382.

Corpe, R. F. (1981). Surgical management of pulmonary disease due to *Mycobacterium avium–intracellulare. Rev. Infect. Dis.* **3**:1064–1067.

Dalovisio, J. R., Pankey, G. A., Wallace, R. J., and Jones, D. B. (1981). Clinical usefulness of amikacin and doxycycline in the treatment of infection due to *Mycobacterium fortuitum* and *Mycobacterium chelonei. Rev. Infect. Dis.* **3**:1068–1074.

Damle, P., McClatchy, J. K., Gangadharam, P. R. J., and Davidson, P. T. (1978). Antimycobacterial activity of some potential chemotherapeutic compounds. *Tubercle* **59**:135–138.

Damsker, B., and Bottone, E. J. (1985). *Mycobacterium avium–Mycobacterium intracellulare* from the intestinal tracts of patients with the acquired immunodeficiency syndrome: Concepts regarding acquisition and pathogenesis. *J. Infect. Dis.* **151**:179–181.

Dautzenberg, B., Legris, S., Truffot, C. H., Mercat, A., and Grosset, J. (1990). Double blind study of the efficacy of clarithromycin versus placebo in *Mycobacterium avium–intracellular* infection in AIDS patients. *Am. Rev. Respir. Dis.* **141**:A615.

Davidson, P. T. (1976a). *Mycobacterium szulgai*. A new pathogen causing infection of the lung. *Chest* **69**:799–801.

Davidson, P. T. (1976b). Treatment and long-term follow-up of patients with atypical mycobacterial infections. *Bull. Int. Union Tuberc.* **51**:257–261.

Davidson, P. T. (1979). Clofazimine (B663) for the treatment of *M. intracellulare* infection in man. *Am. Rev. Respir. Dis.* **119**:398.

Davidson, P. T. (1981). Introduction—International Conference on Atypical Mycobacteria. *Rev. Infect. Dis.* **3**:816–818.

Davidson, P. T. (1985). Atypical mycobacteria. In *Current Pulmonology*, Vol. 6. Edited by D. H. Simmons. Year Book Medical Publishers, Chicago, pp. 115–135.

Davidson, P. T. (1989a). *Mycobacterium avium* complex disease. In *Current Therapy of Respiratory Disease*, Vol. 3. Edited by R. M. Cherniack. BC Decker, Toronto, pp. 65–69.

Davidson, P. T. (1989b). The diagnosis and management of disease caused by *M. avium* complex, *M. kansasii*, and other mycobacteria. In *Clinics in Chest Medicine*, Vol. 10. Edited by D. E. Snider. W. B. Saunders, Philadelphia, pp. 431–443.

Davidson, P. T., and Waggoner, R. (1976). Acquired resistance to rifampicin by *Mycobacterium kansasii*. *Tubercle* **57**:271–273.

Davidson, P. T., Goble, M., Lester, W. (1972). The antituberculosis efficacy of rifampin in 136 patients. *Chest* **61**:574–578.

Davidson, P. T., Khanijo, V., Goble, M., and Moulding, T. (1981). Treatment of disease due to *Mycobacterium intracellulare*. *Rev. Infect. Dis.* **3**:1052–1059.

Dechairo, D. C., Kittredge, D., Meyers, A., and Corrales, J. (1973). Septic arthritis due to *Mycobacterium triviale*. *Ann. Rev. Respir. Dis.* **108**:1224–1226.

D'Esopo, N. D., et al. (1979). Clinical and roentgenographic features of pulmonary nosocomial infection due to *Mycobacterium xenopi*. *Bull. Int. Union Tuberc.* **54**:343–345.

Donta, S. T., Smith, P. W., Levitz, R. E., and Quintiliam, R. (1986). Therapy of *Mycobacterium marinum* infections. *Arch. Intern. Med.* **146**: 902–904.

Dornetzhuber, V., Martin, R., Burjanona, B., Panukova, K., Turzona, M., and Vincurova, M. (1982). Pulmonary mycobacteriosis caused by *Mycobacterium xenopi*: Report of a case. *Eur. J. Respir. Dis.* **63**:293–297.

Dreisin, R. B., Scoggin, C., and Davidson, P. T. (1976). The pathogenicity of *Mycobacterium chelonei* in man: A report of seven cases. *Tubercle* **57**:49–57.

Dutt, A. K., and Stead, W. W. (1979). Long term results of medical treatment in *Mycobacterium–intracellulare*. *Am. J. Med.* **67**:449–453.

Edwards, L. B., and Palmer, C. E. (1955). Epidemiological studies of tuberculin sensitivity. 1. Preliminary results with purified protein derivatives prepared from atypical acid-fast organisms. *Am. J. Hyg.* **68**:231.

Edwards, M. S., Huber, T. W., and Baker, C. J. (1975). *Mycobacterium terrae* synovitis and osteomyelitis. *Am. Rev. Respir. Dis.* **117**:161–163.

Ellner, J. J., Goldberger, M. J., and Parenti, D. M. (1991). *Mycobacterium avium* infection and AIDS: A therapeutic dilemma in rapid evolution. *J. Infect. Dis.* **163**:1326–1335.

Etzkorn, E. T., Aldarondo, S., McAllister, C. K., Matthews, J., and Ognibene, A. J. (1986). Medical therapy of *Mycobacterium avium–intracellulare* pulmonary disease. *Am. Rev. Respir. Dis.* **134**:442–445.

Fauci, A. S. (1984). Acquired immunodeficiency syndrome: Epidemiologic, immunologic and therapeutic considerations. *Ann. Intern. Med.* **110**:92–106.

Fisher, D. A., Lester, W., and Schaefer, W. B. (1968). Infection with atypical mycobacteria. Five years' experience at the National Jewish Hospital. *Am. Rev. Respir. Dis.* **98**:29–34.

Fox, A., Roy, C., Jurado, J., Arteaga, E., Ruiz, J. M., and Moragas, A. (1978). *Mycobacterium chelonei* iatrogenic infection. *J. Clin. Microbiol.* **7**:319–321.

Gangadharam, P. R., Pratt, P. F., Damle, P. B., and Davidson, P. T. (1981). Dynamic aspects of the action of clofazimine (B633) against *Mycobacterium intracellulare*. *Tubercle* **62**:201–206.

Gangadharam, P. R., Edwards, C. K., Murthy, P. S., and Pratt, P. F. (1983). An acute infection model for *Mycobacterium–intracellulare* disease using beige mice: Preliminary results. *Am. Rev. Respir. Dis.* **127**:648–649.

Gangadharam, P. R., Perumal, V. K., Crawford, J. T., and Bates, J. H. (1988). Association of plasmids and virulence of *Mycobacterium avium* complex. *Am. Rev. Respir. Dis.* **137**:212–214.

Graybill, J. R., Silva, J., Fraser, D. W., Lordon, R., and Rogers, E. (1974). Disseminated mycobacteriosis due to *Mycobacterium abscessus* in two recipients of renal homografts. *Am. Rev. Respir. Dis.* **109**:4–10.

Gremillion, D. H., Mursch, S. B., and Lerner, C. J. (1983). Injection site abscesses caused by *Mycobacterium chelonei*. *Infect. Control* **4**:25–28.

Gruft, H., Falkinham, J. O., and Parker, B. C. (1981). Recent experience in the epidemiology of disease caused by atypical mycobacteria. *Res. Infect. Dis.* **3**:990–996.

Harris, G. D., Johanson, W. G., and Nicholson, D. P. (1975). Response to chemotherapy of pulmonary infection due to *Mycobacterium kansasii*. *Am. Rev. Respir. Dis.* **112**:31–36.

Hawkins, C. C., Gold, J. W., Whimbley, E., et al. (1986). *Mycobacterium avium* complex infections in patients with the acquired immunodeficiency syndrome. *Ann. Intern. Med.* **105**:184–188.

Heyworth, F. (1967). B663 in treatment of atypical tuberculosis disease. *Med. J. Aust.* **1**:106–107.

Hoffman, P. C., Fraser, D. W., Robicsek, F., O'Bar, P. R., and Mauney, C. U. (1981). Two outbreaks of sternal wound infections due to organisms of the *Mycobacterium fortuitum* complex. *J. Infect. Dis.* **143**:533–542.

Holton, J., Nye, P., and Miller, R. (1991). *Mycobacterium haemophilum* infection in a patient with AIDS. *J. Infect.* **23**:303–306.

Horadam, V. W., Smilack, J. D., and Smith, E. C. (1982). *Mycobacterium fortuitum* infections after total hip replacement. *South. Med. J.* **75**:244–246.

Hornick, D. B., Dayton, C. S., Bedell, G. N., and Fick, R. B., Jr. (1988). Nontuberculous mycobacterial lung disease. Substantiation of a less aggressive approach. *Chest* **93**:550–555.

Horsburgh, C. R., Jr., and Selik, L. M. (1989). The epidemiology of disseminated nontuberculous mycobacterial infection in the acquired immunodeficiency syndrome (AIDS). *Am. Rev. Respir. Dis.* **139**:4–7.

Horsburgh, C. R., Jr., Mason, U. G., III, Farhi, D. C., and Iseman, M. D. (1985). Disseminated infection with *Mycobacterium avium–intracellulare*. *Medicine* **64**:36–50.

Horsburgh, C. R., Jr., Mason, U. G., III, Heifits, L. B., Southwick, K., Labrecque, J., and Iseman, M. D. (1987). Response to therapy of pulmonary *Mycobacterium avium–intracellulare* infection correlates with results of in vitro susceptibility testing. *Am. Rev. Respir. Dis.* **135**:418–421.

Hoy, J., Mijch, A., Siedland, M., Grayson, L., Lucas, R., and Dwyer, B. (1990). Quadruple-drug therapy for *Mycobacterium–avium–intracellulare* bacteria in AIDS patients. *J. Infect. Dis.* **161**:801–805.

Iseman, M. D., Corpe, R. F., O'Brien, R. F., Rosenzweig, D. Y., and Wolinsky, E. (1985). Disease due to *Mycobacterium avium–intracellulare*. *Chest* **87**:139S–149S.

Izumi, A. K., Hanke, C. W., and Higaki, M. (1977). *Mycobacterium marinum* infections treated with tetracycline. *Arch. Dermatol.* **113**:1067–1068.

Jacobson, M. A., Hopewell, P. C., Yajko, D. M., Hadley, W. K., Lazarus, E., Mohanty, P. K., Modin, G. W., Feigal, D. W., Cusick, P. S., and Sande, M. A. (1991). Natural history of disseminated *Mycobacterium avium* complex infection in AIDS. *J. Infect. Dis.* **164**:994–998.

Jenkins, P. A. (1985). *Mycobacterium malmoense*. *Tubercule* **66**:193–195.

Jost, P. M., and Hodges, G. R. (1991). *Mycobacterium kansasii* infection in a patient with AIDS. *South. Med. J.* **84**:1501–1504.

Jucker, M. T., and Falkinham, J. O., III (1990). Epidemiology of infection by nontuberculous mycobacteria IX. Evidence for two DNA homology groups among small plasmids in *Mycobacterium avium*, *Mycobacterium intracellulare*, and *Mycobacterium scrofulaceum*. *Am. Rev. Respir. Dis.* **142**:858–862.

Kelly, R. (1976). *Mycobacterium marinum* infection from a tropical fish tank. Treatment with trimethoprim and sulfamethoxazole. *Med. J. Aust.* **2**:681–682.

Kemper, C. A., Chiu, J., Meng, T. C., Nussbaum, J., Bartok, A. E., and California Collaborative Treatment Group (1990). Microbiologic and clinical response of patients with AIDS and MAC bacteremia to a four oral drug regimen [Abstract]. *Prog. Abstr. 30th Intersci. Conf. Antimicrob. Agents Chemother.* (Atlanta). American Society of Microbiology, Washington, D.C., Abstr. 1267.

Kim, R. (1974). Tetracycline therapy for atypical mycobacterial granuloma. *Arch. Dermatol.* **110**:229.

Klemens, S. P., and Cynamon, M. H. (1991). In vivo activities of newer rifamycin analogs against *Mycobacterium avium* infection. *Antimicrob. Agents Chemother.* **35**:2026–2030.

Krasnow, I., and Gross, W. (1975). *Mycobacterium simiae* infection in the United States. A case report and discussion of the organism. *Am. Rev. Respir. Dis.* **111**:357–360.

Kuritsky, J. N., Bullen, M. G., Broome, C. V., Silvax, V. A., Good, R. C., and Wallace, R. J., (1983). Sternal wound infections and endocarditis due to organisms of the *Mycobacterium fortuitum* complex. *Ann. Intern. Med.* **98**:938–939.

Kurnik, P. B., Padmanabh, U., Bonatsos, C., and Cynamon, M. G. (1983). *Mycobacterium gordonae* as a human hepato-peritoneal pathogen with a review of the literature. *Am. J. Med. Sci.* **285**:45–48.

Laszlo, A., and Siddiqi, S. H. (1984). Evaluation of a rapid radiometric differentiation test for the *Mycobacterium tuberculosis* complex by selective inhibition with p-nitro-α-acetylamino-β-hydroxypropiophenone. *J. Clin. Microbiol.* **19**:694–698.

Law, S. W. (1965). Surgical treatment of atypical mycobacterial disease: A survey of experience in Veteran Administration Hospitals. *Dis. Chest* **47**:296–303.

Law, S. W., Jenkins, D. E., Chofnas, I., Bahar, D., Whitcomb, F., Barkley, H. T., and DeBakey, M. E. (1963). Surgical experience in management of atypical mycobacterial infections. *J. Thorac. Cardiovasc. Surg.* **46**:689–701.

Lester, W., Moulding, T., Fraser, R. I., McClatchy, J. K., and Fischer, D. A. (1969). Quintuple regimens in the treatment of Battey-type infections. *Trans. 28th Pulmon. Dis. Res. Conf.*, VA-Armed Forces, p. 83.

Lewis, A. G., Lasche, E. M., Armstrong, A. L., and Dunbar, F. P. (1960). A clinical study of the chronic lung disease due to nonphotochromogenic acid-fast bacilli. *Ann. Intern. Med.* **53**:273–285.

Loria, P. R. (1976). Minocycline hydrochloride treatment for atypical acid-fast infection. *Arch. Dermatol.* **112**:517–519.

Lunn, H. F., and Rees, R. J. (1964). Treatment of mycobacterial skin ulcers in Uganda with a riminophenazine derivative (B663). *Lancet* **1**:247–249.

MacKellar, A. (1976). Diagnosis and management of atypical mycobacterial lymphadenitis in children. *J. Pediatr. Surg.* **11**:85–89.

Marks, J., Jenkins, P. A., and Tsukamura, M. (1972). *Mycobacterium szulgai.* A new pathogen. *Tubercle* **53**:210–214.

Meissner, P. S., and Falkinham, J. O. (1986). Plasmid DNA profiles as epidemiologic markers for clinical and environmental isolates of *Mycobacterium avium*, *Mycobacterium intracellulare*, and *Mycobacterium scofulaceum*. *J. Infect. Dis.* **153**:325–331.

Mollahan, C. S., and Romer, M. (1961). Public health significance of swimming pool granuloma. *Am. J. Public Health.* **51**:883–891.

Moran, J. F., Alexander, L. G., Staub, E. W., Young, W. G., and Sealy, W. C. (1983). Long-term results of pulmonary resection for atypical mycobacterial disease. *Am. Thorax Surg.* **35**:597–604.

Narasimhan, S. L., and Austin, T. W. (1978). Prosthetic value endocarditis due to *Mycobacterium fortuitum*. *Can. Med. Assoc. J.* **119**:154–155.

Petrini, B., Hellstriand, P., and Eriksson, M. (1980). Infection with *Mycobacterium chelonei* following injection. *Scand. J. Infect. Dis.* **12**:237–238.

Pitchenik, A. E., Fostel, D., and Bloch, A. B. (1988). Mycobacterial disease: Epidemiology, diagnosis, treatment and prevention. *Clin. Chest Med.* **9**:425–441.

Poropatich, C. O., Labriola, A. M., and Tuazon, C. U. (1987). Acid fast smear and culture of respiratory secretions, bone marrow, and stools as predictions of disseminated *Mycobacterium avium* complex infection. *J. Clin. Microbiol.* **25**:929–930.

Portaels, F., Denef, M., and Larsson, L. (1991). Pulmonary disease caused by *Mycobacterium malmoense*. Comments on the possible origin of infection and methods for laboratory diagnosis. *Tubercle* **72**:218–222.

Reich, J. M., and Johnson, R. E. (1991). *Mycobacterium avium* complex pulmonary disease. Incidence, presentation, and response to therapy in a community setting. *Am. Rev. Respir. Dis.* **143**:1381–1385.

Repath, F., Seabury, J. H., Sanders, C. V., and Domer, J. (1976). Prosthetic value endocarditis due to *Mycobacterium chelonei*. *South. Med. J.* **69**:1244–1246.

Revill, W. D. L., Morrow, R. H., Pike, M. C., and Ateng, J. (1973). A controlled trial of the treatment of *Mycobacterium ulcerans* infection with clofazimine. *Lancet* **2**:873–877.

Robicsek, F., Daugherty, H. K., Cook, J. W., Selle, J. G., Masters, T. N., O'Bar, P. R., Fernandez, C. R., Mauney, C. U., and Calhoun, D. M. (1978). *Mycobacterium fortuitum* epidemics after open-heart surgery. *J. Thorac. Cardiovasc. Surg.* **75**:91–96.

Rose, H. D., Dorff, G. J., Lauwasser, M., and Sheth, N. K. (1982). Pulmonary and disseminated *Mycobacterium simiae* infection in humans. *Am. Rev. Respir. Dis.* **126**:1110–1113.

Rosenzweig, D. Y. (1979). Pulmonary mycobacterial infections due to *Mycobacterium intracellulare–avium* complex. *Chest* **75**:115–119.

Sanfilippo, A., Bruna, C., Marsili, L., Morvillo, E., Pasqualucci, C. R., Schioppacassi, G., and Ungheri, D. (1980). Biological activity of a new class of rifamycins. Spiropiperidyl-rifamycins. *J. Antibiot.* **33**:1193–1198.

Schaad, U. B., Votteler, T. P., and McCracken, G. H., Jr. (1979). Management of atypical mycobacterial lymphadenitis in childhood. A review based on 380 cases. *J. Pediatr.* **95**:356–360.

Schaefer, W. B., Wolinsky, E., Jenkins, P. A., and Marks, J. (1973). *Mycobacterium szulgai* a new pathogen. Serologic identification and report of five new cases. *Am. Rev. Respir. Dis.* **108**:1320–1326.

Schonell, M. E., Crofton, J. W., Stuart, A. E., et al. (1968). Disseminated infection with *Mycobacterium avium*. Part I. Clinical features, treatment and pathology. *Tubercle* **49**:12–30.

Schroder, K. H., and Jaklin, I. (1977). *Mycobacterium malmoense* sp. nov. *Int. J. Syst. Bacteriol.* **27**:241.

Sethi, G. K., Simons, W. J., and Scott, S. M. (1985). *Mycobacterium fortuitum* infections of the mediastinum. *J. Cardiovasc. Surg. (Torino)* **26**:307–309.

Sherer, R., Sable, R., Sonnenberg, M., Cooper, S., Spencer, P., Schwimmer, S., Kocka, F., Muthuswamy, P., and Kallick, C. (1986). Disseminated infection with *Mycobacterium kansasii* in the acquired immunodeficiency syndrome. *Ann. Intern. Med.* **105**:710–712.

Taha, A. M., Davidson, P. T., and Bailey, W. C. (1985). Surgical treatment of atypical mycobacterial lymphadenitis in children. *Pediatr. Infect. Dis.* **4**:664–667.

Tortoli, E., and Simonetti, M. T. (1991). Isolation of *Mycobacterium skimoidei* from a patient with cavitary pulmonary disease. *J. Clin. Microbiol.* **29**:1754–1756.

Valdivia-Alvarez, J. (1973). *Mycobacterium habana*: Clinical and epidemiologic significance. *Ann. Soc. Belg. Med. Trop.* **53**:263.

Wallace, J. M., and Hannah, J. B. (1988). *Mycobacterium avium* complex infection in patients with the acquired immunodeficiency syndrome. *Chest* **93**:926–932.

Wallace, R. J., Jones, D. B., and Wiss, K. (1981). Sulfonamide activity against *Mycobacterium fortuitum* and *Mycobacterium chelonei*. *Rev. Infect. Dis.* **3**:898–904.

Wallace, R. J., O'Brien, R., Glassroth, J., Raleigh, J., and Dutt, A. (1990). Diagnosis and treatment of disease caused by nontuberculous mycobacteria.

Official statement of the American Thoracic Society. *Am. Rev. Respir. Dis.* **142**:940–953.

Wallace, R. J., Glassroth, J., and O'Brien, R. (1991). A plea for clinical trials to resolve the issue of optimal therapy in the treatment of *Mycobacterium avium* infection. *Am. Rev. Respir. Dis.* **144**:3–4.

Watson, B. M., and Smyth, J. T. (1968). B663 and ethambutol in the treatment of Battey disease. *Med. J. Aust.* **1**:261.

Wolinsky, E. (1979). State of the art: Nontuberculous mycobacteria and associated diseases. *Am. Rev. Respir. Dis.* **119**:107–159.

Wolinsky, E., and Rynearson, T. K. (1968). Mycobacteria in soil and their relation to disease-associated strains. *Am. Rev. Respir. Dis.* **97**:1032–1037.

Wolinsky, E., Gomez, F., and Zimpfer, F. (1972). Sporotrichoid *Mycobacterium marinum* infection treated with rifampin–ethambutol. *Am. Rev. Respir. Dis.* **105**:964–967.

Yajko, D. M., Nassos, P. S., Sanders, C. A., and Hadley, W. K. (1989). Killing by antimicrobial agents of AIDS-derived strains of *Mycobacterium avium* complex inside cells of the mouse macrophage line J774. *Am. Rev. Respir. Dis.* **140**:1198–1203.

Yakrus, M. A., and Goad, R. C. (1990). Geographic distribution, frequency, and specimen source of *Mycobacterium avium* complex serotypes isolated from patients with acquired immunodeficiency syndrome. *J. Clin. Microbiol.* **28**:926–929.

Yeager, H., and Raleigh, J. W. (1973). Pulmonary disease due to *Mycobacterium intracellulare*. *Am. Rev. Respir. Dis.* **108**:547–552.

Young, L. S., Inderlied, C. B., Berlin, O. G., and Gottlieb, M. S. (1986). Mycobacterial infections in AIDS patients, with an emphasis on the *Mycobacterium avium* complex. *Rev. Infect. Dis.* **8**:1024–1033.

Young, L. S. (1988). *Mycobacterium avium* complex infection. *J. Infect. Dis.* **157**:863–867.

24

The Epidemiology of Tuberculosis in the Foreign-Born in Canada and the United States

PAMELA HUTCHINS ORR and EARL S. HERSHFIELD

University of Manitoba, Faculty of Medicine
Winnipeg, Manitoba, Canada

I. Introduction

Over the past three decades, the incidence of tuberculosis in North America has declined by 5–6% per year (Snider, 1989). However, the incidence has not decreased uniformly in all segments of the population, and since 1988, the number of new cases has actually increased in both Canada and the United States. The risk of active tuberculous disease remains high in certain subpopulations, including blacks, Hispanics, aboriginals, the urban poor, human immunodeficiency virus (HIV)-infected individuals, and immigrants (Jereb et al., 1991). The latter group brings with them the risk of disease prevalent in their country of origin. Increased morbidity because of microbial drug resistance, especially to isoniazid, is also a common problem in this population (Wang et. al., 1989). Recent efforts to control tuberculosis in the foreign-born have led to a review of immigration medical screening processes and surveillance recommendations in Canada, the United States, Britain, and Australia (MMWR, 1990; Orr et al., 1990; British Thoracic Society, 1990; Streeton, 1987).

This review will focus on the epidemiology of tuberculosis in the foreign-born living in Canada and the United States and on the control measures presently applied to this population.

II. Terminology

Any review of tuberculosis in the foreign-born in North America must take into account the plethora of terms used to described these individuals (Centers for Disease Control [CDC], 1990a; Orr et al., 1990). The terms *immigrant* or *landed immigrant* in the United States and Canada, respectively, refer to noncitizens who have been granted immigrant visas by consular officers. Other immigration categories in the United States include undocumented aliens, nonimmigrants, refugees, entrants, and parolees, and in Canada include visitors, students, "Minister's permits," and refugees. Yearly statistics of tuberculosis cases occurring in the foreign-born, without categorization according to immigration status, are published by the Centers for Disease Control in the United States and Statistics Canada, a department of the Canadian Federal Government. Individual studies have looked at tuberculosis in subpopulations of immigrants, including refugees, and parolees/Minister's permit cases, but national statistics on these groups are not published in either country.

III. Immigration Policy: United States and Canada

In Canada, prospective immigrants with "active" tuberculosis are barred from entry into the country unless, under exceptional circumstances, they have been given a Minister's permit and may be admitted for humanitarian reasons. In the United States, immigrants with active tuberculosis, that is in an infectious state, are barred from entry into the country, and they must receive appropriate treatment and become noninfectious before they are admissible to the United States. Prospective immigrants are routinely examined in their country of origin or country of last residence by local physicians designated by embassies and consulates. A chest radiograph is required before entry for those 15 years or older who wish to enter the United States and for those 11 years or older who wish to enter Canada. Individuals younger than this may be required to have a chest radiograph if clinically indicated, or if they are close contacts of persons with present or past tuberculosis. A tuberculin skin test is required according to U. S. policy for persons younger than 15 years of age if the individual has an illness suggestive of tuberculosis or has a family member with suspected tuberculosis (CDC, 1990a). Tuberculin skin testing has not been routinely required on all prospective immigrants owing to the problems of quality control and cost (CDC, 1990a). Canadian policy allows skin testing at the discretion of the local examining physician (*Medical Officers Handbook*, 1991).

Under Canadian policy, individuals with recent chest radiographs suggestive of pulmonary tuberculosis are reviewed. Previous chest x-rays, if available, are obtained and compared. Sputum, gastric, or laryngeal specimens for smear and culture are requested at the discretion of the examining medical officer.

Those with stable radiographic findings and with negative microbiological cultures for tuberculosis are allowed to proceed with immigration. Preventive chemotherapy is not required before immigration. Individuals with either radiologic or microbiological evidence of active tuberculosis are not admitted to Canada until their condition can be upgraded to inactive status. This upgrading requires evidence of an adequate treatment regimen of at least 6-months duration that must have included isoniazid and rifampin throughout its course. Alternative regimens that do not include either isoniazid or rifampin must be given for at least 12 months or longer. Three sputum cultures incubated for at least 7–8 weeks must be negative for tubercle bacilli; the sputum culture reports must not be more than 6 months old. If results of bacteriological examinations are unavailable, stable or improving chest x-ray films obtained over a minimum of 3 months are required; the last film must not be more than 6 months old.

Under U. S. policy, individuals with clinically active tuberculosis who have one or more positive sputum smear examinations are classified as "class A." Those individuals must be started on the recommended treatment regimen and must become sputum smear-negative on 3 consecutive days before they are allowed to apply for a waiver of excludability and proceed with immigration. Waivers require the signature of a health care provider in the United States who agrees to see the individual for an evaluation of the tuberculous condition within 30 days after arrival. The endorsement of the state or local health department in the location of the individual's intended place of residence is also required for the waiver (CDC, 1990a).

Persons with clinically active tuberculosis, no history of a positive sputum smear, and negative sputum smears on 3 consecutive days are classified as "class B-1" and are allowed to proceed with immigration. Individuals with tuberculosis, not clinically active, are classified as "class B-2" and are also allowed to proceed with immigration. A waiver of excludability is not required for these two categories. When immigrants who have been classified with class A or class B tuberculosis arrive in the United States, a notification is sent from the quarantine officer at the port of entry to the health care provider who agreed to provide follow-up for the class A cases and to the state and local health departments. The immigrant is instructed to report to the health care provider or the health department for prompt assessment. The health departments are required to furnish an evaluation of the immigrant's tuberculous condition to the Centers for Disease Control, U. S. Public Health Service.

IV. Follow-up in the United States and Canada

In the United States a standard national protocol for the investigation of class A or class B persons after arrival does not exist. Similarly, subsequent surveillance of this population is not required by law.

Following arrival in Canada, immigrants with inactive tuberculosis are required by law to comply with surveillance in their province of destination. Surveillance consists of regular visits to designated physicians for 3–5 years, depending on the regulations of the province of final destination, or until discharged from follow-up by the physician. The approach to microbiological and radiologic investigation at the first and subsequent clinic visits is not standardized across Canada (Orr et al., 1990). To encourage compliance with follow-up, outreach programs staffed by public health nurses, using home visits, telephone calls, and physician and community contacts, have been established in most provinces.

V. Patterns of Immigration and Disease

Over the past two decades the total number of immigrants to the United States has increased, whereas immigration to Canada has declined (Table 1). During this period, there has been a major shift in the source of immigrants to both countries. A greater proportion of immigrants are from countries with high endemic prevalence rates of tuberculosis. If one compares the decades 1970–1979 with 1980–1989, the percentage of Asian immigrants has increased from 34.4 to 42.9% in the United States and from 24.8 to 44.7% in Canada. The largest increase in the number of Asian immigrants to both countries occurred between 1978 and 1982, which can be attributed to an increase in the number of persons arriving from Southeast Asia. The number of immigrants from the Americas (North, Central, and South America and the Caribbean) has increased in the United States, but has decreased in Canada, whereas the number and percentage of European immigrants to the United States and Canada have decreased.

These immigration patterns are reflected in the number and distribution of new tuberculous cases in the foreign-born (Table 2). By 1989, 48 and 24.1% of all cases of tuberculosis in Canada and the United States, respectively, occurred in the foreign-born, an increase from 40.6 and 20.5% in 1985. Of the foreign-born Canadian cases, 57.8% occurred in persons from Asia, whereas Asian-born persons accounted for 45.8% of foreign-born cases in the United States (Table 3). In the United States, 44.2% of the cases occurred in persons from countries of the Americas, and only 5.9% in those of European origin. In contrast, only 10.3% of cases in the Canadian foreign-born occurred in persons from the Americas, reflecting low immigration rates from these areas, whereas 24.5% of cases occurred in persons originally from Europe.

A comparison of tuberculosis incidence rates between Canada and various regions of the world is shown in Table 4. Within Canada, the incidence of tuberculosis is three to four times higher in the foreign-born population compared with the rate in the Canadian-born. Similar disparities have been noted in Europe and Australia (Mortensen et al., 1989; Lange et al., 1986; Geographical

Table 1 Immigrants to Canada and the United States by Region of Origin[a]

Region of origin[b]	Canada				USA			
	1970–1979		1980–1989		1970–1979		1980–1989	
	No.	%	No.	%	No.	%	No.	%
Asia	358,050	24.8	562,724	44.7	1,492,586	34.4	2,714,904	42.9
Americas	420,944	29.1	269,445	21.4	1,875,947	43.3	2,742,040	43.3
Europe	565,997	39.2	350,751	27.8	845,246	19.5	665,350	10.5
Africa	64,979	4.5	59,332	4.7	85,627	1.9	170,300	2.7
Oceania	34,928	2.4	17,275	1.4	36,583	0.8	39,477	0.6
Unknown	19	0.001	300	0.02	12	0.0003	147	0.002
Total	1,444,917	100	1,259,827	100	4,336,001	100	6,332,218	100

[a]Statistics refer to aliens admitted for legal permanent residence in Canada and the United States.
[b]U.S. statistics reported by region of birth. Canadian statistics reported by region of last permanent residence. Americas includes North, Central, and South America and the Caribbean. Oceania includes the Pacific Ocean Islands and Australasia.
Source: Statistical Yearbook of the Immigration and Naturalization Service (U.S. Department of Justice, Immigration and Naturalization Service), and Immigration Statistics (Employment and Immigration, Canada).

Table 2 New Cases of Active Tuberculosis in Canada and the USA, by Origin of Birth, 1985–1989

	Canada										USA									
	1985		1986		1987		1988		1989		1985		1986		1987		1988		1989	
New cases of tuberculosis	No.	(%)	No.	(%)	No.	(%)	No.	(%)	No.	(%)	No.	(%)	No.	(%)	No.	(%)	No.	(%)	No.	(%)
Foreign-born	870	(40.6)	865	(40.3)	876	(44.8)	907	(46.2)	976	(48)	4,562	(20.5)	5,155	(22.6)	5,293	(23.5)	5,144	(22.9)	5,666	(24.1)
Canada/USA-born	1,274	(59.4)	1,280	(59.7)	1,081	(55.2)	1,055	(53.8)	1,059	(52)	15,641	(70.5)	17,482	(76.8)	17,039	(75.7)	17,120	(76.3)	17,391	(74)
Unknown											1,998	(9)	131	(0.6)	185	(0.8)	172	(0.8)	438	(1.9)
Total	2,144		2,145		1,957		1,962		2,035		22,201		22,768		22,517		22,436		23,495	

Table 3 Tuberculosis Cases in the Foreign-Born in Canada and the United States by Region of Origin, 1985–1989

Continent of origin	Canada No.	Canada (%)	USA No.	USA (%)
Asia	2,598	(57.8)	11,827	(45.8)
Americas	463	(10.3)	11,427	(44.2)
Europe	1,100	(24.5)	1,521	(5.9)
Africa	263	(5.9)	534	(2.1)
Oceania	9	(0.2)	149	(0.6)
Unknown	61	(1.3)	362	(1.4)
Total	4,494		25,820	

Source: Tuberculosis statistics (1990); CDC (1990b).

Table 4 Incidence of Tuberculosis in Canada, Southeast Asia, Europe, and Africa

	Incidence (per 100,000 population) 1980–1984	Incidence (per 100,000 population) 1985–1989
Canada		
Canadian-born	9	6
Foreign-born	30	28
Asians	120	93
Europeans	14	11
Africans	25	57
Southeast Asia	87	85
Europe	34	33
Africa	57	57

Source: Canadian data from Statistics Canada, using 1981 and 1986 population census. Remaining data from WHO, Tuberculosis Unit, Geneva.

distribution, 1986; Sutherland et al., 1984; McIntyre et al., 1987). The incidence of tuberculosis is lower in individuals living in Canada who were born in Europe and Africa, compared with rates of tuberculosis reported by the World Health Organization (WHO) from these continents (Sudre et al., 1991). The Canadian foreign-born may have a lower incidence of tuberculosis compared with those in their country of origin owing to socioeconomic and medical selection pressures applied during the immigration process, as well as to decreased risk of infection and disease after arrival in Canada (Wang et al., 1989; Enarson et al., 1979). Problems of case detection and underreporting in developing countries may account for the apparent higher tuberculosis rates in Asian-born Canadians compared with WHO reported rates of tuberculosis from Southeast Asia. Also, the two areas are not strictly comparable, as Asian-born Canadians include those born on the Indian subcontinent and in the Middle East.

In the United States, approximately 43% of cases in the foreign-born diagnosed between 1985 and 1989 occurred in those 25–44 years of age, 15% in those 45–64 years of age, and 16% in those older than 65 years (Table 5). In comparison with cases in U. S.-born persons, the foreign-born are significantly more likely to be younger and female (P < 0.001). Similar data are not published in Canada.

In Canada, 20–36% of tuberculosis cases in the foreign-born occur in nonlanded immigrants, which includes students, visitors, refugees, illegal aliens,

Table 5 Age and Sex Distribution of Tuberculosis in the United States by Origin, 1985–1989

	Foreign-born		All U.S. cases	
	No.	(%)	No.	(%)
Age (yr)				
<5	473	(1.8)	3,684	(3.3)
5–14	715	(2.8)	2,423	(2.1)
15–24	3,801	(14.7)	8,525	(7.5)
25–44	11,209	(43.4)	37,904	(33.4)
45–64	5,470	(21.2)	29,735	(26.2)
65+	4,143	(16.0)	31,087	(27.4)
Unknown	9	(0.03)	59	(0.1)
Sex				
Male	15,638	(60.6)	74,045	(65.3)
Female	10,156	(39.3)	39,145	(34.5)
Unknown	26	(0.1)	227	(0.2)

Source: CDC (1990b).

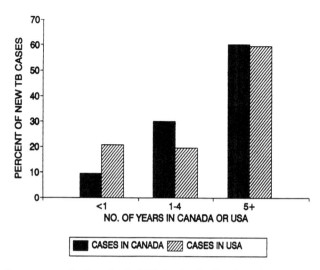

Figure 1 Percentage of tuberculosis (TB) in the foreign-born by years in Canada and the United States: 1985–1989.

and those admitted to the country for humanitarian reasons. (Orr et al., 1990; Enarson et al., 1979). Similar observations have been made in the United States and Australia (Passes, 1981; Streeton, 1987). These persons are at particularly high risk of developing active tuberculosis. Nonlanded immigrants are not necessarily required to undergo an immigration medical screening examination before arrival in the United States, Canada, the United Kingdom, or Australia, and they are not routinely placed on surveillance after arrival in these countries.

Twenty-one percent of American and 10% of Canadian cases of active tuberculosis in the foreign-born are diagnosed within the first year of their arrival, and 20–30% between 1 and 4 years of arrival (Fig. 1). In Canada, the incidence of tuberculosis in foreign-born persons that occurred in the first year of arrival has varied between 55 and 87 cases per 100,000 during the period 1975–1989, except for a dramatic rise in the incidence to 160–165 cases per 100,000 in 1979–1980 owing to an influx of both landed immigrants and refugees from Southeast Asia (Fig. 2). From 1979 to 1980, 36.9% of tuberculosis cases in the foreign-born that were diagnosed within 1 year of arrival in Canada occurred in those from Vietnam, compared to 5.8% of cases from 1975–1978, and 16.5% of cases from 1981–1984.

Some of the persons diagnosed with active tuberculosis in the first year of arrival may have had active disease at the time of their immigration medical screening, with the diagnosis being missed because of physician or laboratory error. Others may have developed disease between the medical examination and

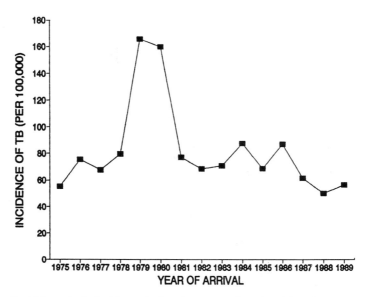

Figure 2   Tuberculosis incidence in immigrants to Canada within the first year after arrival.

the time of arrival, or they may have developed active disease after their arrival in Canada or the United States. Two recent studies in both Canada and the United States have suggested that 3–5% of the foreign-born who are thought to have inactive tuberculosis at the time of immigration were found to have active disease at their first clinic visit after arrival (Orr et al., 1990; Nolan et al., 1989). Those at particularly high risk for active disease were Asians and persons younger than 50 years of age. Both studies emphasized the importance of performing sputum or gastric cultures in addition to chest radiographs in asymptomatic persons referred for surveillance. Reliance on chest radiographs alone could have resulted in failure to diagnose and treat active tuberculosis in 2–5% of immigrants at their first clinic visit. The risks of inadvertently administering isoniazid chemoprophylaxis to these individuals include not only inadequate therapy for active disease but also the development of drug resistance.

The incidence of tuberculosis in cohorts of all immigrants decreased by approximately 50% by the fifth year after arrival in Canada. Similar observations have been made in the United States and Europe (British Thoracic and Tuberculosis Association, 1975; Bloch et al., 1989). In Canada, variations in the rate of decrease in tuberculosis incidence are evident according to year of arrival and continent of origin (Figs. 3 and 4). The increased incidence of tuberculosis

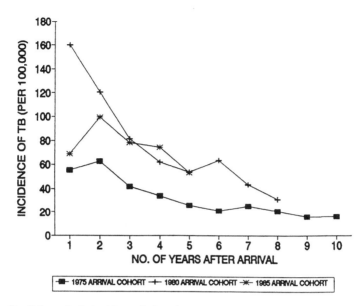

Figure 3 Tuberculosis incidence in immigrant cohorts by year after arrival in Canada.

in the 1980 cohort reflects the large influx of Asian immigrants and refugees. Over the past decade, there has been a decline in the incidence of tuberculosis in successive immigrant cohorts coming to Canada from Asia and Europe, and an increase in the incidence in cohorts arriving from Africa (Figs. 5–7). During this period there has been no significant change in the immigration medical screening process. It is unclear how recent African cohorts immigrating to Canada differ from previous ones in their risk of tuberculous infection and disease, and whether infection with human immunodeficiency virus (HIV) plays a role in these trends.

Of the 9461 cases of tuberculosis occurring in the foreign-born in Canada from 1975 to 1984, 90.6% represented new active cases and 9.4% were relapses (Uygur, A. O., personal communication, 1987). However, many cases may be inappropriately labeled as new active disease, owing to inadequate documentation of previous infection. The frequency of exposure in the foreign-born to infection after immigration, with subsequent development of new active disease, is unknown. Crowded housing, poverty, stress, and problems in accessing health care, all may contribute to high rates of transmission of infection within immigrant groups (Beaujot et al., 1988; Perez-Stable et al., 1986; Joint Tuberculosis

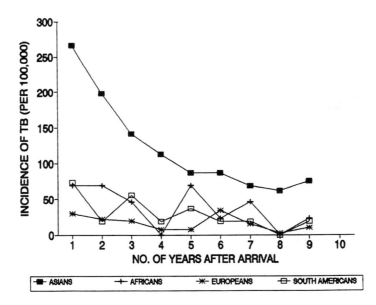

Figure 4 Tuberculosis incidence in 1980 immigrant cohorts by year after arrival in Canada.

Committee, 1978; McNicol, 1983; Powell et al., 1981; Enarson et al., 1979). Immigrants with undetected active disease likely act as important sources of infection for uninfected immigrants, as well as for North American-born children of immigrant parents (Ashley et al., 1974; Mortensen et al., 1989). The high tuberculin conversion rates in the children of immigrants suggests on-going transmission within these households. In a study of American-born children of Latino immigrant parents, the tuberculin conversion rate was 15–30 times higher than that of the United States general population (Perez-Stable et al., 1985).

Infection may also occur in immigrants at the time of return visits to their country of origin. In a study of Asian immigrants in England, it was estimated that over a 5-year period, one-fifth of those who developed tuberculosis were infected during a recent visit to their homeland (McCarthy, 1984).

In North America, Europe, and Australia, the foreign-born are more likely to develop extrapulmonary tuberculosis, compared with the native-born population (Mortensen et al., 1989). Asian immigrants, in particular, have a higher incidence of tuberculous lymphadenitis than the non-Asian native-born population (Ashley et al., 1974; McNicol, 1983; Powell et al., 1981).

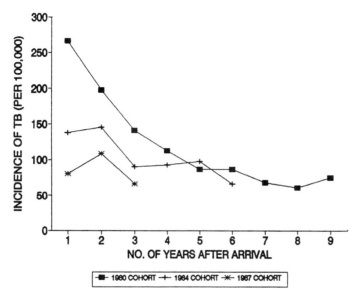

Figure 5   Tuberculosis in Asian immigrant cohorts by year after arrival in Canada.

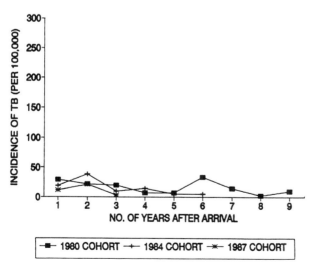

Figure 6   Tuberculosis in European immigrant cohorts by year after arrival in Canada.

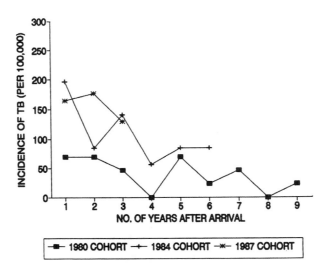

Figure 7 Tuberculosis in African immigrant cohorts by year after arrival in Canada.

VI. Drug Resistance

The frequency of drug resistance is high in the foreign-born, particularly in those from Asia (Snider, 1980; Thomas and Ayres, 1986; Wang et al., 1989). From 1976–1983, 0.62–1% of all isolates of *Mycobacterium tuberculosis* from British-born individuals in Birmingham, England were resistant to one or more antituberculous drugs, compared with 5.1–6.5% of isolates in the foreign-born (Thomas and Ayres, 1986). In the United States, drug resistance is seen in approximately 11% of Latino immigrants and 15–20% of Indochinese refugees with tuberculosis (Snider, 1980; CDC, 1983). In a Canadian study, initial and acquired drug resistance was seen in 6.8 and 19.4%, respectively, of foreign-born individuals with tuberculosis who were from the Philippines, India, China, and Hong Kong, compared with 1.4 and 7.4% of Canadian-born persons (Wang et al., 1989). These resistance rates in the foreign-born were lower than those documented in their country of origin. Initial drug resistance in the foreign-born was significantly more common in those younger than 40 years of age, whereas no age dependency was seen in the resistance patterns among Canadian-born persons. It may be difficult to distinguish between primary and acquired drug resistance in older persons, owing to inadequate documentation of previous cultures and therapy.

In both foreign- and British-born cases in England, resistance to one antituberculous drug was more common than multidrug resistance; however, resistance to multiple drugs was found in a higher proportion of foreign-born subjects (Thomas and Ayres, 1986). Among those with resistance to a single agent, the foreign-born were more likely to demonstrate resistance to isoniazid, and the British-born to streptomycin.

VII. Discussion and Recommendations

The problems associated with immigration medical screening and surveillance programs for tuberculosis in developed countries have been described in several recent reviews (CDC, 1990a; Orr et al., 1990; Streeton, 1987; Nolan et al., 1989). Inappropriate or incorrect diagnoses may be due to failure to obtain appropriate cultures and chest radiographs, or to errors on the part of physicians and laboratories. Individuals seeking immigration status may falsify information. In addition, a medical examination is not required for nonlanded immigrants to Canada, such as students, visitors, and those entering on temporary visas unless they are from a designated country and are staying longer than 6 months. Many of these persons, especially those from high-tuberculosis prevalence countries, have been previously infected with the tubercle bacillus and are at risk of active disease. Those persons who are allowed into Canada and the United States for humanitarian reasons also are at risk of having active tuberculosis at the time of their landing or in the first 4 years thereafter. For those persons coming to Canada, who are diagnosed as having active tuberculosis before immigration, treatment guidelines are provided by the medical regulations to the Canadian Immigration Act. For the United States, treatment schedules are provided by the U. S. Public Health Service Centers for Disease Control. Individual compliance is, however, uncertain. At present it is not possible to ensure that a person with active tuberculosis diagnosed at the time of visa application will adhere to a specific regimen.

Newcomers may develop active tuberculosis during the interval between the medical examination and arrival at the country of destination. Although in the United States and Canada federal health authorities notify state or provincial tuberculosis control officers of the arrival of persons requiring surveillance, contact may not be made owing to clerical error, change of address, or noncompliance with the order on the part of the newcomer. Although complying with surveillance is required by law in North America, in practice, federal action is rarely taken in recalcitrant cases. Language, cultural barriers, poverty, fear, and mistrust of authority, all may contribute to noncompliance and failure to access medical care on the part of immigrants (Peters et al., 1987). For those who are seen by surveillance physicians after arrival, evaluation is often problematic owing to language and cultural barriers, as well as difficulties in obtaining previous chest radiographs and immigration medical records containing accurate documentation of previous investigation and therapy (Orr et al., 1990).

Recommendations for the prevention and control of tuberculosis in the foreign-born include the following: (1) closer regulation and quality control of physicians and laboratories involved in medical screening in the country of birth or country of last residence should be instituted; (2) examinations for nonlanded immigrants from high-prevalence countries should be mandatory; (3) compliance with surveillance and therapy after immigration should be enforced; (4) sharing of medical information between immigration medical officers and local health authorities should be facilitated; (5) culturally appropriate and accessible health care services for these individuals should be provided (Ormerod, 1990; CDC, 1990a; Orr et al., 1990; Streeton, 1987).

Certain subgroups at higher risk of disease, particularly refugees and migrant workers from high-incidence countries, may require more intensive investigations. These might include chest radiographs in children and wider application of tuberculin testing both before and after immigration (CDC, 1990a). The latter may be difficult because of the widespread use of bacille Calmette-Guerin (BCG) vaccination in many developing countries. Systematic tuberculin testing followed by chemoprophylaxis when indicated has been recommended for both foreign-born children and children born to immigrants in Britain and North America (British Thoracic Society, 1990; Perez-Stable et al., 1986). A threshold of a 1% prevalence rate for tuberculin positivity in children younger than 5 years of age has been suggested as a marker for immigrant populations in whom routine skin testing is indicated to trace the transmission of infection to susceptible individuals (Perez-Stable et al., 1985). Indications for BCG vaccination are controversial; the British Thoracic Society has recommended its use in previously unvaccinated immigrant children from high-risk areas, and for children born in Britain of immigrant parent from these areas (British Thoracic Society, 1990).

The extent of the investigation of adult foreign-born individuals performed by physicians in Canada and the United States is variable. Although chest radiographs are usually performed, tuberculin skin tests as well as sputum or gastric cultures are frequently either not requested or not provided by the patient. Uniform guidelines for investigation of these patients would be of benefit (Orr et al., 1990). Suggested guidelines for the investigation of individuals newly arrived in Canada who are under surveillance for tuberculosis have been developed recently (see Appendix).   In the absence of contraindications, chemoprophylaxis is routinely suggested for foreign-born individuals younger than 35 years old who are tuberculin-positive and who do not have evidence of active disease (CDC, 1990a). However, preventive therapy may also be indicated for those at high risk for disease who are 35 or more years of age (CDC, 1990a).

As the number of tuberculosis cases in North America continues to rise, it has become increasingly important to focus on prevention and treatment of high-risk populations, including immigrants. Innovative methods must be used to access these populations after they have arrived in Canada or the United States and to ensure that the provision of culturally appropriate education about tuberculosis, its prevention, treatment, and follow-up are available. Programs involving lay outreach health workers operating in their own ethnic milieu may be helpful here.

Although vigilance in the screening and follow-up of prospective immigrants to North America is necessary and appropriate, only by reducing the risk of infection of tuberculosis in the countries of high prevalence of disease will scourge of worldwide tuberculosis be reduced.

Appendix: Guidelines for the Investigation of Persons Who Were Placed Under Surveillance for Tuberculosis After Arriving in Canada

Individuals newly arrived in Canada may have been placed under surveillance for tuberculosis by the Medical Services Branch of the Department of National Health and Welfare because of a previous history of tuberculosis or an abnormal chest x-ray suggestive of inactive tuberculosis (Orr et al., 1990). Following their arrival in Canada, these persons are required to report to a designated clinic to establish whether active tuberculosis exists.

The following guidelines, jointly prepared by the Canadian Thoracic Society, the Tuberculosis Directors of Canada, and Department of National Health and Welfare in consultation with the provincial/territorial epidemiologists, have been approved by the Canadian Lung Association and the Canadian Thoracic Society (Health and Welfare Canada, 1992).

Although there are no specific regulations, individuals should be followed for at least 3–5 years since the highest incidence of active tuberculosis in recent arrivals to Canada develop within the first 3–5 years of their immigration (Powell et al., 1981; CDC, 1975; Wang et al., 1989, 1991).

First Visit

1. Complete history and physical examination including review of previous treatment of tuberculosis

2. Chest x-ray and/or other appropriate radiological examinations

3. Send at least one, but preferably three, sputum specimens (may be induced) or gastric lavage specimens for smear and culture for *Mycobacterium tuberculosis*

4. Other appropriate laboratory tests, including a tuberculin test if appropriate

5. Medical Services Branch, Department of National Health and Welfare, should be contacted to obtain medical information and chest x-rays (if available)

Follow-up After Initial Assessment

1. If a diagnosis of *active* tuberculosis is established, treatment for at least 6 months with an appropriate regimen should be instituted. The treatment regimen chosen should account for the possibility of drug-resistant tuberculosis being present when the individual has immigrated from a country with a high prevalence of tuberculosis (Wang et al., 1991).

2. If a diagnosis of *inactive* tuberculosis is established and if the individual has had no or inadequate treatment for active tuberculosis in the past, then consideration should be given to initiate appropriate chemoprophylaxis. Follow-up of individuals after completion of a course of chemoprophylaxis will be at the discretion of the jurisdiction involved.

    Trials using alternative chemoprophylaxis regimens are currently being conducted to determine appropriate regimens when multidrug-resistant tuberculosis is suspected. Consultation with a tuberculosis authority is recommended.

3. If a diagnosis of *inactive* tuberculosis is made and the individual has had adequate treatment, then the individual should be followed for at least 3–5 years. Follow-up should occur at approximately 3, 9, and 21 months, and yearly thereafter. An appropriate history, physical examination and x-rays as well as other appropriate laboratory tests should be obtained at each follow-up visit.

References

Ashley, M. J., Anderson, T., and LeRiche, W. H. (1974). The influence of immigration on tuberculosis in Ontario. *Am. Rev. Respir. Dis.* **110**:137–146.

Beaujot, R., Basavarajappa, K. G., and Verma, R. B. P. (1988). *Current Demographic Analysis: Income of Immigrants in Canada. A Census Data Analysis.* Statistics Canada Cat. 91-527E.

Bloch, A., Reider, H., Kelly, G., Canthen, G., Hayden, C., and Snider, D. (1989). The epidemiology of tuberculosis in the United States. Implications for diagnosis and treatment. *Clin. Chest Med.* **10**:297–313.

British Thoracic and Tuberculosis Association (1975). Tuberculosis among immigrants related to length of residence in England and Wales. *Br. Med. J.* **3**:698.

British Thoracic Society (1990). Control and prevention of tuberculosis in Britain: An updated code of practice. Subcommittee of the Joint Tuberculosis Committee of the British Thoracic Society. *Br. Med. J.* **300**:995–999.

Centers for Disease Control (1983). Primary resistance to antituberculosis drugs—United States. *MMWR* **32**:521–523.

Enarson, D., Ashley, M. J., and Grzybowski, S. (1979). Tuberculosis in immigrants to Canada. A study of present-day patterns in relation to immigration trends and birthplace. *Am. Rev. Respir. Dis.* **119**:11–18.

Health and Welfare Canada (1992). Guidelines for investigation, of individuals who were placed under surveillance for tuberculosis post-landing in Canada. *Can. Commun. Dis. Rep.* **18–20**:153–155.

Jereb, J. A., Kelly, G. D., Dooley, S. W., Cauthen, G. M., and Snider, D. E. (1991). Tuberculosis morbidity in the United States: Final data, 1990. CDC Surveillance Summaries, December 1991. *MMWR* **40**(SS-3):23–27.

Lange, P., Mortensen, J., and Viskum, K. (1986). Tuberculosis in a developed country. *Acta Med. Scand.* **219**:481–487.

McCarthy, O. R. (1984). Asian immigrant tuberculosis—the effect of visiting Asia. *Br. J. Dis. Chest* **78**:248–253.

McIntyre, P. B., McCormack, J. G., and Vacca, A. (1987). Tuberculosis in pregnancy—implications for antenatal screening in Australia. *Med. J. Aust.* **146**:42–44.

McNicol, M. (1983). Trends in the epidemiology of tuberculosis—a physician's view. *J. Clin. Pathol.* **36**:1087–1090.

Medical Officer's Handbook (1991). Immigration Medical Services, Medical Services Branch, Department of National Health and Welfare, Ottawa, Sects. 2–4.

Mortenson, J., Lange, P., Storm, H. K., and Viskum, K. (1989). Childhood tuberculosis in a developed country. *Eur. Respir. J.* **2**:985–987.

Nolan, C. M., Telu, B., and Wu, R. (1989). The use of sputum cultures in the evaluation of immigrants classified as tuberculosis suspects. *Am. Rev. Respir. Dis.* **140**:996–1000.

Ormerod, L. P. (1990). Tuberculosis screening and prevention in new immigrants 1983–88. *Respir. Med.* **84**:269–271.

Orr, P. H., Manfreda, J., and Hershfield, E. (1990). Tuberculosis surveillance in immigrants to Manitoba. *Can. Med. Assoc. J.* **142**:453–458.

Passes, H. I. (1981). Isoniazid prophylaxis in new immigrants. *Ann. Intern. Med.* **95**:657.

Perez-Stable, E., Levin, R., Pineda, A., Slutkin, G. (1985). Tuberculosis skin test reactivity and conversions in United States- and foreign-born Latino children. *Pediatr. Infect. Dis.* **4**:476–479.

Perez-Stable, E. J., Slutkin, G., Paz, E. A., and Hopewell, P. (1986). Tuberculin reactivity in United States and foreign-born Latinos: Results of a community-based screening program. *Am. J. Public Health* **76**:643–646.

Peters, D., Hershfield, E. S., Fish, D. G., et al. (1987). Tuberculosis status and social adaption of Indochinese refugees. *Int. Migration Rev.* **21**:845–856.

Powell, K., Meador, M., and Farer, L. (1981). Foreign-born persons with tuberculosis in the United States. *Am. J. Public Health* **71**:1223–1227.

Snider, D. (1980). Tuberculosis in Oriental immigrants. *Chest* **77**:812.

Snider, D. E. (1989). Reorientation of tuberculosis control progams in the USA. *Bull. Int. Union Tuberc. Lung Dis.* **64**:25–26.

Streeton, J. A. (1987). Paradise lost? Is there a case for immigrant health screening? *Med. J. Aust.* **146**:1–3.

Sudre, P., ten Dam, G., Chan, C., Kochi, A. (1991). Tuberculosis in the present time: A global overview of the tuberculosis situation. Tuberculosis Unit, Division of Communicable Diseases, World Health Organization, Geneva, p.26.

Sutherland, I., Springett, V. H., Nunn, A. J. (1984). Changes in tuberculosis notification rates in ethnic groups in England between 1971 and 1978/79. *Tubercle* **65**:83–81.

The geographical distribution of tuberculosis notifications in a national survey of England and Wales in 1983. (1986). *Tubercle* **67**:163–178.

Thomas, H., and Ayres, J. (1986). The Birmingham tuberculosis drug resistance register, 1956–1983. *Tubercle* **67**:179–188.

Centers for Disease Control (1990a). Tuberculosis among foreign-born persons entering the United States, recommendations of the Advisory Committee for Elimination of Tuberculosis. *MMWR* **39**:1–21.

Joint Tuberculosis Committee (1978). Tuberculosis among immigrants in Britain. Memorandum from the Joint Tuberculosis Committee. *Br. Med. J.* **1**:1038–1040.

Tuberculosis statistics (1986–1990). Morbidity and mortality. Statistics Canada, Health Division, 1985–1989.

Centers for Disease Control (1990b). Tuberculosis statistics in the United States. U.S. Department of Health and Human Services, Public Health Service, Division of Tuberculosis Control, 1985–1989.

Wang, J. S., Allen, E. A., Chao, C. W., Enarson, D., Grzybowski, S. (1989). Tuberculosis in British Columbia among immigrants from five Asian countries, 1982–85. *Tubercle* **70**:179–186.

25

Tuberculosis in Correctional Facilities

M. MILES BRAUN*

The Johns Hopkins University School of Hygiene and Public Health
Baltimore, Maryland

I. Introduction

Jail and prison populations in the United States may now be more vulnerable to tuberculosis than at any time in the last decade. At least three factors are exacerbating the tuberculosis problem. First, human immunodeficiency virus (HIV) infection, often linked to intravenous drug use, is prevalent in many correctional systems. The HIV-infected persons are at greatly increased risk of progressing from tuberculous infection to active disease and then infecting others—effectively amplifying tuberculosis. Second, increases in prison populations that result in greater numbers of inmates sharing the same amount of air have put more inmates and staff at risk for tuberculosis. Third, the recent appearance of difficult-to-treat multidrug-resistant tuberculosis in this environment is providing a monumental challenge to tuberculosis prevention and control efforts.

The problem of tuberculosis control in correctional facilities is not restricted to any single geographic area. The Centers for Disease Control (CDC) noted 11 tuberculosis outbreaks in eight states in the period 1985–1989. Annual tuberculosis rates of greater than 100 cases per 100,000 persons—approximately tenfold higher than the national rate—have been noted in correctional systems in several states. Moreover, the population at risk is large. Each year more than

Present affiliation: National Cancer Institute, National Institutes of Health, Bethesda, Maryland.

8 million inmates are discharged from local jails in the United States. The cross-sectional population in jails and prisons has recently been estimated to total 1.2 million (Centers for Disease Control [CDC], 1989c, Bureau of Justice Statistics, 1992).

Tuberculosis in correctional facilities has wider scope than just the correctional setting. First, tuberculosis in jail or prison inmates puts the staff who work with them at risk of acquiring tuberculosis. In addition, inmates exposed to tuberculosis in correctional facilities, but who develop the disease after their release, can become a source of infection for the community at large (Stead, 1978; Braun et al., 1989; King and Geis, 1977; Abeles et al., 1970; Pelletier et al., 1991).

II. Epidemiology of Human Immunodeficiency Virus Infection and Acquired Immune Deficiency Syndrome in Correctional Facilities (See also Chapter 17)

A. Overview

The acquired immune deficiency syndrome (AIDS) epidemic has progressed rapidly in the United States during the late 1970s and 1980s, and it has concurrently become a major public health problem in many correctional facilities (National Commission on AIDS, 1991). Through October 1989, 5411 (5%) of the 110,333 cases of AIDS in the United States were reported from correctional facilities (Hammett, 1990).

In Maryland, a study in the state prison system showed that AIDS became the leading cause of death in 1987 (Salive et al., 1990b). In the New York state prison system, as early as 1984–1985, more that 50% of the deaths were due to AIDS; through February 1990, 729 inmates had died with AIDS (Morse, in press).

B. Human Immunodeficiency Virus Seroprevalence Studies and Risk Factors for HIV Infection

Although inmates with HIV infection may be in any AIDS risk group, HIV infection in inmates is most frequently associated with intravenous drug use before incarceration. For example, in New York from 1980 to 1988 and in Maryland in 1987, 95 and 85%, respectively, of inmates with AIDS had been intravenous drug users (Morse et al., 1990; Vlahov, 1992). Intravenous drug use is also linked to illicit behaviors that result in arrest and detention. Therefore, correctional facilities concentrate persons who have acquired HIV infection through intravenous drug use, and the prevalence of HIV seropositivity in correctional facility entrants correlates with the HIV seroprevalence in intravenous drug abusers in the areas from which the entrants come. Large regional differences in HIV seroprevalence in intravenous drug users have been shown (U. S. Dept. Health and Human Services, 1990), and these differences may generally be reflected in correctional system entrants (Table 1). Sexually acquired HIV infec-

Table 1 Human Immunodeficiency Virus Seroprevalence in Selected Correctional Facilities

State	Year	Number tested	Percent HIV seropositive	Comment	Ref.
California	1988	5372	2.5	Male entrants	Singleton et al., 1990
California	1988	807	3.1	Female entrants	Singleton et al., 1990
Iowa	1986	859	0.0	Entrants	Glass et al., 1988
Michigan	1987–1988	802	1.0	Entrants	Patel et al., 1990
New York	1988	450	18.9	Female entrants	Smith, 1991
New York	1988	494	17.4	Male entrants	Smith, 1991
Ten states	1988–1989	9080	2.1–7.6	Male entrants	Vlahov et al., 1991
Ten states	1988–1989	1914	2.5–14.7	Female entrants	Vlahov et al., 1991
Maryland	1987	1488	7.0	Entrants	Vlahov, 1992

tion is now generally less common in inmates, but may become increasingly common (CDC, 1989a).

C. Intraprison Transmission of Human Immunodeficiency Virus

Situational homosexuality as well as use of intravenous drugs occurs in prison (Vlahov, 1992) and can lead to intraprison transmission of HIV infection. However, epidemiological studies have found the risk of HIV seroconversion in prison to be relatively low and proportional to the prevalence of HIV infection in entrants. Three such seroconversion studies found from none to 4.2 cases of new HIV infection per 1000 prisoner-years (Brewer et al., 1988; Kelly et al., 1986; Horsburgh et al., 1990).

D. Human Immunodeficiency Virus Testing, Segregation of Seropositive Inmates, and the Potential for Tuberculosis Outbreaks

Although policies on screening inmates for HIV infection vary among correctional facilities, and some inmates have expressed concerns about testing for HIV in prisons (Starchild, 1989), the states with the largest numbers of

HIV-seropositive inmates generally do not routinely screen for HIV infection. Therefore, in these states, inmates with asymptomatic HIV infection are not and generally cannot be segregated from the general prison population. However, when inmates become ill with HIV-associated disease or AIDS, they sometimes are grouped together in segregated living situations, including infirmaries. If an inmate with active pulmonary tuberculosis lives in close proximity to other HIV-infected inmates, those contacts will be at high risk for acquiring tuberculous infection and then progressing to active tuberculosis. Nosocomial outbreaks of this pattern have been described in settings that have some similarities to correctional facilities (Di Perri et al., 1989; CDC, 1989b, 1991c; Daley et al., 1992). These outbreaks have shown that symptomatic HIV-seropositive persons newly infected with *Mycobacterium tuberculosis* can, in a period of months, progress to smear-positive pulmonary tuberculosis and then transmit infection to others. Therefore, the potential for the amplication of tuberculosis in this setting by further rounds of transmission is clear. Outbreaks of this type caused by multidrug-resistant tuberculosis (which may continue to be infectious after initiation of standard short-course chemotherapy) pose a particularly serious threat (Pitchenik et al., 1990; CDC, 1991a; Stead and Lofgren, 1991).

III. Correctional Facilities Are a High-Risk Environment for Tuberculosis Transmission

A. A Model for Tuberculosis Transmission

A model useful to understanding the epidemiology of tuberculosis transmission in a closed environment, such as a correctional facility, has recently been discussed by Riley and Nardell (Riley and Nardell, 1989; Nardell et al., 1991; Nardell, 1990). In a mathematical formula, this model states essentially that the number of new *M. tuberculosis* infections or active tuberculosis cases among susceptibles in an environment increases with the number of persons with infectious tuberculosis, the numbers of viable tubercle bacilli passed into the environment by these infectious cases, and the duration of exposure of susceptible persons. The model also states that the number of new *M. tuberculosis* infections or active tuberculous cases *decreases* as the fresh-air ventilation of the environment *increases*.

B. Prison Conditions and Overcrowding

Approximately 1.2 million persons are incarcerated in prisons and jails in the United States. It is unfortunate for tuberculosis control that recent growth in the incarcerated population in the United States has often surpassed growth in the facilities to house inmates. Between 1980 and 1989, 18 states, the District of

Columbia, and the federal prison system have more than doubled their prison populations (Dubler and Sidel, 1989). "As of 1990, 37 states, the District of Columbia, Puerto Rico, and the Virgin Islands operate prisons under court orders pursuant to findings of poor conditions, overcrowding, or lack of medical care serious enough to violate constitutional protections" (National Commission on AIDS, 1991).

One effect of overcrowding on tuberculosis is to allow each inmate case to expose more contacts. In addition, overcrowding makes the logistics of tuberculosis prevention, detection, and treatment much more difficult.

In some correctional facilities, effects of overcrowding may be compounded by poor ventilation. Such a situation was demonstrated in an investigation of an outbreak of 46 cases of invasive pneumococcal disease in an overcrowded and underventilated county jail in Texas. The jail housed 6800 inmates, although its capacity was 3500. Mean outside airflow to cells with four-person sleeping areas was 4.6 ft^3/min (CFPM) per person, although the investigators stated that airflow should have been at least 20 CFPM. Seventy percent of cases had underlying conditions such as asplenism or a history of intravenous drug abuse (Hoge et al., 1990). Such an environment would also be highly conducive to the transmission of tuberculosis, although the longer incubation period of tuberculosis, its relatively low attack rate (in the absence of HIV infection), and the high turnover of inmate populations can make tuberculosis transmission difficult to demonstrate.

C. Risk Factors for Tuberculosis Among Inmates

Infection with HIV is clearly the strongest risk factor for the progression of latent *M. tuberculosis* infection to active tuberculosis. In addition, intravenous drug use, a major HIV risk factor of inmates, was shown, before the AIDS epidemic, to be an important risk factor for tuberculosis (Reichman et al., 1979). Intravenous drug users with HIV infection and latent tuberculous infection (documented by positive tuberculin skin tests) in one study developed 7.9 cases of tuberculosis per 100 person-years of follow-up, an extremely high risk of tuberculosis (Selwyn et al., 1989). Because inmates infected with HIV probably have at least a 10–20% prevalence of latent tuberculous infection in the United States, it is clear that they too are at greatly elevated risk for developing tuberculosis. Moreover, the risk of developing tuberculosis when tuberculous infection occurs at the time of symptomatic HIV infection may be even higher than the risk of reactivation tuberculosis noted in the study by Selwyn and coworkers. Di Perri et al. (1989) reported that 7 of 14 tuberculin skin test-negative HIV-infected persons developed tuberculosis within 60 days of exposure to an infectious case in a hospital setting. Similarly, Daley and co-workers reported that 11 (37%) of 30 residents of a housing facility for HIV-infected persons developed active tuberculosis after exposure to a resident with sputum smear-positive pulmonary tuberculosis (Daley et al., 1992).

The proportion of inmates with positive tuberculin skin tests has ranged from 10 to 20% in correctional systems recently publishing such data (Table 2). In contrast, it has been estimated that approximately 5% of the U. S. population is tuberculin-positive (CDC, 1990b). Several factors may explain this large difference. Demographically, inmates are not representive of the general population. Inmates are preponderantly men, and males' risk of tuberculosis exceeds females'. Blacks and Hispanics are overrepresented among inmates, and these two groups have tuberculous infection prevalences and tuberculosus disease rates that exceed those of the white population (CDC, 1987; Reichman and O'Day, 1978; Snider et al., 1989). These differences in prevalence of tuberculous infection by race and ethnicity may reflect low socioeconomic status—long recognized as a tuberculosis risk factor (Stead and Bates, 1988). However, in a controversial study, Stead has recently presented data from contact investigations of tuberculosus cases in nursing homes and prisons. He concludes that blacks are more likely to acquire tuberculous infection than whites under similar exposure conditions; however, further study is needed to confirm these findings (Stead et al., 1990).

D. New Increased Potential for Outbreaks

As shown in the foregoing, HIV infection can have a large impact on the magnitude of the tuberculosis problem in a correctional system. For example, in the New York State prison system, a study among entrants found 18.8% of women and 17.4% of men to be HIV-seropositive in 1988 (Smith, 1991). Meanwhile, from 1978 to 1988, with progression of the AIDS epidemic, the incidence of tuberculosis in the New York State prison system had risen from 15.4:100,000 in 1976 to 136:100,000 in 1988, a 7.8-fold increase. Of inmates with tuberculosis diagnosed in 1985–1988, 65% had AIDS or were HIV-seropositive; the HIV test results of the remainder were unavailable. In addition, one investigation showed that at least one cluster of three inmates with tuberculosis could be linked in space and time. Their *M. tuberculosis* isolates were also of the same phage type, thereby suggesting the possibility of intraprison tuberculosis transmission (Braun et al., 1989; Morse et al., 1990).

E. Multidrug-Resistant Tuberculosis

In 1991, several nosocomial outbreaks of multidrug-resistant tuberculosis associated with HIV infection were reported (CDC, 1991a). Recent reports in 1991 have also described deaths of multidrug-resistant tuberculosis in 13 HIV-infected inmates and 1 prison guard (who had previously been diagnosed with cancer) in the New York State prison system (McFadden, 1991). These

Table 2 Tuberculin Skin Test Positivity in Selected Correctional Facilities

State	Year	Number tested	Tuberculin positive, (%)	Sex	Comment	Ref.
Maryland	1988	698	12.7	M	Prison entrants	Salive et al., 1990a
New Mexico	1986–1987	2240	10.3	M and F	Prison record review	Spencer and Morton, 1989
Washington	1983	4269	12.5	M	Prison entrants	Anderson et al., 1986
Nassau Co., New York	1990	1855	20.0	M and F	Jail inmates	Pelletier et al., 1991
DeKalb Co., Georgia	1990	5096	18.0	M & F	Jail entrants	Braun, unpublished data

developments are particularly serious for the following reasons. First, HIV-seroprevalence is often high in prison systems, and AIDS patients can serve to accelerate and amplify tuberculosis transmission (Stead and Lofgren, 1991). Second, falsely negative tuberculin skin tests occur commonly in HIV-infected persons, making it difficult to identify persons newly infected with *M. tuberculosis*. Third, at the time of diagnosis, multidrug-resistant tuberculosis may be clinically indistinguishable from non–multidrug-resistant tuberculosis. Fourth, there is little experience with tuberculosis preventive therapy in persons exposed to *M. tuberculosis* resistant to both isoniazid and rifampin (Snider et al., 1991). Fifth, *M. tuberculosis* resistant to isoniazid and rifampin often responds slowly, incompletely, or not at all to antituberculosis chemotherapy (Goble et al., 1988). Therefore, although patients with multidrug-resistant tuberculosis may be isolated, and their contacts identified and tuberculin skin tested, quickly resolving such outbreaks will be extremely difficult.

IV. Tuberculosis Prevention and Control

Tuberculosis prevention and control activities in correctional facilities share many similarities with such activities in other populations (Barnes et al., 1991a). This section will focus on issues that are unique or particularly important to correctional facilities.

A. Importance of Length of Stay

When considering tuberculosis prevention and control in correctional facilities, it can be helpful to distinguish between prison systems and jails. A major difference between them is the length of stay, generally longer than 1 year in prison systems (although inmates may be transferred among facilities within prison systems) and less than 1 year (and often hours to days) in jails. This is important to consider because the diagnosis of tuberculosis, and the ruling out of active tuberculosis in those with tuberculous infection, may in practice take days to weeks to complete—often exceeding an inmate's length of stay. Moreover, the recommended durations of both tuberculosis treatment and preventive therapy are at least 6 months.

B. Screening for Tuberculosis Infection and Disease

The tuberculin skin test is used to screen inmates for tuberculous infection at correctional system entry, in contact investigations, and in periodic screening. The test is underutilized in correctional facilities. For example, in 1983, a CDC survey found that, only 33 (66%) of the 50 states reported that prison inmates were screened routinely for tuberculosis on admission, and only 6 (12%)

states reported routine periodic screening (Snider et al., 1984; Snider and Hutton, 1989).

Whom to Screen at Entry

Rapid inmate turnover in jails often results in incomplete diagnostic evaluations for tuberculosis and tuberculous infection. Similarly, courses of tuberculosis preventive therapy may be terminated by discharge. These conditions have been taken into account in the Centers for Disease Control recommendations stating that correctional facilities need not necessarily tuberculin skin test inmates "unlikely to remain in the system or in that facility for more than seven days" (CDC, 1989c). When the likely length of a person's incarceration is difficult and time-consuming to determine, it is simple and prudent to initiate tuberculosis screening on all entrants.

Because persons with HIV infection are prone to falsely negative tuberculin skin tests, consideration should be given to routinely performing chest x-ray examinations, in addition to the tuberculin skin test, on HIV-infected entrants, especially those with any symptoms of tuberculosis.

Frequency of Periodic Screening

An important policy question for each facility or system is how frequently to screen inmates (prisons) and staff (prisons and jails) with tuberculin skin tests. Because, as noted earlier, inmates generally represent a group at increased risk of tuberculosis, a recommendation for annual screening of tuberculin skin test-negative inmates and staff is reasonable. Therefore, correctional facilities choosing less frequent screening schedules would be prudent to document an absence of cases of active tuberculosis, a low prevalence of HIV infection, and a low risk of tuberculous infection (e.g., less than 0.5% annual incidence of skin test conversions) in screenings undertaken every 2 or 3 years (CDC, 1989c).

Diagnosis of Tuberculosis

A critical part of tuberculosis control in correctional facilities is identifying cases of active pulmonary tuberculosis. When inmates are initially incarcerated with active pulmonary tuberculosis, the entry point into the correctional system (often a jail) is the optimum point for the diagnosis of tuberculosis. Otherwise, when tuberculosis develops after incarceration, diagnoses are made in the jail or prison through medical care or periodic screening.

Policies for diagnosis of tuberculosis may need to be tailored to specific correctional facilities' epidemiological circumstances. In general, cough of longer than 2-weeks duration is cause to suspect tuberculosis (even in a smoker), especially when other signs of tuberculosis or HIV infection are present. The sputum smear for acid-fast bacilli, although imperfect, is a very useful tool to gauge roughly and relatively quickly the infectiousness of tuberculosis suspects (Manoff et al., 1988). A basis for diagnosing tuberculosis and determining a patients' infectivity can be established using history and physical examination, tuberculin skin test, chest x-ray films, sputum smear, and sputum culture. Definitive diagnosis of tuberculosis can be made only by culture of *M. tuberculosis*. Whenever *M. tuberculosis* is first cultured from a patient from a correctional facility, drug susceptibility testing should be performed to ensure that an appropriate chemotherapy regimen is instituted.

C. Diagnostic and Therapeutic Issues Related to Human Immunodeficiency Virus

Anergy Testing and the Tuberculin Skin Test Cutoff

Depending on HIV infection status, different cutoffs for determining positivity of the tuberculin skin test may be used in routine screening for tuberculous infection. According to the CDC, if a person is HIV-infected, the cutoff for tuberculin skin test positivity is 5 mm; for other inmates and staff (in the absence of other risk factors), the cutoff is 10 mm. However, HIV infection status will often be unknown, and correctional facilities at which the prevalence of HIV infection is high may consider employing a cutoff of 5 mm for inmates with risk factors for HIV infection.

For persons who are known to be HIV-seropositive, CDC has recommended that those with negative tuberculin skin tests and with anergy to delayed-type hypersensitivity antigens should be considered for isoniazid preventive therapy if their risk of tuberculous infection is estimated to be 10% or more (CDC, 1991b). Inmate populations may frequently have prevalences of tuberculous infection this high; for example in Table 2, all of the inmate populations exceeded 10% prevalence of tuberculous infection.

Some investigators have proposed even more liberal criteria for prescribing preventive therapy, although these criteria may be logistically difficult to implement in the correctional setting. Graham and co-workers have suggested a cutoff of 2 mm for tuberculin skin test positivity in HIV-seropositive intravenous drug users and also have advocated concomitant anergy testing to assess the possibility of false-negative skin tests (Graham et al, 1992). Jordan and co-workers performed a decision analysis to determine when isoniazid should be prescribed in HIV-seropositive intravenous drug users. They concluded that a net benefit from the use of isoniazid could be shown for all intravenous drug users (except black women), even *without* tuberculin skin testing or anergy testing (Jordan et al., 1991). Further study of these issues should help resolve the different views and guide new policies on the tuberculin skin test cutoff and anergy testing.

Diagnosing Tuberculosis in Human Immunodeficiency Virus-Seropositive Persons Who Have Negative Tuberculin Skin Tests

Because HIV infection increases the probability of false-negative tuberculin skin tests, even in patients with tuberculosis (CDC, 1991b), these patients must have procedures for the diagnosis of tuberculosis initiated on the basis of signs and symptoms of the disease. Unfortunately, in the correctional setting, the situation is further complicated because many times an inmate's HIV infection status is unknown. Therefore, use of chest x-ray films, sputum smear, and sputum culture take on particular importance for the diagnosis and prompt treatment of tuberculosis in persons with symptoms of the disease. The clinical threshold should be especially low for ordering these diagnostic tests in inmates with known or suspected HIV infection.

Duration of Preventive Therapy

For persons found to have tuberculous infection, 6 months of tuberculosis preventive therapy has been recommended for HIV-seronegative persons and 12 months for HIV-seropositive persons (CDC, 1989d).

When HIV serological status is unknown, a decision on the length of therapy will have to be made. Six- and 12-month tuberculosis preventive therapy regimens have not been compared in HIV-infected persons with tuberculous infection. Because 6 months of chemotherapy shows good results in HIV-infected patients with *active tuberculosis*, and because preliminary results suggest that 6 months of chemoprophylaxis in patients with HIV infection reduces the incidence of tuberculosis by 89%, one could infer that 6 months could be considered adequate for prevention of tuberculosis in HIV-infected persons (Small et al., 1991; Devendra et al., 1991). A 6-month regimen has the advantage of being less expensive and logistically more simple than longer regimens. However, there is a spectrum of opinion on this issue. Some experts favor longer regimens because they could also be expected to protect against new tuberculous infections by susceptible bacilli (Barnes et al., 1991b). Others have even proposed lifelong preventive therapy to provide continuously some protection against tuberculosis as HIV infection incrementally destroys immunity (Di Perri et al., 1991).

D. Assuring Adequate Therapy

Directly Observed Preventive Therapy

Tuberculosis preventive therapy in correctional facilities is ideally administered by directly observed therapy; when daily directly observed therapy is not feasible, twice-weekly directly observed therapy is a satisfactory alternative (CDC, 1989c). If therapy is not directly observed, pills are less likely to be ingested and may even be kept by inmates for representation as other substances that are sold or traded.

Preventive Therapy Often Not Completed

A study in a large New York City jail highlighted some of the difficulties there with tuberculosis prevention. Mean compliance with the preventive therapy regimen was only 37%. Compliance was related to the convenience of the tuberculosis prevention program's site of dispensing medication as well as the inmate's knowledge of tuberculosis. An interesting finding was that inmates who had tuberculous infection, but believed that they were diagnosed with active tuberculosis had increased compliance with preventive therapy (Alcabes et al., 1989). Although these findings should not be construed as an advocation of misinforming asymptomatic inmates that they have tuberculosis, the data do show that compliance with preventive therapy is related to an individual's perceptions of disease.

The recommended course of tuberculosis preventive therapy is at least 6 months, but jail stays frequently are of shorter duration. When jail inmates are transferred to prison, good communication of medical records to the prison is essential for appropriate continuation of preventive therapy. When inmates are released to the community, it frequently becomes their own responsibility to follow-up with the local health department or physicians to continue preventive therapy. The author observed in a Georgia county where he worked that former inmates often were lost to follow-up by the tuberculosis control program after release from jail. Because few other data are available on this subject, is it unknown how common this situation is elsewhere.

Although preventive therapy in jails is often incomplete, such regimens may represent the only practical chance many individuals have to reduce their risk of tuberculosis. It is unfortunate, therefore, that preventive therapy regimens of less than 6 months have suboptimal effectiveness (American Thoracic Society–CDC, 1986; Comstock and Ferebee, 1970; Ferebee, 1970). New preventive therapy regimens of shorter duration (e.g., 2- and 4-months duration) are currently being investigated.

The relation of incomplete isoniazid preventive therapy regimens to the emergence of drug resistance has not been extensively studied. However, because of relatively low body burdens of *M. tuberculosis* in persons with asymptomatic tuberculous infection, their risk of developing an isoniazid-resistant strain during incomplete therapy may be much lower than in tuberculosis patients who harbor orders of magnitude more tubercle bacilli. Nonetheless, this area deserves future study.

Therapy Refusal

On occasion, patients with active tuberculosis may refuse medication for their disease. If such a patient has HIV infection, it is very likely that the tuberculosis will be fatal or at least contribute to death. If a patient is not infected with HIV, tuberculosis may also be fatal, but survival is more likely. Both types of patients will potentially spread tuberculosis. In any event, the infectious tuberculous patient in a correctional facility must be kept in *respiratory* isolation until no longer infectious. In many states, laws give public health officials the authority to deal with recalcitrant individuals with infectious tuberculosis. In such cases, correctional officials and state tuberculosis control officers should determine what legal authority may be invoked to protect public health within the correctional facility.

Importance of Continuation of Therapy for Active Tuberculosis

For inmates diagnosed with active tuberculosis, it is most important that a full course of therapy (preferably directly observed) be delivered, regardless of whether the inmate stays in the correctional system or is released to the community. Inmates released to the community should be referred to a local health department or health care provider for continuation of therapy. Otherwise, there is an increased risk of the inmate's experiencing life-threatening tuberculosis or developing drug-resistant tuberculosis—as well as infecting others. Accordingly, it seems reasonable to consider making postrelease continuation of antituberculosis chemotherapy a part of an inmate's release planning process.

E. Coordination of Tuberculosis and Infection Control

Central Reporting

Reporting of cases of tuberculosis to a central office is extremely important in multi-institutional correctional systems. If a chief health officer takes responsibility for tracking cases, central reporting can facilitate continuity of tuberculosis treatment by helping prevent lapses in therapy when inmates are transferred among facilities. In addition, central reporting gives an epidemiologic overview of the entire system. This overview may be useful in initiating contact investigations and in identifying outbreaks that may otherwise be obscured from recognition by frequent inmate transfers throughout the system. Such a reporting system should track drug susceptibility testing results of *M. tuberculosis* isolates, and can provide early warning of the emergence of drug resistance. Central reporting can also be useful to monitor the process and outcomes of tuberculosis therapy and preventive therapy.

Respiratory Isolation

To contain tuberculosis in the correctional setting, respiratory isolation should be available and used for cases of suspected or confirmed tuberculosis (CDC, 1990a). Respiratory isolation rooms should have negative-pressure relative to the hallway (i.e., airflow from the hallway to the rooms). Doors to these rooms should be kept closed as much as possible, and air should be vented directly outside the building—not recirculated (CDC, 1990a).

Although respiratory isolation rooms need not exist within every correctional facility, each facility should have an agreement with another facility or a nearby hospital to provide isolation when needed. Respiratory isolation is not synonomous with solitary confinement because air, potentially containing *M. tuberculosis* from solitary cells, may be recirculated to other parts of a facility. It is advisable that respiratory isolation of cases of active tuberculosis should continue until patients are receiving appropriate therapy and have at least three consecutive daily negative sputum smears (CDC, 1989c).

Infection Control

When persons who have HIV infection are gathered together in the correctional setting, there is a significant risk of a person's developing tuberculosis and infecting others who will then quickly progress to active tuberculosis. Rapid isolation, diagnosis, and treatment of cases of active tuberculosis should significantly decrease transmission. In addition, some experts have suggested that for environments that may have similarities to certain parts of correctional facilities, the use of ultraviolet lights for upper-air sterilization or the use of air filtration through a high-efficiency particulate air filter (HEPA) should be considered for prevention of tuberculosis transmission (Riley and Nardell, 1989; Nardell et al., 1991; Nardell, 1990; Stead et al., 1991; CDC, 1990a).

F. Role of the Health Department

The local and state health departments in whose jurisdiction the correctional facility is located can provide consultation concerning tuberculosis prevention and control. When cases of active tuberculosis are identified, the health department can provide advice and, in some cases, resources, to implement contact investigations and to initiate control measures. Achievement of smooth cooperation between a correctional system and health department may be facilitated by the designation of a correctional staff member whose responsibilities specifically include serving as a liaison with the health department. This should probably be the same individual responsible for maintaining the central reporting system as well as for monitoring treatment and preventive therapy.

V. Conclusions

As the year 2000 approaches, enormous challenges will confront correctional institutions in their efforts to prevent and control tuberculosis. The HIV-seropositive prisoners will constitute a subgroup at extremely high risk for reactivation tuberculosis. In addition, they also are at high risk for developing active tuberculosis subsequent to acquiring tuberculous infection within the correctional setting. This latter process can be facilitated by crowding. In addition, the emergence of multidrug-resistant tuberculosis can greatly complicate tuberculosis control by reducing the efficacy of tuberculosis therapy and preventive therapy.

Barring a technological breakthrough, tuberculosis prevention and control must rely on careful and thorough tuberculosis screening programs; preventive therapy programs with high completion rates, focusing when possible on persons with or at elevated risk for HIV infection; a low threshold for investigating respiratory symptoms compatible with tuberculosis, especially in persons with or at elevated risk for HIV infection; and perhaps most importantly, rapid isolation, diagnosis, and treatment of persons with active tuberculosis. Tuberculosis control should be made an integral part of all correctional health care programs, and should be coordinated with HIV–AIDS health care.

Acknowledgments

The author thanks Drs. George Comstock and David Vlahov for thoughtful reviews of this chapter.

References

Abeles, H., Feibes, H., Mandel, E., and Girard, J. A. (1970). The large city prison—a reservoir of tuberculosis. *Am. Rev. Respir. Dis.* **101**:706–709.

Alcabes, P., Vossenas, P., Cohen, R., Braslow, C., Michaels, D., and Zoloth, S. (1989). Compliance with isoniazid prophylaxis in jail. *Am. Rev. Respir. Dis.* **140**: 1194–1197.

American Thoracic Society–Centers for Disease Control (1986). Treatment of tuberculosis and tuberculous infection in adults and children. *Am. Rev. Respir. Dis.* **134**:355–363.

Anderson, K. M., Keith, E. P., and Norsted, S. W. (1986). Tuberculosis screening in Washington state male correctional facilities. *Chest* **89**:817–821.

Barnes, P. F., Bloch, A. B., Davidson, P. T., and Snider, D. E. (1991a). Tuberculosis in patients with human immunodeficiency virus infection. *N. Engl. J. Med.* **324**:1644–1650.

Barnes, P. F., Bloch, A. B., Davidson, P. T., and Snider, D. E. (1991b). Tuberculosis and HIV infection. *N. Engl. J. Med.* 325:1884.

Braun, M. M., Truman, B. I., Maguire, B., DiFerdinando, G. T., Wormser, G., Broaddus, R., and Morse, D. L. (1989). Increasing incidence of tuberculosis in a prison inmate population: Association with HIV infection. *JAMA* **261**:393–397.

Brewer, T. F., Vlahov, D., Taylor, E., Hall, D., Munoz, A., and Polk, B. F. (1988). Transmission of HIV-1 within a statewide prison system. *AIDS* **2**:363–367.

Bureau of Justice Statistics (1992) *National Update*. U.S. Department of Justice, Washington, D.C. Vol.1, No.3.

Centers for Disease Control (1987). Tuberculosis in minorities—United States. *MMWR* **36**:77–80.

Centers for Disease Control (1989a). Heterosexual transmission of AIDS and HIV infection—U. S. *MMWR* **28**:423–434.

Centers for Disease Control (1989b). *Mycobacterium tuberculosis* transmission in a health clinic—Florida, 1988. *MMWR* **38**:256–258,263–264.

Centers for Disease Control (1989c). Prevention and control of tuberculosis in correctional institutions: Recommendations of the Advisory Committee for the Elimination of Tuberculosis. *MMWR* **38**:313–325.

Centers for Disease Control (1989d). Tuberculosis and human immunodeficiency virus infection: Recommendations of the Advisory Committee for the Elimination of Tuberculosis. *MMWR* **38**:236–238, 243–250.

Centers for Disease Control (1990a). Guidelines for preventing the transmission of tuberculosis in health-care settings, with special focus on HIV-related issues. *MMWR* **39**(RR-17):1–29.

Centers for Disease Control (1990b). The use of preventive therapy for tuberculous infection in the United States. *MMWR* **39**(RR-8):9–12.

Centers for Disease Control (1991a). Nosocomial transmission of multidrug-resistant tuberculosis among HIV-infected persons—Florida and New York, 1988–1991. *MMWR* **40**:585–591.

Centers for Disease Control (1991b). Purified protein derivative (PPD)-tuberculin anergy and HIV infection: Guidelines for anergy testing and management of anergic persons at risk of tuberculosis. *MMWR* **40**(RR-5):27–32.

Centers for Disease Control (1991c). Tuberculosis outbreak among persons in a residential facility for HIV-infected persons—San Francisco. *MMWR* **40**:649–652.

Comstock, G. W., and Ferebee, S. H. (1970). How much isoniazid is needed for prophylaxis? *Am. Rev. Respir. Dis.* **101**:780–782.

Daley, C. L., Small, P. S., Schecter, G. F., Schoolnik, G. K., McAdam, R. A., Jacobs, W. R., and Hopewell, P. C. (1992). An outbreak of tuberculosis with accelerated progression among persons infected with the human immunodeficiency virus. *N. Engl. J. Med.* **326**:231–5.

Devendra, W., Hira, S., Mwansa, N., Tempo, G., and Perine, P. (1991). Preventive tuberculosis chemotherapy in persons infected with human immunodeficiency virus infection [Abstract]. In *Proc. Seventh Int. Conf. AIDS*, Book 3. Florence, Italy. Istituto Superiore di Sanita, Rome, p. 246.

Di Perri, G., Cruciani, M., Danzi, M. C., Luzzati, R., De Checchi, G., Malina, M., Pizzighella, S., Mazzi, R., Solbiati, M., Concia, E., and Bassetti, D. (1989). Nosocomial epidemic of active tuberculosis among HIV-infected patients. *Lancet* **334**:1502–1504.

Di Perri, G., Vento, S., Cruciani, M., Micciolo, R., Concia, E., and Bessetti, D. (1991). Tuberculosis and HIV infection. *N. Engl. J. Med.* **325**:1882–1883.

Dubler, N. N., and Sidel, V. W. (1989). On research on HIV infection and AIDS in correctional institutions. *Milbank Q.* **67**:171–207.

Ferebee, S. H. (1970). Controlled chemoprophylaxis trials in tuberculosis. A general review. *Adv. Tuberc. Res.* **17**:29–106.

Glass, G. E., Hausler, W. J., Loeffelholz, P. L., and Yesalis, C. E. (1988). Seroprevalence of HIV among individuals entering the Iowa prison system. *Am. J. Public Health* **78**:447–449.

Goble, M., Horsburgh, R., Waite, D., Madsen, L., and Iseman, M. (1988). Treatment of isoniazid and rifampin-resistant tuberculosis. *Am. Rev. Respir. Dis.* **137** (Suppl.):24.

Graham, N. H., Nelson, K. E., Solomon, L., Bonds, M., Rizzo, R. T., Scavotto, J., Astemborski, J., and Vlahov, D. (1992). Prevalence of tuberculin positivity and skin test anergy in HIV-1-seropositive and -seronegative intravenous drug users. *JAMA* **267**:369–373.

Hammett, T. M. (1990). *Update 1989: AIDS in Correctional Facilities*. National Institute of Justice, Washington, D.C.

Hoge, C., Reichler, M., Mastro, T., Elliott, J., Facklam, R., Bremer, J., Hendricks, K., Dominguez, E., and Breiman, R. (1990). Outbreak of invasive pneumococcal disease in a jail [Abstract]. *Progr. Abstr.* 30th *ICAAC*, Atlanta, p. 171, Abstr. 510.

Horsburgh, C. R., Jarvis, J. Q., McArthur, T., Ignacio, T., and Stock, P. (1990). Seroconversion to human immunodeficiency virus in prison inmates. *Am. J. Public Health* **80**:209–210.

Jordan, T. J., Lewit, E. M., Montgomery, R. L., and Reichman, L. B. (1991). Isoniazid preventive therapy in HIV-infected intravenous drug abusers. *JAMA* **265**:2987–2991.

Kelley, P. W., Redfield, R. R., Ward, D. L., Burke, D. S., and Miller, R. N. (1986). Prevalence and incidence of HTLV-III infection in a prison. *JAMA* **256**:2198–2199.

King, L., and Geis, G. (1977). Tuberculosis transmission in a large urban jail. *JAMA* **237**:791–792.

Manoff, S. B., Cauthen, G. M., Stoneburner, R. L., Bloch, A. B., Schultz, S., and Snider, D.E. 1988. TB patients with AIDS: Are they more likely to spread TB? In *Fourth Int. Conf. AIDS.* Stockholm, Abstr. 4621, p. 216.

McFadden, R. D. (1991). *New York Times* Nov. 17, p. 39.

Morse, D. L., Truman, B. I., Hanrahan, J. P., Mikl, J., Broaddus, R. K., Maguire, B. M., Grabau, J. C., Kain-Hyde, S., Han, Y., and Lawrence, C. E. (1990). AIDS behind bars. Epidemiology of New York State prison inmate cases, 1980–1988. *N. Y. State J. Med.* **90**:133–138.

Morse, D. L. (in press) The epidemiology of HIV/AIDS in the New York State correctional system. *Criminal Justice Policy Rev.*

Nardell, E. A. (1990). Dodging droplet nuclei. Reducing the probability of nosocomial tuberculosis transmission in the AIDS era. *Am. Rev. Respir. Dis.* **142**:501–503.

Nardell, E. A., Keegan, J., Cheney, S. A., and Etkind, S. C. (1991). Airborne infection. Theoretical limits achievable by building ventilation. *Am. Rev. Respir. Dis.* **144**:302–306.

National Commission on AIDS (1991). HIV disease in correctional facilities. National Commission on AIDS, Washington, D.C.

Patel, K. K., Hutchinson C., and Sienko, D. G. (1990). Sentinel surveillance of HIV infection among new inmates and implications for policies of corrections facilities. *Public Health Rep.* **105**:510–514.

Pelletier, A. R., DiFerdinando, G., Greenberg, A., Sosin, D., Jones, W., and Bloch, A. (1991). Tuberculosis in a county jail, New York. In *Abstracts of Epidemic Intelligence Service Conference*, Atlanta.

Pitchenik, A. E., Burr, J., Laufer, M., Miller, G., Cacciatore, R., Bigler, W. J., Witte, J. J., and Cleary T. (1990). Outbreaks of drug-resistant tuberculosis at AIDS centre. *Lancet* **336**:440–441.

Reichman, L. B., and O'Day, R. (1978). Tuberculosis infection in a large urban population. *Am. Rev. Respir. Dis.* **117**:705–712.

Reichman, L. B., Felton, C. B., and Edsall, J. R. (1979). Drug dependence, a possible new risk factor for tuberculosis disease. *Arch. Intern. Med.* **139**:337–339.

Riley, R. L., and Nardell, E. A. (1989) Clearing the air. *Am. Rev. Respir. Dis.* **139**:1286–94.

Salive, M., Vlahov, D., and Brewer, T. F. (1990a). Coinfection with tuberculosis and HIV-1 in male prison inmates. *Am. J. Public Health* **105**:307–310.

Salive, M. E., Smith, G. S., and Brewer, T. F. (1990b). Death in prison: Changing mortality patterns among male prisoners in Maryland, 1979–1987. *Am. J. Public Health* **80**:1479–1480.

Selwyn, P. A., Hartel, D., Lewis, V. A., Schoenbaum, E. E., Vermund, S. H., Klein, R. S., Walker, A. T., and Friedland, G. H. (1989). A prospective study of the risk of tuberculosis among intravenous drug users with human immunodeficiency virus infection. *N. Eng. J. Med.* **320**:545–550.

Singleton, J. A., Perkins, C. I., Trachtenberg, A. I., Hughes, M. J., Kizer, K. W., and Ascher, M. (1990). HIV antibody seroprevalence among prisoners entering the California correctional system. *West. J. Med.* **153**:394–399.

Small, P. M., Schechter, G. F., Goodman, P. C., Sande, M. A., Chaisson, R. E., and Hopewell, P. C. (1991). Treatment of tuberculosis in patients with advanced immunodeficiency virus infection. *N. Engl. J. Med.* **324**:289–94.

Smith, P. F., Mikl, J., Truman, B. I., Lessner, L., Lehman, J. S., Stevens, R. W., Lord, E. A., Broaddus, R. K., and Morse, D. L. (1991). HIV infection among women entering the New York State correctional system. *Am. J. Public Health* **81S**:35–40.

Snider, D. E., Anderson, H. R., and Bentley, S. E. (1984). Current tuberculosis screening practices. *Am. J. Public Health* **74**:1353–1356.

Snider, D. E., Salinas, L., and Kelly, G. D. (1989). Tuberculosis: An increasing problem among minorities in the United States. *Public Health Rep.* **104**:646–653.

Snider, D. E., and Hutton, M. D. (1989). Tuberculosis in correctional institutions. *JAMA* **261**:436–437.

Snider, D. E., Cauthen, G. M., Farer, L. S., Kelly, G. D., Kilburn J. O., Good, R. C., and Dooley, S. W. (1991). Drug-resistant tuberculosis. *Am. Rev. Respir. Dis.* **144**:732.

Spencer, S. S., and Morton, A. R. (1989). Tuberculosis surveillance in a state prison system. *Am. J. Public Health* **79**:507–509.

Starchild, A. (1989). Testing for HIV in federal prisons. *N. Engl. J. Med.* **320**:315.

Stead, W. W. (1978). Undetected tuberculosis in prison. Source of infection for community at large. *JAMA* **240**:2544–2547.

Stead, W. W., and Bates, J. H. (1988). Epidemiology and prevention of tuberculosis. In *Pulmonary Diseases and Disorders*. Edited by E. P. Fishman. McGraw-Hill, New York.

Stead, W. W., and Lofgren J. P. (1991). Tuberculosis and HIV infection. *N. Engl. J. Med.* **325**:1882.

Stead, W. W., Senner, J. W., Reddick, W. T., and Lofgren, J. P. (1990). Racial differences in susceptibility to infection by *Mycobacterium tuberculosis*. *N. Engl. J. Med.* **322**:422–427.

U.S. Department of Health and Human Services, Public Health Service, Centers for Disease Control. (1990). National HIV Seroprevalence Surveys. Data from serosurveillance activities through 1989. Washington, D.C., HIV/CID/9–90/006.

Vlahov, D. (1992). HIV-1 infection in the correctional setting. *Criminal Justice Policy Rev.* (in press).

Vlahov, D., Brewer, T. F., Castro, K. G., Narkunas, J. P., Salive, M. E., Ullrich, J., and Munoz, A. (1991). Prevalence of antibody to HIV-1 among entrants to U. S. correctional facilities. *JAMA* **265**:1129–1132.

Part Four

TUBERCULOSIS CONTROL IN THE WORLD

26

National Tuberculosis Control Programs

KAREL STYBLO

International Union Against Tuberculosis and
   Lung Disease
Paris, France

M. ANGÉLICA SALOMÃO

Ministry of Health
Maputo, Republic of Mozambique

I. Main Factors Influencing the Course of Tuberculosis in a Community

It was widely believed that three factors could favorably influence the course of tuberculosis in a community:

1. Improvement of the general socioeconomic situation and of hygiene

2. Mass bacille Calmette-Guérin vaccination (BCG)

3. Case-finding and treatment

A. Improvement of the General Socioeconomic Situation and of Hygiene

In some developed countries, tuberculosis started to decrease during the second half of the 19th century, before the discovery of the tubercle bacillus in 1882. In England and Wales, nearly 600:100,000 children from newborn to 4 years of age died annually from tuberculosis in the early 1850s. It took some 55 years to reduce mortality by 50%. The decrease was much steeper (approximately 5% annually) between 1905 and 1940, in spite of World War I and the serious economic depression in the late 1920s and early 1930s. A similar distinct decrease in tuberculosis rates was observed in many developed countries between the two World Wars.

It should be stressed that improved socioeconomic conditions and hygiene were not the only factors that accelerated the decrease in tuberculous mortality during the first four decades of this century. Another factor in the more distinct decrease in tuberculous mortality (and incidence) in the prechemotherapy era must be related to the isolation in sanatoria of an increasing number of patients with infectious tuberculosis. Since a larger proportion of highly infectious cases were isolated and treated for many months in sanatoria, the risk of tuberculous infection in the community must have been to some extent reduced.

Little is known about tuberculosis situation and trend of tuberculosis in developing countries in the prechemotherapy era. It is most unusual for such countries to have reliable information on the epidemiological situation or on calender trends in tuberculosis. However, experience from the last four decades indicates no improvement of tuberculosis in developing countries without a well-run national tuberculosis program (NTP).

B. Mass BCG Vaccination

It became evident in the mid-1970s that mass BCG vaccination of children and young adults cannot substantially improve the epidemiological situation of tuberculosis (Styblo and Meijer, 1976). The main reason is that more than 95% of reported tuberculous cases among children are smear-negative, of those with infection in the 15 to 29-year age group and reported as clinical tuberculous, 75% are smear-negative. It has been shown that smear-negative patients are much less infectious than those whose smears are positive. Furthermore, the protection afforded by BCG vaccination is of limited duration.

Despite this, there is a valid argument in support of BCG vaccination of infants in countries with a high risk of infection (World Health Organization [WHO], 1991a). This approach has been greatly facilitated by WHO policy, which shifts responsibility for BCG vaccination from the tuberculosis control program to the Expanded Program on Immunization.

C. Case-Finding and Treatment

In the early 1950s, it became evident that adequate chemotherapy is one of the most important tools needed to influence the course of tuberculosis in a community. Crofton (1962) had shown in 1953 that isoniazid, streptomycin and p-aminosalicylic acid (PAS) could cure virtually all patients however severe their disease, provided that their bacilli were initially sensitive to these drugs. Although antituberculosis drugs were introduced in technically advanced countries soon after their discovery, it took 6–10 years to persuade tuberculosis specialists to discontinue artificial pneumothorax and surgical treatment, replacing them with adequate chemotherapy and, thereby, achieving a high cure rate, as demonstrated by Crofton in the early 1950s. Curiously enough, antituberculous drugs were considered for many years merely as a welcome means of support for "classic" methods of treatment and not as the sole tool for treatment of tuberculosis.

II. The Tuberculosis Situation in the World After the Discovery of the Tubercle Bacillus in 1882, and Its Trend

A. The Prechemotherapy Era

Before the introduction of antituberculous drugs, tuberculous mortality rates provided fairly satisfactory data for evaluation of the epidemiological situation of tuberculosis and its trend. Reliable information on mortality rates from tuberculosis are available in most European and North American countries, dating from the turn of this century. Mortality figures were high (frequently between 200:100,000 and 400:100,000) but even during the first four decades of this century, they showed a distinct downward trend of a similar order in each country, approximately 4–5% annually.

As early as the mid-1930s, Frost (1937) argued that the decreasing mortality rates from tuberculosis demonstrated that each infectious case of tuberculosis was giving rise to less than one new infectious case. Continuation of the conditions producing this sequence would obviously lead some day to the eradication of the disease. Among specific prevention procedures, Frost gave first priority to isolation of infectious cases. His second priority was preventive treatment of noninfectious cases, and the third was early case-finding.

Little is known about the tuberculosis situation and its trend in developing countries during the first half of this century owing to the absence of reliable data on prevalence of infection and on mortality from tuberculosis. The main sources of information for the study of certain aspects of the natural history of tuberculosis in developing countries are found in the results of tuberculosis surveys carried out by WHO teams in the 1950s and 1960s, mostly in Africa (Roelsgaard et al., 1964). Further sources are the results of tuberculin testing in a few developing countries preceding mass BCG vaccination carried out by the International Tuberculosis Campaign (WHO, 1954). Valuable data on tuberculosis in Eskimos were collected by the U.S. Public Health Service in the 1930s (Fellows, 1934).

B. The Chemotherapy Era

In the chemotherapy era, adequate chemotherapy accelerated the decrease in the risk of tuberculous infection in many developed countries, from 4–5% to 10–14% each year. Consequently, the risk of infection (and disease in children and young adults) decreased by 50% in these countries every 5–7 years during the last four decades (Styblo, 1984).

Figure 1 shows the risk of infection in several developed countries from 1950 to 1975 (Styblo and Meijer, 1978). It is seen that the risk of infection was low in 1975, ranging between 30 and 200 infections per 100,000 population, and

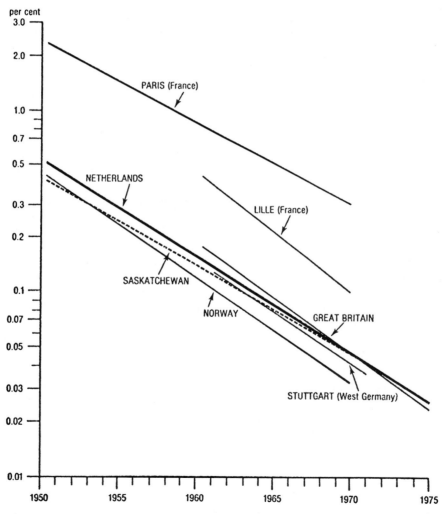

Figure 1 Annual risks of tuberculous infection and their trends in low-prevalence countries, 1950–1975. (From *IUATLD Bull.* **53**:283–294, 1978.)

was decreasing by more than 10% each year. The current (1990) risk of infection in most developed countries is low (approximately 0.1%) or very low (under 0.01%). It is obvious that such a major decrease in risk resulted in profound changes in the prevalence of tuberculous infection in the population. Consequently, the prevalence of infection in those aged 20–50 years is now relatively low (e.g., in the Netherlands, the prevalence of tuberculous infection is under 0.4% in those aged 20 years, and approximately 12% at the age of 50 years; Fig. 2). In 10 years in the future, the figures will be approximately 0.1% and 4%, respectively (Styblo, 1990).

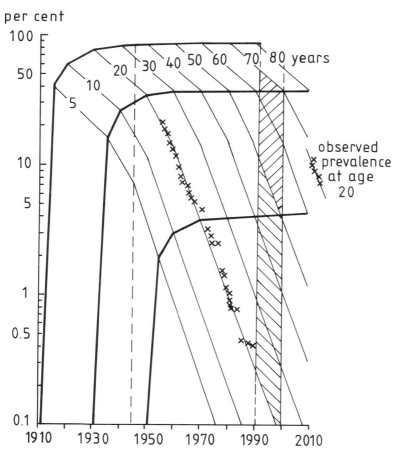

Figure 2 Estimated prevalence of tuberculous infection in the Netherlands in cohorts born in 1910, 1930, and 1950. (From *IUATLD Bull.* **66**:27–32, 1991.)

Figure 2 also explains why elimination of tuberculosis (less than 1% infected persons among the general population) is such a slow process. In the Netherlands, the cohort born in 1910 was exposed to a very high risk of infection during the first 20 years of its life (11.3% in 1910, 6.7% in 1920, and 3.9% in 1930). The prevalence of infection reached about 77% at the age of 20 years in 1939, and 85% at the age of 35 in 1945. It is understandable that the 1910 cohort could benefit little from the large decrease in the risk of infection of 13.8% each year after 1945.

The cohort born in 1930 was exposed to a much lower risk than that born in 1910. The risk of infection was 3.9% in 1930, 2.1% in 1940, and 0.53% in 1950. The prevalence of infection reached about 36% at the age of 20 years (compared with 77% in the cohort born in 1910). The estimated prevalence of the 1930 cohort at the age of 80 years (in 2010) will be about 40% (see Fig. 2).

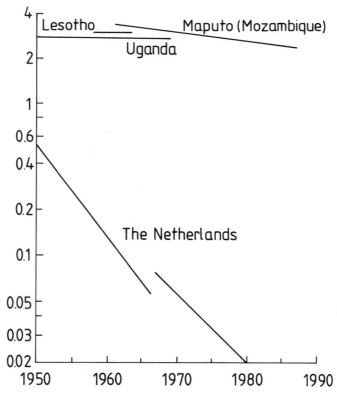

Figure 3 Annual risks of tuberculous infection and their trends in high-prevalence countries and in the Netherlands, 1950–1987. (From *IUATLD Bull.* **66**: 27–32, 1991.)

Finally, in the cohort born in 1950, the prevalence of infection was slightly above 3.5% at the age of 20 years in 1970 and less than 4% at the age of 40 years in 1990. The cohort will barely reach an overall prevalence of 5%.

In the Netherlands, the level of 1% of the prevalence of infection in those aged 10 years was achieved in 1970; 20 years in 1977, and 30 years in 1992. For persons aged 50 years, the 1% level is expected to be reached in 2002, and for those aged 60 years in 2012.

As opposed to developed countries, in developing countries the annual decrease in the risk of tuberculous infection was very slow during the last four decades, and in some of them only 1 or 2% (Uganda, Lesotho, Mozambique), compared with 10–14% in developed countries (Fig. 3). A similar decrease has been observed in Tanzania (Bleiker et al., 1987). In many developing countries, it became evident soon after the introduction of antituberculosis drugs that, despite the availability of powerful and effective drugs, tuberculosis programs under field conditions have not been very successful. The concept of a comprehensive control program on a countrywide scale, integrated into the existing health infrastructure, was formulated by the eighth WHO Expert Committee on Tuberculosis in 1964 and is referred to in section IV.

III. Epidemiological Indices for Planning, Surveillance, and Evaluation of the National Tuberculosis Program

Two epidemiological indices are currently considered the most relevant for measuring the epidemiological situation of tuberculosis and its trend in a given community:

A. Incidence of Tuberculous Patients Excreting Tubercle Bacilli Demonstrable by Direct Smear Examination

The foregoing epidemiological index cannot be used in most developing countries, since case-finding of smear-positive tuberculosis is usually deficient. There is evidence that, as few as one-third of smear-positive cases, the transmitters of the disease, are diagnosed. The reported incidence of tuberculosis, positive by direct smear, is closely related to the quality and extent of case-finding based on a microscopy network.

Note: Although a well-conducted prevalence survey gives reliable information on the magnitude of the pool of infectious sources in the community, this does not imply that the prevalence survey is a reliable index of the epidemiological situation of tuberculosis and its trend. It can be influenced either way by the extent of case-finding and the quality of chemotherapy. Moreover, a prevalence survey is expensive and needs a highly qualified staff.

B. The Risk of Tuberculous Infection

The average annual risk of infection indicates what proportion of the population will be infected; it is usually expressed as a percentage or a rate. Unlike mortality and notification rates, it is not directly influenced by the extent and efficiency of the tuberculosis program.

The risk of infection can be derived from tuberculin test results in a representative sample of non–BCG-vaccinated schoolchildren. It has been determined that a 1% annual risk of tuberculous infection corresponds to an incidence of approximately 50 smear-positive cases of pulmonary tuberculosis per 100,000 general population in areas where prevalence of human immunodeficiency virus (HIV) infection is low (Styblo, 1985; Murray et al., 1990).

Note: It is not easy to conduct a reliable tuberculin survey, since it must be representative for the country or the area under study, and it must be carried out by trained staff using standard procedures for testing and reading.

To evaluate the trend of the epidemiological situation of tuberculosis, at least two tuberculin surveys in representative samples of non–BCG-vaccinated children or young adults, of the same age or age groups, and tested by the same technique, should be carried out at intervals of approximately 5 years.

The average annual risk of tuberculous infection is now the most useful epidemiological index for planning, surveillance, and evaluation of national tuberculosis programs in developing countries.

IV. The National Tuberculosis Program

The WHO National Tuberculosis Program (NTP), as established in 1964, was reaffirmed by a WHO expert committee in the ninth report in 1974 (WHO, 1974). The committee formulated four principles for an NTP in developing countries.

A. The World Health Organization Principles for the National Tuberculosis Program

The Program Must Be Countrywide

Numerous studies in technically advanced and developing countries have shown that tuberculous infection and disease are usually fairly evenly distributed between villages and towns. In developing countries in which the population is rural, the bulk of the tuberculosis problem is found in the rural areas.

The Program Must Be Permanent

In developing countries, most of the adult population has been infected with tubercle bacilli. The current high risks of infection and their slow decrease in many developing countries are due to (1) shortcomings in the implementation of NTPs; (2) a high and increasing prevalence of HIV infection in Africa, America, and Asia; (3) a relatively high prevalence of primary and acquired resistance to the major antituberculosis drugs; (4) the population explosion; and (5) a deteriorating economic situation. All these elements point us toward preparing for a long struggle against the tubercle bacillus that will last for several generations.

The Program Must Be Adapted to the Expressed Demands of the Population

The program should be in consonance with the current attitudes and behavior of the community, should meet the public demand and, in particular, be convenient for the consumer, rather than merely for those providing the services. Accessibility and acceptability of the program are important basic aims. The public will have confidence in the services if they are effective.

The Program Must Be Integrated Within the Community Health Structure

The program must be integrated within the community health structure to meet these requirements. It should be developed as a well-balanced component of the country health program, within available resources. Attempts to establish a specialized tuberculosis service in developing countries are irrational, as such a service would absorb a disproportionate share of the limited resources available, at the expense of other essential health services.

A critical element of the overall program strategy must be the development of the NTP as an integral part of the primary health care (PHC) system in developing countries. Diagnosis and treatment of tuberculosis should be conducted wherever possible through the PHC system at the district level, with supervision, training, monitoring, and leadership provided by the NTP (WHO, 1991a). The community health worker provides a link between the community and the health services and could be expected to play a significant role in tuberculosis control.

B. Rationale for a National Tuberculosis Program

The rationale for an NTP is based on the following (Styblo, 1986):

1. Unlike many other infectious diseases seen in developing countries, tuberculosis can be controlled with the currently available tools under any socioeconomic condition because the infectious agent is almost exclusively found in the diseased patient who can be quickly rendered noninfectious.

2. Since a balance exists, both in developed and developing countries, between the tubercle bacillus and humans in the absence of man-made

interference (i.e., case-finding and chemotherapy), any reduction in the sources of infection will inevitably improve the epidemiological situation. If all (or nearly all) smear-positive cases of pulmonary tuberculosis now diagnosed in any developing country could be rendered noninfectious, the risk of infection would immediately start to fall.

3.   Case-finding of infectious cases (mainly smear-positive) and their cure are the key to any effective control of the disease, both in developed and developing countries. In addition, they reduce suffering and, if adequately applied, considerably lower the tuberculosis death rate.
     Note: BCG vaccination has a limited epidemiological effect, but reduces human suffering, especially among children.

4.   Reliable diagnostic tools enabling detection of almost all smear-positive cases of pulmonary tuberculosis, and highly efficient chemotherapy regimens that can cure nearly all discovered cases of tuberculosis are available.

C. Objectives of the National Tuberculosis Program

The objectives of the NTP in developing countries are twofold:

1.   To diagnose and cure as many tuberculous patients as possible. It should be stressed that alleviation of recognized human suffering must have a higher priority than preventing future human suffering.

2.   To gradually reduce the transmission of tuberculous infection in a community by at least 4–5% annually. This would reduce the risk of infection and the disease in children and young adults by 50% in about 15 years.

D. Structure of the National Tuberculosis Program

The establishment and implementation of the NTP in a country demands a continuous and long-term commitment by the government.

Central Level

At the central level there must be a single directing authority with responsibility (e.g., central tuberculosis unit; CTU). The main CTU's functions are

1.   Planning of the operational steps in implementing, monitoring, and evaluating the NTP

2.   Coordination and supervision of the NTP: at intermediate and peripheral levels, and with other sections of the ministry of health (especially

with those responsible for general laboratories, the expanded program of immunization [EPI] and primary health care [PHC] systems

3. Acquisition and distribution of supplies needed for the NTP, in particular: drugs, in collaboration with the central medical store (to check whether drugs are ordered, delivered, stored, and distributed to the intermediate and the peripheral levels); laboratory equipment (microscopes, slides, and stains) in collaboration with the laboratory services of the ministry of health; and documentation of case-finding, treatment, and administration

4. Training of the personnel involved in the NTP

Intermediate Level

At the intermediate (regional or provincial) level, the regional (provincial) director of health is responsible for carrying out the NTP in the region (province). The regional (provincial) director of health, in consultation with the CTU, appoints an officer known as the regional (provincial) tuberculosis coordinator (RTC or PTC), a medical officer or a nurse.

The functions of the RTC (PTC) are

1. To work closely with the CTU in the performance of his or her duties.

2. To coordinate tuberculosis control in the districts and supervise the personnel involved in case-finding and treatment of tuberculosis. The RTC (PTC) is expected to visit each district at least every 6 months. Districts with a poor performance should receive special attention. The RTC (PTC) will discuss deficiencies in treatment and case-finding observed during his or her visit to the respective district with the district chief medical officer (DCMO) and propose improvements.

3. To organize training programs in the region (province) in collaboration with the CTU and the DCMO, and to give on-the-job training to district and peripheral workers.

4. To ensure that requested quarterly reports on case-finding and on results of chemotherapy are made in each district and sent to him or her. The RTC (PTC) checks and comments on the reports received from the DTCs and produces a report covering the whole region (province) for the attention of the TCU. (A regional [provincial] report is not produced by the RTC [PTC] if the evaluation of the quarterly reports is computerized at the central level.)

5. The RTC (PTC) ensures close cooperation between the staff involved in case-finding and treatment of tuberculosis and with the network of microscopy services.

District Level

At the district level, the DCMO is responsible for carrying out the NTP in his or her district. The DCMO, in consultation with the RTC (PTC), appoints a full-time or part-time district tuberculosis coordinator, a medical assistant or a nurse.

Responsibilities and tasks of the district tuberculosis coordinator (DTC) are

1. To implement the NTP through the staff of district health services

2. To supervise treatment throughout the district and particularly ensure that: (1) the NTP regimens are prescribed; (2) patients under treatment are closely supervised by the health workers; (3) regimens are given for the required period, and that cured patients are discharged from treatment; (4) sputum is examined for tubercle bacilli at the requested intervals; and (5) patients are referred to the DCMO or RTC (PTC) for possible retreatment following failure of chemotherapy for any given reason

3. To assist health workers in the extension of case-finding of tuberculosis in all existing facilities in the district

4. To visit the district microscopy centers regularly and check whether all newly diagnosed smear-positive cases are receiving adequate chemotherapy

5. To supervise updating and accuracy of the district tuberculosis register and check that the documentation on case-finding and treatment is properly filled in

6. To be responsible for procuring supplies, such as drugs, laboratory reagents, sputum containers, and forms for the district, and for distributing them to the health units in the district

Health Centers and Health Posts

At the level of health centers and health posts, all health units should be involved in tuberculosis activities. In addition to other day-to-day medical work, the staff is responsible for case-finding and treatment of tuberculosis, including tracing of irregular attenders. They are also responsible for obtaining drugs and other supplies, keeping accurate records, and giving health education to patients and the community.

E. Planning and Programing the National Tuberculosis Program

Currently, many developing countries in Africa, Asia, and Latin America have poorly developed and inadequately funded NTPs. The weakest point in such an NTP is usually the lack of a regular supply of antituberculosis drugs. It goes without saying that such "treatment" is disastrous, creating chronic tuberculous excretors harboring resistant bacilli and discouraging health workers responsible for the NTP.

A relatively cheap, but inefficient, approach of many public health authorities in developing countries coping with the NTP in the 1960s and 1970s was to focus on mass BCG vaccination of young children. A justification for such an approach might have been based on the section in the ninth expert committee report (WHO, 1974) dealing with the selection of technical policies. In the report it is stated that "the components to be considered are case-finding, treatment, and BCG vaccination." The key to any effective tuberculosis control is case-finding of smear-positive patients and their cure, and not mass BCG vaccination.

Unfortunately, despite its tremendous global magnitude, tuberculosis has probably been the most neglected of all health problems for the past 10–15 years. Dr. Hiroshi Nakajima, Director-General of WHO, identified two reasons for this in his address at the World Conference on Lung Health in Boston in May 1990: First, tuberculosis has become politically "invisible" in the industrialized world, despite that it is still a major infectious disease there. Second, in many developing countries, tuberculosis control programs do not show tangible achievements within a short time. This tends to create pessimism and often also an atmosphere of indifference to the problem (Nakajima, 1990). The situation is changing: first, because of the rapidly deteriorating tuberculosis situation in acquired immune deficiency syndrome (AIDS) epidemic areas; second, because a tuberculosis elimination program has been initiated in the United States; and third, because it has been shown that an NTP can produce tangible results, even in the difficult environment of resource-poor countries (Nakajima, 1990).

It is very encouraging that the World Health Assembly passed the WHO Resolution 44.8 in May 1991 on the tuberculosis control program. It is hoped that the governments of many developing countries will focus on the WHO NTP described in the foregoing in the near future. It must be emphasized that the political will of each country is of the utmost importance for realizing a strong NTP.

The second factor for planning and programing an efficient NTP is adequate funding. Low-income developing countries (with a GNP per capita under 300 U.S. dollars) are unable to run a NTP in which retreatment cases would be adequately treated, and new smear-positive cases would be enrolled on an adequate short-course regimen. In many resource-poor countries, the development of political will must be matched and supported by a coordinated external assistance.

Finally, the third factor for planning and programing a well-run NTP is the availability of national personnel, particularly committed leadership.

To plan an efficient NTP, it is also important to have a reasonable idea of the extent of the tuberculosis problem in the country. The annual risk of tuberculous infection is considered the most useful epidemiological index for planning, programing, and evaluation of the NTP.

F. Technical Policies

Since BCG vaccination is under the responsibility of the Expanded Program on Immunization, reference is made to chemotherapy and case-finding only.

Chemotherapy

Although a case-finding and treatment program must be developed as an entity, case-finding being preliminary to treatment and cure, the first step to be taken in any inefficient NTP is to ensure that the cure rate under routine field conditions of all diagnosed cases is raised to exceed approximately 80%. This rate, with about 4–5% deaths from tuberculosis during the first weeks of treatment (owing to late diagnosis), will result in the elimination of sources of infection in diagnosed cases in about 85% of cases. The remaining 15% failure cases will not substantially increase the pool of infection. If the success rate is low, say, 50% or less, a high number of chronic excretors harboring drug-resistant bacilli will ensue, with all the consequences.

As has been seen over the last three to four decades, it is difficult to achieve improvement of chemotherapy in new smear-positive patients in developing countries. However, it has recently been shown to be possible by several International Union Against Tuberculosis and Lung Diseases (IUATLD)-assisted NTPs (in Tanzania, Malawi, Mozambique, Nicaragua, and Benin). The primary reason for the failure of the commonly employed treatment regimen of 12–18 months [isoniazid and amithiazone (thioacetazone), supplemented by streptomycin during the first 2 months], is the delay in smear conversion from positive to negative. During the initial phase of treatment, patient adherence to the regimen may be good while symptoms persist, and treatment with daily injections permits full supervision. However, at the end of 2 months, when streptomycin is stopped, about 50% of the patients are still smear-positive. To counter this problem, close supervision of treatment for at least the first 5 months is required, but this is not feasible in rural areas in many developing countries.

There is no doubt that the patient complies best when he or she is seriously ill. This is true in most smear-positive patients in developing countries, as the disease is discovered only in those who consult a health unit for complaints. The short-term compliance of the patient, lasting often only a few weeks, must be exploited by giving all patients an efficient chemotherapy under *close supervision* to kill almost all tubercle bacilli in the body as quickly as possible (e.g., isoniazid, rifampicin, pyrazinamide, and streptomycin for the first 2 months). The continuation phase after sputum conversion can be based on self-administration of the drugs if indicated. It should also be stressed that patients previously treated with antituberculous drugs for more than 1 month (smear-positive relapses, smear-positive failure cases) must be suspected of harboring drug-resistant bacilli, and a retreatment regimen ought to be prescribed.

Case-Finding

In the context of developing countries, *case-finding* refers to the diagnosis of sputum smear-positive disease. Undiagnosed smear-positive tuberculosis limits life expectancy to 2 years or so, and is responsible for virtually all transmission of infection. Despite this, undiagnosed smear-positive tuberculosis is very much the normal state of affairs in developing countries, where only one out of every two or three of such cases ever reaches diagnosis.

In developing countries, passive case-finding is the method of choice: the first move toward diagnosis is made by the patient, who seeks medical aid for complaints. Whatever other symptom or sign may accompany smear-positive tuberculosis, one is particularly frequent: persistent cough for 3 weeks or more with sputum. Such a history categorizes any such patient as a tuberculous suspect, and the sputum must be examined bacteriologically for tubercle bacilli.

Bacteriological examination of sputum is a direct way of diagnosing tuberculosis, since the demonstration of tubercle bacilli is conclusive. From the point of view of their value in an NTP, bacteriological techniques may be prioritized in the following order: examination of direct smears, culture, and sensitivity testing.

The highest priority of a bacteriological service in developing countries should be to perform sputum examination by microscopy on a large enough scale to permit the accurate bacteriological diagnosis of every smear-positive case and to monitor results of chemotherapy. Bright-field microscopy (usually using Ziehl–Neelsen staining) is most suitable for peripheral laboratories. Fluorescence microscopy would be preferable in larger laboratories, because it allows more specimens to be examined in the same amount of time and is economical.

The examination of cultures in addition to smear examination will add to the number of patients with a confirmed diagnosis of tuberculosis, especially those who are not excreting large numbers of bacilli. It might also be of value as a check on the effectiveness of diagnosis by direct microscopy. The extension of culture examination to symptomatic suspects may result in more frequent and earlier diagnosis of tuberculosis. This question is, however, controversial, and it would be of value to explore the feasibility of introducing culture examination for symptomatic subjects and its influence on the effectiveness of case-finding. The question of whether symptomatics should be selected for sputum culture by prior radiographic examination is complex and requires operational research (WHO, 1982).

Sensitivity tests are mainly of value for epidemiological purposes, to determine primary and acquired resistance. They may also be useful for guiding retreatment if first-line chemotherapy has failed. Steps should be taken to prevent infection of the staff working in laboratories. The risk of infection is higher in laboratories undertaking culture and sensitivity tests than in those carrying out smear examination only.

Implementation of the National Tuberculosis Program

Development of the program usually proceeds by areas. It should be started in the best-performing district of two or three regions (provinces) having a favorable logistic situation. The main aim of these training and demonstration districts is to provide opportunities for practical field experience and training for the other districts in which the NTP will be introduced. The feasibility and the actual flow of the NTP under field conditions ought to be evaluated from the outset of the program.

V. Definitions of Tuberculosis Cases and Choice of Chemotherapy Regimens

A. Case-Definitions

An *active case* of tuberculosis refers to symptomatic disease from *Mycobacterium tuberculosis* complex (*M.tuberculosis, M.africanum*, or *M.bovis*). The following case-definitions were adapted to chemotherapy guidelines (WHO, 1991b).

Site of Disease
Pulmonary Tuberculosis

Smear-Positive Patient. A patient with at least two sputum specimens positive for acid-fast bacilli (AFB) by microscopy: *or* a patient with one sputum specimen positive for AFB *and* radiographic abnormalities consistent with active pulmonary tuberculosis: *or* a patient with at least one sputum AFB smear-positive and culture positive for *M.tuberculosis*.

Smear-Negative Patient. A patient with at least two sputum specimens negative for AFB by microscopy *and* radiographic abnormalities consistent with active pulmonary tuberculosis *and* decision by a physician to treat with a full curative course of antituberculosis chemotherapy: or a patient with AFB smear-negative sputum that is culture-positive for *M.tuberculosis*.

Extrapulmonary Tuberculosis

A patient with histological or clinical evidence consistent with active tuberculosis *and* decision by a physician to treat with a full curative course of antituberculosis chemotherapy: *or* a patient with one culture specimen from an extrapulmonary site positive for *M.tuberculosis*.

History of Prior Tuberculosis Chemotherapy

Patients who have taken antituberculous drugs for 1 month or more at any time in the past have an increased chance of having drug-resistant tuberculosis. Therefore, it is essential that all patients, especially smear-positive patients, be carefully questioned about previous antituberculosis treatment before current treatment is started. Cases are, therefore, further defined by treatment history as:

New Case. A patient who has never taken antituberculous drugs for more than 1 month.

Relapse. A patient declared cured in the past, who again has active tuberculosis, meeting the foregoing definitions.

Smear-Positive Failure Case. A patient who remains sputum smear-positive 5 months or more after the start of chemotherapy: *or* a patient who interrupted the treatment after 1 to 5 months of chemotherapy and is subsequently found to be smear-positive.

Chronic Case. A patient who remains AFB smear-positive after completing an adequate retreatment regimen (e.g., that given in Sec. V.B), under close supervision.

Although smear-negative pulmonary or extrapulmonary cases may also be failure, relapse, or chronic, this should be a rare event. When there is proven evidence of active tuberculosis, these cases should be treated as smear-positive cases with the retreatment regimen.

B. Choice of Regimens (see also Chapter 11)

The WHO tuberculosis unit has recently recommended the use of short-course chemotherapy both in developed and developing countries, and to discontinue— wherever possible—12- to 18-month regimens (WHO, 1991b). Economic analyses indicate that, even though drug costs are higher, 6-month or 8-month therapy is more cost-effective than 12–18 months of outmoded treatment (Murray et al., 1990). There are few health interventions that are as cost-effective as tuberculosis treatment with short-course chemotherapy.

The CTU of a developing country must categorize patients according to the priority for treatment and determine the regimens to be used in the country for each category nationwide. Short-course chemotherapy consists of the 2 (3)-month intensive initial phase, and 4 (6)-month continuation phase. It is also very useful to introduce in the NTP a fixed-dose drug combination of isoniazid–rifampin of high quality and bioavailibility. The intensive initial phase should be fully supervised.

Highest Priority

The highest priority must be given to new smear-positive cases (i.e. to newly discovered patients who have never taken antituberculous drugs for more than 1 month).

Recommended Regimens

Initial Intensive Phase. 2HRZS(E); that is isoniazid (H), rifampin (R), pyrazinamide (Z), and either streptomycin (S) or ethambutol (E), given preferably daily for 2 months (8 weeks). *Note*: If the budget is limited, the drugs can be given intermittently during the second month.

When the patient has completed the 2-month intensive initial phase and the sputum is AFB smear-negative, the continuation phase will start. If sputum is smear-positive at 2 months, the initial intensive phase of four drugs daily is continued up to 4 more weeks; then the continuation phase is started, regardless of sputum test results.

Continuation Phase. 4HR or 4H3R3; that is, isoniazid and rifampin for 4 months daily, or three times a week.

Alternative Continuation Phase. 6HE(T); that is, isoniazid and ethambutol or isoniazid and thioacetazone daily for 6 months. *Note*: in proved or suspected HIV-infected patients, ethambutol should be used in place of thioacetazone. *Note*: The high-priority recommended regimen is also given to other newly diagnosed seriously ill patients with severe forms of tuberculosis (e.g., tuberculous meningitis, disseminated tuberculosis, tuberculous pericarditis, spinal disease with neurological complications, and such). For patients with tuberculous meningitis, disseminated tuberculosis, or spinal disease with neurological complications, isoniazid and rifampin should be given daily for 6–7 months (i.e., a total of 8–9 months of therapy).

High Priority for Relapse and Failure Smear-Positive Patients

The relapsed or failure patients must be suspected of having isoniazid- or streptomycin-resistant disease. Furthermore, they are at increased risk of developing multidrug-resistant disease and should receive fully supervised chemotherapy until sputum conversion is documented or until they are classified as a chronic case.

Recommended Regimen

Initial Intensive Phase. 2HRZES/1HRZE, that is, isoniazid combined with rifampin, pyrazinamide, and ethambutol for 3 months, supplemented with streptomycin for the first 2 months.

When the patient has completed the 3-month intensive initial phase and the sputum is AFB smear-negative at 3 months, the continuation phase is started. If sputum is positive at 3 months, the four oral drugs are continued daily for another 1 month. If the patient is still smear-positive at the end of the fourth month, all drugs are stopped for 2 or 3 days, and a sputum specimen is sent to the laboratory for culture and susceptibility testing (if available). The patient should then start the continuation phase.

If pretreatment studies show resistance to isoniazid or rifampin alone, the patient should start the continuation phase fully supervised (preferably in a referral hospital). In this case the chance of achieving sputum conversion, provided that all doses of drugs are taken until the end of the treatment, is good.

If the pretreatment studies show resistance to both isoniazid and rifampin, or isoniazid–rifampin-resistance is found in a patient remaining smear-positive, the chance of achieving sputum conversion is limited.

Continuation Phase. 5H3R3E3, or 5HRE, that is, 5 months of isoniazid, rifampin, and ethambutol, either three times a week under supervision or daily if supervised treatment is not possible. If the patient remains smear-positive after the completion of the continuation phase he or she is no longer eligible for the retreatment regimen.

Relatively High Priority

A relatively high priority should be given to smear-negative tuberculosis cases in children whose pulmonary disease is almost always smear-negative. Another important group is young persons infected during adolescence who develop primary tuberculosis, usually appearing as pleural effusion or small parenchymal lesions in the lungs. Symptomatic adult cases with smear-negative pulmonary tuberculosis also benefit from treatment, because a proportion of these patients will become smear-positive if not treated.

Recommended Regimens

Initial Intensive Phase. 2HRZ or 2H3R3Z3, that is 2 months of daily or three-times weekly isoniazid, rifampin, and pyrazinamide.

Continuation Phase. 2HR or 2H3R3, that is, 2 months of daily or three-times weekly isoniazid and rifampin. *Note*: In pulmonary tuberculosis with parenchymal involvement exceeding a total of 10 cm^2 on chest radiograph, or in extrapulmonary tuberculosis with incomplete remission of signs and symptoms, the continuation phase should be extended by administering isoniazid alone for an additional 4 months.

Alternative Continuation Phase. 6HE(T), that is, isoniazid and ethambutol or isoniazid and amithiozone (thioacetazone) daily for 6 months. *Note*: If resources are very limited, the patient is suspect or proven HIV-positive, and is smear-negative at the beginning of the fifth month of treatment, isoniazid alone may be given daily for the last 4 months (i.e., 2HE/4H).

Chronic Cases

Chronic cases have a low priority because they have a high likelihood of multidrug-resistant tuberculosis (i.e., resistance to at least isoniazid and rifampin).

It must be stressed that the intensive, short-course regimens are not, in themselves, the answer to the cure. To build an effective tuberculosis treatment system, drugs must always be available to the patients. Moreover, the initial intensive phase must be closely supervised to achieve sputum conversion close to 100% during the first 8–12 weeks of treatment.

VI. Recording, Reporting, and Evaluation of Case Finding and Results of Treatment

Accurate record keeping on all individual patients, and periodic reporting with statistics on patients and activities, is essential to the management of any NTP in developing countries. Unfortunately, systems introduced in developed countries in the last four decades cannot be used in developing countries.

The reporting of new and relapse cases of tuberculosis in developed countries is based on notification of individual patients by physicians to a central unit that is responsible for compilation of the data. In developing countries this is usually very difficult to carry out. In certain developing countries tuberculosis registers were introduced in the past, enabling collection of information on cases detected in the respective area, for instance, at the district level. We make reference to a built-in recording and reporting system on case-finding, case-holding, and evaluation of chemotherapy of tuberculosis developed in the IUATLD-assisted NTPs over the last 10 years. The data on case-finding and evaluation of treatment results covering an entire country are analyzed by cohort analysis. *Cohort analysis*, as used in this text, indicates the identification of consecutive patients registered during a defined time period (usually one calendar quarter) for determining rates of case-finding and the results of treatment after completion of the chemotherapy regimens. Procedures and forms used for recording and reporting in NTP are presented in the Appendix.

VII. Evaluation of Case Finding and Treatment

The following items were chosen for **evaluation** of case-finding and treatment:

1. *Case-finding*. The detected cases are grouped by sex into new smear-positive cases, smear-positive relapses, smear-negative cases, and extrapulmonary cases. New smear-positive cases are also grouped by age.

2. *Treatment*. New smear-positive cases and smear-positive relapses are evaluated separately by cohort analysis every 3 months. New cases are separately evaluated for those on short-course chemotherapy and 12-month chemotherapy (if the latter is still applied to some smear-positive cases).

VIII. Human Immunodeficiency Virus and the National Tuberculosis Program (see also Chapters 17 and 18)

It is evident that persons infected with tubercle bacilli and with HIV have an increased risk of tuberculosis (Pitchenik et al., 1984; Chaisson et al., 1987; Murray et al., 1987; Sunderam et al., 1986; Slutkin et al., 1988). Consequently, worldwide tuberculosis elimination will be seriously affected by HIV infection, particularly in Africa, and also in Asia and Latin America. The extent of the deterioration of the tuberculosis situation as caused by HIV infection cannot yet be reliably estimated, since the natural history of HIV infection is not well understood, neither in humans nor in the community.

However, it is evident that in countries where both tuberculous and HIV infections are prevalent, there is already an increase in new smear-positive, smear-negative, and extrapulmonary tuberculous cases. There is no doubt that the tuberculosis situation will continue to deteriorate for a number of years.

A. Effect of Human Immunodeficiency Virus Infection on the Epidemiological Situation of Tuberculosis

The progressive immunodeficiency caused by HIV infection may lead to an increase in tuberculosis incidence in three ways: first, by the multiplication of tubercle bacilli in quiescent foci after a remote tuberculous infection; second, through progression of a recent tuberculous infection to the disease among HIV-positive subjects whose progressive immunodeficiency substantially increases the breakdown rate to tuberculous disease; third, through superinfection with tubercle bacilli. This is less likely than the first two.

In contrast to developed countries, the last two causes for the excess incidence of tuberculosis in developing countries may result in a considerable number of tuberculous cases among HIV-infected subjects. Even so, in such countries, most of the tuberculosis in HIV-infected individuals is attributable to endogenous reactivation of a remote tuberculous infection.

Technically Advanced Countries

The decrease in the risk of tuberculous infection during the last 50 years has been so rapid in these countries that a steadily increasing number of persons up to the age of 50 are free from tuberculous infection. The current risk of tuberculous infection is low and continuously decreasing. Consequently, HIV infection, acquired mostly by those aged 20–50 years, will occur in a relatively small proportion of persons infected with tubercle bacilli. Therefore, HIV infection will not cause the epidemiological situation in these countries to deteriorate.

Developing Countries

In developing countries, most notably those in sub-Saharan Africa in which the prevalence of tuberculous infection in persons aged 20–50 years is relatively high (40–50%) and HIV infection is also prevalent (more than 2% HIV-infected in the general population), the excess incidence of tuberculosis caused by HIV infection is evident and continuously increasing (Styblo and Enarson, 1991). In several African countries, one-quarter to one-third of smear-positive cases detected in the entire country could be due to HIV infection.

Although a sharp increase in tuberculosis incidence has been observed in several developing countries with the prevalent dual infection, it is very probable that the transmission of tuberculosis will not increase accordingly. However, if the current risk of tuberculous infection is high and the annual decrease in the risk is low, the extra infectious tuberculous cases attributable to HIV will gradually increase the risk of infection. If a substantial decrease in the risk of infection is achieved by an efficient case-finding program and by a high cure rate for smear-positive cases, the increase in the risk of infection caused by HIV infection might be contained or considerably reduced.

B. Curtailing the Effect of Human Immunodeficiency Virus Infection on the Epidemiological Situation of Tuberculosis

There are two methods of curtailing the effect of HIV infection on the epidemiological situation of tuberculosis: (1) prevention of tuberculosis in HIV-infected persons by preventive chemotherapy, and (2) curtailing transmission of tuberculous infection in the community by an efficient case-finding and treatment program. The latter item will be discussed first.

Curtailing Transmission of Tuberculous Infection in the Community

Currently, the most important tool required to curtail the impact of HIV infection on the epidemiological situation of tuberculosis is scrupulous maintenance of a high detection and cure rate of smear-positive cases of tuberculosis. Tuberculous patients who have been infected with HIV usually respond well to short-course chemotherapy and can be cured as quickly as HIV-negative patients. However, their clinical improvement is frequently a great deal less pronounced than that of HIV-negative tuberculous patients. The HIV-infected tuberculous patients are more likely to die while receiving treatment for tuberculosis than are patients without HIV. Thus, in countries with a high prevalence of dual infection, the fatality rate for tuberculosis is rising. In reviewing patients with dual infection, it is frequently observed that those who die while receiving treatment do so after sputum conversion, when their tuberculosis has improved bacteriologically and clinically (Mohammed et al., 1990).

Among patients who survive treatment, response to therapy does not appear to differ, whether the patient is infected with HIV or not (Chaisson et al., 1987). In IUATLD-assisted NTPs in which HIV prevalence has been rapidly rising, rates of sputum conversion have not changed and appear to be the same in districts with a high prevalence of HIV infection as in districts where HIV infection is uncommon. Since the life expectancy after completion of treatment of patients with HIV infection is relatively short, the likelihood of relapse is necessarily reduced.

While receiving treatment for tuberculosis, adverse reactions to medications have been noted to be more common among those who are HIV-positive. This is especially true in developing countries in which resources are limited and programs must use amithiozone (thioacetazone).

The safety of staff and of other patients is a matter for consideration when HIV infection is common. It is extremely important when injections (for example, streptomycin) are given, or when blood from such patients is handled, that proper sterilization and disposal procedures for hazardous materials be strictly practiced.

Diagnosis of tuberculosis in HIV-infected persons may be difficult in other than smear-positive cases. The principal presenting features of patients with AIDS are relatively nonspecific. However, in most cases, there is pulmonary involvement, and in a high proportion of cases this is infectious (sputum smear-positive). Such cases can be diagnosed, by smear microscopy and form the most important group of tuberculous patients resulting from HIV infection, because of their infectious potential. Among smear-negative cases, some studies from developed countries have indicated that atypical radiographic appearances are more frequent (Reichman, 1988).

Since many smear-negative tuberculous cases among HIV-infected persons are culture-positive or culture-negative, it is necessary, whenever possible, to improve case-finding of smear-negative tuberculous cases. At present, the most suitable method is screening patients suspected of having tuberculosis by x-ray films of the chest, and to examine those with a positive x-ray film by sputum microscopy and, if possible, by culture for the tubercle bacilli. It is probable that the transmission of infection can be considerably curbed in a well-run case-finding and treatment program.

Prevention of Tuberculosis in Human Immunodeficiency Virus–Infected Persons

Since HIV infection is the greatest risk factor in the development of tuberculosis, this group should benefit from preventive chemotherapy. Although the efficacy of preventive chemotherapy with isoniazid has been well established in non–HIV-infected subjects in numerous controlled trials, there is virtually no evidence on the efficacy of preventive chemotherapy for tuberculous infection in dually infected subjects. A consultation on preventive chemotherapy among HIV-infected persons was held by WHO in Geneva early in 1990, and guidelines for efficacy study protocols were promulgated. However, even if preventive chemotherapy can be shown to be efficacious in preventing tuberculosis in HIV-infected individuals, the likelihood that it could be implemented efficiently in the poorest developing countries, where HIV infection is common, is questionable. The increasing burden of patients with tuberculosis caused by HIV infection requiring treatment, is beginning to put stress on the limited capacity of even well-organized treatment programs. Moreover, the screening of the population for HIV infection is likely to be prohibitive in cost, manpower, and logistics.

Management of Excess Tuberculous Cases Caused by Human Immunodeficiency Virus Infection

In the developing countries with a high prevalence of HIV infection, proper management of excess tuberculous cases is very difficult in large cities. The personnel dealing with tuberculous patients, and especially with those enrolled on outpatient chemotherapy, have become overstretched.

Operational research is urgently needed to explore how to cope with the substantial and continuing increase in tuberculous cases in large cities, until the epidemic of HIV infection in a given population eventually stabilizes or starts to decrease.

Appendix

Recording and Reporting

1.   The most important document in the system is the *District Tuberculosis Register*, which is kept by the district tuberculosis coordinator. The register contains:

The type of tuberculosis (pulmonary, extrapulmonary)

Classification of the case (new, relapse, transferred in from elsewhere, treatment after return from defaulting, other)

Results of sputum smear examinations and laboratory numbers of the examinations: at 0, 2 (3 months for retreatment cases), 5, and 8 months in patients enrolled on the 8-month short-course regimen for new cases and retreatment cases [and at 0, 5 (8), and 12 months in patients put on the 12-month regimen].

Results of treatment:

Cured (smear-negative at 5 and 8 months in patients enrolled on short-course chemotherapy; at 8 and 12 months in those enrolled on the 12-month regimen)

Treatment completed (no bacteriological results)

Died while receiving treatment

Smear-positive at 5 months or later during treatment

Lost to follow-up (defaulter)

Transferred out to another district

2.   The *tuberculosis treatment card* is kept at every health unit at which treatment is given. It is kept for every patient under treatment within the framework of the NTP. The card includes type of treatment and dosage of drugs during the intensive and continuation phases; records on injections of streptomycin (record should be entered on the card immediately after the injection has been given); dates of drug collection; and clinical notes.

3.   The *patient's identity card* is kept by the patient. It should contain name, age, sex, and address of the patient; name of health unit; health unit identification number; Tuberculosis Register number; type of tuberculosis and initial bacteriology; start of treatment (date); regimen used; and space for dates of appointments.

4.   The *tuberculosis laboratory register* is kept at laboratories carrying out sputum examination for tubercle bacilli. For every smear examined, the required information must be entered by the microscopist or technician who carries out the smear examination. The register should contain the serial number of the sputum smear; the date of examination; the name and address of the patient; the name of the health unit requiring the examination; information on whether the examination is requested for diagnosis or for follow-up of chemotherapy; and the result of examination.

The register gives information on the number of suspects examined, the number of smear-positive cases detected, and the number and results of smear examinations for follow-up of treatment. The district tuberculosis coordinator must regularly check (every 2 weeks the district laboratory and every month the chest clinic laboratories) to determine if all cases with positive smears in the tuberculosis laboratory register have been enrolled on chemotherapy and entered in the District Tuberculosis Register.

5. *Request form for sputum examination* is kept at all health units. It contains name of the health unit requesting examination and date of the request; patient's name, age, sex, address, type of tuberculosis (pulmonary, extrapulmonary); reason for the examination (diagnosis or follow-up of chemotherapy); specimen identification number and health unit identification number (sputum for diagnosis) or District Tuberculosis Register number (sputum for follow-up of treatment); data of sputum collection and results of examination (to be completed by a laboratory technician).

6. *Request form for culture and sensitivity tests of M.tuberculosis*: This form is kept in hospitals and is usually designed by the central tuberculosis unit and the reference laboratory.

7. The *quarterly report on new cases and relapses* is kept by the district tuberculosis coordinator.

8. The *quarterly report on results of treatment of smear-positive cases of pulmonary tuberculosis registered 12–15 months earlier* is kept by the district tuberculosis coordinator.

The quarterly reports are completed by district tuberculosis coordinators and collected and checked by regional tuberculosis coordinators who submit these 3-month summary statistics to the CTU. The forms are computerized at the CTU for easy retrieval and for production of reports on national, regional, and district occurrence of tuberculosis, as well as program performance indices on treatment in regions and nationwide.

References

Bleiker, M. A., Chum, H. J., Nkinda, S. J., and Styblo, K. (1987). Tanzania National Tuberculin Survey, 1983–1986. In *Tuberculosis and Respiratory Diseases*. Professional Postgraduate Services, Singapore.

Crofton, J. (1962). The contribution of treatment to the prevention of tuberculosis. *Bull. Int. Union Tuberc.* **32**:643–653.

Chaisson, R. E, Schecter, G. F., Theurer, C. P., et al. (1987). Tuberculosis in patients with the acquired immunodeficiency syndrome. *Am. Rev. Respir. Dis.* **136**:570–574.

Fellows, D. S. (1934). Mortality in the native races of the Territory of Alaska, with special reference to tuberculosis. *Public Health Rep.* **49**:289–299.

Frost, W. H. (1937). How much control of tuberculosis? *Am. J. Public Health* **271**:759–766.

Mohammed, A., Lwechungura, S., Chum, H. J., Styblo, K., and Broekmans, J. F. (1990). Excess fatality rate after sputum conversion of new smear-positive patients enrolled on short-course chemotherapy in a country with prevalent HIV infection. Presented at the *World Conference on Lung Health*, Boston.

Murray, C. J. L., Styblo, K., and Rouillon, A. (1990). Tuberculosis in developing countries: Burden, intervention and cost. *Bull. Int. Union Tuberc.* **65**:1–20

Murray, J. F., Garay, S. M., Hopewell, P. C., et al. (1987). Pulmonary complications of the acquired immunodeficiency syndrome: An update. *Am. Rev. Respir. Dis.* **135**:504–509.

Nakajima, H. (1990). Address at the World Conference on Lung Health, Boston 1990. *Bull. Int. Union Tuberc.* **65**:8–9.

Pitchenik, A. E., Cole, C., Russel, B. W., et al. (1984). Tuberculosis, atypical mycobacteriosis and the acquired immunodeficiency syndrome among Haitian and non-Haitian patients in South Florida. *Ann. Intern. Med.* **101**:641–645.

Reichman, L. B. (1988). HIV infection—a new face of tuberculosis. *Bull. Int. Union Tuberc.* **63**:19–26.

Roelsgaard, E., Iversen, W. E., and Blocher, C. (1964). Tuberculosis in tropical Africa. *Bull. WHO* **30**:459–518.

Slutkin, G., Leowski, J., and Mann, J. (1988). The effects of the AIDS epidemic on the tuberculosis problem and tuberculosis programmes. Presented at the *First International Conference on the Global Impact of AIDS*. London.

Styblo, K. (1984). Epidemiology of tuberculosis. In: *Infektionskrankheiten und ihre Erreger, Band 4/VI. Mykobakteria und mykobakteriellen Krankheiten.* Edited by G. Meissner, Gustav Fischer Verlag, Jena, pp. 78–161. [Slightly revised and expanded. In *Selected Papers* (1991). Edited by the Royal Netherlands Tuberculosis Association. P.O. Box 146, 2501 CC The Hague, Netherlands.]

Styblo, K. (1985). The relationship between the risk of tuberculosis infection and the risk of developing infectious tuberculosis. *Bull. Int. Union Tuberc.* **60**:117–119.

Styblo, K. (1986). Tuberculosis control and surveillance. In *Recent Advances in Respiratory Medicine*, Vol. 4. Edited by D. S. Flenley and T. L. Petty. Churchill-Livingstone, Edinburgh, pp. 77–108.

Styblo, K. (1990). The elimination of tuberculosis in the Netherlands. *Bull. Int. Union Tuberc.* **65**:49–55.

Styblo, K., and Enarson, D. A. (1991). The impact of infection with human immunodeficiency virus on tuberculosis. In: *Recent Advances in Respiratory Medicine*. Edited by D. M. Mitchell. Churchill-Livingstone, Edinburgh.

Styblo, K., and Meijer, J. (1976). Impact of BCG vaccination programmes in children and young adults on the tuberculosis problem. *Tubercle* **57**:17–43.

Styblo, K., and Meijer, J. (1978). Recent advances in tuberculosis epidemiology with regard to formulation or readjustment of control programmes. *Bull. Int. Union Tuberc.* **53**:283–294.

Sunderam, G., McDonald, R. J., Maniatis, T., et al. (1986). Tuberculosis as manifestation of the acquired immunodeficiency syndrome (AIDS). *JAMA* **256**:362–366.

World Health Organization (1954). *Mass BCG Vaccination Campaigns, 1948–1949.* WHO, Copenhagen, Denmark.

World Health Organization (1974). WHO Expert Committee on Tuberculosis. Ninth report. *Tech. Rep. Ser.* **552**, WHO, Geneva.

World Health Organization (1982). Tuberculosis control. Report on a joint IUAT/WHO study group. *Tech. Rep. Ser.* **671**, WHO, Geneva.

World Health Organization (1991a) Tuberculosis control programme. Report of the first meeting of the coordination, advisory and review group. WHO, Geneva. WHO/TB/Carg(C1)/91.

World Health Organization (1991b). Guidelines for tuberculosis treatment in adults and children in national tuberculosis programmes. WHO, Geneva.

27

Evaluation of Applied Strategies of Tuberculosis Control in the Developing World

Pierre Chaulet and Noureddine Zidouni

Hôpital de Beni Messous
Centre Hospitalier Universitaire d'Alger-Ouest
Algiers, Algeria

I. Introduction

In 1991, the World Health Organization (WHO) developed a new strategy for global tuberculosis (TB) control that centers on targets for case finding and treatment.

Case finding: to detect on average 70% of all sputum smear-positive cases worldwide by the year 2000, with targets of 60 and 85% for low- and intermediate-income countries, respectively.

Treatment: to cure at least 85% of all sputum smear-positive cases detected worldwide by the year 2000. In low-prevalence countries the target is set at 95% (Kochi, 1991).

However, health programs, especially national tuberculosis programs, vary from country to country and within countries. This is partly explained by the considerable differences in the financial resources available for health programs worldwide. (World Bank, 1990, 1991) (Table 1). The differences in gross national product (GNP) and governmental expenditure per capita for health are, in part, responsible for the unevenness of public health services and are why, in spite of the simplification and the relatively low cost of standardized technical

Table 1 Governmental Health Expenditure per Capita in Different Groups of Countries Classified by GNP per Capita

Groups of countries	Population per millions 1989[a]	GNP per capita in USD 1989[a]	Governmental health expenditure per capita in USD 1988[b]
Low-income countries			
Total	2,948.4	330	2
China	1,113.9	350	3
India	832.5	340	1
Others	1,002	300	1.9
Intermediate-income countries			
Total	1,104.5	2,040	23
Lower part	681.8	1,360	8.5
Upper part	422.7	3,150	43
High-income countries	830.4	18,330	612

Source: [a]World Bank (1991); [b]World Bank (1990).

measures recommended against tuberculosis, the targets set in the new WHO strategy will be different country by country.

In each country, program managers must have the ability to evaluate the results of case-finding and treatment activities of national tuberculosis programs (NTP) according to fixed or expected objectives. To offer optimal health coverage to the population, to direct these activities toward the most exposed population groups, to choose the most adaptable technical organizational measures, to provide the necessary staff, adequate financial resources must be made available to meet these goals. Therefore, the evaluation of the strategies of a NTP must be constantly adapted to the real and prevailing conditions of the NTP. Thus, there may not be one, but many, evaluation methods that can be selected according to the objectives, the epidemiological situation, and the historical development of the program to be examined.

II. Evaluation of Applied Strategies for Tuberculosis Treatment

A. Basic Method: The Patient Cohort Analysis

The fundamental method that can be applied is the cohort analysis of patients with pulmonary tuberculosis. Cases of extrapulmonary tuberculosis do not form a homogeneous enough group because the criteria for diagnosis and cure are different according to the localization of the disease.

Cases of pulmonary tuberculosis are classified according to the bacteriological status before and after treatment for those who are still available for analysis. Comparison of the bacteriological data at the beginning and the end of treatment will assist in the evaluation of the results of the applied treatment strategy.

Prerequisite Conditions for a Cohort Analysis

Registration of All Tuberculosis Cases by Chronologic Order in Each Health District of the Country

The tuberculosis register, which is standardized at the national level, must identify new cases and previously treated cases in each district according to their initial bacteriological status.

Laboratory Services

Each district where tuberculosis treatment is applied must have access to a laboratory for microscopy and if possible culture. The procedures within these laboratory services must be standardized and quality-controlled from a central source. If quality control of routine procedures used in these laboratories cannot be assured, the evaluation will lose its validity. For the cohort to be assessed, it is better to have a reference laboratory at the district level to control the microscopic examinations made and to eventually perform cultures. A single control reference laboratory is needed to analyze treatment results according to the initial sensitivity of strains isolated from the patient. These results will greatly influence the evaluation of the program (Bignall, 1979).

What Is a Cohort?

Among pulmonary tuberculosis patients, a *cohort* may be defined by the initial bacteriological status and the past tuberculosis treatment history of each patient. The following groups can be included:

1. All new smear-positive cases (this is the cohort most often selected).

2. All new cases analyzed according to three subpopulations: smear-positive, culture-positive cases only, cases without initial bacteriological confirmation; old cases (previously treated) with new positive bacteriological smears or cultures are another group. In this latter group when retreatment is undertaken, it must be analyzed separately from the other groups because the chemotherapeutic regimen is usually different from the regimen given to new cases, often because of the measured or presumed bacterial resistance.

Patient cohorts may be defined for all patients recorded consecutively, or by a representative sample of these patients.

Strategy for Cohort Analysis

The analysis of patient cohorts may be made at the end of an allocated period of chemotherapy or after a defined period of the assessment of relapses that might have occurred during the posttreatment phase.

Whatever the selected date for the final analysis, the essential criteria include the final bacteriological status of these patients according to the duration and type of chemotherapy actually received by them.

The patient cohort may be divided into six main groups the definition of which is in line with the definition of WHO (Tuberculosis Unit, WHO, 1991b). These are the following:

1. Patients who have received an adequate treatment regimen and who have two bacteriologically negative sputum specimens (microscopy or culture) at the end of the treatment period or at the end of a defined period of follow-up after treatment.

2. Patients known to be alive who received a complete course of chemotherapy without bacteriological control (or with a single negative result) at the end of treatment or a defined period of follow-up.

3. Patients who have two positive bacteriological results beyond the fifth month of treatment.

4. Patients who died during chemotherapy or after the end of chemotherapy (of tuberculosis, another, or an unknown cause).

5. Patients lost during treatment; that is, those who have failed to adhere to their treatment regimen for more than 1 month or those who did not take their monthly supply of medications for 2 months consecutively. Among these patients, those who are traced later and treated again are analyzed separately.

6. Patients transferred out during treatment to another health facility or to another district.

B. Methods of Evaluation

Several methods of evaluation may be used, such as retrospective or prospective studies. Retrospective studies may provide an accurate picture of treatment results in routine practice, but this implies the existence of a recording system of basic information about the diagnosis and the treatment in all districts of the country under evaluation. Prospective studies are more accurate because they allow a description of all the desired information and the method for collecting and analyzing this information before the onset of the study.

Retrospective Studies

Two types are useful: exhaustive or study on a sample.

The Exhaustive Study

The exhaustive study is the simplest procedure and is applied in national programs supported by the International Union Against Tuberculosis and Lung Disease (IUATLD) (Styblo, 1987a,b) and is now recommended for monitoring tuberculosis programs by WHO (Tuberculosis Unit WHO, 1991a). It consists of collecting data, from each district, on results recorded for patients admitted for treatment during the corresponding quarter of a preceding year. This allows a sufficient delay to occur between the presumed date of the end of treatment and the time that the necessary information is gathered to classify patients according to their respective status at the end of the treatment. The cohort of patients assessed at the end of treatment must be consistent so that the original criteria for assigning an individual patient to a particular cohort were the same at the beginning and at the end of treatment.

This type of evaluation is the easiest and simplest to undertake. Nevertheless, numerous biases limit its validity. The first bias may be introduced when data are collected from district registers. Errors may creep in during the listing of the individual patient, including demographic data and dates of the beginning and the end of treatment. There may be errors in patient selection, distribution to the various cohorts, overestimation of smear-positive cases, underestimation of smear-negative cases and those without bacteriological examination. Confusion may exist between patients who are cured and those who have received a complete course of treatment, but without bacteriological confirmation at the end of treatment and between those who are lost from follow-up or have transferred out.

These errors are more frequent when the evaluation might be perceived to have an influence on health staff activities and eventual professional promotion. This risk can be reduced when the data are collected by independent inquirers or supervisors coming from a higher administrative level (Chaulet and Zidouni, 1989).

The second bias might be introduced when information about treatment actually received by patients is placed on their individual files. Accurate information may often be absent or incomplete. The treatment card does not always prove that the drugs, as recorded, have been distributed or taken by the patients. The risk of inadequate dosages or errors in recording, omission or loss of medication can be reduced by regular supervision (Pan-American Health Organization, 1986).

The third bias may be due to the unequal quality of the results provided by the microscopy laboratory in the districts. This bias can be reduced by centrally organizing a permanent quality control system of laboratories.

Results of one 8-month chemotherapy regimen given to new smear-positive pulmonary tuberculosis cases were assessed in six national programs supported by IUATLD between 1983 and 1985. The cure rate was usually higher than 85% when patients who died or transferred out were excluded from the analysis (Table 2) (Styblo, 1991; Gninafon, 1989; Idukitta and Bosman, 1989; Arguello, et al. 1989). (See Table 2.)

The Retrospective Study on a Sample

The retrospective procedure is a variation of the previous one. It is applied when monitoring that is based on a quarterly report is not possible. Here, the patient cohort comprises a representative sample of patients treated in the health services of a country or a province; for example, all new pulmonary tuberculosis cases, consecutively recorded during a quarter in each of the districts, randomized from lists of urban and rural districts, and classified according to the population covered (IUAT, 1978; Bignall, 1979).

By analyzing between 500 and 1500 patients in a limited number of districts, independent inquirers from a central health center staff are able to collect these data by themselves, thereby reducing the first bias mentioned previously. Such a procedure may underline differences between districts. For example, in a study in 1985 in Algeria, 52 districts covering 6.6 million people, the cure rate was higher in the 27 districts (covering 3.4 million individuals) where activities were regularly supervised, compared with the other 25 districts (covering 3.2 million individuals) where activities were not supervised (Berkani et al., 1985) (Table 3).

Prospective Studies

The main advantages of prospective studies are as follows:

1. Centralization of bacteriological samples before, during, and after treatment, allowing the investigators to obtain realistic comparative and complete results including culture and sensitivity testing

2. The permanent collection of information at the beginning, during, and at the end of treatment by independent investigators

3. Centralized reading of chest x-ray films made before and after treatment by an independent reader

4. The assessment of the proportion of smear-positive, culture-positive, smear- or culture-negative cases admitted for study

5. The presence of bacteriological resistance, either primary or acquired

6. The status of patients 1 year after treatment or later according to actual treatment and sensitivity-testing reports received

Table 2 Treatment Results Evaluation of Smear-Positive New Cases Initially Treated By an 8-Month Chemotherapy Regimen Applied in National Tuberculosis Programmes Between 1983 and 1988

Countries	Patients analyzed	Cured	Completed treatment	Still positive cases	Deaths	Lost	Transferred out	Ref.
			Distribution of cases at 8th month (%)					
Tanzania	28,110	77		2	7	10	4	Styblo, 1991
Malawi	6,920	87		2	7	2	2	Styblo, 1991
Mozambique	4,220	78		1	2	11	8	Styblo, 1991
Bénin	1,259	82		2	6	9	1	Gninafon, 1989
Kenya (nomads)	996	57	13.5	0.5	3.5	16	9.5	Idukitta and Bosman, 1989
Nicaragua	1,156	56	20	2	2	16	4	Arguello et al., 1989

Table 3 Treatment Results Evaluation of a National Representative Sample of 719 Tuberculosis Cases Treated by a 6-Month Short Course Chemotherapy Regimen in Algeria: Influence of Supervision on Treatment Results

	Patients analyzed	Patients status at 6 mo after end of treatment (%)					
		Cured	Completed treatment	Still positive cases	Deaths	Lost	Transferred out
Total analyzed	719	63.3	16	2.3	2.2	8.2	8
Districts supervised	503	69.8	13	2.5	2.2	6.5	6
Districts not supervised	216	48.5	22.2	2	2.3	12	13

Source: Berkani et al. (1985).

Prospective Study on a Sample

A representative sample of districts where patient cohorts are admitted, may be randomly selected. The only difference from the retrospective study is that the number of districts selected to be representative at provincial or national level and other criteria are fixed before the study. The criteria include duration of time patients are entered into the study, according to the number of expected patients, which will be based on the sputum specimens that can be obtained during the fixed time and analyzed by a central laboratory.

This method has been applied at regular intervals every 10 years in the same districts in Tanzania (Tanzania–British MRC Collaborative Study, 1985) and in Kenya (East African–British MRC Cooperative Investigation, 1978, 1979; Kenyan–British MRC Cooperative Investigation, 1989). Differences found in these successive studies have been used to assess the evolution of treatment regimens applied in a particular program. In Kenya between 1964 and 1974, an improvement in the results was observed because of the reduction of lost or transferred-out patients and the number of relapses.

The same method, using a simplified protocol, especially without organized chest x-ray examinations and independent readings was tried in three countries in a cooperative study of the IUATLD (Bignall et al., 1979; Leal Gonsalves et al., 1979; Anastasatu et al., 1979; Chaulet et al., 1979).

In spite of their precision and objective nature, prospective studies on a sample have a minor inconvenience. Bias may be introduced in program evaluation by a temporary improvement in the working methods of health staff during the study.

Exhaustive Prospective Study

To reduce the bias as just described, an alternative method of evaluation has been tried (Algerian Working Group–British MRC Cooperative Study, 1991). The cohort to be studied consisted of all new cases of tuberculosis reported over several years in districts of several provinces under regular supervision. Sputum samples from patients were collected, not only before treatment and at the end of treatment, but also for 2 years after the cessation of the prescribed regimen.

Periodic supervision of the activities in the districts during the study permits an evaluation of whether the cohort selected is representative and allows measuring the compliance of patients and physicians. This is accomplished by analyzing the information that has been collected locally concerning what treatment the patient has actually taken. The extension of the follow-up period after treatment may confirm recovery and will assess the number of failures or relapsed cases for those in whom a new course of chemotherapy was thought to be necessary. Centralization of bacteriological samples examination in a single reference laboratory and chest x-ray film readings before and after treatment may help meet the objective criteria for assessment.

In Algeria, to evaluate two short-course chemotherapy regimens of different durations (6 and 8 months) applied under routine conditions of the health services, the bacteriological data collected in a single laboratory were analyzed. This continued for 4 consecutive years in 30 districts covering about 4 million people (Chaulet, 1991; Zidouni and Chaulet, 1991). The cure rate following the 2 years after cessation of treatment of 2218 patients was 86.5% without any major difference between the two short-course regimens used. The percentage of patients who needed an additional course of chemotherapy was 2.3% and the rate of persistent positive cultures (chronic cases) was only 1.5% (Table 4).

Depending on various factors, including the working conditions of the health staff in an intermediate-income country like Algeria, this type of study is limited by some constraints:

1.   The districts must be situated less than 200 km from the reference central laboratory.

Table 4   Treatment Results Evaluation of Smear-Positive New Cases Initially Treated by Short-Course Chemotherapy Regimens in National Program Conditions (6 mo and 8 mo)

Results 2 yrs after end of chemotherapy	Regimen initially prescribed				Patients analyed	
	6 mo		8 mo			
	N	%	N	%	N	%
Negative cultures						
After 18th mo	678 (16)	69	810 (18)	66	1488 (34)	67
Between end of treatment and 18th mo	174 (3)	18	258 (4)	20	432 (7)	19.5
Completed treatment without control since end of treatment	66	7	101 (1)	8	167 (1)	7.5
Positive cultures when last seen after end of treatment	13 (2)	1	22 (7)	2	35 (9)	1.5
Deaths	46	5	50	4	96	4.5
Total	977 (21)	100	1241 (30)	100	2218 (51)	100

Numbers in parenthesis refer to patients who have received additional course of chemotherapy for failure, relapse, or development of a nonpulmonary lesion.
Source: Adapted from Algerian Working Group–British Medical Research Council Cooperative Study (1991).

2. A research team of two or three persons must be specially constituted to ensure supervision of tasks during the entire study, and a special budget is needed.

C. Results of the Evaluation of the Treatment of New Pulmonary Tuberculosis Cases

Whatever strategies are used, the results of the evaluation of the treatment of new cases of pulmonary tuberculosis depends on the quality of chemotherapy applied in the national program. Since the early 1980s, the introduction of rifampin in association with other drugs in initial treatment regimens has strengthened all chemotherapy regimens. All evaluation studies agree; cure rates between 80 and 87% can be reached in antituberculous programs in low- and intermediate-income countries (Chaulet, 1990). A cure rate of 85% of new cases of sputum smear-positive pulmonary tuberculosis is now an attainable target in every program when the following two conditions are met:

1. Widespread implementation of short-course chemotherapy regimens of either 6 or 8 months for all new cases of pulmonary tuberculosis.

2. A simultaneous undertaking to develop measures to ensure the compliance of patients and physicians during the treatment phase. This includes standardization of working procedures, regular supervision of health staff activities, dissemination of information, and health education of patients and families.

III. Problems Encountered in Cohort Analysis of "Old" Cases

With the introduction of the more extensive use of rifampin in association with isoniazid in the initial treatment of tuberculosis, failures are less common. When acquired bacterial resistance of previously treated patients is measured, it is now less frequent than in the past, but it may be more serious for the particular subpopulation affected, especially if the organisms are resistant to both isoniazid and rifampin.

A. Bacterial Resistance of "Old" Cases

This situation has been observed in Korea during national prevalence studies (Kim and Hong, 1991). In a 1990 study, the acquired resistance rate was 38.5%. Patients with resistant bacilli to both isoniazid and rifampin represented 15.4% of previously treated patients (Table 5).

In Algeria after 10 years of initial treatment based on 6-month regimens containing isoniazid and rifampin, the acquired resistance rate was 21% for the

Table 5 Evolution of Acquired Bacterial Resistance During National Prevalence Studies in Korea (1965–1990)

Year of prevalence study	Old cases tested	Resistant strains to at least one drug		Resistant strains rate (%)	
		N	%	to INH	to INH and RIF
1965	29	16	55.2	37.9	0
1970	40	28	70	70	0
1975	81	60	74.1	72.8	1.2
1980	69	52	75.4	72.5	4.3
1985	86	48	55.8	47.7	19.8
1990	52	20	38.5	36.5	15.4

Source: Kim and Hong (1991).

most recent period (Boulahbal et al., 1989, 1991). In this cohort, patients with bacilli resistant to both isoniazid and rifampin represented 11.5% of the previously treated patient cohort (Table 6). Similar trends were observed in Tanzania after the introduction of an initial standardized 8-month regimen with rifampin during the first 2 months (Chonde, 1989) (Table 6). Therefore, among previously treated patients who require retreatment, three groups can be identified for whom the retreatment regimen may have to be altered.

1. The patient whose organisms are still sensitive to both major antibiotics, isoniazid and rifampin
2. Patients whose organisms are still sensitive to rifampin but resistant to isoniazid
3. Patients whose organisms are resistant to both isoniazid and rifampin

In a review of relapsed cases in Algeria, records from one clinic were reviewed. The source of patients to this clinic came from several provinces of the country. All of these patients received a second course of chemotherapy containing isoniazid and rifampin, according to applied national standards. Among patients previously treated with isoniazid and rifampin, acquired bacterial resistance is more frequent and more severe according to the number of courses of treatment that the patients have undergone (Table 7) (Mazouni et al., 1992) (Table 7).

In developing strategies for the treatment of tuberculosis, acquired resistance can be prevented by better organization of primary chemotherapy, based on the most efficient drugs available, and ensuring patient compliance.

Table 6 Evolution of Acquired Bacterial Resistance According to Chemotherapy Applied Routinely in Algeria (1965–1990)

Period	Analyzed cases tested strains	Resistant strains to at least one drug		% of resistant strains to at least isoniazid and rifampin
		N	%	
1965–67 Chemotherapy not standardized	858	703	81.9	0
1975–80 Chemotherapy standardized (rifampin reserved to retreatment)	1480	917	61.5	2.7
1981–85 Chemotherapy standardized (rifampin for all patients)	406	145	35.7	11
1986–90 Chemotherapy standardized (rifampin for all patients)	408	86	21	11.5

Source: Adapted from F. Boulahbal et al. (1989); and Boulahbal, F., personal communication, 1991.

B. Evaluation of Standardized Chemotherapy Strategies for Previously Treated Patients

Old Cases

Those patients who have undergone one previous course of chemotherapy are considered *old patients*. The WHO guidelines for tuberculosis treatment (Tuberculosis Unit, WHO, 1991a) recommend a realistic strategy for the standard retreatment of old cases to limit acquired resistance. The standardized retreatment protocol includes a regimen consisting of isoniazid, rifampin, and ethambutol for 8 months, given daily for the first 3 months and then every day or three-times per week for the last 5 months. There should be an initial supplement of pyrazinamide for the first 3 months and streptomycin for the first 2 months.

The strategy of standardized retreatment chemotherapy has been evaluated in Tanzania (Chum, 1989), in Mozambique (Salomao and Parkalli, 1989), in Malawi (Salaniponi, 1989), and in Benin (Gninafon, 1989). The cure rate of patients still under follow-up appears to be higher than 80% in these studies (Table 8).

Table 7 Frequency and Severity of Acquired Bacterial Resistance in 81 Patients Previously Treated by One or Several Short-Course Chemotherapy Regimen with Isoniazid and Rifampin (Algeria, 1992)

Number of chemotherapy courses received by patients	Number of analyzed cases	Resistant strains to at least one drug		Specific resistance of strains					
		N	%	SM	INH	INH + SM	At least INH + RIF	
							N	%
One course	27	9	33	1	0	2	6	22
Two course	22	14	64	1	1	0	12	55
Three or more	32	32	100	0	0	1	31	97
Total	81	55	68	2	1	3	49	60

Source: Mazouni, L., 1992.

Table 8 Results of 8-m Standardized Retreatment in Smear-Positive Patients Previously Treated by a First Short-Course Chemotherapy Regimen

Country	Author (yr)	Patients analyzed	% Patients according to their bacteriological status					
			Negative cured	Completed treatment	Still positive	Deaths	Lost	Transferred out
Tanzania	Chum (1989)	2074	73		4	6	14	3
Mozambique	Salomao (1989)	1137	70		3	3	16	8
Malawi	Salaniponi (1989)	772	88		1	5	2	4
Bénin	Gninafon (1989)	135	85		3	3	9	
Nicaragua	Arguello (1989)	259	44	10	10	4	29	3

Chronic Cases

The prognosis is poor for cases of tuberculosis who have received more than two complete courses of antituberculous chemotherapy containing isoniazid and rifampin. In these cases, the risk of acquired resistance to isoniazid and rifampin is extremely high. In truth, however, there are very few developing countries in which reliable sensitivity testing can be performed and in which available resources to purchase second-line drugs are likely (Tuberculosis Unit WHO, 1991a).

Although cases that have been treated with two or more chemotherapy courses are infrequent, their epidemiological significance is important. Therefore, their number must always be measured so that all technical and organizational aspects of a program are implemented to prevent the emergence of these cases and to prevent the spread of resistant organisms in the community.

IV. Evaluation of Tuberculosis Case-Finding Strategies

Because of the diversity of the socioeconomic and epidemiological situations in developing countries, evaluation methods for tuberculosis case-finding strategies are necessarily different. Whatever the situation, evaluation of tuberculosis case-finding is based on gathering three pieces of accurate data: the total number and the demographics of the population; the number of new cases of pulmonary tuberculosis notified; and the annual risk of infection.

Demographic Data

Statistics for the average population by sex and age act as denominators to calculate rates. These data must be collected for every district. Additional information such as the makeup of ethnic minorities, the socially underprivileged, the number of migrant workers and refugees, and the part-time workers is usually very useful.

Tuberculosis Register

The tuberculosis register of each district is the essential support for the epidemiological information. All tuberculosis cases identified and living in the district must be recorded. This information may be easier to obtain when private medical services are underdeveloped or absent, as the recording of a case by the public health service will be the only way the patient has of obtaining free treatment. In urban areas of some developing countries in which the private medical and pharmaceutical sectors are active, the significance of recorded data will be limited to the population covered by the public health service. According to the WHO Tuberculosis Unit, a tuberculosis register must identify the following:

1. New cases of pulmonary tuberculosis (i.e., those who have never been previously treated or have been treated for less than 1 month who are either smear-positive or culture-positive only, or smear-negative).

2. New cases of extrapulmonary tuberculosis.

3. Pulmonary and extrapulmonary tuberculosis cases transferred to the district during treatment, and whose treatment was begun in other districts.

4. Old cases of pulmonary tuberculosis previously treated for whom a new course of chemotherapy was begun and whether they were smear- or culture-positive or both. Old cases may be one of the following:

   a. False-failures: those who received more than 1 month but less than 5 months of chemotherapy and who interrupted their treatment before a fixed completion date. These cases should be recorded once more as "treatment taken again after interruption."

   b. True-failures: those cases observed beyond the fifth month of treatment in the last months at the end of the first chemotherapy course.

   c. Relapses: these are usually observed during the 3 years following the end of treatment in patients considered as cured at the end of the first chemotherapy course.

   d. Chronic cases: those who have received at least two complete chemotherapy courses.

Discrimination between these different groups of patients is important because alternative therapeutic decisions must be taken for each group. It is also important for the epidemiological analysis, since the declared incidence of smear-positive pulmonary tuberculosis cases directly reflects on the results of applied case-finding strategies.

Annual Risk of Infection

The method of calculating the annual risk of tuberculous infection has been described previously (Bleiker et al., 1989; Bleiker, 1991). It has been agreed that for an annual risk of infection of 1%, the average annual incidence of smear-positive pulmonary tuberculosis is 49 cases per 100,000 population, with a confidence limit of 95% (Murray et al., 1990). This enables one to calculate an expected incidence and compare it with the observed incidence. In spite of the apparent simplicity of this method, the relation between the annual risk of infection and the incidence of notified cases is not always easy to establish, since the calculated annual risk of infection is not always representative of the real situation. In addition, when the risk is less than 1%, the relation with the incidence of tuberculosis is not always constant. Finally, this relation cannot be used in high-HIV infection prevalence countries (Tuberculosis Unit WHO, 1991b).

A. Evaluation of Case-Finding Results in High Tuberculosis Prevalence Countries

In high tuberculosis prevalence countries for which the annual risk of infection is higher than 1%, the evaluation method that compares the incidence of expected contagious tuberculosis cases and the incidence of notified cases is theoretically easiest to apply. Nevertheless, various factors make this evaluation difficult.

Influence of Health Services Coverage

Access of the population to health services for tuberculosis case-finding is very uneven. It is estimated that, in developing countries, available health services for the diagnosis and treatment of tuberculosis covers only 46% of the population on average; 24% in Africa and 88% in the Western Pacific (Table 9). Whether health service coverage of the population for tuberculosis case-finding is adequate depends on several factors that are difficult to control. These include the extension and quality of basic health services to the periphery, the competence of the health staff working in these services, and the ability of outpatient

Table 9 Estimate of Tuberculosis Service Coverage in Developing Countries (1988–1989)

Region	Service coverage (%)
Africa	24
Americas[a]	42
Eastern Mediterranean	70
South East Asia	44
Western Pacific[b]	88
Total	46

[a]Excluding United States and Canada
[b]Excluding China, Australia, Japan, and New Zealand
Source: Kochi (1991)

clinics to select persons for examination who are suspected of having active tuberculosis. In addition, the trust of the population in the health service staff, and the competence of the microscopy laboratory staff to identify the tubercle bacilli are also important. Without quality control of the laboratories, the development of communications, and the means of transport of medications to the periphery, there will be difficulty in ensuring widespread and equal health service coverage. The relation of the number of notified cases to the number of expected cases, therefore, is proportional to the real health services coverage of the population.

Estimation of the Annual Risk of Infection

When tuberculin prevalence studies based on representative samples of schoolchildren are not available, national or provincial risks cannot be calculated. In the same country, considerable differences may exist between rural and urban areas (Table 10). Important errors of evaluation are often made in programs of developing countries when the annual risk of infection is calculated in schoolchildren living in the capital city and adopted as a basic estimation of the annual risk of infection for the entire country.

Table 10 Annual Risk of Tuberculous Infection in Developing Countries Based on Tuberculin Surveys

Countries	Year	Area	Survey	Annual risk of infection
Gambia	1958–59	Bathurst	Sample survey	
			Urban strata	4.43
			Rural strata	1.74
Tanzania	1983–87	18 areas	Sample survey	1.11
		among them:	of schools	
		Kilimanjaro,		0.48
		Mtwara		2.20
Indonesia	1986	Sambas in		1.83
		West Kalamenta;		
		Padany Parvaman		3.07
		in West Sumatra		
	1985	Ogan kamering		3.48
		Illis in South Sumatra		
		Gowain South Sulawesi		3.92

Source: Cauthen et al. (1988).

Table 11   Influence of Supervision Activities of Health Staff on Case-Finding Results

	Health districts ($n=52$)	
	With periodic supervision of activities ($n=27$)	Without periodic supervision of activities ($n=25$)
General population	3.4 million 100,000	3.2 million 100,000
Outpatients attending health service per year	68,578	65,713
Number of smears performed in suspected persons	1,910	1,302
Number of smear-positive pulmonary tuberculosis cases identified	47	24

Source: Berkani et al. (1985).

Supervision activities

In the application of a national tuberculosis program, regular supervision of service activities influences case-finding results considerably. During a retrospective study on a representative national sample of 52 districts in Algeria for the year 1984, case-finding results were compared. Twenty-seven districts covering 3.4 million persons where case-finding activities were regularly supervised during the previous 5 years were compared with 25 districts covering 3.2 million persons where case-finding activities were not supervised. Since 1980, the health staff of these 52 districts used the same technical guide in applying the national program (Berkani et al., 1985). It was observed that the public health services were delivered in out-patient clinics at the same rate to patients in both groups; but, in the supervised group, individuals with suspect tuberculosis were selected at a much greater rate, the number of smear examinations was 46% higher, and the number of cases identified was twice that of the districts where case-finding activities were not supervised (Table 11).

Strategy Target

Whereas the target of the treatment strategy is to a single goal (i.e., a cure rate of 85%), the target of case-finding strategies is dependent on several variables, including the centralization of the health structure, the level of case-finding services available, and the means of communications (Table 12). An estimated case-finding rate of 60–65% of expected cases was fixed as a target in countries

Table 12 New Tuberculosis Control Strategy Targets

	Targets	
Countries	Cure rates (%)	Detection rates (%)
Low-income developing countries with poorly developed health services	85	60–65
Middle-income developing countries with relatively well-developed health service system	85	85
Low tuberculosis prevalence countries	95	NA

NA, Because of the lack of a method to estimate the incidence of tuberculosis when the annual rate of infection becomes low, it is impossible to monitor the case-finding coverage rate.
Source: Adapted from Kochi (1991).

where health services are the least developed and of 85% of expected cases in countries where health services are the most developed.

B. Evaluation of Case-Finding Results in Low- and Intermediate-Prevalence Tuberculosis Countries

In some intermediate-prevalence countries (Middle East, North Africa, South America), the annual risk of tuberculous infection is less than 1%, and health services ensure a total or near complete health coverage of the population. In this context, tuberculin testing studies constitute an element of tuberculosis surveillance, but cannot be used as a basis to evaluate results of case-finding, except in areas or in population groups for which the risk is higher than 1%. Therefore, it is necessary to have several indicators that, taken together, will show whether case-finding for new contagious cases is effective. These include the integration of tuberculous case-finding into the routine activities of the health services. The relative scarceness of tuberculosis in this situation may make integration of tuberculous case-finding a real problem.

The selection of patients suspected of having active tuberculosis depends on the health education of the population and on the confidence and competence of the health care staff, including nurses, auxiliary physicians, and general practitioners. Indeed, the staff must be specially trained to take care of all patients with respiratory symptoms. They must be able to identify and treat those who have acute respiratory symptoms caused by acute respiratory infections of the upper or lower respiratory tract. They must also be able to identify, treat, and eventually refer those who have chronic respiratory diseases, such as asthma, chronic bronchitis, bronchiectasis, occupational lung disease, and so on. Between these groups they must be able to select the few suspected cases of tuberculosis. For these persons, sputum must be collected and examined in the laboratory. The microscopic diagnosis of tuberculosis must be done in the nearest laboratory. But this laboratory must be accessible and reliable; that is, populations of each district of 50,000–300,000 inhabitants must have a laboratory in which quality and working procedures are regularly controlled. X-ray facilities may improve the selection of suspected persons when radiologic facilities are available. Performance indicators must be established, collected, and analyzed in a predetermined time frame.

The simplest indicators to collect are as follows:

1. The number of persons seen in the health services of each district by age and sex

2. The number of sputum examinations made for tuberculosis case-finding in persons who present with suspicious symptoms

3. The number of new pulmonary cases of tuberculosis identified

These three indicators, collected annually in each district and reported per 100,000 population, can measure the eventual increase or decrease of case-finding activities, thereby allowing appropriate corrective measures to be taken (Chaulet, 1975; Pan-American Health Organization, 1986).

Notification of case surveillance at the district level provides a useful item for evaluation when the annual incidence of notified smear-positive cases is fewer than 40:100,000. When program activities are permanently managed over several years, the epidemiological situation progresses slowly in the same district. Inequalities between districts or provinces were observed in some high-income countries (Medical Research Council, Tuberculosis and Chest Diseases Unit, 1986; Center for Disease Control, 1987, 1989, 1991). These differences actually appear in developing countries where the prevalence of tuberculosis is relatively low and where the annual risk of infection is less than 1%.

A proposed pragmatic approach, relying on the results of monitoring, may set an annual target of identifying more than 90% of observed cases during the preceding year, especially in high-prevalence groups that may exist in low-prevalence countries.

V. Evaluation of Strategies and Strategies for Evaluation

Because of the extraordinary diversity in the socioeconomic and epidemiological situations in developing countries, it is necessary to adapt tuberculosis control strategies to the national context of each country.

A. Process for Evaluation

Evaluation strategies measure results reached according to fixed targets. To be objective, they must be performed by individuals who were not involved in the execution of the activities under study and must rely on the data given to them by the health service staff themselves. Thus, the validity of the evaluation methods depends upon the way the activities were supervised. The purpose of supervision is to check on the quality of the activities in the health services and the laboratories in the district (Pan-American Health Organization, 1986).

On the other hand, evaluation gives important data for tuberculosis surveillance in a country. Accurate evaluation of case-finding and treatment results help establish and define epidemiological data-gathering for tuberculous case notification, mortality rates for tuberculosis, incidence of tuberculous meningitis in children younger than 5 years of age, as well as primary and acquired bacterial resistance. But evaluation can be done only if accurate targets are fixed with the help of program surveillance, especially national tuberculin prevalence studies and the evaluation of the incidence curves of smear-positive new cases in each province.

B. Combining Evaluation Methods

To assess results of tuberculosis control strategies applied in a developing country, it is necessary to combine several evaluation methods, according to the level of health service development. Basic data are provided by new tuberculous case notification from the tuberculosis register of each district and by the calculation or the estimation of the annual risk of infection at the national level.

Calculation of case-finding coverage of contagious cases by district, the cure rate of new cases of pulmonary tuberculosis, and relapse cohorts are easy monitoring methods for national program activities. Exhaustive retrospective analysis of whole cohorts or a randomized representative sample of pulmonary tuberculosis in previously untreated cases may help develop strategies to supervise case-finding activities and may help in assessing results of routine case-finding and treatment strategies.

However, in reality, only the prospective analysis of a patient cohort consisting of individuals who were diagnosed and treated, with bacteriological examinations made before and after treatment, will allow the objective assessment of case-finding and cure rates of contagious cases with minimal bias. This procedure will control the validity of the local bacteriological results and may identify the respective proportions of pulmonary tuberculosis smear-positive and smear-negative cases diagnosed and treated by health services. This evaluation should identify treatment failures and suggest what appropriate measures to take.

VI. Conclusion

To undertake a national evaluation of a tuberculosis program in a developing country two steps are required.

There must be permanent monitoring of program activities on the basis of quarterly and annual reports transmitted by the health services of a district to the national authority. This will allow retrospective assessment of case-finding coverage and cure rates. As this is perfected in a single district the process must then be extended progressively to all of the districts of the country for which the program is applied. This procedure often takes place over several years.

Monitoring must be permanently in place and pursued on a regular basis. It will be accomplished by prospective evaluation studies on a representative sample of patients at greater intervals such as every 5–7 years, because the time needed for the preparation and the analysis of each particular study. It is the repetition of such prospective studies that permits the accurate measurement of the effect of strategies on the tuberculous situation in a particular country. The analysis of objective data collected by reliable staff and analyzed by an independent team, using the same methods, will ensure adequate and complete coverage by a national tuberculosis program (Chaulet and Zidouni, 1989).

References

Algerian working Group–British Medical Research Council Cooperative Study (1991). Short course chemotherapy for pulmonary tuberculosis under routine programme conditions: A comparison of regimens of 28 and 36 weeks duration in Algeria. *Tubercle*, **72**:88–100.

Anastasatu, C., Mihailescu, P., Gartner, A., et al. (1979). Enquête nationale d'évaluation de la chimiothérapie de la tuberculose en Roumanie. *Bull. Int. Union Tuberc.* **54**:40–44.

Arguello L., Castillo, O., Chavarria, J., Cuadra, I., and Heldal E. (1989). Chimiothérapie de courte durée de la tuberculose. L'expérience du Nicaragua 1984–1987. *Bull. Int. Union Tuberc.* **64**:48–50.

Bignall, J. R. (1979). Enquête nationale sur les résultats du traitement de la tuberculose en pratique quotidienne. *Bull. Int. Union Tuberc.* **54**:37–38.

Berkani, M., Ait Khaled, N., and Bouchahda, K. (1985). Les mesures techniques de la lutte antituberculeuse. In *L'organisation de la Lutte Antituberculeuse en Algérie*, Vol. 1. Edited by P. Chaulet. Société Algérienne de Pneumo-Phtisiologie, pp. 75–77.

Bleiker, M. A., Sutherland, I, Styblo, K., ten Dam, H. G., and Misljenovic, O. (1989). Règles pour l'estimation des risques d'infection tuberculeuse d'après les résultats du test tuberculinique dans un échantillon représentatif d'enfants. *Bull. Int. Union Tuberc.* **64**:7–14.

Bleiker, M. A. (1991). Le taux annuel d'infection tuberculeuse, l'enquête tuberculinique, et le test tuberculinique. *Bull. Int. Union Tuberc.* **66**: 55–59.

Boulahbal, F., Khaled S., and Tazir, M. (1989). Intérêt de la surveillance de la résistance du bacille tuberculeux pour l'évaluation d'un programme. *Bull. Int. Union Tuberc.* **64**:23–25.

Boulahbal, F., et al. (1991). Personal communication.

Cauthen, G. M., Pio, A., and ten Dam, H. G. (1988). Annual risk of tuberculous infection. WHO/TB/88–154, Geneva.

Centers for Disease Control (1987). Tuberculosis in the United States, 1985–86. CDC, Division of Tuberculosis Control, Atlanta.

Centers for Disease Control (1989). Tuberculosis statistics in the United States 1987. CDC, Division of Tuberculosis Control, Atlanta.

Centers for Disease Control (1991). Tuberculosis statistics in the United States, 1989. CDC, Division of Tuberculosis Control, Atlanta.

Chaulet, P. (1975). L'évaluation pratique d'un réseau de dépistage et de traitement de la tuberculose. *Bull. Int. Union Tuberc.* **50**:57–69.

Chaulet, P., et al. (1979). Les résultats du traitement de la tuberculose pulmonaire en Algérie. *Bull. Int. Union Tuberc.* **54**:44–48.

Chaulet, P. (1990). La lutte antituberculeuse dans le monde: Stratégies et actions sur le terrain. *Respiration* **57**:145–159.

Chaulet, P. (1991). Implementation of short course chemotherapy in Algeria. In *Short Course Chemotherapy for National Tuberculosis Control Programmes in Developing Countries* Vol. 1. Edited by Medicine Publishing Foundation Symposium Series 30, The Medicine Group, Oxford, pp. 15–21.

Chaulet, P. and Zidouni, N. (1989). Methodological problems in evaluating tuberculosis treatment programmes. In *Tuberculosis Surveillance Research Unit of the IUATLD, Progress report 1989*, Vol. 1. Royal Netherlands Tuberculosis Association, The Hague, pp. 66–85.

Chonde, T. M. (1989). Le rôle des services bactériologiques dans le programme national contre la tuberculose et la lèpre en Tanzania. Bull. *Int. Union Tuberc.* **64**: 37–40.

Chum, H. J. (1989). Dix ans de fonctionnement du programme national contre la tuberculose et la lèpre en Tanzanie. Bull. *Int. Union Tuberc.* **64**:34–37.

East African and British Medical Research Council Co-operative Investigation (1970). Tuberculosis in Kenya: A follow-up of a national, sampling survey of drug resistance and other factors. *Tubercle* **51**:1–38.

East African and British Medical Research Council Cooperative Investigation (1979). Tuberculosis in Kenya: Follow-up of the second (1974) national sampling survey and a comparison with the follow up data from the first (1964) national sampling survey. *Tubercle* **60**:125–149.

Gninafon, M. (1989). Evolution du dépistage et du traitement de la tuberculose au cours des 3 dernières années après l'introduction de la chimiothérapie antituberculeuse de courte durée de 8 mois au Bénin. *Bull. Int Union Tuberc.* **64**:43–44.

Idukitta, G. O., and Bosman, M. C. J. (1989). Le projet des Manyattas de la tuberculose pour les nomades du Kenya. *Bull: Int. Union Tuberc.* **64**: 45–48.

International Union Against Tuberculosis and Lung Diseases (1989). Type of collaboration provided by IUATLD national tuberculosis programmes in developing countries. In *Tuberculosis Surveillance Research Unit of the IUATLD Progress report 1989*, Vol 1. pp. 138–140.

International Union Against Tuberculosis and Lung Diseases (1991). *Tuberculosis Guide for High Prevalence Countries*, Vol. 1. Edition de l'Aulne, Paris, 72 pp.

Kenyan–British Medical Research Council Cooperative Investigation (1989). Tuberculosis in Kenya 1984: A third national survey and a comparison with earlier surveys in 1964 and 1974. *Tubercle* **70**:5–20.

Kim, S. J., and Hong, V. P. (1991). Drug resistance of *M. tuberculosis* in Korea. In *Tuberculosis Surveillance Research Unit of the IUATLD, Progress report 1991*, Vol. 1. Royal Netherlands Tuberculosis Association; The Hague, pp. 87–95.

Kochi, A. (1991). The global tuberculosis situation and the new control; strategy of the World Health Organization. *Tubercle* **72**:1–6.

Leal Gonsalves, L., and Cabral, J. (1979) Evaluation du mode de diagnostic et du résultat du traitement au douzième mois dans la pratique de routine au Portugal. *Bull. Int. Union Tuberc.* **54**:38–40.

Mazouni, L., et al. (1992). Treatment of failure and relapse cases of pulmonary tuberculosis within a national programme based on short course chemotherapy. In *Tuberculosis Surveillance Research Unit of the IUAT, Progress report, 1992*, vol. 1, p. 36.

Medical Research Council Tuberculosis and Chest Diseases Unit (1986). The geographical distribution of tuberculosis notifications in a national Survey of England and Wales in 1983. *Tubercle* **67**:163–178.

Murray, C. J. L., Styblo, K., and Rouillon, A. (1990). La tuberculose dans les pays en développement: importance, stratégies de lutte et coût. *Bull. Int. Union Tuberc.* **65**:6–26.

Pan-American Health Organization (1986). *Tuberculosis Control: A Manual on Methods and Procedures for Integrated Programs*. Scientific publication No 498. PAHO, Washington D.C.

Salomão, and M. A. Parkalli, L. M. (1989). Evaluation des résultats de la chimiothérapie de courte durée au Mozambique 1985–1987. *Bull Int. Union Tuberc.* **64**:31–24.

Salaniponi, F. L. M. (1989). Le programme national de lutte contre la tuberculose du Malawi. *Bull. Int. Union Tuberc*. **64**:41–42.

Styblo, K. (1987a). IUATLD. Assisted National tuberculosis programmes in developing countries. In *Tuberculosis Surveillance Research Unit of the IUAT. Progress report, 1987*, Vol. 2. p. 101.

Styblo, K. (1987b) Recording and reporting system on tuberculosis in control programmes in developing countries. In *Tuberculosis Surveillance Research Unit of the IUAT Progress Report* 1987, Vol. 2. pp. 102–105.

Styblo, K. (1991). L'impact de l'infection par le VIH sur l'épidémiologie de la tuberculose dans le monde *Bull. Int. Union Tuberc*. **66**:27–33.

Tanzanian–British Medical Research Council Collaborative Study (1985). Tuberculosis in Tanzania. A National Survey of newly notified cases. *Tubercle* **66**:161–178.

Tuberculosis Unit, WHO (1991a). Guidelines for tuberculosis treatment in adults and children in national tuberculosis programmes WHO/TUB/91.161, Geneva.

Tuberculosis Unit, WHO (1991b). Tuberculosis surveillance and monitoring. Report of a WHO Workshop. WHO/TB/91.163, Geneva.

Union Internationale Contre la Tuberculose, Commission du Traitement (1978). *Méthode d'évaluation des résultats du traitement de routine de la tuberculose pulmonaire dans un pays*. Imprimerie Nord Africaine, Alger, 45 pp.

World Bank (1990). *World Development Report 1990*. Oxford University Press, New York.

World Bank (1991). *World Development Report 1991*. Oxford University Press, New York

Zidouni, N., and Chaulet, P. (1991). Evaluation of the treatment results of pulmonary tuberculosis in a community survey in Algeria including the comparison of 2 (6 month and 8 month) short course chemotherapy regimens. In *Tuberculosis Surveillance Research Unit of the IUATLD Progress Report 1991*, Vol. 1. Royal Netherlands Tuberculosis Association, The Hague, pp. 29–44.

28

The Plan to Eliminate Tuberculosis in the United States

JOHN A. SBARBARO

University of Colorado Health Sciences Center
Denver, Colorado

I. Introduction

The history of tuberculosis is the history of mankind. The tubercle bacillus has participated in our explorations, our quests, and our crusades. It has been our constant companion through the early eras of ignorance and fear; through the Renaissance with its advances in art, music, and poetry; through the Industrial Revolution; and throughout our wars. It lays in rest with the mummies of Egypt; gave Camille the translucent skin and waning frailty so enchanting to poets; and provided the setting for the intellectual drama of *The Magic Mountain* (Mann, 1927).

Together we advanced man's knowledge of our world—creating a challenging environment that led scientists, such as Koch, to advance our understanding of infectious agents and establish principles of cause and effect (Daniel, 1982). Our relationship gave surgeons the opportunity to further explore the functioning of the human body through procedures, such as thoracoplasty, that removed the upper ribs collapsing diseased lung; but resulting in permanent human disfigurement. Others repeatedly injected air into the thoracic cavity or implanted Ping-Pong ball-like "plombages" in their effort to crush tuberculous cavities, thereby providing further insight into lung and circulation dynamics (Gaensler, 1982).

At the beginning of the 20th century, almost every family in the United States found itself affected by tuberculosis. This relation led to a vast industry of tuberculosis-related health care services. Sanatoriums were built as islands of rest and solitude; places of comfort for the sick and the dying. At the peak of that effort, in 1942, over 97,500 sanatorium beds had been established in the contiguous 48 states (Sbarbaro, 1982).

Our companion for over 5000 years, and now we seek to eliminate tuberculosis! Dream? Possibility? or Reality?

A review of epidemiological statistics reveals that we began to part company shortly after the turn of the century (Frost, 1937; Styblo, 1989). Having thrived in an environment of hunger, poverty, and miserably crowded living conditions, the tubercle bacillus did not do well in an environment of relative luxury—where grandmothers and grandfathers were beginning to live apart from grandchildren; where diseased individuals were removed from the home and housed in isolated sanatoriums or sent West to benefit from high altitudes and bountiful sunlight (while simultaneously lessening their contact with uninfected individuals).

After a steep decline in the first half of the century, the annual number of tuberculosis cases in the United States began to steadily decrease at a rate of 5% per year (from 84,304 cases in 1953 to 22,255 in 1984). At this rate, assuming a continued steady decline of 5% per year, tuberculosis would have reached the point of *elimination* by the year 2076—having caused disease in an additional 665,000 individuals during the 82-year span between 1990 and 2072 (Centers for Disease Control [CDC], 1989).

II. Elimination: A Case Rate of Fewer than One per Million

With the number of tuberculosis cases in the United States at an all time low (1984), Dr. James Mason, newly appointed as Director of the Centers for Disease Control challenged the health community to eliminate tuberculosis within the boarders of the United States (CDC, 1989). That challenge set in motion the development of both a conceptual plan and the operational capacity to support such a national effort. Unfortunately, apathy and disinterest in this declining disease had left the once-feared "Captain of the Men of Death" to be challenged by diagnostic tools of the late 1800s and early 1900s and an array of treatment alternatives ranging widely in duration and potency. Inadequate professional care and high rates of patient noncompliance had already created significant numbers of drug-resistant organisms, once believed to be less contagious, but now recognized to be equally transmissible (CDC, 1991). Public monies, originally committed to the care of tuberculosis patients were already being diverted to other more visible health problems.

To add to the challenge, the steady decline in the national rate of tuberculosis in the United States unexpectedly stopped, remaining level in 1985 and increasing 2.6% in 1986 (CDC, 1989) This change was considered to be highly significant, for even the massive influx of people from war-ravaged Southeast Asia had only been associated with a 0.3% increase in tuberculosis during 1980 (CDC, 1989) In fact, the 1986 increase of tuberculosis was signaling the entrance of the acquired immune deficiency syndrome (AIDS), with its explosive impact on the immune system. Many of those who, in the absence of infection with the human immuno-deficiency virus (HIV), would have been able to contain their latent–dormant tuberculosis infection were now at high risk to become disseminators of the disease. A strategic plan to eliminate tuberculosis suddenly assumed increased importance (CDC, 1989).

A three-pronged national effort was envisioned, focusing on

1. The intensified use of existing prevention, treatment, and tuberculosis control methods and procedures

2. The development of new diagnostic techniques and treatments for tuberculosis

3. The capability of rapidly transferring new knowledge, skills, and technology into the daily practices of private and public health care providers

Scientific and community "advisory committees" were established at the national and state levels, drawing expertise from all segments of the community.

The goal of these efforts was to effect tuberculosis elimination—a case rate of one per *million* population—by the year 2010. Confronted with a 1987 United States' tuberculous case rate of 9.3:100,000 population, an interim target of 3.5 cases per 100,000 population was established for the year 2000 as a means of monitoring the progress of the program (CDC, 1989).

III. Step 1 of the Strategic Plan: Effectively Using Existing Technology

As the epidemic tide of tuberculosis recedes from the shores of America, small tidepools of disease remain behind; pools populated by minorities, immigrants, the elderly and the immunocompromised.

Michael D. Iseman, M.D.
(personal communication)

An epidemiological analysis of the United States' tuberculous cases gave both stimulus and direction to the more effective use of existing prevention, treatment, and control methods and procedures as the first step toward the elimination of tuberculosis. Nearly two-thirds of tuberculous cases were occurring among minorities, including those of Hispanic heritage. Twenty-five percent of the total cases were to be found among immigrants, refugees, and migrant workers from countries in which tuberculosis was prevalent; and half of these cases were occurring within 2 years of entry into the United States (CDC, 1989). Of note, fewer than 4% of the nations 3138 counties accounted for most of preventable tuberculous cases among racial and ethnic minorities.

Reflecting the high rates of infection that had occurred during the early decades of the 20th century, significant disease was also found among the elderly. The homeless appeared to be another high-risk group. But the highest rates of disease were found among those infected with the HIV virus, whose resulting impaired immune status provided fertile ground for the reactivation of once dormant bacilli.

Improved case detection and surveillance efforts among these high-risk groups, combined with prompt and thorough treatment of those found to be diseased or infected, assumed a high priority in the drive to eliminate tuberculosis.

A. Screening for Tuberculosis and Tuberculous

Infection in High-Risk Populations

The strategic plan calls for the following population groups and subgroups to be carefully screened for tuberculosis and tuberculous infection:

1. Persons infected with HIV
2. Close contacts of persons known or suspected to have tuberculosis, sharing the same household or other enclosed environments
3. Persons with medical factors known to increase the risk of disease once infection has occurred (i.e., silicosis, chronic renal failure, gastrectomy, jejunoileal bypass, 10% underweight, diabetes, malignancies, and high-dose corticosteroid treatment or other immunosuppressive therapy)
4. Foreign-born persons from countries with high prevalence of tuberculosis
5. Medically underserved low-income populations including high-risk racial or ethnic minority populations
6. Residents of long-term care facilities, correctional institutions, mental institutions, and other long-term nursing homes and residential facilities
7. Alcoholics and intravenous drug users

Until more accurate diagnostic procedures are developed, the tuberculin skin test remains the only method to identify persons infected with *Mycobacterium tuberculosis*. However, chest radiography or sputum smear are the screening methods of choice when the objective is to identify persons with current (active) pulmonary disease or when the population is transient or highly mobile (e.g., the homeless).

Note: In any screening program, all persons with signs or symptoms suggestive of pulmonary or pleural tuberculosis should have a standard chest radiograph, regardless of the tuberculin skin test result. Numerous studies confirm the observation that 20–25% of individuals with active disease will not react to a tuberculin test—presumably secondary to an overwhelming abundance of antigen being produced endogenously.

In addition to the focus on these known risk groups, the plan calls for health departments to periodically assess the prevalence, incidence, and socio-demographic characteristics of the cases and infected persons within their communities. Given the findings of these studies, tuberculin-screening programs are then to be specifically targeted to each community's high-risk groups. (CDC, 1989; Sbarbaro, 1980).

B. Control and Prevention of Tuberculosis

Once identified, each sputum-positive patient should fully complete a recommended course of treatment. This goal assumes primary importance. The 1988 statistics from the Centers for Disease Control reveal that over 25% of sputum-positive patients were not known to have converted from a positive- to a negative-sputum culture within 6 months—yet over 95% of patients receiving adequate treatment will convert within the first 2 months of therapy. Moreover, almost 12% of patients were not known to be currently receiving therapy; and more than 17% did not take their medication continuously (CDC, 1989) Up-to-date bacteriological information was available for only 57% of patients (CDC, 1990).

To achieve elimination, the strategic plan (CDC, 1989) calls for this potent source of continued spread of infection to be contained through the assignment of a specific health department employee to each case. Each employee will then be responsible for ensuring that adequate treatment is not only prescribed, but is taken by the patient. Although care through a private provider is certainly acceptable, monitoring the effectiveness of that care remains a health department responsibility. Furthermore, the plan recognized that there is real need for a nationwide network of computer-to-computer reporting, along with the establishment of a national record system to permit ongoing evaluation and quality assessment of tuberculosis control programs.

When patient compliance with treatment is questionable, direct administration of the medications to the patient by a third responsible party becomes essential. Patients failing to adhere to an adequate treatment regimen should be removed from the community through the implementation of quarantine measures. No citizen has the right to infringe on the civil rights of others through wanton spread of an infectious agent. The discovery of antituberculous medications in 1950 permitted the replacement of physical isolation by "chemical isolation," but when that control measure fails to be effective, physical isolation through institutionalization is required. For program evaluation purposes, a specific treatment and monitoring plan should be developed and begun within 4 days of diagnosis (CDC, 1989).

The strategic plan noted that preventable cases of tuberculosis continue to occur within the United States. By definition, a *preventable case* is one in whom a currently recommended intervention should have been employed, but was not, with subsequent progression to disease. Ranking very high among these possible interventions is the use of preventive therapy—for most, single-drug treatment directed at dormant intracellular organisms—identical with the continuation phase of treatment for active disease. The detection and treatment of infected persons before disease emerges is without question a most critical element in the plan for tuberculosis elimination. (See Chapters 7 and 12.)

To assist the early identification of newly infected individuals, the plan (CDC, 1989) calls for all United States residents to have the results of at least one tuberculin skin test recorded in their medical records. Such information would enhance the effectiveness of case-contact identification and evaluation. The need for repeat skin testing would be determined by the likelihood of exposure to infectious tuberculosis. All tuberculin-negative persons in high-risk groups should be retested if exposure to an infectious case occurs. In some institutional and group-living environments, the risk of exposure is probably high enough to justify repeat testing at 6- to 24-month intervals. (See Chapter 7.)

In addition to these activities, the strategic plan calls for health departments to routinely monitor the time between the diagnosis of tuberculosis and the date the case is reported to the department. Delays of more than 3 days should be investigated and action taken to prevent similar delays in the future. Periodic reviews of selected record systems, such as laboratory and pharmacy reports, AIDS registries, and death certificates, should be performed to validate the surveillance system and to detect any failure to report cases.

C. High-Risk Groups and Environments

As noted earlier, the first step in the strategic plan to eliminate tuberculosis is the effective and efficient application of existing technology to those environments and subgroups within our population who contribute significantly to the risk of tuberculosis.

Specific tuberculosis control surveillance and containment measures have been developed for the following population subgroups:

HIV infected

Foreign-born

Homeless

Minorities

Intravenous substance abusers

and for the following high-risk environments:

Correctional institutions

Nursing homes for the elderly

Tuberculosis surveillance and containment programs can be similarly designed to meet the unique characteristics of any occupational, geographic, or life-style group identified as being at high risk for infection or disease (e.g., migrant farm workers). Such programs require only curiosity, investigative stamina, and creativity in those committed to the elimination of tuberculosis (American Thoracic Society, 1989; Sbarbaro, 1979).

IV. Step 2 of the Strategic Plan: Development of New Diagnostic and Treatment Technologies

Stimulated by the recommendations of a National Conference on Future Research in Tuberculosis (American Thoracic Society, 1986), efforts have been initiated to clarify the metabolic functions of the tubercle bacillus and their interaction with various drugs. Treatment trials are underway to identify shorter and more potent preventive therapy regimens. New and more accurate methods for identifying those who are infected and those who are diseased are being developed. In essence, the knowledge and techniques that have been focused in other field of science and medicine are now being directed at improving the methods for identifying and treating those infected or diseased by the tubercle bacillus.

In addition, the potential for developing a truly potent vaccine is being reassessed, along with other methods of preventing infection, including control of the environment. The skills of epidemiologists and social scientists are being incorporated into a wide array of studies directed at making our present and future techniques more effective in their daily application.

If this momentum is maintained, these scientific efforts could have phenomenal impact far beyond the tuberculosis elimination program.

V. Step 3 of the Strategic Plan: The Transfer and Incorporation of Newly Identified Technology into Clinical and Public Health Practices

The incorporation of new diagnostic tools and diagnostic procedures into medical practice is seldom difficult. However, the past 30 years have clearly demonstrated the difficulty in achieving change when introducing new approaches to therapy. It took almost 20 years after the introduction of ambulatory chemotherapy for the last tuberculosis sanatorium in the United States to close its doors (Moulding et al., 1968). Intermittent therapy, introduced into the United States in 1968 (Sbarbaro and Johnson, 1968), is still underutilized. Ten years after repeated evidence that a 6-month short-course chemotherapy was effective, such regimens had not been incorporated into the routine practices of health departments and infectious disease–pulmonary experts.

To address this problem of slow professional change, the plan emphasizes the need to develop professional consensus on the appropriateness of new advances and the need to identify those groups who will be using the new technology and to enlist their aid (CDC, 1989). Rather than await a technical or scientific breakthrough, supporters of the program to eliminate tuberculosis have already introduced the concept of elimination into key elements of federal, state, local, and volunteer components of our nations's scientific, governmental, media, business, and community sectors. To date, the response has been most supportive.

The support both of national and state voluntary associations and of advocacy groups, especially those committed to minorities and the disadvantaged, will be vital if the plan is to be effective.

VI. Problems that Must Be Addressed If Elimination Is to Be Achieved

A. Resistant Disease

Inadequately or partially treated individuals, instead of dying and removing themselves as a continuing source of infection, tend to live and become chronic spreaders of disease. This is often the situation for individuals whose personal or social situation has led to frequent interruptions in treatment and deficient chemotherapy regimens. The end result is the emergence of contagious organisms completely resistant to any medication.

It is becoming clear that until new technologies or medications are developed, we, as a society, must reestablish one or more chronic care institutions. Such residential treatment facilities would provide supportive care for those whose contagious condition is untreatable, while ensuring their isolation from the general community. The specter of a wave of new infections, with the emergence of new cases of totally resistant, but transmissible disease, is frightening.

The noncontrolled availability of antituberculous antibiotics within many countries, especially those in the early stages of socioeconomic development, has accelerated both their misuse and the emergence of resistant organisms and chronically diseased individuals (Aitken et al., 1984; Iseman et al., 1990). The improving relations between countries of the world, with its enhanced opportunities for immigration, tourism, and student exchange, combined with the ease and quickness of travel, exacerbate this potential problem. Although the strategic plan addresses the early identification of disease among the foreign-born, effective containment will require long-term isolation until new technologies become available.

B. Community Interest

Ten years after the discovery of effective treatment, two of the giants in the fight against tuberculosis, Palmer (the head of tuberculosis research division of the CDC; Palmer, 1958) and Perkins (managing director of the American Lung Association—then the national Tuberculosis Association; Perkins, 1959) recognized the need to redirect our nation's efforts toward the eradication of the disease. Anticipating the present strategic plan, Palmer emphasized that success would be dependent upon "pinpointing and eradicating" the last remaining reservoirs of infection.

In response, Dr. Soper, from the Office of Surgeon General, recalling his wide experience with other eradication projects, noted that many problems would have to be solved: psychological, technical, administrative, educational, and financial (Soper, 1962). He felt that although the problems seemed many, success would depend upon four basic points:

1. The absolute acceptance of tuberculosis eradication as an urgent objective by national and state health authorities and interested voluntary agencies

2. The recognition that tuberculosis was no longer a social and economic problem, but rather a public health disease, in which the community had a responsibility for the infected, *and* the infected had a responsibility to protect the uninfected

3. Preparation of a national plan for tuberculosis eradication; establishment of a national coordination authority; and the necessary financial, technical, and administrative support

4. Adequate training of staff (Soper, 1962)

In essence, Soper noted that the transition from "control" to "eradication" will require a profound change in thinking and attitude by both professionals and by the community. Interest and commitment to the goal of eradication will have to be intensified as the incidence of the disease diminishes—momentum that is very difficult to maintain.

To emphasize that success will ultimately depend upon the full cooperation of each individual in the community, Soper suggested consideration of legal obligations and even tax incentives to maximize personal responsibility. Challenging thoughts, but directly on target. Traditionally, public concern, funding, and interest wanes as personal risk diminishes, and with it diminishes the opportunity for eradication. To be successful, those committed to the elimination of tuberculosis must keep a declining disease in the focus of public attention. That will be the real challenge.

VII. Conclusion

The elimination of tuberculosis in the United States is possible. However, it will require the dedicated efforts of all segments of the health care community fully applying the knowledge and technology that is presently available and the rapid development and deployment of effective new diagnostic and therapeutic options.

Progress toward these advances is already underway. And if our society is able to put in place, *and maintain*, the appropriate surveillance and containment programs directed at the infected or diseased subgroups within our population, the strategic plan can become reality.

References

Aitken, M. L., Sparks, R., Anderson, K., and Albert, R. K. (1984). Predictors of drug-resistant *Mycobacterium tuberculosis. Am. Rev. Respir. Dis.* **130**:831–833.

American Thoracic Society–Centers for Disease Control (1983). Control of tuberculosis. *Am. Rev. Respir. Dis.* **128**:336–42.

American Thoracic Society, Centers for Disease Control, National Institutes of Health, Pittsfield Antituberculosis Association (1986) Future research in tuberculosis: Prospects and priorities for elimination. *Am. Rev. Respir. Dis.* **134**:401–420.

Centers for Disease Control (1989). A strategic plan for the elimination of tuberculosis in the United States. *MMWR.* **38**(suppl.):1–25.

Centers for Disease Control (1990). Update: Tuberculosis elimination—United States. *MMWR* **39**:153–156.

Centers for Disease Control (1991). Nosocomial transmission of multidrug-resistant tuberculosis among HIV-infected persons—Florida and New York, 1988–1991. *MMWR* **40**:585–591.

Daniel, T. (1982). Robert Koch: Tuberculosis, and the subsequent history of medicine. *Am. Rev. Respir. Dis.* **125**:1–3.

Frost, W. H. (1937). How much control of tuberculosis? *Am. J. Public Health* **27**:759–766.

Gaensler, E. A. (1982). The surgery for pulmonary tuberculosis. *Am. Rev. Respir. Dis.* **125**:73–84.

Iseman, M. D., Manalo, R., Tan, P., and Sbarbaro, J. A. (1990). Community based short-course treatment of pulmonary tuberculosis in a developing nation: Initial report of an 8-month, largely intermittent regimen in a population with a high prevalence of drug resistance. *Am. Rev. Respir. Dis.* **142**:1301–1305.

Mann, T. (1927). *The Magic Mountain*. Alfred A. Knopf, New York.

Mason, J. O. (1986). Opportunities for the elimination of tuberculosis. *Am. Rev. Respir. Dis.* **134**:201–203.

Moulding, T. S., Sbarbaro, J. A., Bauer, H., Chapman, P. T., and Moodie, A. A. (1968). Treatment pays off, a discussion. *Bull. Natl. Tuberc. Respir. Dis. Assoc.* **64**:3–8.

Palmer, C. (1958) Tuberculosis: A decade in retrospect and in prospect. *Lancet* **78**:257–260.

Perkins, J. (1959). Global tuberculosis eradication. *Am. Rev. Respir. Dis.* **80**:138–139.

Sbarbaro, J. A. and Johnson, S. (1968). Tuberculosis chemotherapy for recalcitrant outpatients administered directly twice weekly. *Am. Rev. Respir. Dis.* **99**:895–903.

Sbarbaro, J. A. (1979). Compliance: Inducements and enforcements. *Chest* **76S**:750S–756S.

Sbarbaro, J. A. (1980). Public health aspects of tuberculosis: Supervision of therapy. *Clin. Chest Med.* **1**:253–263.

Sbarbaro, J. A. (1982). Tuberculosis: A portal through which to view the future. *Am. Rev. Respir. Dis.* **125**:127–132.

Soper, F. L. (1962). Problems to be solved if the eradication of tuberculosis is to be realized. *Am J. Public Health* **52**:734–745.

Styblo, K. (1989). Eradication of tuberculosis in developed countries in the HIV era. *Bull. Int. Union Tuberc. Lung Dis.* **64**:5864

29

Evaluation of Applied Strategies in Low-Prevalence Countries

JAAP F. BROEKMANS

Royal Netherlands Tuberculosis Association
The Hague, The Netherlands

I. Introduction

Elimination of tuberculosis has been planned in the United States by the year 2010 (Dowdle, 1989) and predicted for The Netherlands by the year 2025 (Styblo, 1990). However, in these countries, as in most industrialized countries, the steady decline in tuberculosis incidence observed for many years appears to have leveled off, or even to have reversed.

In The Netherlands, the average decline in notification rates was about 11% (1951–1960), 9% (1961–1970), and 5% (1981–1987). During the period 1988–1990, the rate leveled off at 9:100,000. In new bacillary pulmonary cases (foreigners excluded) from 1973–1976 to 1981–1984 the decline was approximately 4% per year (van Geuns et al., 1987).

In the United States, an average 5.7% annual decline in notification rates was observed between 1975 and 1984. This downward trend halted in 1985 and reversed in 1986, resulting in about 28,000 cumulative excess cases of tuberculosis in the period 1985–1990 (Centers for Disease Control, [CDC], 1990). During the period 1984–1990, the rate leveled off at 9:100,000 to 10:100,000.

The impact of immigration from high-prevalence countries [and other factors, such as human immunodeficiency virus (HIV) infection] on the tuberculosis incidence in low-prevalence countries should be carefully evaluated. This will enable health authorities to adjust currently applied strategies in the elimination phase of tuberculosis.

Section II of this chapter summarises the epidemiology of tuberculosis in low-prevalence countries. Section III describes the characteristic features of a tuberculosis program in low-prevalence countries as far as a relevant background for a detailed description of the evaluation of applied strategies. The evaluation of applied strategies is summarised under two headings: epidemiological surveillance (Sec. IV) and monitoring of program performance (Sec. V).

II. Epidemiology of Tuberculosis in Low-Prevalence Countries

In most industrialized countries, tuberculosis control efforts have been applied successfully. The tremendous impact of these measures on the tuberculosis situation in The Netherlands is graphically represented in Figure 1. The figure shows the estimated prevalence of infection with *Mycobacterium tuberculosis* by age in the indigenous population of The Netherlands in 1945, 1975, and 2005. This figure is based on calculations of Styblo, using the Dutch army recruit data meticulously collected by Bleiker and Misljenovic of NIPG/TNO in The Hague (Bleiker, 1984) and it demonstrates that, with an approximate 90% case-detection rate and an almost 100% cure rate, a country can indeed move from a high- to a low-prevalence country.

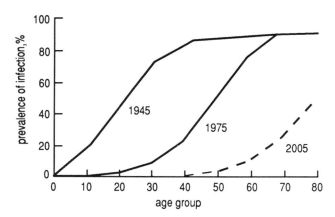

Figure 1 Estimated prevalence of tuberculous infection by age: The Netherlands, 1945, 1975, 2005. (From Bleiker, 1984.)

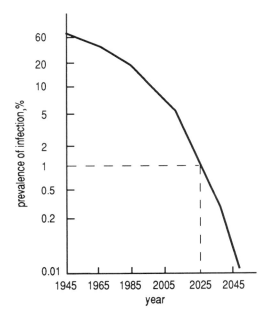

Figure 2 Estimated prevalence of tuberculous infection in the general population: The Netherlands, 1945–2045. (From Styblo, 1990.)

At the same time, this figure predicts a relatively high prevalence of infection in the older aged groups in the decades to come. In 1990, more than 2 million indigenous Dutch people (approximately 15% of the total population) carried potentially live tubercle bacilli in their bodies, most of them acquired before 1950. This is the major reason elimination of tuberculosis in The Netherlands, with the present intervention strategies, cannot be expected before the year 2025 (Fig. 2). In the year 2025 the prevalence of infection in the indigenous Dutch population will be below 1%, and the incidence of smear-positive tuberculosis is expected to be below 1:1 million, the conventional limit of elimination (Styblo, 1990).

In low-prevalence countries, almost all new cases result from exacerbation of latent tuberculous infection and not from recent transmission.

Less accurate data are available on the potential effect of the immigration from high-prevalence countries of persons already infected with *M. tuberculosis* on the prevalence of infection in the general population of The Netherlands. In 1990, an estimated 700,000 persons in The Netherlands were of foreign extraction. If we assume that 50% are infected with *M. tuberculosis*, this would increase the prevalence of infection in 1990 from the estimated 15% by 2.4% to become approximately 17%. Continued immigration from countries with a high incidence of tuberculosis to The Netherlands would delay elimination of tuberculosis for several years.

The notification rate of tuberculosis in 1990 for The Netherlands is 9.2:100,000. Foreigners or foreign-born constituted 541 (41%) of 1369 patients diagnosed in The Netherlands in that year.

The effect of HIV transmission on the elimination of tuberculosis in low-prevalence countries will depend on the ''overlap'' between the prevalence of tuberculous and that of HIV infection in the population studied. Figure 1 shows that in The Netherlands tuberculous infection is an increasingly rare phenomenon in the age groups most vulnerable for HIV transmission. Although excess cases of tuberculosis will occur owing to HIV transmission, this will not result in a subsequent distinct deterioration of the epidemiological situation for tuberculosis in The Netherlands.

In 1990, the Tuberculosis Unit of the World Health Organization (WHO) in Geneva estimated the prevalence of infection with *M. tuberculosis* for the entire Western Europe to be 28.04% (Fig. 3). The higher the prevalence of infection with *M. tuberculosis* in those younger than about 50 years in a particular country, the greater the potential effect of HIV transmission.

In The Netherlands, the general population younger than aged 50 years is virtually free of tuberculous infection. The prevalence of tuberculous infection for those aged 15–54 years was 7.1% in 1985 and will be 2.7% in 1995. Besides the continued importance of passive case-finding among suspects, active case-finding in risk groups (contacts, foreign-born, HIV infected) and the containment of microepidemics around sources of infection become relatively more important (Broekmans, 1991).

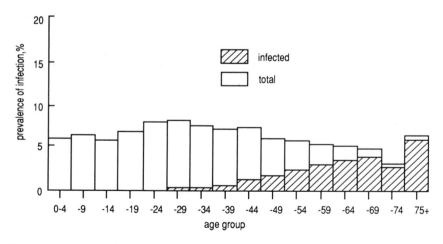

Figure 3 Estimated prevalence of tuberculous infection and population composition in 1990. Western Europe, population total 237.9 million. (From WHO Tuberculosis Unit, 1989.)

At an International Union Against Tuberculosis and Lung Disease (IUATLD)–WHO workshop held in March 1990 at Wolfheze, The Netherlands (Clancy et al., 1991), it was proposed to define a low-prevalence country when the incidence of all forms of active tuberculosis would fall below 10:100,000. Strict adherence to the Wolfheze definition implies that actually very few industrialized countries belong to this category: Australia, Canada, Denmark, Iceland, The Netherlands, Norway, Sweden, and a few others. With an increase in the notification rate from 9.5 in 1989 to 10.3 in 1990, the United States appears to move outside this category (CDC, 1990). Indeed, a more appropriate definition is needed. It is tentatively proposed to define low-prevalence countries when the notification rate of *bacteriologically confirmed* pulmonary tuberculosis would fall below 10:100,000. With this definition, most European countries would be included. However, several countries in Europe (for instance Portugal, Rumania, and Yugoslavia) have notification rates that are substantially higher than 10 bacillary cases per 100,000.

III. The Tuberculosis Program in Low-Prevalence Countries

The characteristic features of a tuberculosis program in low-prevalence countries are to be distinguished from the characteristics of a tuberculosis control program in the era of high incidence of disease. From an analysis of the situation in The Netherlands (Broekmans, 1991), the main characteristics are presented in Table 1. From this analysis it is concluded that it is difficult to maintain a viable and effective tuberculosis program in a low-incidence environment

With the disappearance of expertise among physicians

To be delivered by a multifunctional service

Under less secure financial conditions

With a shift in the nature of surveillance and control strategies

Against the background of the emergence of HIV infection

and that it constitutes a considerable challenge for the public health community. It actually asks for a reorientation of service delivery and for a critical readjustment of the concepts of tuberculosis control of earlier decades.

Although this analysis was based on the experience in The Netherlands, ample evidence has recently been presented and published (Reichman, 1991; Tala and Kochi, 1991; Brudney and Dobkin, 1991) that its basic tenets are valid for the epidemiological situation and tuberculosis program in the great majority of industrialized low-prevalence countries.

Table 1 Characteristic Features of a Tuberculosis Program in a Low-Prevalence Country: The Netherlands

1. Expertise		
Tuberculosis becomes a rare disease	▷	Disappearance of expertise among physicians
2. Program		
Categorical service	▷	Multifunctional service
3. Finance		
Central government subsidy	▷	Nonearmarked budget from local government
4. Surveillance		
Passive case-finding	▷	Screening of risk groups (e.g., foreign-born) and containment of microepidemics; surveillance of recent infections
5. HIV infection		
Emergence of HIV infection	▷	Effects on risk groups with relative high prevalence of tuberculous infection

Source: Broekmans (1991).

IV.   Epidemiological Surveillance

A.   Surveillance of Infection

The annual tuberculosis infection rate is the best single indicator for evaluating the tuberculosis problem and its trend in developed and developing countries. It is an index that expresses the attacking force of tuberculosis within a given population and, unlike disease notification rates, is not linked directly to the case-finding and treatment measures of the tuberculosis program (Styblo, 1991).

Figure 4 presents the annual infection rate in The Netherlands from 1910 to 1979. Since 1956, these rates were derived from the prevalence of infection in Dutch army recruits. The decline of the risk of infection was 13.7% annually between 1956 and 1965, 10.4% annually between 1966 and 1979 (Sutherland et al., 1979), and about 8% between 1980 and 1990 (Sutherland, preliminary data, personal communication). It is estimated that the annual rate of infection in The Netherlands in 1990 was about 10:100,000 or slightly lower (Sutherland, personal communication).

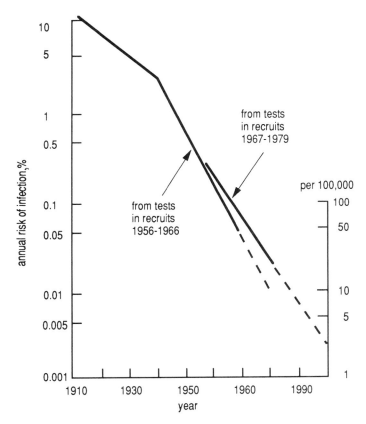

Figure 4 Annual risk of tuberculous infection: The Netherlands 1910–1979. (From Sutherland, 1979.)

Rieder et al. (1989) extrapolated the rate of infection among navy recruits in the United States of the 1950s to a rate of infection of 6.1:100,000 population in 1986. In an independent comparison, derived from an analysis of contact investigations reported in 1985 and 1986, Rieder (1989) derived an estimated annual infection rate of 8.5:100,000 population. Comstock estimated the rate of infection in 1990 in the United States to be approximately 10:100,000 (Comstock, personal communication).

Table 2 presents the prevalence of infection in Dutch army recruits, as obtained by the tuberculin team of NIPG/TNO in collaboration with the Army Medical Services in the years 1980–1991, and Figure 5 shows the prevalence of

Table 2   Results of Tuberculin Testing in Unvaccinated Recruits,
Aged 20 years: The Netherlands (1980–1991)

Year	Number tested	Induration > 9 mm	
		No.	%
1980	45,895	392	0.85
1981	45,893	386	0.84
1982	42,155	335	0.79
1983	44,331	325	0.73
1984	41,161	292	0.71
1985	43,265	196	0.45
1986	44,365	209	0.47
1987	45,737	189	0.41
1988	44,393	215	0.48
1989	43,801	175	0.40
1990	41,040	172	0.42
1991	39,956	176	0.44

Source: Bleiker et al. (1956–1991).

infection for the entire 35-year period of observation (1956–1991). It suggests that the tuberculin surveys in unvaccinated Dutch army recruits give reliable information on the prevalence of infection until its level falls to approximately 0.4%. This corresponds to an annual risk of infection of 0.01% (10 infections per 100,000 population annually).

It appears useless to begin tuberculin surveys at regular intervals in low-prevalence countries at this time. The prevalence of infection becomes so low (in most age groups) that it becomes difficult to distinguish a meaningful trend. In some countries, the widespread use of bacille Calmette-Guérin (BCG) vaccination or the presence of "atypical" mycobacteria may hamper the interpretation of the survey results.

It has been suggested that disease surveillance be expanded in low-prevalence countries to include recent infections detected by contact tracing. It may very well be that systematic notification of recent converters detected by contact-tracing procedures by age group (children aged 0–4, 5–9, and 10–14, and young adults eligible for preventive chemotherapy) will yield a sensitive indicator of the tuberculosis problem in very low-prevalence countries.

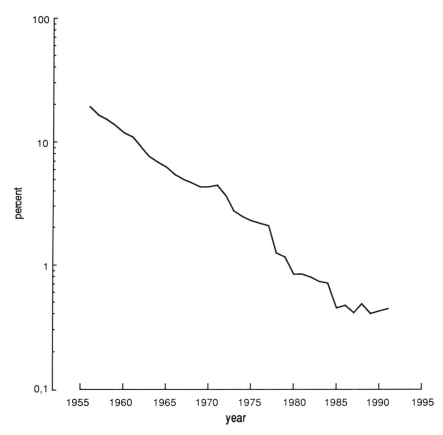

Figure 5 Prevalence of tuberculous infection (army recruits: The Netherlands, 1956–1991). (From Bleiker, 1956–1991.)

B. Surveillance of Disease

Notification Rates of New and Relapsed Cases

The notification rates of new and relapsed cases in low-prevalence countries are of the greatest value in evaluating the overall epidemiological situation. Figure 6 presents the notification rates (per million) of tuberculosis in The Netherlands from 1951 to 1990. Figure 7 presents the notification rates of tuberculosis (all cases) in the United States from 1980 to 1990 (CDC, 1990).

In general, significant intracountry differences in the trend and level of notification rates can be observed. Figure 8 and Table 3 document these differences for Central Harlem, New York City, and the United States (Brudney and

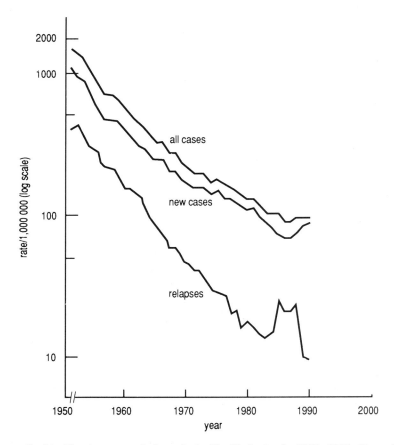

Figure 6 Notification rates of tuberculosis: The Netherlands, 1951–1990. (From Chief Medical Officer, 1951–1990.)

Dobkin, 1991). Resurgent tuberculosis in Central Harlem was attributed to the effects of HIV transmission on tuberculosis, to homelessness, and to the disintegration of the tuberculosis program.

Even in such a small and sociologically homogeneous country as The Netherlands, notification rates of new cases may differ from 11:100,000 to 25:100,000 in the major metropolitan areas such as Rotterdam and Amsterdam, and 5:100,000 to 8:100,000 in rural areas (1990 figures).

Notification Rates for Bacteriologically Confirmed Pulmonary Tuberculosis

Notification rates for bacteriologically confirmed pulmonary tuberculosis provide a sensitive measure for the occurrence of sources of infection in the

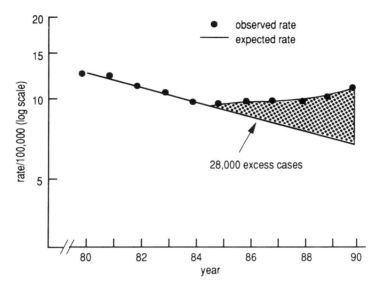

Figure 7 Notification rates of tuberculosis (all cases): United States 1980–1990. (From CDC, 1990.)

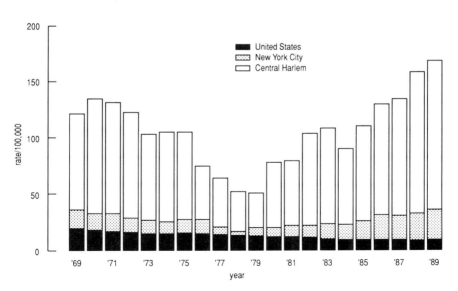

Figure 8 Tuberculosis case rates for the United States, New York, and Central Harlem from 1969 to 1989 per 100,000 population. (From Brudney and Dobkin, 1991.)

Table 3 Notification Rates of Tuberculosis[a]: Central Harlem, New York City, and the United States (1969–1989)

Year	Central Harlem	New York City	United States
1969	121.2	36.4	19.37
1970	135.0	32.8	18.22
1971	131.7	32.6	17.07
1972	123.0	28.8	15.79
1973	103.3	26.6	14.77
1974	105.5	25.6	14.25
1975	105.5	27.2	15.95[b]
1976	75.4	27.3	14.96
1977	64.2	21.1	13.93
1978	52.2	17.2	13.08
1979	50.9	20.1	12.6
1980	78.6	19.9	12.2
1981	79.9	22.4	11.9
1982	104.0	22.5	11.0
1983	109.0	23.4	10.2
1984	90.7	23.0	9.4
1985	110.9	26.0	9.3
1986	130.4	31.4	9.4
1987	134.9	31.1	9.4
1988	158.9	32.8	9.1
1989	169.2	36.0	9.5

[a]New cases per 100,000 population.
[b]National reporting criteria changed, effective from 1975.
Source: Brudney and Dobkin (1991).

population. The bacteriological confirmation of diagnosis improves the reliability of this indicator. Two examples (albeit from the period 1973–1984) are presented, derived from the study by van Geuns et al. (1987). Table 4 presents the notification rates of new bacteriologically confirmed pulmonary tuberculosis (foreigners excluded) by sex for the period 1973–1984 in The Netherlands: 4.9:100,000 for 1973–1976, 3.9:100,000 for 1977–1980, and 3.5:100,000 for

Table 4 Average Annual Notification Rates of Bacteriologically Confirmed Pulmonary Tuberculosis (Foreigners Excluded) per 100,000 Population: The Netherlands (1973–1984)

	1973–1976	1977–1980	1981–1984
Male	4.9	3.9	3.5
Female	2.6	2.4	2.0
All	3.7	3.2	2.7

Source: van Geuns et al. (1987).

1981–1984 (van Geuns et al., 1987). Derived from the same study, Figure 9 presents the notification rates of bacillary pulmonary tuberculosis (foreigners excluded) by age and sex. Figure 9 and Table 4 suggest that the disease will continue to decrease, in particular in those aged 50 years or older in whom the prevalence of infection has been considerably decreasing from the mid-1980s.

Against the background of the leveling off (and even reversal) of notification rates of tuberculosis in new or in all cases in low-prevalence countries, the trend in the notification rate of bacillary-confirmed tuberculosis may become a more sensitive measure of the epidemiological situation. This is

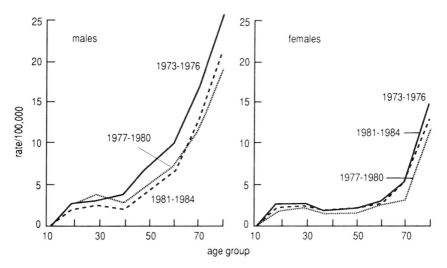

Figure 9 Annual rates of bacillary pulmonary tuberculosis (foreigners excluded), by age and sex: The Netherlands, 1973–1984. (From van Geuns et al., 1987.)

especially valid if rates are calculated separately for the indigenous population (by age and sex) and for the foreign-born or other minorities.

Surveillance of Initial and Acquired Resistance

The issue of multidrug resistance in relation to the immigration of persons from high-prevalence countries to low-prevalence countries and outbreaks of multidrug resistant tuberculosis under special circumstances, such as in large cities among homeless people, drug addicts, HIV infected, or alcoholics (CDC, 1990), may be of importance. Systematic surveillance of the initial drug resistance in new cases with pulmonary tuberculosis and surveillance of acquired resistance in retreatment (relapsed and treatment failure) cases with pulmonary tuberculosis in such places become important, both for epidemiological surveillance as well as an indication of program performance.

An example of a continuous surveillance of initial resistance carried out nationwide is presented from the tuberculosis program in Japan. Table 5 indicates the level of initial resistance in Japan in 1977, 1982, and 1987 (Aoki, 1991).

Notification by Country of Origin, Ethnicity, or Race

In low-prevalence countries, the tuberculosis problem is increasingly a problem of foreign-born or specific risk groups. Accordingly, separate surveillance of tuberculosis by country of origin, ethnicity, or race is particularly important. Two examples are presented, one from The Netherlands and one from the United States.

Figure 10 shows the absolute number of tuberculosis cases in The Netherlands from 1974–1990 as well as the absolute number among Dutch and foreign-born residents. It appears from this figure that the leveling off in the decline of tuberculosis in The Netherlands since 1987 can be largely attributed to tuberculosis disease among foreign-born residents.

The frequency distribution (Fig. 11) of tuberculosis cases by age, race, and ethnicity in the United States, for 1989, is also revealing here. Most cases in the

Table 5 Prevalence of Initial Resistance in Japan (Reference Laboratory)

	1977	1982	1987
Streptomycin	3.4%	5.2%	4.7%
Isoniazid	2.8%	1.5%	1.4%
Rifampin		0.7%	0.8%
Ethambutol		0.7%	0.3%
Kanamycin		0%	0.3%

Source: Aoki (1991).

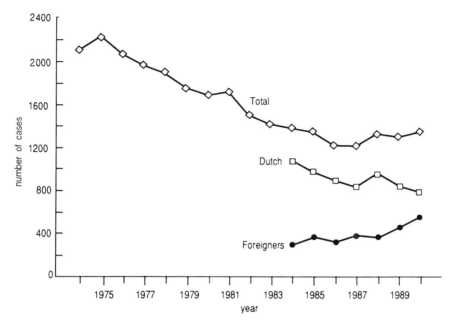

Figure 10 Annual notifications of tuberculosis (all cases, new cases, and relapses): The Netherlands, 1974–1990. (From Chief Medical Officer, 1951–1990.)

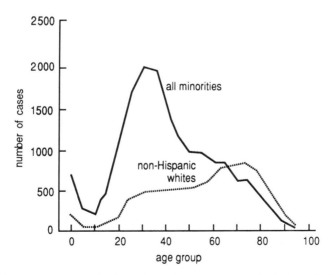

Figure 11 Frequency distribution of cases by age, race, and ethnicity: United States, 1989. (From CDC, 1989.)

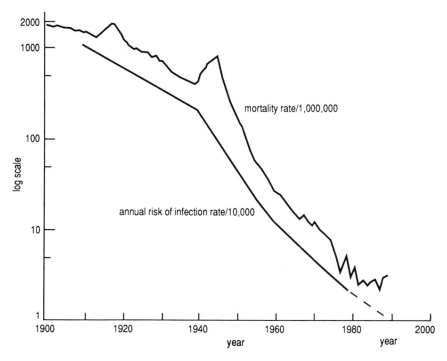

Figure 12 Tuberculosis mortality rates and annual risk of infection: The Netherlands, 1901–1989. (From Chief Medical Officer, 1951–1990.)

non-Hispanic whites occur in persons older than 55 years. The majority of cases in all minorities occur in persons younger than 50 years (CDC, 1989).

C. Surveillance of Mortality

In low-prevalence countries, mortality rates are of only historical value in indicating the extent of the tuberculosis problem and its trend. With the introduction of effective chemotherapy after World War II, mortality rates have been reduced to very low levels. As an illustration, the mortality rates for The Netherlands are presented from 1901 to 1989 (Fig. 12).

V. Monitoring of Program Performance

A. Surveillance of Diagnostic Measures

In addition to the epidemiological indexes discussed in the section on disease surveillance (see Sec. IV.B.), specific diagnostic measurements are

Table 6 Patients' and Doctors' Delays: The Netherlands (1973–1984)

Patients' and doctors' delays (months)	Smear-positive			Culture-positive		
	1973–1976 N(%)	1977–1980 N(%)	1981–1984 N(%)	1973–1976 N(%)	1977–1980 N(%)	1981–1984 N(%)
1–2	639(57)	552(52)	526(53)	707(51)	584(52)	470(56)
3–4	248(22)	249(23)	234(23)	465(33)	352(31)	235(28)
5 or more	242(21)	270(25)	238(24)	226(16)	188(16)	136(16)
Total	1129(100)	1071(100)	998(100)	1398(100)	1124(100)	841(100)
No information	40(3)	22(2)	44(4)	38(3)	30(3)	33(4)

Source: van Geuns et al. (1987)

of increasing importance to monitor program performance in low-prevalence countries.

Patients' and Doctors' Delays

Patients' and doctors' delays in the diagnosis of sources of infection prolong the infectious period and may enhance the occurrence of microepidemics (Veen, 1991). As an illustration of routine surveillance of patients' and doctors' delay, reference is made to the study by van Geuns et al. (1987). Table 6 suggests that in 21% of smear-positive patients detected during 1973–1976, in 25% of patients reported during 1977–1980, and in 24% of cases diagnosed in 1981–1984, more than 4 months elapsed before tuberculosis was diagnosed. For culture-positive cases the corresponding proportions were 16, 16, and 16%, respectively. Over the whole study period (1973–1984), the average duration between the appearance of the first symptoms attributable to tuberculosis disease and the onset of treatment (combined patients' and doctors' delays) was about 2.5 months in bacillary pulmonary cases.

Death Before the Onset of Treatment

The proportion of patients who die of tuberculosis before diagnosis (and onset of treatment) may become a relevant indicator in low-prevalence countries, especially if postmortem examinations are carried out frequently. In the study by van Geuns et al. (1987), the available data for 1982–1984 indicate that in 19 (1.3%) of 1414 patients with bacteriologically confirmed tuberculosis, the disease was diagnosed after death. Subsequent detailed analysis revealed that 9 of the 19 patients died of tuberculosis. However, in The Netherlands, postmortem examinations are not carried out frequently and, therefore, this study cannot give reliable information on the total proportion of tuberculosis patients whose disease is diagnosed after death.

In the "Kolin" study (Styblo et al., 1967), in 21 (4.3%) of 473 cases of tuberculosis detected between 1961–1964, tuberculosis was a postmortem diagnosis. In Scotland, in 20 (2.5%) of 790 patients with pulmonary tuberculosis notified in 1968 the disease was diagnosed after death (Heffernan et al., 1976). Rieder et al. (1991) reported that in 5.1% of tuberculosis cases reported in the United States from 1985 through 1988, the disease was diagnosed at death.

Mode of Detection

In low-prevalence countries, in addition to passive case-finding among self-reporting suspects, active case-finding by screening of risk groups and the containment of microepidemics become progressively more important. The proportion of patients detected by screening the risk groups will probably increase. Although no information on the actual proportion of cases detected by active case-finding in specific risk groups is available from low-prevalence countries, it appears worthwhile to further investigate this indicator.

Surveillance of Microepidemics

In The Netherlands, the indigenous population younger than 50 years is virtually free of tuberculous infection (Fig. 13). In such a "virgin" population, microepidemics may occur and are more easily detected. Specific host factors such as a prolonged infectious period because of an excessive patients' or doctor's delay or an increased susceptibility for disease among contacts owing to HIV infection, may enhance transmission. Environmental factors (poor ventilation or confined spaces) are other factors that may contribute to increased transmission.

A *microepidemic* is defined as an outbreak in which one index case infects 20 or more contacts. In The Netherlands, on average 1 of every 25–30 bacillary cases causes a major outbreak of infections (and disease). On average, 50 persons are infected in these microepidemics (Veen, 1991). Outbreak investigation under these circumstances follows the "stone-in-the-pond principle," or ripple effect (Veen, 1992), in which persons belonging to the inner circle of contacts are examined first. The results of contact investigation are presented according to the closeness of contact and duration of exposure. Table 7 illustrates the findings in such a microepidemic caused by one index case (Veen, 1991).

B. Surveillance of Treatment Measures

The first aim of a tuberculosis program is to cure all (or nearly all) sources of infection. To what extent the treatment results achieved in a tuberculosis

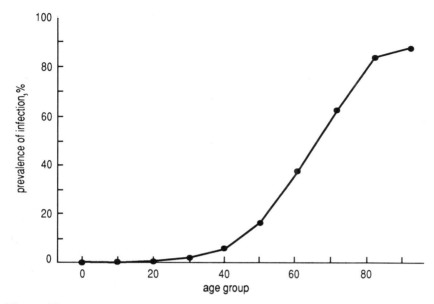

Figure 13 Estimated prevalence of tuberculous infection in The Netherlands in 1990 by age. (From Veen, 1991.)

Table 7 Tuberculous Infections (Active Tuberculosis Included) in a Micro-epidemic Caused by One Index Case and Grouped According to the Closeness of Contact and Duration of Exposure (all aged Between 14 and 22 Years)

	Circle	Total examined	Number with infection	Observed prevalence of infection (%)
Employees dancehall	A	40	5	12.5
Youth center	B	192	8	4.2
Dancehall	B	2748	101	3.8
Schools	C	3646	14	0.4
Total		6626	128	1.9

Source: Veen (1991).

program under routine program conditions approximate the results obtained in controlled clinical trials is the most important issue of the surveillance of treatment measures.

For tuberculosis programs in low-prevalence countries contemplating the routine surveillance of treatment measures, it is suggested that sputum conversion in all bacteriologically confirmed pulmonary patients be monitored by smear microscopy at the end of the intensive phase of treatment and that the cure rate be determined at the end of treatment by smear and culture examination.

Results of Treatment in All Consecutive Bacteriologically Confirmed Pulmonary Cases

The study by van Geuns et al. (1987) extensively addressed this issue. Table 8 presents the results of treatment in all consecutive bacteriologically confirmed pulmonary cases (new and relapsed) in The Netherlands who were notified between 1975 and 1984. The patients are divided into patients who completed treatment and those with incomplete treatment. The division into the "completed" and "incompleted" treatment groups was applied to avoid underestimation of the items concerning the evaluation of treatment measures (in particular owing to deaths of causes other than tuberculosis, range 10.2–13.1%).

The duration of chemotherapy in the incomplete treatment group was considerably shorter than the duration of treatment for those in the completed treatment group. Sputum conversion (see Sec. V.B.) was evaluated for both groups together.

The completed treatment group (range 83.5–86.8% of all patients) included those who were considered by attending physicians to have completed the prescribed treatment regimen and were alive at 24 (18) months, those who died of tuberculosis, and those for whom no information was available. The proportion of patients in this group who completed treatment and were alive ranged from 80.1% (in 1983–1984) to 85.0% (in 1977–1978).

Results of Bacteriological Examination in Bacteriologically Confirmed Pulmonary Tuberculosis During and at the End of Chemotherapy

From the study by van Geuns et al. (1987) the frequency of sputum conversion in patients with bacteriologically confirmed pulmonary tuberculosis in The Netherlands was analyzed for all consecutive patients (both with completed as well as incomplete chemotherapy) notified between 1975 and 1984 (Table 9).

Sputum conversion was very satisfactory during the whole observation period. Of patients with available culture results at completion of chemotherapy, fewer than 1% remained culture-positive. However, there is some concern about the increasing proportion of patients from whom no culture examination was obtained at completion of treatment nor was available at 18 months. An increase

Table 8 Complete and Incomplete Chemotherapy in Patients with Bacteriologically Confirmed Tuberculosis (New and Relapse Cases) Notified in The Netherlands During the Periods 1975–1983

	1975–1976 1331 N(%)	1977–1978 1224 N(%)	1979–1980 1023 N(%)	1981–1982 981 N(%)	1983–1984 935 N(%)
Number of patients					
Completed chemotherapy					
Alive at 24 months (18 months from 1979 onward)	1096(82.3)	1040(85.0)	851(83.2)	822(83.8)	749(80.1)
Death of tuberculosis	10(0.8)	19(1.6)	21(2.1)	22(2.2)	33(3.5)
No information, no treatment	6(0.5)	3(0.2)	13(1.3)	5(0.5)	9(1.0)
Total	1112(83.5)	1062(86.8)	885(86.5)	849(86.5)	791(84.6)
Incomplete chemotherapy					
Death of causes other than tuberculosis	174(13.1)	125(10.2)	109(10.7)	118(12.0)	112(12.0)
Side effects of drugs	16(1.2)	13(1.1)	13(1.3)	5(0.5)	15(1.6)
Uncooperative				3(0.3)	13(1.4)
Left the country	29(2.2)	24(2.0)	16(1.6)	6(0.6)	4(0.4)
Total	219(16.5)	162(13.2)	138(13.5)	132(13.5)	144(15.4)

Source: van Geuns et al. (1987).

Table 9 Frequency of Sputum Conversion in Patients with Bacillary Pulmonary Tuberculosis: The Netherlands (1975–1984)

Culture-negative after treatment (months)	1975–1976 N(%)	1977–1978 N(%)	1979–1980 N(%)	1981–1982 N(%)	1983–1984 N(%)
3	881(78.7)	746(76.7)	552(77.3)	429(77.2)	306(69.5)
6	1045(93.4)	929(95.6)	670(93.8)	517(93.0)	376(85.5)
12	1103(98.6)	959(98.7)	708(99.2)	550(98.9)	409(93.0)
18	1108(99.0)	967(99.5)	710(99.4)	552(99.3)	437(99.3)
24	1109(99.1)	968(99.6)			
Culture-positive at 2 years[a]	10(0.9)	4(0.4)	4(0.6)	4(0.7)	5(0.7)
Subtotal	1119(100.0)	972(100.0)	714(100.0)	556(100.0)	442(100.0)
Death due to tuberculosis	10(0.8)	19(1.6)	21(2.1)	22(2.2)	33(3.5)
No information on bact. status at 2 years[a]	100(7.5)	160(13.1)	197(19.3)	315(32.1)	349(37.4)
Not applicable[b]	102(7.7)	73(6.0)	91(8.9)	88(9.0)	111(11.9)
Total	1331(100.0)	1224(100.0)	1023(100.0)	981(100.0)	935(100.0)

[a]At 18 months from 1979 onward.
[b]Deaths of causes other than tuberculosis before the end of treatment.
Source: van Geuns et al. (1987).

was observed in the proportion of patients without information on the bacteriological status at 2 years from 7.5% in 1975–1976 to 37.4% in 1983–1984. Analyzed in combination with the results presented in Section V.B., the overall results of treatment, however, are very good.

Inpatient Versus Outpatient Care

From the study by van Geuns et al., 1987, results are available of the proportion and average duration of initial inpatient care. Table 10 presents the overall data for smear-positive and culture-positive pulmonary patients. The proportion of patients with completed treatment who had initial hospitalization fluctuated between 48 and 56%. The proportion of smear-positive patients (range 67–71%) who received initial hospitalization was higher than the proportion of culture-positive patients (range 23–35%) (van Geuns et al., 1987; not shown in table). The average duration of inpatient treatment decreased from 5 months in 1975–1976 to 2.3 months in 1983–1984. It was observed that many of the patients were elderly and several suffered from associated disease.

Hospitalization in the intensive phase of treatment may very well be an important contributing factor to achieve successful treatment results under routine program conditions in HIV-infected, homeless, and other (drug abusers, alcoholics) patients.

Adherence to Recommended Treatment Regimens

Surveillance of adherence to (nationally) recommended treatment regimens is, as such, a process indicator in the monitoring of treatment measures. In the study by van Geuns et al. (1987), it was observed that in bacteriologically confirmed pulmonary patients who had completed treatment, the total duration of chemotherapy gradually declined from 16.2 months in 1975–1976 to 10.3 months in 1983–1984. This duration of chemotherapy was close to the recommended treatment regimen of 9 months of the National Tuberculosis Policy Committee in The Netherlands. At that time, most patients received no pyrazinamide during the initial phase of chemotherapy.

In a similar study by the British Thoracic Society Research Committee (1991), it was reported that 97% of patients were prescribed rifampin and isoniazid. Pyrazinamide was prescribed for 80%, which represented a substantial increase from the 19% recorded in a similar survey of patients notified in 1983. Of the patients who were prescribed pyrazinamide, only 29% received therapy approximating the schedule recommended as standard in the United Kingdom. According to the authors, the findings of this survey highlight the nonuniformity of prescribing practices and some of the difficulties of ensuring that patients with pulmonary tuberculosis complete an appropriate course of therapy.

Table 10 Proportion of Smear-Positive and Culture-Positive Patients Having Completed Chemotherapy Who Did and Did Not Follow the Initial Inpatient Treatment: The Netherlands (1975–1984)

	1975–1976 N(%)	1977–1978 N(%)	1979–1980 N(%)	1981–1982 N(%)	1983–1984 N(%)
Number of patients	1112	1062	885	849	791
Inpatient (and outpatient)	531(48)	544(51)	465(53)	427(50)	446(56)
Outpatient only	573(51)	506(48)	399(45)	408(48)	323(41)
No information, no treatment	8(1)	12(1)	21(2)	14(2)	22(3)
Average duration of inpatient chemotherapy					
Number of patients	531	544	465	427	446
Average duration of inpatient treatment (months)	5.0	4.2	3.3	2.7	2.3
Inpatient treatment > 6 months	156(29)	111(20)	50(11)	32(4)	21(5)

Source: van Geuns et al. (1987).

Case-Fatality

The *case-fatality* records the proportion of patients who died of any cause during the course of treatment. In the study by van Geuns et al. (1987) (see Table 9), death of tuberculosis was listed separately from death of causes other than tuberculosis. Deaths were recorded during the first 2 years after diagnosis. It is remarkable that the case-fatality attributable to tuberculosis steadily increased from 0.8% in 1975–1976 to 3.5% in 1983–1984.

C. Surveillance of BCG Vaccination

It is inevitable that in low-prevalence countries the time will come (and already has in some countries) when cessation of mass BCG vaccination, especially at birth, will have to be considered because, quite apart from economic considerations, the complications of BCG vaccination will outweigh the benefits obtained (Styblo, 1991). For example, Sweden discontinued BCG vaccination in 1975, and the former Federal Republic of Germany in 1983. Waaler and Rouillon estimate that in an epidemiological situation, in which the annual risk of tuberculous infection fell to 0.02%, two to four cases of primary tuberculosis are prevented during a 15-year period in a cohort of 100,000 subjects vaccinated at birth, assuming 100% coverage, 80% protection by BCG vaccine, and 15-year duration of protection (Waaler and Rouillon, 1974).

D. Surveillance of Chemoprophylaxis

A selective search for tuberculin converters in high-risk groups, such as among contacts of bacillary index cases and active case-finding in specific risk groups, is an important intervention for preventing tuberculosis by supplying chemoprophylaxis. It has been suggested that disease surveillance be expanded in low-prevalence countries by the surveillance of recent infections detected by contact tracing. It may very well be that systematic notification of recent converters detected by contact-tracing procedures (and eligible for preventive chemotherapy) by age group (children and young adults) will yield a sensitive measure of the tuberculosis problem in low-prevalence countries (see Sec. IV.B.).

Although no objective indicator exists, it is suggested that an operational indicator be introduced to monitor side effects and to measure chemoprophylaxis completion rates.

References

Aoki, M. (1991). Surveillance of tuberculosis in low prevalence countries where tuberculosis is in decline. *Bull. Int. Union Tuberc.* **66**:201–202.

Bleiker, M. A. (1984). Tuberculine en tuberculine-onderzoek. In *Leerboek der Tuberculosebestrijding KNCV*, The Hague, pp. VI.1–19.

Bleiker, M. A., Misljenovic, O., Broekmans, J. F., and Blijker I. C. F. (1956–1991). Annual reports, International Tuberculosis Surveillance Centre, NIPG/TNO.

British Thoracic Society Research Committee and the Medical Research Council Cardiothoracic Epidemiology Group (1991). The management of pulmonary tuberculosis in adults notified in England and Wales in 1988. *Respir. Med.* **85**:319–323.

Broekmans, J. F. (1991). The point of view of a low prevalence country: The Netherlands. *Bull. Int. Union Tuberc.* **66**:179–183.

Brudney, K., and Dobkin, J. (1991). Resurgent tuberculosis in New York City. Human immunodeficiency virus, homelessness, and the decline of tuberculosis control programs. *Am. Rev. Respir. Dis.* **144**:745–749.

Centers for Disease Control (1989). Summary of notifiable diseases, United States. *MMWR* **38**:45.

Centers for Disease Control (1990). Tuberculosis morbidity in the United States: Final data. *MMWR*, **40**(SS-3):23–27.

Chief Medical Officer (1951–1990). Ministry of Welfare, Health and Culture, The Netherlands. Annual reports.

Clancy, L., Rieder, H. L., Enarson, D. A., and Spinaci, S. (1991). Tuberculosis elimination in the countries of Europe and other industrialized countries. Based on a workshop held at Wolfheze, Netherlands, 4–9 March 1990, under the joint auspices of the IUATLD (Europe region) and WHO. *Eur. Respir. J.* **4**:1288–1295.

Dowdle, W. R. (1989). A strategic plan for the elimination of tuberculosis in the United States. *MMWR* **38**:S-3:1–25.

Heffernan, J. F., Nunn, A. J., Peto, J., and Fox, W. (1976). Tuberculosis in Scotland: A national sample survey (1968–70). 2. A two-year follow-up of newly-diagnosed respiratory tuberculosis notified in 1968. *Tubercle* **57**:161–175.

Reichman, L. B. (1991). [Editorial]. The U-shaped curve of concern. *Am. Rev. Respir. Dis.* **144**:741–742.

Rieder, H. L., Cauthen, G. M., Comstock, G. W., and Snider D. E., Jr. (1989). Epidemiology of tuberculosis in the United States. *Epidemiol. Rev.* **11**:79–98.

Rieder, H. L., Kelly, G. D., Bloch, A. B., Cauthen, G. M., and Snider, D. E., Jr. (1991). Tuberculosis diagnosed at death in the United States. *Chest* **100**:678–681.

Styblo, K. (1990). The elimination of tuberculosis in The Netherlands. *Bull. Int. Union Tuberc.* **65**:49–55.

Styblo, K. (1991). Epidemiology of tuberculosis. *Selected Papers* **24** KNCV, The Hague.

Styblo, K., Dankova, D., Drapela, J., Galliova, J., Jezek, Z., Krivanek, J., Kubik, A., Langerova, M., and Radkovsky, J. (1967). Epidemiological and clinical study of tuberculosis in the District of Kolin, Czechoslovakia. *Bull. WHO* **37**:819–874.

Sutherland, I., Bleiker, M. A., Meijer, J., and Styblo, K. (1984). The risk of tuberculous infection in The Netherlands from 1967 to 1979. Report of the Tuberculosis Surveillance Research Unit (TSRU) established by the International Union Against Tuberculosis (IUAT) in collaboration with the World Health Organization (WHO). *Selected Papers* **22**:75–92, KNCV, The Hague.

Tala, E., and Kochi, A. (1991). [Editorial]. Elimination of tuberculosis from Europe and the world. *Eur. Respir. J.* **4**:1159–1160.

van Geuns, H. A., Hellinga, H. S., Bleiker, M. A., and Styblo, K. (1987). Surveillance of diagnostic and treatment measures in The Netherlands. *TSRU Progr. Rep.* **1**:60–81.

Veen, J. (1991). Tuberculosis in a low prevalence country: A wolf in sheep's clothing. *Bull. Int. Union Tuberc.* **66**:203–205.

Veen, J. (1992). Microepidemics in tuberculosis: The stone-in-the-pond principle. *Tuberc. Lung Dis.* **73**:73–76.

Waaler, H. T., and Rouillon, A. (1974). BCG vaccination policies according to the epidemiological situation. *Bull Int. Union Tuberc.* **49**:166–189.

World Health Organization (1989). Tuberculosis Unit, Division of Communicable Diseases, WHO, Geneva.

30

The Role of Nongovernmental Organizations

ANNIK ROUILLON

International Union Against Tuberculosis
and Lung Disease
Paris, France

FRANCES R. OGASAWARA

American Lung Association
New York, New York

I. Introduction

In the fight against tuberculosis, a partnership exists among three important sectors: the public, the health professionals, and the government. This chapter will deal with two of these three partners: the public and the health professionals.

Previous chapters have shown that our present weapons against tuberculosis are effective, are acceptable by the population, are affordable by governments, are able to be assimilated by less sophisticated health personnel and, therefore, can be evaluated. They can be coordinated into national tuberculosis control programs in developed countries as well as in developing countries. A simple relationship between a patient and the doctor as individuals through community-oriented national tuberculosis programs is part of the global fight against tuberculosis. The responsibility for having a national program rests with the government; it is up to the health authorities to design, staff, implement, assess, and orient the program. Although this is generally accepted and would seem fully logical today, it is remarkable that the first organized effort against tuberculosis (which in many instances led the way to other public health measures) originated from the voluntary combination of the energy of physicians and the public in an attempt to relieve suffering, prevent disease, and disseminate information. Thus were created at the end of the past century and the beginning of this century, voluntary associations that gather together lay individuals and professionals to develop the first elements for the concerted effort to fight tuberculosis. In most countries, even though governments have taken the responsibility for providing health services in relevant programs, the success of any governmental program continues to depend on the competence and attitudes of professionals who are delivering the programs and on the active and understanding participation by the people in the measures offered them.

Voluntary nongovernmental organizations are the best means of ensuring high standards in the application of the professional and governmental measures and the widespread participation of the public in any control program. This includes lobbying for improvements and acting as a "watchdog" for the program.

A. What Is a Volunteer?

Since nongovernmental organizations (NGO) originate from the grass roots level, that is, from ordinary citizens, it is necessary to define a *volunteer*. Volunteers are persons from any walk of life, who are ready to devote, freely and without remuneration, part of their time and effort to a special cause or task to which they feel motivated to commit themselves.

Volunteers should not be expected nor requested to work more than a few hours each week (or to give a very sustained effort for more than a limited time). They must know exactly what they have to do and should receive proper training in their approach to the task and to other people, and in the procedures to be followed if they will have to apply specific means.

Members of an organization are the first level of voluntarism: they are persons who took the step to enlist themselves or to register and who contribute; they are supposed to follow the development of the activities toward the relevant aim and, when necessary, to give their moral, then possibly financial and physical support to action, thereby becoming more and more an active volunteer. The work of volunteers is organized and backed by an association, and these exist at the local, national, and international levels.

B. What Is a Nongovernmental Organization?

An NGO is an organization or association formed by a group of persons with a common interest, a shared experience, or a similar goal. The NGOs may also be called nonprofit organizations or philanthropic organizations; voluntary or community councils; neighborhood groups; women's organizations; or economic and social development groups. They may be organized for a particular purpose, such as—in the field of health—disease-specific organizations or disability-specific organizations. They may be groups of patients, families, and friends suffering from the same disease or condition. Also included are professional so-cieties organized by members of the health professions, such as physicians, nurses, or other public health workers, or charitable organizations, such as church-related groups who contribute to needy causes.

The NGO can be purely local or may have national or international scope. Often a national or international organization may function as a federation of corresponding local or national NGOs.

It is at the local level that the association should prove its efficacy and worth. The national body has the role of assisting a local association by pro-viding proper information, training, guidance, and backing.

The NGOs are generally directed by the members themselves, The mem-bers select a group from the membership to provide leadership and determine how the organization will achieve its goals. Throughout the organization, vol-unteers do much of the work of leadership and program implementation. When budget allows, staff is hired to carry out the program of the organization and to give administrative support. NGOs are funded by one or a combination of the following sources: membership dues, contributions, service fees, and contracts or grants from private and government sources. Fund-raising, however, is a per-manent problem for most associations.

Because they are independent, NGOs can function in any political climate and usually maintain a neutral position on political matters. They are free to pur-sue the policies and programs that the governing body, whether it be a board of directors, executive committee, or governing council, has determined will best achieve the mission of the organization. The NGO may determine membership criteria and may have several classes of members, including a category of mem-bership open to any interested person.

The NGO is a group with specific interest, experience, commitment, and expertise. They have the ability and willingness to respond to the needs of a par-ticular community in innovative and creative ways. Depending on the problem addressed, the community to be served, and the expertise of the NGO, it may have an important role in the formulation of strategies, in planning implemen-tation, and in providing service.

In dealing with health issues NGOs are a source of ideas and manpower. They can cooperate with, participate in, help to publicize and to influence pub-lic opinion in support of a government health program. They can also pressure governments to address unmet health needs. Grass roots NGOs, activists repre-senting victims or patients, can vociferously call attention to the needs of the consumers. Those NGOs that are professional societies may provide important technical advice on the scientific aspects of a health program. They may also play an important role in educating professional colleagues about new methods and concepts in treating and controlling disease (NGO, 1981).

Although so very diverse in their aims, structure, operation, and size, NGOs are sometimes considered as falling into one of the three following categories (Broadhead, 1989; Moerkek, 1989):

1. Service delivery (such as running of facilities for diagnosis, treatment, or rehabilitation)

2. Innovation (such as developing new approaches to yet unmet or new needs, for example, AIDS)

3. Advocacy (campaigning on a specific issue such as smoking)

In fact, many NGOs actually address all three aspects, simply focusing more on one, rather than the others; this also depends on the issue at stake.

Nongovernmental organizations are by no means new (Lee, 1988). Trade-groups existed in the Roman empire and in ancient Eastern, as well as in pre-Columbian, cultures. In Europe, the late Middle Ages saw the establishment of various guilds of merchants or artisans to protect their interests, rule prices, wages and procedures, and introduce codes of ethics. The Industrial Revolution saw the decline of these guilds in Europe, while at the same time, Americans started to show a propensity to band together. By 1900, 100 associations were in existence in the United States, 1000 by the end of World War I in 1918 and currently 21,000 exist, of which 3200 have their headquarters in Washington D.C.; 2300 have an office in New York; and 900 in Chicago; 1000 are being created every year.

Voluntary health organizations have played an important role in the health programs in most of the countries of Europe and North America (Holm, 1972). They started to emerge over 100 years ago, at a time when the social conditions and the health situation were quite different from what they are today; the countries of Europe and North America were in a process of socioeconomic development, influencing the rural populations that formed the greatest part of the countries' population at that time. Social and health services were hardly developed; self-reliance was a characteristic feature in most places. The first voluntary associations were founded to fight the most important and feared diseases; tuberculosis was first among these.

The tuberculosis or lung associations are nonprofit organizations. Basic financial support for the organizations comes from membership dues, voluntary contributions, and grants. In some countries associations receive grants from governments to carry out special programs. Some associations may have government contracts to provide medical services, and often hire staff to administer and carry out the day-to-day activities.

At the international level, the International Union Against Tuberculosis and Lung Disease (IUATLD) is the nonprofit, nongovernmental voluntary organization working in the tuberculosis and lung field. Among its constituent members are the national voluntary tuberculosis and lung associations world-wide. In the United States, the constituent member is the American Lung Association which, in turn, has constituent and affiliate associations throughout the country. The medical section of the American Lung Association, the American Thoracic Society, is also a professional society.

II. National Tuberculosis Associations

A. North America

American Lung Association

The American Lung Association (ALA) was founded in 1904 as the National Association for the Study and Prevention of Tuberculosis. It was the first national, voluntary health agency in America dedicated to fighting a single disease. It was also the first to combine the energies of physicians and lay persons in fighting a public health problem. The association was founded on the idea that something could be done about tuberculosis by citizens (Shryock, 1957).

A few local voluntary societies had been formed to fight tuberculosis as early as 1892. The founders of the national association were leading practitioners of medicine and active in broad projects for social betterment. They formed the new association to study tuberculosis in all its forms; to disseminate knowledge about the causes, treatment, and prevention of tuberculosis; and to encourage the prevention and scientific treatment of tuberculosis.

Widespread social organization, actions taken by an informed citizenry, was an important factor in the evolution of the modern public health campaign. A public education program was launched to inform people of the dangers of tuberculosis and the steps required to fight the disease. Pressure was put on lawmakers to build sanatoriums to provide rest, fresh air, and good food—the therapy advocated in 1904. When tuberculosis was recognized as being a contagious, rather than in inherited, disease, the need for sanatoriums to isolate the source of infection from the community became an important public health measure.

Tuberculosis control as a public health function was new in 1904, and most communities in the United States did not have organized health departments. Local tuberculosis associations pressured for the establishment of public health departments with tuberculosis control programs in every community. Lawmakers were also urged to fund these services with tax money so tuberculosis care would be available to all without cost to the patient.

The national association organized state and local associations all over the country to carry out this educational and legislative program at the community level. By 1956, there were about 2700 local associations; hence, programs and fund raising could be conducted in the local community. The Christmas Seal Campaign became the primary source of funds to conduct these activities. The first nationwide Christmas Seal Campaign was conducted in 1908. By 1920 the national association had shortened its name to National Tuberculosis Association (NTA).

In the prechemotherapy era, the National Tuberculosis Association, its constituents (state associations) and affiliates (local associations), conducted educational programs to dispel myths about tuberculosis, to encourage early detection and prompt treatment, and lobbied for adequate services and facilities and the means to finance them. The associations conducted tuberculin testing and mass chest X-ray services, provided rehabilitation services for persons with arrested disease, conducted school health education programs to promote good nutrition and healthy living to build up resistance. These programs were conducted in cooperation with official agencies (health departments, social welfare departments, education departments) and with private and professional societies, such as medical associations.

The medical section of the National Tuberculosis Association, the American Trudeau Society, was originally the American Sanatorium Association, founded in 1905. Its members included the physicians who were leaders in the field of tuberculosis. The organization supported research to study the tubercle bacillus, to find a cure for the disease, and to study the epidemiology of the disease so that it could be prevented. Through its annual meeting and other conferences, the American Trudeau Society provided the forum during which research results could be described, and successful treatment regimens could be shared. The American Trudeau Society also set standards for treatment.

After the discovery of effective chemotherapy for tuberculosis, the association promoted its widespread use and changes in services that were needed for outpatient care. The National Tuberculosis Association also changed its goal to the eradication of tuberculosis and, together with other agencies and organizations, devised nationwide plans to achieve that goal. As the tuberculosis problem declined, other lung diseases, especially smoking-related diseases were increasing. The National Tuberculosis Association expanded its program to include all respiratory diseases and changed its name to National Tuberculosis and Respiratory Disease Association in 1968 and to American Lung Association (ALA) in 1973. The Trudeau Society became the American Thoracic Society (ATS) in 1960.

In the post chemotherapy era, the lung associations, in cooperation with the U.S. Public Health Service and state and local health departments and other agencies and organizations, conducted tuberculosis eradication projects throughout the United States, promoting the use of chemotherapy and chemoprophylaxis. These projects were not only to cure an individual patient, but were viewed as public health measures: to prevent new infections by removing the source of tubercle bacilli and to prevent the infected from becoming infectious. Associations had programs to address problems in high-incidence and low-incidence communities and to meet the needs of multicultural communities and non-English-speaking persons.

As the tuberculosis problem declined in magnitude, programs were targeted to specific high-incidence groups of high-risk individuals, such as unemployed alcoholic men, migrant farmers, and recent immigrants. The American Thoracic Society issued statements and position papers on numerous aspects of tuberculosis treatment and control to promote optimum treatment and to change attitudes about what constitutes modern tuberculosis care. These statements have usually been issued jointly with the U.S. Public Health Service. They are used for professional education and as a guide to communities in planning tuberculosis services.

The increase in immigration of persons from high-incidence countries provided a source of infected persons at risk of becoming infectious and slowed the downward trend of morbidity. The appearance of the acquired immune deficiency syndrome (AIDS) and human immunodeficiency virus (HIV) infection, especially in large cities, has resulted in a reversal in the decline of the tuberculosis problem. The American Lung Association is still committed to the elimination of tuberculosis and is placing continued emphasis on solving the difficult blocks to reaching the goal.

The mission of the American Lung Association today is the conquest of lung disease and the promotion of lung health; the goals are the prevention of lung disease, the cure of lung disease, and the control of lung disease. The program includes lung disease care and education, which includes all lung diseases, with emphasis on asthma, influenza, and pneumonia prevention, and on tuberculosis. Also included in the program is air conservation; combating air pollution, both outdoors and indoors; smoking cessation, prevention, and education; control of occupational hazards to the lungs; and promotion of school health education.

The American Lung Association–American Thoracic Society conducts its program through education, advocacy, and the support of research. Examples of educational activities include programs directed to the public about steps they can take to fight air pollution; helping in the design of educational materials on asthma for the public, patients, and school personnel; conferences for the media to discuss new reports on lung health issues; conducting a study of a comprehensive school health curriculum; helping new parents learn of the harm to babies and children of passive smoking; and information for workers at risk for occupational lung disease.

In its advocacy activities, the American Lung Association and American Thoracic Society provide spokespersons to provide expert testimony before the U.S. Congress on lung health issues, such as indoor and outdoor air pollution; the need to increase funding of the lung research program of the National Institutes of Health (NIH); the importance of grants to state and local communities to support the tuberculosis control programs; and the health effects of second-hand smoke on airlines.

The ALA and ATS work through coalitions of other like-minded health organizations. Sometimes ALA and ATS bring together a coalition or invite the participation of other interested organizations to solve problems they have in common and to conduct joint programs.

The research program of the ALA and ATS awards "seed money" research grants to young investigators. It encourages the training and development of future research scientists. The professional education program includes the publication of two journals; the *American Journal of Respiratory and Critical Care Medicine* (formerly *American Review of Respiratory Disease* and the *American Journal of Respiratory Cell and Molecular Biology*. The ALA–ATS international conference is an annual meeting during which papers on original research, symposia, major lectures, and numerous other educational sessions are presented. Conferences and workshops on specialized subjects are conducted during the year to develop policies or to discuss issues, or to increase the medical community's knowledge about a particular disease and its treatment.

An important part of the American Lung Association is its communications program. Working through all media, television, radio, and publications, it disseminates information and educates the public on all aspects of the lung disease problem and what can be done about it. As a voluntary organization, with expertise, it is perceived by the public as having credibility and being a source of valid scientific knowledge and accurate information.

The American Lung Association is governed by a volunteer board of directors. Volunteers also serve on the council and on numerous committees, both administrative and program, that guide the operation and program of the organization. The national paid staff, directed by the Managing Director, is made up of competent trained professionals in all aspects of association management, health education, communications, fund raising, business management, and organizational development.

Serving all communities through the United States are 122 state and local lung associations. Each is independently incorporated, affiliated with the national association through a legal agreement, and is governed by a volunteer Board of Directors. Each is staffed by an Executive Director and other staff members to carry out the activities of the association. The Board of Directors of each association sets the policies for that association and, working with the staff, develops its program and fund raising following the policies and guidelines of the national association. The number of associations has been declining in recent years, as boards see economies of scale and cost savings in staff and office sharing, leading to total mergers of programs and then associations.

Public financial support comes from many sources: the traditional Christmas Seal Campaign, other direct-mail efforts, special events, major corporate and individual gifts, workplace giving, planned gifts, memorials, grants, and in kind contributions. Membership fees and service fees also help fund activities.

Because program is determined by each association, there is some variation in the particular activities carried out. Programs are planned according to the needs identified, and priorities are set, and activities chosen according to the resources available. Through expansion of the mission and changes in objectives, the association has continued its role of leading and enlisting citizen action to help solve a health problem. It works with all groups and all sectors of society to identify what needs to be done, to influence those in a position to make changes, and to educate and encourage those whose participation or individual action is required. It emphasizes individual responsibility as well as concerted community action.

Canadian Lung Association

The Canadian Lung Association (CLA) was founded in 1900 as that country's national NGO dealing with tuberculosis. In 1969, the emphasis was changed to include lung diseases under its mandate, and the organization was changed to Canadian Tuberculosis and Respiratory Disease Association. Finally, in 1977, at its annual meeting in Moncton, New Brunswick, Canada, the association changed its name to the Canadian Lung Association. The medical arm is called the Canadian Thoracic Society. The major role of the CLA in its relation to the International Union Against Tuberculosis and Lung Disease has been to spearhead international activities through the IUATLD's Mutual Assistance Program in the form of grants to various projects in developing countries (Hershfield, 1981, 1987). This program was instituted at the time of the IUAT's World Conference held in Toronto in 1961. It consisted primarily of maintaining an IUAT's office in Kuala Lumpur, Malaysia for the Far Eastern region, in developing regional seminars in the Far East, and to assist in developing provincial and district offices in various countries in the Far East. The Canadian Lung Association has also contributed heavily to tuberculosis educational seminars in various Far Eastern countries, including Sri Lanka, Pakistan, Malaysia and Nepal, Indonesia, India, Thailand, Bangladesh, and the Republic of Korea. In more recent years the CLA has supported the establishment of an international course in tuberculosis microbiology in Ottawa for individuals from developing countries. It has also assisted these countries in establishing and equipping tuberculosis laboratories.

Similar to its counterpart, the American Lung Association, the association is divided into provincial associations who raise funds through a national Christmas Seal campaign. These funds are directed toward education in tuberculosis and lung disease, research in these areas, and to assisting the IUATLD in its operating and mutual assistance budgets. The members of CTS are active in provincial, national, and international organizations, including the IUATLD.

B. Latin America

In Latin America, especially in areas where there is not yet full medicosocial protection of the population, "tuberculosis leagues," as they are most often called, have long been striving to assist poor patients and their families, to run outpatient clinics, and to trigger government interest for the establishment of modern national programs. An extreme case is the Comision Honoraria para Tuberculosis of Uruguay.

The Comision has full technical, financial, and operational responsibility for all antituberculosis activities in the country. Through carefully applied treatment, they were able 10 years ago to cure all the 350 then existing chronic tuberculosis patients in the country. The Comision also carries on research, mostly epidemiological. It is also responsible for all vaccinations (against any disease) with vaccines provided by the government. Funds necessary for these activities come from a tax on alcoholic beverages and from lotteries.

C. Europe

National tuberculosis associations were formed in Austria in 1890, in France in 1891, in Great Britain and Belgium in 1898, and in Portugal and Italy in 1899.

A survey of 25 (practically all) European national tuberculosis or lung disease associations (Trnka, 1984) showed that, by the mid-1980s, tuberculosis had remained the sole concern of only two associations; 18 others kept tuberculosis as their main priority; so 23 out of 25 now include other lung diseases or cardiovascular diseases and, in one, aging, in another malnutrition, and another, malaria. Their approach to dealing with their objectives is through counseling, assessment of control (in 18), and postgraduate education (in 17); 10 have research activities and 7 social and welfare activities. All except 3 hold regular meetings, conferences and symposia. Almost 90% issue regular journals, yearbooks, selected papers, or other publications. Membership consists mainly of physicians and other medical or paramedical personnel, 8 also enroll lay persons, and 5 enroll institutions. Their source of income is usually membership fees; however, 13 carry out fund-raising campaigns, 10 receive support from official authorities, and 4 manage their own property.

No single European association intends to restrict its activity in the future. On the contrary, more than half envisage extension. In the field of tuberculosis, they recommend the promotion of research activities in tuberculosis surveillance, in solving problems with foreign workers and immigrants, and in dealing with nontuberculous mycobacterial diseases.

A comparison of associations in two European countries, which are approaching elimination of tuberculosis, illustrate the differences.

The Royal Netherlands Tuberculosis Association

The Royal Netherlands Tuberculosis Association (KNCV) is an advocate of one single disease, tuberculosis, and it has been preparing for its new role in the tuberculosis elimination phase: it has progressively donated to the government the whole network of specialized facilities that its branches had been operating; these facilities and their corresponding staff are now being integrated into the general health services; at the same time it has expanded its capacity for preserving the existing knowledge about tuberculosis and providing expert consultations on public health and clinical aspects of the disease; it has increased its educational and quality assurance activities. It is recognized by the Ministry of Health, the Municipal Health Services, and the Netherlands association for specialists in pulmonary diseases and tuberculosis.

Meanwhile and, in fact for 30 years, the Netherlands association from its privileged low-prevalence situation has felt direct concern for high-prevalence countries (Broekmans, 1991), and it was one of the initiators and first contributors with the Canadian Lung Association to the Mutual Assistance Program installed within the IUATLD. Like Canada, it contributed to seminars in developing countries and to the first projects of assistance to newly created tuberculosis associations in developing countries, in particular to a program of sputum smear case-finding and ambulatory treatment in a sparsely populated area in Mali, entirely relying on the work of a male nurse. Later on, when the IUATLD Mutual Assistance Program ran essentially full national programs in collaboration with governments, the KNCV contributed, and still does contribute, technical and material help to Tanzania, Malawi, Benin, Mali, and Kenya.

Norway

Norway, another European country that will also see the elimination of tuberculosis in the early part of the 21st century, has witnessed the transformation of its Tuberculosis and Public Health Association (founded in 1910) toward one dealing with cardiovascular diseases, elderly care and welfare, and healthy lifestyles (Rouillon, 1987; Wilberg, 1987). It kept a small subcommittee on tuberculosis and maintained a constant concern for making others benefit from their efforts and experience in combating tuberculosis, including international advanced training courses; since 1976, the tuberculosis subcommittee has been instrumental in obtaining from the government of Norway substantial support of the IUATLD for its structures and its activities; a first seminar was organized in 1983 in Zimbabwe, gathering 100 delegates from ten countries of Eastern Africa: it was the first time that the countries of that part of the world had a seminar on tuberculosis. The Norwegian association, together with another national voluntary agency, and the Norwegian government support technically and financially the IUATLD collaborative national programs in Nicaragua, Mozambique, Malawi, Benin, and Senegal.

Following the example of the Netherlands and Norwegian associations, other European associations now also promote special drives for developing countries through the IUATLD and also provide it with the support of their governments; such as Switzerland, Finland, France, and Germany. The Belgian association has provided special donations from closed former sanatoriums, and the British association together with the French association assisted the IUATLD to establish its nontuberculosis respiratory program.

D. Middle East

Tuberculosis associations in the Middle East, besides working for their respective country, are also contributing to international activities. Examples are the following:

1. The Syrian association for many years has been reprinting relevant parts of the *IUATLD Bulletin* into Arabic and distributing it in the region.

2. In 1950, the first International Training and Demonstration Centre for Tuberculosis was established in Istanbul and run by the tuberculosis association. Besides its own national tasks (Ozgen, 1987) the association has hosted the 15th World Conference of the IUATLD in 1959, its Annual Meetings in 1970 and 1977 and, in 1985, the IUATLD Middle East Regional Meeting.

3. The Egyptian association has also been supporting international activities of the IUATLD: two regional meetings, a regional seminar, and the Conference on Tuberculosis in Animals in Africa and the Middle East in 1992, promoted by the Tuberculosis in Animals Scientific Committee of the IUATLD. The regional meeting was held in Cairo in 1992.

4. Through the IUATLD, the Kingdom of Saudi Arabia is supporting the whole National Tuberculosis Program of Yemen.

E. Africa

After independence, in western and eastern Africa as well as in North Africa, most of the associations dating from the colonial period reorganized themselves. Lack of funds and the many problems with which those countries are confronted, as well as the disaster of the HIV epidemic, render their work in sub-Saharan Africa especially difficult, although especially needed.

1. In Ivory Coast (Bretton, 1986), the association has been instrumental in promoting the government's program, disseminating instructions and infor-

mation to the staff and to the population and in filling gaps in the procurement of drugs and products or repairing vehicles.

2.   In Togo and in Senegal support has been given by more affluent European associations for their issuing of Christmas seals and conducting education and fund-raising campaigns. The Mali association with the support of the Netherlands association ran a pilot project of sputum smear case-finding and ambulatory treatment.

3.   The old Tunisian Antituberculosis League, which had mainly been creating dispensaries, was reorganized in 1957, 1965, and 1975 to become in 1981 the National League Against Tuberculosis and Respiratory Disease (Tunisian League, 1987). The association is active in giving clothing, food, and travel assistance to patients in underprivileged districts, in many activities of health education for the public, and in contributing to the efforts of the government in training microscopists and in refresher sessions for physicians. After its 1965 relaunching, it conducted with the IUAT an important pilot project of case detection by sputum smear examination and twice-weekly supervised treatment in a remote area. These principles, demonstrated in different ways and settings in Mali and in Tunisia, were to appear in the further resolutions of the World Health Assembly and of the Alma-Ata Primary Health Care Conference of 1978.

4.   In Algeria, the Comité Algérien de Lutte contre la Tuberculose (CALT) founded in 1965 (Larbaoui, 1987) has conducted several seal campaigns, giving as much material support as possible to the national program through the publication of technical guidelines, registers, educational material, the granting of awards to motivate microscopists and treatment supervisors, and through a particularly important activity: the "supervision and evaluation seminars" held once a year in almost every province, in which all members of the team with a group from the capital city examine what succeeded and what failed in the application of the program.

The CALT is a member of the Tuberculosis Surveillance Research Unit (TSRU), an advanced research unit linked to the IUATLD (see below): indeed the National Algerian Program, which was systematically developed on modern bases, is able to provide information for epidemiological and operational analysis useful to assess its own program as well as to assist other countries in their own approaches. It is also supporting the WHO/IUATLD/Algerian government international training course in tuberculosis control methods held every year in Algeria (Perdrizet, 1988).

F.   Far East

Most countries in Asia possess a tuberculosis association and many of them are quite active in running facilities, organizing courses and meetings, and informing the public. Almost all keep tuberculosis as their sole or prominent focus.

Asia

In Asia, the association with the broadest scope in its work is no doubt the Japan Antituberculosis Association (JATA) (Shimao, 1987). Its five major activities are:

1. Distribution of information on tuberculosis, respiratory disease, and smoking-related problems in its *Bulletin*, in books, pamphlets, leaflets, films, slides, and video.

2. Promotion of public concern on tuberculosis and related problems through public assemblies; awards to cities, towns, and villages achieving good results; and cooperation with the Antituberculosis Women's Society.

3. Research activities through the operation of the Research Institute of Tuberculosis, including basic, immunologic, clinical, epidemiological, and operational research.

4. Training activities on both tuberculosis and respiratory disease, with series of courses for medical doctors, students, X-ray technicians, laboratory technicians, public health nurses, administrative staff, as well as one yearly 2-day seminar for each of the seven regions of Japan.

5. International cooperation with courses

Since 1963, a yearly International Course on Tuberculosis jointly with WHO and the government of Japan

Since 1973, a senior training course on tuberculosis control

Since 1977, an international course on laboratory work

From 1965 to 1974, a course on chest surgery

Individual training

People from 53 countries participated in those various international courses.

Participation in bilateral technical assistance provided to developing countries by the Japanese government (Tanzania, Thailand, Nepal, Yemen)

Cooperation with WHO by sending JATA staff members to work for WHO

Cooperation in the United States–Japan Cooperative Medical Science Program

JATA hosted the 22nd World IUATLD Conference in 1973.

India

The Tuberculosis Association of India was established in 1939 (Pamra, 1984). One of the first steps the association took was to evolve a practical approach to the care of tuberculosis patients. The New Delhi Tuberculosis Center, established in 1940, was upgraded with the help of the government, WHO, and United Nations International Emergency Children's Fund (UNICEF; now the United Nations Children's Fund) as a training and demonstration center. In 1948, the association formed its technical committee consisting of 15 senior tuberculosis workers from over the country; the committee acts as a nonofficial advisory body to the government. The National Tuberculosis Program launched in 1962 is periodically revised by the technical committee. The association has a wide program of health education through the production of films, posters, slides, flip charts, and school health brochures. These are distributed through state associations and other voluntary agencies and the government.

The *Indian Journal of Tuberculosis*, a quarterly publication of the association, is the only journal devoted exclusively to tuberculosis in the country. The association also issues textbooks for physicians, blue prints, and the *Handbook of Tuberculosis*, which covers, in simple language, the essential facts about clinical, epidemiological, and social aspects of the disease, and lays special stress on aspects concerning nurses, health visitors, and lay social workers in their day-to-day work. A regular program of the association is holding the annual conferences for tuberculosis and chest disease workers, and the organization, together with the Indian Medical Association, holds periodic 1-day refresher courses for general practitioners.

Funds (some US $80,000 yearly) come from interest on investment, publication sales, donations, and shares on Tuberculosis Seal collections. There are 25 state tuberculosis associations that are affiliated with the central association; most of them also have tuberculosis associations at the district level. They assist official services in the distribution and administration of drugs. They also organize case-finding and immunization camps in remote areas where tuberculosis services are deficient. Many of them hold conferences on the same pattern as the yearly national conference. The 14th World Conference of the IUAT in 1957 was held in New Delhi, the first time the Union left Western capitals.

Bangladesh

The Bangladesh Tuberculosis Association deals with a population of some 120 million in a country under the handicap of enormous flood and typhoon disasters. Education, information and demonstration projects are carried out.

Indonesia, Thailand, Singapore

Such is also true of the Indonesian association (Kusnadi, 1987), also dealing with a vast population; it received a special award from the IUATLD in 1986. The association of Thailand is a 58-year-old institution. The Singapore association hosted the 26th World Conference of the IUATLD in 1986.

Korea

The Korean National Tuberculosis Association (KNTA) was founded in 1953 and evolved as the technical arm of the National Tuberculosis Programme (NTP) (Hong, 1990). For the launching of the NTP in 1962, the KNTA recruited, trained, and posted supervisory medical officers and nurses for the city and provincial governments and follow-up workers and microscopists for health centers. They became government employees in 1967. The KNTA established a Central Tuberculosis Laboratory and nine city or provincial tuberculosis laboratories. Health centers do microscopy only. In 1988, 400,000 microscopy examinations were done at health centers for case-finding, 160,000 cultures were done at the city and provincial and central laboratories and 5000 drug-sensitivity and 4400 identification tests were performed. Contributions to the nationwide random sample epidemiological surveys started in 1965 and are repeated every 5 years.

In 1970, the KNTA established the Korean Institute for Tuberculosis (KIT) within its structure, to strengthen its role as technical arm of the national program. Various surveys, trials, assessment of results, and operational research are thus carried out jointly. The production of freeze-dried bacille Calmette-Guerin (BCG) vaccine is also entrusted to the KIT. The training sessions for all categories of health workers provided by the KNTA, up to 1981, were then transferred to the National Institute of Health, but the staff of the KIT still participates actively. The KNTA has been a member of the international Tuberculosis Surveillance Research Unit (TSRU) since 1984. It has an important health education program, with a monthly magazine, films, videotapes, and slides, distributed to health centers, schools, and relevant agencies. A seal campaign takes place every year. The Korean seals are famous for their design and grace and have almost every year won the first prize at the "Seal of Year International Contest" of the IUATLD.

III. The International Union Against Tuberculosis and Lung Disease

The International Union Against Tuberculosis and Lung Disease (IUATLD) (Rouillon, 1982, 1984) is the federation of national tuberculosis and lung disease associations and of individual persons interested in the fight against these diseases from all over the world. It is one of the oldest voluntary international organizations dealing with health.

Shaped in its present form in 1920 at a Paris Congress on Tuberculosis, it in fact originated at the Berlin International Tuberculosis Congress of 1902, which decided on the creation of a Central Bureau for the Prevention of Tuberculosis (further called the International Antituberculosis Association). Even this central bureau was the result of international concern for tuberculosis, which can be traced back to 1867 when, at the first International Medical Congress, in Paris, several sessions were devoted to this disease and the classic work of Villemin demonstrating the contagion of tuberculosis was presented (Chretien, 1992).

Subsequent international congresses on tuberculosis were held in Paris in 1888, 1891, 1893, and 1898; in Berlin in 1899, when for the first time official representatives from various governments and voluntary agencies were present; in London in 1901; then in Berlin again for the 1902 congress just referred to. It was also at this Berlin congress that, on the proposal of Dr. Gilbert Sisteron, the Secretary General of the federation of the French Antituberculosis Associations, the double-barred red cross was adopted as the emblem of the fight against tuberculosis.*

The international bureau organized conferences in Paris, The Hague, Vienna, Philadelphia (in 1908); Stockholm, Brussels (in 1910, where the death of Robert Koch was announced); Rome and Berlin (1912); it was to take place in Bern, Switzerland, when World War I broke out in 1914 and put a stop to the activities of the international association. The experience and suffering of the war had brought maturity to certain concepts and, when representatives from 31 nations met in October 1920 in Paris, they moved in an impressive procession in the large lecture hall of the Sorbonne and pledged one by one their wholehearted collaboration in the campaign against tuberculosis and declared their belief in an organization that would impose obligations on its members and centralize all the experience of the disease. The words that Leon Bernard, Secretary of the French Association, pronounced on that occasion remain extraordinarily valid today:

> It is necessary for all countries wishing to eradicate tuberculosis to decide among themselves on the methods, to agree on the most effective weapons, and to forge and implement them jointly against the common enemy . . . Anti-tuberculosis measures must some day be standardised but first it is necessary for the research workers to make a thorough investigation of the problem in order to provide governments with the necessary information . . .

These words were no doubt prophetic and during the almost three-quarters of a century of its modern existence, the "Union"—as its members call it—remained faithful to this description of its mission.

---

*The double-barred cross, the origin of which can be traced back to the second Century, was added in 1099 on the banner of the Prince of Lorraine, of France, who raised the first crusades. It thus became the emblem of an enlistment in the service of an ideal, of the rallying of all those committed to an imposing idea. Over the years, certain countries have replaced this emblem with others that they felt corresponded more closely to their countries' traditions and culture. Some have thus chosen the double red crescent (Islamic countries) or the red lion and sun.

In 1973 the IUAT decided to enlarge from tuberculosis to cover other lung diseases and community health but it added "and Lung Disease" (LD) to its name to become the IUATLD only in 1986; actually in this enlarged field it is cautious not to overlap with others (such as mucoviscidosis or cancer) while focusing on lung diseases with both a global and public health significance (acute respiratory infections, a number of aspects of asthma, the fight against smoking, occupational lung diseases, the consequences of natural disaster on the lung, and so on).

Sharing knowledge and efforts while backing national associations is its very essence and it materialized in a permanent program of activities against tuberculosis as well as in various achievements of global practical significance which will be described in the following sections.

A. Program of Activities

Dissemination of Knowledge

Knowledge dissemination is accomplished through meetings, seminars and courses, and publications.

1. World conferences are perhaps the most visible part of the program. They were organized initially every second year, now every fourth year; the next, the 28th of the series, is to take place in Mainz, Germany, in 1994. The preceding conference was in Boston in 1990, held jointly with the American Lung Association and the American Thoracic Society. Over 10,000 participants from 86 countries attended—the largest attendance at any international conference on tuberculosis and lung disease.

2. Regional conferences are held every second year in each of the six regions of the Union (Africa, Far East, Europe, Latin America, Middle East, North America). Some 70 such meetings have taken place.

3. Several regional or national seminars gather from 50 to 300 participants each year.

4. Four international regular yearly courses on tuberculosis are held in English, French, Spanish or Portugese, geared to epidemiology and the delivery of national control programs (Perdrizet, 1988).

5. Since 1920, 66 volumes of the *Bulletin of the IUATLD* were issued giving in their English, French, and Spanish versions the papers presented at the various Union's conferences as well as other original articles. The *Bulletin* and the well-known British international journal on tuberculosis *Tubercle* have recently merged (1992) to become a single publication, *Tubercle and Lung Disease* focusing in greater

part on practical issues in the delivery and assessment of programs (against tuberculosis or lung diseases).

6. Technical guides and manuals for field workers have been developed and printed in English, French, Spanish, Portuguese, Arabic, and Vietnamese. They are adapted to the specific structure of the health services and the measures decided by each national program. A prototype is the *Tuberculosis Guide for High Prevalence Countries* (IUATLD, 1991).

Applied Research

In its concern to try and grasp, and answer needs at the "consumer level" in 1951 the Union organized itself into six regions to adapt activities to local circumstances.

At the same period it also constituted a number of scientific committees (Rouillon, 1973, 1984). They were composed of the best experts in various fields and they began a number of surveys and studies. Among these are two studies on the chemotherapy of tuberculosis, grouping centers in 17 and 21 countries, respectively (Rist and Crofton, 1960; IUAT, 1964); the reading of 1100 X-ray films by 100 readers in ten countries (Springett, 1968); the assessment of treatment results in routine practice in 5 countries (Bignall, 1979); the study on the chemoprophylaxis of fibrotic lesions of the lung (Krebs, et al., 1979) with 25,000 participants followed 5 years in seven countries; and the international survey on BCG complications (Lotte, et al., 1987). These various works were the first international multicentric collaborative studies in the world, soon introduced in other fields of health as well.

At the same time, an international unit for advanced epidemiological studies, the Tuberculosis Surveillance Research Unit (TSRU), was created, jointly with the World Health Organization and four constituent members in 1965 (Rouillon, 1978; Styblo, 1991). The work of this unit, directed by Dr. Karel Styblo, has resulted in the development of a single epidemiological index, the risk of infection, to follow the level and the trend of the tuberculosis situation. A separate unit is operating in The Hague (the International Tuberculosis Surveillance Centre; Bleiker, 1978) to train teams and assist countries in collecting data and calculating their risk of infection (Bleiker, et al., 1989). It has also made important contributions to the understanding and quantification of the natural history of the disease and to the mode of action of our means, thus providing new information, often shaking long-accepted concepts, deep-rooted dogmas, and vested interests. Such long-standing programs were assessed and placed in their proper significance and perspective: the epidemiological role of BCG; the yield of mass X-ray examinations and of regular tuberculin testing of school children; the degree of transmission of the disease; the indefinite systematic follow-up of former patients; the effect of treatment on the epidemiological situation; the defects in diagnosis; the role of the migrant workers' presence on tuberculosis in a country; the proportion of cases diagnosed only after death; the degree of application of the new effective means and approaches; and now the relation between HIV and tuberculosis.

Several countries such as The Netherlands, Sweden, Germany, and Switzerland changed various aspects of their tuberculosis policy following the TSRU findings.

Collaborative National Control Programs

The Mutual Assistance Program of the IUATLD, which started in 1961, represents one further step for the Union in addressing practical problems and trying to remain as close as possible to the "periphery" (Rouillon, 1991). It was initially aimed at strengthening the voluntary part of the tuberculosis programs in resource-poor developing countries, and it was to be implemented by support from affluent member associations giving through the Union. But it appeared more and more that, to be really effective, more had to be done than only assist voluntary associations to become and remain true partners of their government, and that it would be more rewarding and more efficient if the Union would back governments directly. At that period, national and international interest in tuberculosis had decreased significantly and even WHO had considerably reduced its worldwide support for tuberculosis activities.

The Union thus started to work with the governmental tuberculosis units of some developing countries. A few of the Union's members, essentially the Netherlands Tuberculosis Association at the beginning, and the international cooperation departments of a few governments (essentially the Swiss and the Norwegian governments) provided substantial support to these national efforts. Others joined (such as the associations of Finland, France, Norway, Belgium, and the governments of Saudi Arabia, Finland, and France). From 1 million dollars spent in total over the first 15-year period (1961–1976) ("seed" money given to promote association's work), the Mutual Assistance Program now spends 3 million dollars per year. It currently covers directly eight countries in Africa, the Middle East, and Latin America, all resource-poor, and most of them with further impediments in terms of war or political turmoil, nomadic situation, or other demographic problems.

The work consists in the organization of a system of diagnosis delivery (with sputum smear examination of suspects) and chemotherapy (with the least expensive short-course regimen, proper supervision of treatment, proper recording, and proper assessment of results). Over the last 10 years, some 300,000 patients have been diagnosed and treated, and there is a documented assessment of cure rates, which reach 85–90% (a level never reached nationwide before in developing countries) in both new and retreatment cases. Currently, mutual assistance deals with 6 or 7% of the estimated annual total of cases in Africa south of the Sahara. It was thus demonstrated that tuberculosis programs could be conducted under various adverse circumstances, that they could nevertheless be successful in terms of relief of human suffering (decrease in deaths, definitive cure of patients), and be fully documented and permanently assessed through built-in evaluation (Enarson, 1991; Herman van Geuns Symposium, 1991). It was the first time that a system was evolved that would be reproducibly successful with high levels of treatment results that could be maintained over the years and were easily assessable, and that would entail a progressive decrease of the problem.

Moreover, at the same time as this demonstration of efficacy was made, a quite independent analysis by the World Bank, Harvard University, and WHO within the framework of the "Health Sector Priority Review" came to the conclusion that these national programs conducted along the IUATLD prototype *ranked among the most cost-effective health interventions, competing, in cost per year of life saved, with measles immunization and oral rehydration for infantile diarrhea.* (Murray, et al., 1990; Murray, 1991). This system of delivery of effective and efficient tuberculosis programs is relevant for some 30–40 high-prevalence countries with insufficiently developed health infrastructures.

As a consequence of its efficacy and efficiency, governments are induced to undertake such programs; also these programs attract donors, such as international intergovernmental agencies, including the United Nations Development Plan; international cooperation and development departments of governments of the more affluent countries; foundations and all types of nongovernmental organizations.

The method of delivery of tuberculosis programs, as well as the work of TSRU, represent a considerable input in the preparation of the new global strategy against tuberculosis presently being developed by WHO (Kochi, 1991a,b) (see Chapter 31). The importance of first treating already known and diagnosed cases and then only expanding case-finding was confirmed in the various national programs. Also, the levels of cure rates and detection rates obtained in the programs constituted useful practical bases for calculating the targets proposed in the Resolution on Tuberculosis adopted in the World Health Assembly in May 1991 (WHO, 1991).

Moreover, partial results from Africa tend to indicate that the correct application of proper national programs may even be sufficient to contain excess transmission of tuberculous infections caused by smear-positive tuberculous cases induced by HIV infection in dually infected individuals.

Liaison with Other Organizations

The IUATLD has had an official relationship with the WHO since its creation in 1947. It is also in liaison with UNICEF. As we also have seen, the IUATLD works directly with several governments that entrust to it part of their international collaboration funds (Norway, Switzerland, France, Saudi Arabia). It is "registered" with United States Aid For International Development (US-AID) a privilege rarely given by US-AID to a non-U.S. voluntary agency. It also maintains collaborative links with many official research institutions such as the U.S. Centers for Disease Control (CDC) in Atlanta, Georgia, the Medical Research Council of Great Britain, or relief institutions (such as Misereor in Germany and the International Leprosy Association), or NGOs such as the International Union Against Cancer, or teaching bodies such as the International Children's Center.

B. Structure and Budget

The headquarters of the IUATLD are in Paris. Its Executive Committee is composed of eight members at large and six representatives of the regions. The council comprises two counselors per constituent member, whatever the size and wealth of the constituent (which now comprises 118 national entities in as many countries in the world, compared with 31 when the Union was created in 1920).

Funds come from a quota share from constituent members and from individual members' fees. This makes about 40% of the operating cost of headquarters and liaison with the members. The rest is covered by gifts and grants. To run the field projects, seminars, and courses, extra support is often given voluntarily by constituents as well as by departments of governments of several affluent countries who entrust the IUATLD with the use of the grants in underprivileged countries.

C. Finally

It appears that, among international NGOs, the IUATLD stands, to a great extent, as a unique organization in many respects:

1. It is made up of both national entities—the lung associations and other national bodies—and individual persons in 118 countries. It thereby provides a remarkable tool to spread the word rapidly.

2. It is truly international and apolitical, which often means immense good will, tolerance, and understanding on the part of its members; it has meetings and members everywhere (for instance, the two Vietnams, the two Germanies, the two Yemen were members when they were split, and the two Koreas are members).

3. It has always counted among its members, voluntarily and spontaneously, the highest authorities in the field of tuberculosis and lung diseases.

4. As an independent and flexible organization, the Union can and does do pioneering work and pioneering approaches to delivery of health services; as a nongovernmental agency, it can even more easily afford to fail than can a government or an intergovernmental agency, and this is one of the reasons its pioneering activities and programs are so important and precious, worldwide.

5. Among the pneumological societies, the Union is the only one that is concerned with the Third World countries in direct assistance and for training of personnel in an effort at collaboration and solidarity the aim of which is to induce final technical and material self-sufficiency. It also encourages not only a north–south dialogue, but a south–south dialogue, which is another form of its vanguardism.

6. It has a permanent work program, and it has succeeded in several difficult undertakings entailing international collaborative work. The most recent and spectacular is the conduct and success of the National Tuberculosis Programs.

7. It has official ties with all the main intergovernmental and nongovernmental international agencies and is recognized by them as a worthwhile partner and adviser in its field of intervention for health.

8. It fulfills a rather difficult and unrewarding, ungratifying, but very useful, role; namely, that of reconciling the often conflicting interests of the government, the medical profession, and the public, and of integrating clinical and public health aspects.

9. It addresses the whole spectrum of situations in the world, ranging from those in the most sophisticated countries to those in the least affluent. It is trying to create among all types of nations, with widely different tuberculosis and respiratory disease problems, a constant interchange and stream of ideas, of opportunities, and of solidarity.

For all these reasons, the IUATLD provides a unique forum for discussion; it facilitates exchange between clinicians, research workers, and specialists in the same and other disciplines of health and social welfare. In this respect the Union is an important element for international collaboration, friendship, esteem and stimulation, mutual education, and attenuation of prejudices.

IV. Other International Nongovernmental Organizations with Some Tuberculosis or Mycobacterial Activity

As with local and national NGOs, international ones represent a wide spectrum of interests, from health science and technology, to community involvement.

The few examples that follow refer to well-established international NGOs (WHO, 1990).

A. League of Red Cross and Red Crescent Societies

Probably the best- and longest-known of international nongovernmental organizations, this league was created in 1919 in Paris, on the initiative of one of the leaders of the American Red Cross, Henry P. Davidson, with the aim of federating national societies. Currently, 114 national Red Cross societies and 23 Red Crescent societies are members, with a total of 230 million individual members in 137 countries.

The object of the league is to prevent and alleviate suffering and to contribute to peace. It encourages the creation of national societies and assists in the development of their services for the community; it organizes international relief for victims of natural disasters and refugees, often launching worldwide appeals for aid; it also promotes the adoption of national disaster preparedness plans.

As early as 1922, in its 21st Resolution, the General Council of the league underlined the collaboration that existed between the International Union Against Tuberculosis and the league (IUATLD, 1962). In 1924, 1930, 1946, and 1950, the highest authorities of the league defined, in a series of resolutions, the principles and possibilities for the national societies' participation in the campaign against tuberculosis. There is no standard program, but the league lends its full cooperation to back or supplement or to provisionally substitute for the efforts of existing associations and governments' plans. Examples range from assistance to the families of patients, recreational therapy, creation of outpatient clinics, running of training courses, health education, to the well-known "joint enterprise" at the end of World War II, when the Scandinavian Red Cross Societies started an international tuberculosis campaign in the war-stricken countries of middle Europe. UNICEF soon joined in what became the first organized international effort in the health field comprising both BCG vaccination and the training of local teams. The work expanded to other continents, was taken up by WHO in 1951, and progressively entrusted to the respective national governments to pursue a permanent program. The initial phase 1946–1951 covered 23 countries, with an army of personnel comprising 205 doctors, 281 nurses; 40 million tuberculin tests and 17 million vaccinations were effected during this initial period, over 1 billion thereafter.

B. The International Leprosy Association

The International Leprosy Association was created in 1931 in Manila and now has individual members in 100 countries. Its objectives are to facilitate dissemination of knowledge of leprosy and promote its control; for so doing, it cooperates with any other institution or organization.

It organizes frequent international meetings of experts and is maintaining close contacts with WHO in many global or regional activities, in particular research into immunologic, microbiological, and epidemiological aspects, as well as treatment, control, and training.

Most important are the WHO/Immlep and Thelep groups with the WHO Tropical Disease Research Group (for the development of a vaccine and for improvement of treatment). A landmark was the coordinating meeting with WHO in 1984 on implementation of multidrug therapy in leprosy control, a quite important step in the cure and control of leprosy.

There is a collaboration of the leprosy researchers and workers with the IUATLD on topics of immunology and vaccines as well as in service programs in underprivileged countries.

V. Present Trends: Irreplaceable Partners

The NGOs have played a most important role in many nations of the industrial world as the first promoters of concerted, organized actions for health, which were then taken up by governments and official sociomedical schemes. Consequently, in many of these countries, with the main needs taken care of, the influence of NGOs had tended to somewhat diminish. This was particularly true of NGOs dealing with tuberculosis, the concern for which, in these countries, had almost disappeared among the public as well as in the professionals. In developing countries, national NGOs have had difficulties in emerging, in managing, and in finding funds and, here, it is mostly NGOs from developed countries that are taking the first steps to strengthen their counterparts. In recent years, however, NGOs have received increasing prominence. This is the result of an increased understanding of their role and an increased awareness of their potentials: in responding to the needs of people, in being credible to them, in translating messages in simple terms, in pioneering new approaches, in complementing governments' efforts, in advocating, and in bringing financial and manpower support.

More and more governments are recognising NGOs as essential partners in health programs. Some still have some mistrust, and NGOs, on their own side, in general are a bit shy of interference—and want to ensure their complete independence. In fact, it is not a matter of governments using NGOs, and their multifaceted resources, but rather, it is a matter of governments facilitating the work of NGOs.

In our pneumology field, the resurgence of tuberculosis (Chretien, 1991) and a clearer appreciation of the problems it entails and also the occurrence of the HIV pandemic—the consequences of which have been initially, and are still in greater part, tackled by voluntary organizations (WHO, 1989a)—have reawakened the interest in the work of NGOs dealing with tuberculosis.

In fact, in early 1976, the International Union Against Tuberculosis invited the nongovernmental organizations in official relations with the World Health Organization to attend a meeting in Geneva at the time of the 29th World Health Assembly. It called this meeting to exchange views on (1) the role that NGOs may and should play in primary health care (PHC) programs, and (2) the coordination of NGOs' activities in PHC. Some 18 NGOs took part in that initial meeting and resolved to continue meeting to pursue their common interest in PHC. The group set out to promote PHC as a concept within their affiliated NGOs at the national level, to promote the national debate in those countries, and to assist its national expression and implementation. During 1977 and early 1978, the NGO group assisted in the preparation of a position paper on the role of NGOs in PHC. This paper was later presented at the Joint WHO/ UNICEF International Conference on Primary Health Care, held at Alma-Ata in September 1978 (NGO, 1981).

Following the Alma-Ata Conference, four emphases emerged in the discussions of this NGO group. A series of meetings focused on the promotion of people's *participation*, strengthening the means of *communications* at all levels, encouraging *joint planning* among the NGOs within countries, and working for a new style of *coordination* at the local, regional, and international levels.

In 1985, during the 38th World Health Assembly in Geneva, technical discussions took place between WHO and NGOs (over 500 representatives were present) to examine the mechanisms of closer collaboration, to identify and tackle the obstacles to this collaboration, and to indicate the best method of action for the immediate future. The technical discussions resulted in a series of recommendations for NGOs, for governments and for WHO (WHO, 1985, 1987).

VI. Summary

The situation of tuberculosis has worsened and will worsen still more (WHO, 1989b, 1992) if drastic decisions are not taken everywhere to urgently and energetically apply the means we have:

1. It has been demonstrated that they work and if properly and widely applied, they may even be able to curb the damage caused by HIV to the transmission of tuberculous infection.

2. There are able, dedicated, a bit enthusiastic people, but keeping their feet on earth who can apply the means thoroughly.

3.   There are donors who wish to invest in productive areas, including research, to make our means still more effective and easier to apply.

The future is in the hands of governments of individual countries and the international community to decide whether to have a tuberculosis program. A high responsibility lies with WHO and IUATLD together and, for the latter, together with its national affiliates. They must keep the momentum and maintain the international and national communities closely united to undertake the most formidable battle ever against tuberculosis: the enemy has now enrolled two most dangerous allies, HIV and drug resistance.

The conduct and success of the IUATLD collaborative National Tuberculosis Programs has shown that what was considered unfeasible is feasible; what was considered insurmountable is surmountable. This is true because mutual assistance is an example of something that is more than only the direct help provided, the reproducible method, or the documented facts. Behind mutual assistance is a spirit of mutual understanding, mutual esteem, and mutual stimulation and solidarity toward progress. The NGOs constitute irreplaceable partners in the national and global fight against tuberculosis.

References

Bignall, J. R. and international coordinators (1979). Cooperative international study of the IUAT on evaluation of treatment in routine practice. *Bull. Int. Union Tuberc.* **54**:35–46.

Bleiker, M. A. (1978). International Tuberculosis Surveillance Center (ITSC). Its history and objective. *Bull. Int. Union Tuberc.* **53**:122–124.

Bleiker, M. A., Sutherland, I., Styblo, K., ten Dam, H. G., and Misljenovic, O. (1989). Guidelines for estimating the risks of tuberculous infection from tuberculin test results in a representative sample of children. *Bull. Int. Union Tuberc. Lung Dis.* **64**:7–12.

Bretton, R. (1986). The Ivory Coast Committee and its assistance to the state in tuberculosis control. *Bull. Int. Union Tuberc. Lung Dis.* **61**:53–54.

Broadhead, T., and O'Malley, J. (1989). NGOs and Third-World development: Opportunities and constraints. World Health Organization, mimeographed document GPA/GMC (2) 89.5 Add. 1).

Broekmans J. (1991). The point of view of a low prevalence country: The Netherlands. *Bull. Int. Union Tuberc. Lung Dis.* **66**:179–183.

Chrétien J. (1991). Once upon a time there was tuberculosis. *Bull. Int. Union Tuberc. Lung Dis.* **66**(Suppl 90/91):63–67.

Chrétien J. (1992). Commémoration du Centenaire de la mort de Jean-Antoine Villemin (1829–1892). *Bull. Acad. Nathe Med.* **176**(7):1017–1022.

Enarson, D. (1991). Principles of IUATLD collaborative tuberculosis programs. *Bull. Int. Union Tuberc. Lung Dis.* **66**:195–200.

Herman van Geuns International Union Against Tuberculosis and Lung Disease Memorial Symposium on ''10 year collaboration in National Tuberculosis Programs'' (1991). *Bull. Int. Union Tuberc.* **66**(Suppl.):41–58.

Hershfield, E. (1981). If preventable, why not prevented. *Bull. Int. Union Tuberc.* **56**:75–78.

Hershfield, E. (1987). The Canadian Lung Association and international health. *Bull. Int. Union Tuberc. Lung Dis.* **62**:12–16.

Holm J. (1972). Mimeographed Documents, International Union Against Tuberculosis and Lung Disease, Paris.

Hong, Y. P. (1990). The Korean National Tuberculosis Association. *Bull. Int. Union Tuberc. Lung Dis.* **65**:69.

International Union Against Tuberculosis and Lung Disease (1962). The participation of international organizations in the campaign against tuberculosis. Document prepared for the discussion at the IUAT 1962 Annual Meeting, Paris.

International Union Against Tuberculosis (1964). An international investigation of the efficacy of chemotherapy in previously untreated patients with pulmonary tuberculosis. *Bull. Int. Union Tuberc.* **34**:1–191.

International Union Against Tuberculosis (1982). The double-barred cross symbol of the IUAT. Some information on its origin [extract of the proposal of Dr. G. Sisteron in 1902, and historical background of the cross by Dr. B. Fäh and F. Ehrler]. *Bull. Int. Union Tuberc.* **57**:192–195.

International Union Against Tuberculosis and Lung Disease (1991). Tuberculosis Guide for High Prevalence Countries, 2nd ed. IUATLD, Paris.

Kochi, A. (1991a). WHO's role for tuberculosis control in the world. *Bull. Int. Union Tuberc. Lung Dis.* **65**:94.

Kochi, A. (1991b). The global tuberculosis situation and the new control strategy of the World Health Organization. *Tubercle* **72**:1–6.

Krebs, A., Farer, L. S., and Snider, W. E. (1979). Five years of follow up of the IUAT trial of isoniazid prophylaxis in fibrotic lesions. *Bull. Int. Union Tuberc.* **54**:65–69.

Kusnadi, H. (1987). Some notes about the activities of the PPTI or Indonesian Tuberculosis Control Association. *Bull. Int. Union Tuberc. Lung Dis.* **62**:17–18.

Larbaoui, D. (1987). The participation of the Comité Algérien de lutte Contre la Tuberculose in twenty years of tuberculosis control in Algeria. *Bull. Int. Union Tuberc. Lung Dis.* **62**:18–20.

Lee, L. (1988). A nation of associations. In *Leadership* (the magazine for volunteer association leaders). Edited by Ann I. Mahoney. American Society of Association Executives, Washington, D.C., pp. 17–21.

Lotte, A., Wasj-Höckert, O., and Poisson, N. (1988). Second IUATLD study on complications induced by intradermal BCG vaccination. *Bull. Int. Union Tuberc. Lung Dis.* **63**:47–59.

Moerkek, H. (1989). The role of non-governmental organizations in AIDS education. Presented at the World Conference on Lung Health. Boston, May 20–24, 1990 (ALA/ATS/IUATLD).

Murray, C. J. L. (1991). Social, economic and operational research on tuberculosis: Recent studies and some priority questions. *Bull. Int. Union Tuberc. Lung Dis.* **66**:149–156.

Murray, C. J. L., Styblo, K., and Rouillon, A. (1990). Tuberculosis in developing countries: Burden, cost and intervention. *Bull. Int. Union Tuberc. Lung Dis.* **65**:6–24.

NGOs' Group on Primary Health Care (1981). The role of nongovernmental organizations in formulating strategies for health for all by the year 2000 (position paper). [Can be obtained from the Christian Medical Commission, World Council of Churches, 150 route de Ferney, CH-1211 Geneva 20, Switzerland].

Özgen, Z. S. (1987). The role of charitable organizations in tuberculosis control in Turkey. *Bull. Int. Union Tuberc. Lung Dis.* **62**:21.

Pamra, P. N. (1984). The Tuberculosis Association of India. *Bull. Int. Union Tuberc.* **59**:217–218.

Perdrizet, S. (1988). International training courses in tuberculosis control methods. The WHO/IUATLD/France, Algeria course in French. *Bull. Int. Union Tuberc. Lung Dis.* **63**:39–40.

Rist, N., and Crofton, J. (1960). Drug resistance in hospitals and sanatoria. *Bull. Int. Union Tuberc.* **30**:2–45.

Rouillon, A. (1973). Evaluation of the work of the scientific committees. *Bull. Int. Union Tuberc.* **48**:10–21.

Rouillon, A. (1978). The Tuberculosis Surveillance Research Unit (TSRU). *Bull. Int. Union Tuberc.* **53**:117–112 [includes a list of references].

Rouillon, A. (1982). The International Union Against Tuberculosis. *Tubercle* pp. 247–253.

Rouillon, A. (1984). The structure of the IUAT, its budget and its scientific committees. *Bull. Int. Union Tuberc.* **59**:64–66.

Rouillon A. (1986). Address for the official ceremony of the 75th anniversary of the NNHA. *Bull. Int. Union Tuberc.* 76–79.

Rouillon, A. (1991). The IUATLD and its role. *Bull. Int. Union Tuberc.Lung Dis.* **65**:95–96.

Shimao, T. (1987). Five major activities of the Japan Antituberculosis Association. *Bull. Int. Union Tuberc. Lung Dis.* **62**:22–24.

Shryock, R. H. (1957). *National Tuberculosis Association 1904–1954*. National Tuberculosis Association, New York.

Springett, V. H. (1968). Results of the study on x-ray readings of the ad hoc committees for the study of classification and terminology in tuberculosis. *Bull. Int. Union Tuberc.* **41**:107–131.

Styblo, K. (1991). Epidemiology of tuberculosis. *Selected Papers* **24**: 136 pp. [published by the Royal Netherlands Tuberculosis Association, The Hague].

Trnka, L. (1984). European constituent members of the IUAT. Their activities in the early eighties. *Bull. Int. Union Tuberc.* **59**:219–220.

Tunisian League against Tuberculosis and Respiratory Disease (1985). Defeat tuberculosis now and forever. *Bull. Int. Union Tuberc.* **60**:78–79.

Wilberg V. G. (1986). History and development of the Norwegian National Health Association. *Bull. Int. Union Tuberc.* **61**(1-2):75–76.

World Health Organization (1985). Conclusions and recommendations arising out of the plenary and group discussions of 10 May 1985 on the collaboration with non-governmental organizations in implementing the global strategy for health for all. A38/Technical Discussions/WP.1, 10 May 1985.

World Health Organization (1987). Resolution WHA 40.25 of 15 May 1987 on the collaboration with non-governmental organizations: Principles governing relations between WHO and non-governmental organizations.

World Health Organization (1989a). Resolution of 19 May 1989 on nongovernmental organizations and the global AIDS strategy.

World Health Organization (1989b). Statement on AIDS and tuberculosis. World Health Organization in collaboration with International Union Against Tuberculosis and Lung Disease, WHO/GPA/INF/89.4.

World Health Organization (1990). *Directory of Non Governmental Organizations in Official Relations with the World Health Organization.* [Copies can be ordered from the Documents Service, World Health Organization, 1211, Geneva 27, Switzerland.]

World Health Organization (1991). Resolution WHA44.8 of 13 May 1991 on the Tuberculosis Control Program.

World Health Organization (1992). Current and future dimensions of the HIV/AIDS pandemic. Capsule summary. WHO/GPA/Res/SFI/92.1.

31

The Role of the World Health Organization

ARATA KOCHI

World Health Organization
Geneva, Switzerland

I. Introduction

A specialized agency of the United Nations, the World Health Organization (WHO) is an intergovernmental organization the objective of which is the attainment of the highest possible level of health by all peoples. WHO's mandate includes acting as a coordinating authority on international health work; assisting governments in strengthening health services; stimulating and advancing work to eradicate epidemic, endemic, and other diseases; promoting and conducting research; and providing information, counsel, and assistance in the field of health.

The policies of WHO are determined by the World Health Assembly (WHA), which is composed of representatives of all member states and meets at least once a year. They are put into effect by the executive board and the secretariat. For tuberculosis, the first WHA in 1948, resolved that WHO would set up a section on tuberculosis and recommended that governments take preventive, curative, legislative, social, and other measures necessary for tuberculosis control. Accordingly, WHO developed the Tuberculosis Program with the objective of reducing mortality and morbidity caused by tuberculosis.

In 1964, the basis of WHO's modern tuberculosis control policy was formulated through the Seventh Expert Committee of Tuberculosis; it comprised case-finding and treatment, with priority on sputum-positive, infectious cases, and mass bacille Calmette-Guerin (BCG) vaccination. It was based on a relatively comprehensive understanding of the natural history and epidemiology of the disease and on the availability of relatively effective and simple intervention technologies. Since then, no major policy changes have occurred, except that it was found that the epidemiological effect of mass BCG vaccination had been grossly overestimated. Although BCG prevents childhood tuberculosis, particularly its most severe forms, its preventive effect on the infectious types of adult tuberculosis is limited. Therefore, BCG vaccination does not contribute significantly to reduction of transmission. Otherwise, this policy is basically sound from a scientific perspective and remains the basis for achieving objectives for countries where the risk of infection remains substantial. Nevertheless, emphasis is now placed on vaccination of the newborn.

This control policy was successfully implemented in the industrialized countries and in some middle-income developing countries, leading to the rapid decrease of the tuberculosis problem. For example, in Western European countries after the implementation of modern tuberculosis control, the annual decline in the rate of disease reached 10–15%, compared with 4–5% as a result of the improvement in general socioeconomic conditions (housing, nutrition, etc.) and the isolation of tuberculous patients in sanatoriums in the precontrol era. Unfortunately, the rapid decline of tuberculosis in industrialized countries had created the general impression that the disease had been conquered and, at the international level, interest in tuberculosis control and research dwindled under the pressure of new health priorities.

Although the incidence in these industrialized countries had reached a very low level, the rate of decline in the incidence has recently slowed down, and in many countries the incidence has started increasing, partly because many cases now originate from the still large pool of persons infected in the past, and partly because of the increasing number of tuberculosis cases among the foreign-born. Also, the recent human immunodeficiency virus (HIV) epidemic is contributing to the upsurge of tuberculosis, particularly in the United States. Thus, it can be said that these countries are at a new stage of tuberculosis control in which the once very effective control strategy no longer can have the same effect. To achieve elimination of tuberculosis (the working definition of elimination of this disease is to achieve an incidence of less than 1 case per million population) in the future, a new strategy is needed.

On the other hand, the implementation of this policy in most developing countries has not been successful. For example, it is estimated that less than half the existing tuberculosis cases are detected, and that less than half of the cases detected are cured. This is probably due to the combination of the following factors:

1. Technical policies are largely concentrated on "what should and could be done" in relatively well-developed health service systems or under special research settings, and often lack the component of "how to do it" under more difficult operational settings.

2. Some of the intervention technologies that are effective, simple, and affordable in well-developed health service systems, are not necessarily so effective, simple, and affordable in poorly developed health service systems.

3. Some of the technical policies appear to have been taken as a dogma (i.e., tuberculous patients should not be hospitalized) so that result-oriented and locally specific innovative approaches have tended to be discouraged.

However several developing countries (Tanzania, Malawi, Mozambique, and Nicaragua) assisted by International Union Against Tuberculosis and Lung Disease (IUATLD) have been successful in implementing this policy by applying existing technologies, achieving a cure rate of more than 80% and a case-detection rate of more than 65%. These programs clearly demonstrated on a countrywide scale that tuberculosis can be effectively controlled by applying the existing technologies, even under very difficult conditions. Furthermore, cost analysis of these programs indicates that successful tuberculosis control is one of the most cost-effective available health interventions.

II. The World Health Organization's New Tuberculosis Control Strategy

With 2.9 million deaths and 8 million new cases per year, tuberculosis remains a major global public health problem that is not being adequately addressed. In addition, because of the HIV pandemic and rising drug resistance, the tuberculosis situation is now rapidly worsening, and there is an urgent need to bring it under control. Against this background, in 1991, the WHA requested the Director-General of WHO to develop a new tuberculosis control and research strategy by taking the successful experience of the IUATLD-assisted programs into consideration and to implement the strategy as quickly as possible to significantly reduce the mortality and morbidity associated with the disease and to rapidly decrease tuberculosis. In response to this, WHO has developed a new strategy for global tuberculosis control with the following targets and approaches:

A. Targets

Treatment. To cure 85% of all sputum smear-positive cases detected worldwide by the year 2000. In industrialized countries, this target will be 95%.

Case-Finding. To detect 70% of all sputum smear-positive cases worldwide by the year 2000, with targets of 60% and 85% for low and middle-income developing countries respectively.

Since the current major obstacle to achieving the program's goals is the very low cure rate (estimated at less than 50% worldwide) of detected sputum smear-positive cases, the initial *primary target* of the program, is to achieve the 85% cure-rate among detected cases.

B. Approaches

Three major approaches are identified to achieve these targets:

Implementation of the Technical Strategy

1. Improvement in the quality of case-finding, with expansion of coverage once an acceptable cure rate has been achieved.

2. Improvement of the cure rate among smear-positive cases through implementation of standardized short-course therapeutic regimens, application of standardized case definitions, provision of adequate drug supply, assurance of regular drug intake, use of combined tablets with demonstrated appropriate dose bioavailability and routine monitoring, and evaluation of treatment outcomes.

3. Development of new approaches in service delivery and program management, and development and assessment of new diagnostic, treatment, and prevention technologies.

Tuberculosis Control and the Primary Health Care System

The diagnosis and treatment of tuberculosis should be conducted wherever possible through the primary health care (PHC) system at the district level, with supervision, training, monitoring, and leadership provided by national tuberculosis control programs (NTPs). These activities should help strengthen the local health infrastructure and, in some countries, may serve as a spearhead for the development of the curative component of PHC.

Global Coalition Building

To be successful, this effort will require that member states take the initiative in developing and improving their NTPs. International or bilateral agencies, nongovernmental organizations, the medical community, and scientists should do all in their power to assist member states in this effort. WHO should provide overall leadership for these coalitions.

III. Organizational Structure

To successfully implement the foregoing strategy, in 1992, WHO developed an organizational structure for its tuberculosis program that aims to mobilize necessary resources and to coordinate the use of resources in the most effective and efficient manner toward achieving the global target through building a broad political and scientific coalition. Its underlying philosophy is that (1) enhanced tuberculosis control globally can be achieved only through effective national initiatives and (2) the program should be able to effectively support the national initiatives. The organizational structure is shown in Figure 1. It comprises:

A. An Administrative Arm

The administrative arm comprises the Coordination, Advisory, and Review Group (CARG), with members representing tuberculosis "endemic" countries, financial contributors, NGOs, and permanent members (United Nations Development Program, the World Bank, and WHO), which will be supported by:

1. A Standing Committee, comprised of United Nations Development Program, the World Bank, WHO, the CARG chairperson and one other CARG member

2. A Technical and Research Advisory Subcommittee (TRAC), comprised of individuals serving in a personal capacity, to review and advise on the program from a scientific and technical viewpoint, as a subcommittee of the CARG.

The terms of reference of the CARG, the CARG Standing Committee, and the Technical and Research Advisory Subcommittee (TRAC) are shown in the chapter Appendix.

B. A Technical Arm

The technical arm consists of the following:

1. A Steering Committee on Operational Research, to oversee and advise on both global and country-specific operational research projects

2. A Steering Committee on Mycobacterial Research, jointly sponsored with the Special Program for Research and Training in Tropical

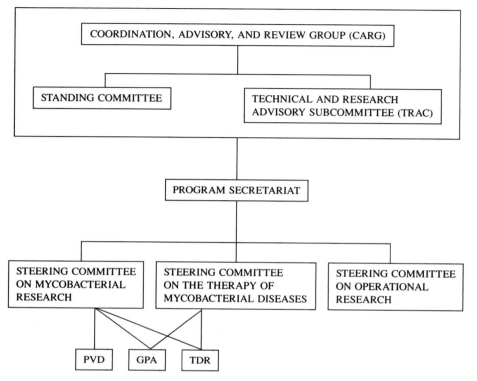

Figure 1   Organizational structure of the tuberculosis program.

Diseases (TDR), the Program on Vaccine Development (PVD), and the Global Program on AIDS (GPA)

3.   A Steering Committee on the Therapy of Mycobacterial Diseases, jointly sponsored with TDR and GPA.

C. The Program Secretariat

The Headquarters' structure of the Program Secretariat consists of two interacting operational ''units''—Operations Support (comprising national program support and operational research activities) and Research and Development—under overall Program Management and Coordination as shown in Figure 2.

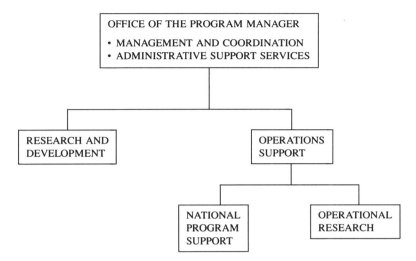

Figure 2 Organizational structure of the tuberculosis program at headquarters.

IV. Tuberculosis Program Activities

The World Health Organization recognizes, from the experience of other successful programs, that national initiatives are likely to arise only where the magnitude of the problem is recognized (including awareness in the general population), where its social and economic effect is fully understood, where there is national commitment to disease control, and where sufficient resources (staff and funds) are made available (either from national or external sources) for program implementation.

Current expenditures for treatment of sputum smear-positive tuberculosis cases are estimated at 320 million US dollars annually. The estimated incremental annual resources needed to achieve the year 2000 targets are 175–200 million US dollars, of which at least 75–100 million dollars will be needed from sources external to the developing countries carrying out tuberculosis control. To achieve the program goals and meet the established targets by the year 2000, a sustained commitment by donors up to the year 2000, and beyond, will likely be required. In addition, the most critical element will be the commitment of resources by member states themselves to their own tuberculosis control efforts. Some countries will need to commit specified resources for the first time to start control efforts, whereas others will focus on expanding existing commitments to achieve the global targets.

Key elements in national initiatives will be

Creation of political support through advocacy

Assessment of existing programs or program needs

Selection of appropriate national policies and strategies

Planning, including drug selection and procurement

Mobilization and coordination of financial resources

Training of personnel

Implementation, including monitoring

Problem-solving through operational research

Evaluation and analysis

Thus, the program is undertaking as the support to those national initiatives activities that will, in both the short- and the longer-term, foster, sustain, and strengthen NTPs.

Fostering strong national initiatives will require advocacy (at all levels nationally and internationally) to create the political and public awareness of the needs for developing or strengthening NTPs. Mobilization of resources for NTPs will also require advocacy to national governments and potential external sources of support, and coordination among providers of resources.

Launching enhanced national efforts in tuberculosis control can be facilitated by making available *technical cooperation* [i.e., access to information and guidance on the effectiveness of various policy, strategy, and program options for tuberculosis control (to be adapted locally)]. Strengthening national initiatives will require operational research that can help solve a wide range of operational problems that confront NTPs and prevent the achievement of the objectives. Development of new and more effective technologies and knowledge will reinvigorate existing and stimulate new national initiatives in tuberculosis control.

The major categories of activities to foster and sustain national initiatives are outlined in the following sections.

A. National Program Support

The philosophy underlying such support will be facilitating access by NTPs to technical cooperation, materials, and training to best serve the requirements of the strategy the country selects as most appropriate for its situation (i.e., making available a ''menu'' of support, rather than providing a monolithic prescription). National program support may be required in the following areas:

1. Development of critical tools for NTP implementation (e.g., training modules, treatment guidelines)

2. Training

3. Monitoring and evaluation (including surveillance)

4. Ensuring regular supplies of affordable antituberculosis drugs

5. Technical cooperation (including planning support)

6. Resource mobilization and coordination

Tool Development and Training

On specific technical subjects WHO issues guidelines that are usually based on the recommendations of expert groups. Recent examples are guidelines on tuberculosis surveillance and monitoring and guidelines on treatment. Since the classic definition of a *case* of tuberculosis (a patient excreting *Mycobacterium tuberculosis*) had been too restrictive, a revised case definition was proposed, with a breakdown according to type of disease and patient history. The treatment guidelines still follow the principle of standard regimens (of short-course chemotherapy) but propose different regimens for different types of patients and, moreover, allow adjustments to be made according to the patient's response to treatment.

Training of national staff, especially at the district level, is of crucial importance in national programs. To assist in this matter, WHO has prepared a series of detailed training modules on the various aspects of program management, such as ensuring identification of suspect patients, registering patients, monitoring treatment, quarterly reporting of case-finding and of treatment results, maintaining regular drug supplies, supervising laboratory services, and conducting supervisory visits. These modules will be used in WHO-sponsored training courses for key staff of national programs, together with modules for course facilitators so that the staff trained will be able to conduct training courses for midlevel managers in their own country. Technical training for senior national staff, for instance in bacteriology, is supported through WHO Collaborating Centers. These centers also provide special services (e.g., typing of strains) on request.

Monitoring and Evaluation

The introduction at a national level of rational registration and monitoring methods has made it possible for WHO to collect information that is indicative of program performance. The information collected annually now includes the number and proportion of cases diagnosed (by type), the treatment outcome as assessed by cohort analysis, the BCG vaccination coverage, treatment regimens used, drug supply issues, and some basic organizational questions.

A method is being developed for the evaluation of national tuberculosis programs by WHO staff, jointly with national program personnel. Evaluation is based on a comprehensive program review according to a detailed manual.

Antituberculosis Drug Supplies

A successful NTP requires the uninterrupted supply of four or more antituberculosis drugs of assured quality, at affordable prices, and the distribution of these drugs on time to patients in need. Drug costs represent 20–40% of the budget of most NTPs. Drug shortages can be caused by (1) unexpected variations in consumption (2) the late purchasing of drugs (3) the unavailability of supplies on the pharmaceutical market and (4) delays in the drug distribution chain. Each of these potential problems needs to be addressed by NTPs, with external technical assistance and financial support if required.

To address these problems, the program is conducting and planning a range of activities to improve antituberculosis drug supplies as part of its national program support activities: (1) developing a data-base on global antituberculosis drug production capacity; (2) assessing current drug procurement and distribution practices in developing countries; (3) developing models for forecasting drug requirements; (4) addressing drug supply and distribution issues in training, monitoring, and program review activities; (5) conducting relevant operational research; (6) facilitating drug financing and procurement; (7) assessing the feasibility and efficient approaches for joint procurement and revolving funds; (8) supporting bioavailability testing and improving low-cost methods of drug quality assurance in developing countries; and (9) coordinating with related programs at the international level, especially WHO's Action Program on Essential Drugs.

Intensified Support

In addition to basic support, intensified support will be provided in a few instances for which a range of factors are favorable. Factors influencing the extent to which intensified support will occur include

1. Political commitment to PHC and to strengthening of national tuberculosis control
2. The availability of national personnel, particularly committed leadership
3. The level of the existing infrastructure
4. The likelihood that the country could serve as a demonstration model of effective NTP implementation for other countries (geographic and language considerations will need to be taken into account here)
5. The availability of collaborating parties—nationally and externally (e.g., nongovernmental organizations, donors)–to support the envisaged efforts.

Some large countries (China, India, Bangladesh, Philippines, Madagascar) are already proceeding, with World Bank support, to plan or implement expanded NTPs. Some of these programs have called upon WHO to a considerable extent for technical cooperation. It is anticipated that others will also call upon WHO for such cooperation.

It is also anticipated that, for various other countries, the opportunities for NTP development and intensified technical cooperation with WHO may be favorable, but external financial support may not be immediately available. In these instances, the program must have the resources (financial and human) to be in a position to respond appropriately. However, intensified technical cooperation is envisaged with only a small number of countries (five to ten) in the first phase of the program. This is an important step in the initial phase of implementing the technical strategy, since strong "model" NTPs do not yet exist in Asia, French-speaking Africa, and Latin America. The length of the first phase will depend, to some extent, on the speed with which adequate resources are provided for national program support.

In the subsequent phase(s), wider support to NTPs can be provided through utilizing model countries, as part of the process of illustrating how tuberculosis control can be successfully implemented, for example, by using them as demonstration sites for training managers from neighboring countries.

B. Operational Research

Generic and Global Operational Research Issues

Certain generic issues, common to many NTPs, will need addressing through operational research. Such work should be coordinated globally, but conducted in collaboration with NTPs when conditions are favorable for such research. Activities of this program component will also include development of methods for operational research and analysis of issues relating to integration of tuberculosis control as part of primary health care.

Locally Specific Operational Research Issues

Operational research to solve problems identified in the implementation of particular NTPs will also be required. Such research clearly needs to be under the auspices of NTPs, with cooperation, as desired, from external experts in relevant operational research methods. Where possible it is desirable that NTPs make financial provisions within their overall budgets for such problem-solving activities and their design and monitoring, perhaps by small national operational research panels that could draw on the broader global community of operational research experts.

Organization of Operational Research Activities

Operational research, to be truly relevant to country needs, must be conducted as an integral part of NTPs. It is most logical, therefore, that the closest possible links be maintained between those in the program responsible for operational research, those program staff responsible for liaison with and support of NTPs, and the NTPs themselves. Indeed country-specific operational research is essentially a national activity, but may need some provision for external (WHO) funding, if the need for funding from other NTP sources has not been anticipated.

C. Research and Development

The need to backup WHO's tuberculosis program with focused research was realized right from the start. In 1949, the WHO Tuberculosis Research Office was created, first to solve the many practical problems encountered in the BCG vaccination campaigns, but also to study some basic issues, such as nonspecific tuberculin sensitivity, and then to measure the extent of the tuberculosis problem, notably in tropical Africa and Southeast Asia, by means of sample surveys. In the late 1950s, systematic research on chemotherapy was started in the WHO-sponsored chemotherapy centers in Madras and Nairobi and in several European countries. WHO actively directed development work on (freeze-dried) BCG vaccines and, together with the U. S. Public Health Service, supported the large-scale community trial of BCG vaccines in India. When, by 1980, the results of this trial proved disappointing, WHO initiated a series of case-control and contact studies to determine the effectiveness of BCG vaccination of the newborn. In addition, studies on the molecular biology of mycobacteria were started and a Program for Vaccine Development was set up. Current studies in the area of diagnosis include assessment of polymerase chain reaction (PCR) and restriction fragment length polymorphism (RFLP), and in the area of chemotherapy studies on sparfloxacin and long-acting rifamycins.

For the last several years, WHO has mainly addressed various problems related to the association of tuberculosis and HIV infection. In the area of epidemiology, WHO supports two seroprevalence surveys among tuberculosis patients: in Tanzania and Uganda. The project in Tanzania provides for a comprehensive, countrywide sample of tuberculosis patients obtained by studying all patients in one-third of the country's districts each year for a 6-month period. The study results will be compared with longitudinal data from the program, prior and current results of tuberculin surveys in all districts, as well as data from community HIV serosurveys. Thus, the study has the potential for providing the most complete epidemiological description of the effect of HIV on tuberculosis in Africa yet undertaken. In Uganda, sentinel surveillance is being conducted among tuberculosis patients diagnosed in hospitals, the results being compared with data from community HIV serosurveys in the same areas. WHO also supports a second national tuberculin survey in Tanzania among 10-year-old children who had not been previously immunized with BCG. With these data, one can calculate the annual risk of infection and, by comparison with earlier information and with data from the national program and the HIV seroprevalence study, determine to what extent the HIV epidemic is influencing tuberculosis transmission and future case rates. In Rwanda, support has been given for a prospective study of a cohort of approximately 1600 women of childbearing age who have been diagnosed with HIV infection. During a 2-year period, the annual risk of tuberculosis was approximately 5% among those who were tuberculin-positive at the time HIV infection was diagnosed. These results are similar to those from other studies, indicating that the risk of tuberculosis among coinfected persons ranges from 5 to 8% per year. In a study of childhood tuberculosis in Zambia, 37% of nearly 300 pediatric patients with diagnosed tuberculosis had HIV infection, compared with the prevalence in a control group of approximately 10%. This is the first study of its kind to demonstrate a high risk of tuberculosis in pediatric HIV infection, comparable with that seen among adults.

With a view toward developing diagnostic guidelines, WHO is supporting a study of pulmonary complications of HIV in Tanzania. Adults hospitalized with smear-negative, pulmonary disease, not caused by asthma or bronchiectasis, undergo a series of diagnostic studies, including HIV testing and fiber-optic bronchoscopy with bronchoalveolar lavage. Preliminary results indicate that perhaps as many as three-quarters of these patients have bacteriologically confirmed tuberculosis.

For chemotherapy, the study in Tanzania will be following up patients with diagnosed pulmonary tuberculosis for 4 years to help provide additional data on the efficacy of short-course therapy in persons with HIV infection. The clinical pattern and the response to treatment in children are being studied in a project in the Dominican Republic. The study of pediatric tuberculosis and HIV infection in Zambia also collects information on the response to therapy. An alarming finding was the high incidence of Stevens–Johnson syndrome. Results from this and other studies have led to WHO's strong warning against the use of amithiozone (thiacetazone) in persons at increased risk of HIV infection. WHO is supporting a study in Haiti comparing the outcome of 6-month therapy in HIV-positive and HIV-negative tuberculosis patients.

In the area of prevention, WHO has supported a BCG study in Uganda to better define the safety of neonatal BCG given to children at risk of perinatally acquired HIV infection. Data on children with BCG-induced adenitis indicate that this complication does not appear to be significantly increased among those with HIV infection. These data have helped to support WHO's continuing recommendation that BCG be given to asymptomatic newborns in areas of high tuberculosis prevalence, even when HIV infection is common. The highest priority has been given to studies of tuberculosis preventive chemotherapy. One topic, the feasibility of isoniazid preventive therapy for HIV-infected, tuberculin-positive persons, is being studied in Uganda. WHO is supporting two efficacy studies of short-course preventive therapy with rifampin–pyrazinamide, compared with standard isoniazid and with placebo controls.

Appendix: Terms of Reference for the CARG, a CARG Standing Committee, and a Technical and Research Advisory Subcommittee of the Tuberculosis Control Program

A. Functions, Composition and Operation of the Coordination, Advisory and Review Group

The Coordination, Advisory, and Review Group (CARG) shall represent the interests and responsibilities of the parties collaborating with WHO in its Tuberculosis Program. It acts as an advisory body to the Director-General of WHO, on matters of policy, strategy, finance, management, monitoring and evaluation of the programs.

1. Functions
   The CARG shall have the following functions:

   1.1 To monitor the planning and execution of the program. For this purpose it shall keep itself informed of all aspects of the program and review reports submitted to it by the WHO Secretariat (hereinafter referred to as secretariat), the CARG Standing Committee (referred to in Sec. 5), and any scientific and technical advisory groups as may be established by the Director-General (referred to in Sec. 1.7)

   1.2 To review a work plan and proposed program budget prepared by the secretariat for the coming financial period in light of a report on anticipated income

   1.3 To review longer-term plans of action and their financial implications

   1.4 To review annual financial statements submitted by the secretariat

   1.5 To evaluate progress in program implementation, particularly in the effectiveness of support to national tuberculosis programs

   1.6 To advise on the organization of periodic external evaluations that will assess the achievements and make suggestions for future directions of the program

1.7 To advise on the establishment of scientific advisory groups and steering committees through which the program will obtain guidance on its scientific and technical aspects

1.8 To advise on ways to promote the adoption by countries collaborating in global tuberculosis control of appropriate methods for ascertaining progress toward national and global targets for cure rates and case detection

2. Membership

2.1 The CARG shall consist of up to 24 members, drawn from among the collaborating parties as follows:

2.1.1 *Government representatives* of up to 11 countries in which tuberculosis is a major health problem and whose governments are actively engaged in tuberculosis control. Such representatives shall be chosen in the first instance by the Director-General and, thereafter, by the Director-General on the basis of recommendations made by the standing committee (which shall take into account suggestions made by the regional directors), from among those countries indicating to WHO their commitment to tuberculosis control and interest in membership. Selection of such representatives shall take into account the need for appropriate geographic representation and turnover in membership.

2.1.2 *Representatives of financial contributors*: Up to nine government representatives from the countries that were the largest financial contributors to the program in the previous biennium.

2.1.3 *Nongovernmental organizations*: Representatives of the International Union Against Tuberculosis and Lung Disease (IUATLD) and one nongovernmental organization to be selected by the Director-General from among those indicating to the program manager their interest in membership;

2.1.4 *Permanent members*: UNDP and the World Bank.

2.2 *Terms*: The terms of office of CARG members selected under paragraphs 2.1.a and 2.1.c shall be 3 years. They shall be eligible for reappointment, provided that members selected under paragraphs 2.1.a and 2.1.c shall not normally serve more than two terms consecutively. The initial terms of office of members selected under paragraph 2.1.a shall be chosen to provide a staggering of membership.

2.3 *Observers*: Upon written application, observer status for CARG meetings may be granted by the Director-General, who may delegate this function. Observers shall make their own arrangements to cover expenses incurred in attending sessions of the CARG.

3. Operation

3.1 WHO shall provide reasonable support services and other facilities for the CARG.

3.2 The CARG shall meet at least once a year and, subject to the agreement of the Director-General, in extraordinary sessions, if required.

3.3 The CARG shall elect from among its members a chairman who shall serve for a term of 2 years. The chairman shall be eligible for reelection, but shall not serve more than two consecutive terms.

3.4 The chairman shall:

Preside over CARG sessions

Be a member of the CARG Standing Committee

Undertake such additional duties as may be necessary in agreement with the Director-General

3.5 At each meeting the CARG shall elect from among its members a vice-chairman and rapporteur.

3.6 Subject to any special arrangements that may be suggested by the CARG, members of the CARG shall make their own arrangements to cover expenses incurred in attending sessions of the CARG.

4. Procedures

4.1 The CARG should, whenever possible, adopt its conclusions by consensus.

4.2 In consultation with the standing committee, the secretariat shall prepare an annotated agenda for each session.

4.3 A report, prepared by the rapporteur, with the assistance of the secretariat, shall be circulated as soon as possible after the conclusion of the session for the approval of the members.

5. CARG Standing Committee

The purpose of the CARG Standing Committee is to provide to the

Director-General such advice on the program as may be needed between CARG sessions.

5.1 *Composition*

The CARG Standing Committee shall comprise representatives of UNDP, the World Bank, the CARG Chairman, and one other member of the CARG to be elected by the CARG. The standing committee may suggest to the Director-General other individuals to be invited to attend as advisers.

5.2 *Functions*

The CARG Standing Committee shall have the following functions:

5.2.1 To review work plans and the proposed program budget for the coming financial period prepared by the secretariat and reviewed by such scientific and technical advisory bodies as may be established by the Director-General, in time for presentation to the annual session of the CARG

5.2.2 To make proposals to the CARG for the financing of the program for the coming financial period

5.2.3 To review and make recommendations on the reallocation of resources during a financial period

5.2.4 To review reports submitted by the secretariat and such scientific and technical advisory bodies as may be established by the Director-General, and to transmit these with comments as appropriate to the CARG

5.2.5 To review particular aspects of the program, including those that may be referred to it by the CARG, and present findings and recommendations to the CARG

5.2.6 To prepare an annual report of its activities for the CARG

5.3 *Operation*

5.3.1 The standing committee shall normally meet once between sessions of the CARG. If more frequent communication between the standing committee members is needed, it shall be done by means of correspondence. The standing committee should, whenever possible, adopt its conclusions by consensus.

5.3.2 WHO shall provide reasonable support services and facilities for the standing committee.

5.3.3   Subject to special arrangements that may be suggested by the standing committee, members of the standing committee shall make their own arrangements to cover the expenses incurred in participating in standing committee meetings.

6. Technical and Research Advisory Subcommittee (TRAC)

   6.1 *Functions*

   As a subcommittee of the CARG, the Technical and Research Advisory Subcommittee shall have the following functions:

   6.1.1   To review from a scientific and technical viewpoint the program's collaboration with, and support of national tuberculosis programs, including policy, strategy and procedural guidance, and the provision of technical support assistance

   6.1.2   To review from a scientific and technical standpoint, the content, scope, and dimensions of the operational research and research and development activities of the program, their relevance to NTPs, and approaches to be adopted

   6.1.3   To review and make recommendations on the establishment of steering committees and other means through which scientific and technical matters are addressed

   6.1.4   To recommend priorities between areas of possible program activity

   6.1.5   To provide to the CARG and the standing committee independent evaluation of the scientific and technical aspects of the program

   6.1.6   To review work plans and the proposed program budget for the coming financial period prepared by the program's secretariat and make proposals to the standing committee for possible reallocation of resources within the scientific and technical components of the program during the financial period

   For these purposes the TRAC may propose and present for consideration to the secretariat, the standing committee, or the CARG, as appropriate, such technical documents and recommendations as it deems necessary.

6.2 *Composition*

   6.2.1   The TRAC shall have up to ten members, who shall serve in their personal capacities to represent the range of disciplines relevant to tuberculosis control, operational research and research and development necessary to properly advise on areas outlined in 6.1.1 and 6.1.2.

   6.2.2   Members of the TRAC, including the chairman, shall be selected by the Director-General on the basis of scientific and technical competence after taking into account the view of the standing committee and the CARG.

   6.2.3   Members of the TRAC shall not be members of other committees of the program and the chairman and members of the TRAC shall not be eligible to receive research funds from the program.

   6.2.4   Members of the TRAC, including the chairman, shall be appointed to serve for a period of 3 years and shall be eligible for reappointment; but may not serve more than two consecutive terms. The initial terms of office of members should be chosen to provide a staggering of membership.

6.3 *Operation*

   6.3.1   The TRAC shall usually meet at least once each year.

   6.3.2   The chairman of the CARG (or their designee) shall attend meetings of the TRAC.

   6.3.3   WHO shall provide any necessary scientific, technical and other support for the TRAC.

   6.3.4   The TRAC shall elect for each meeting a vice-chairman and rapporteur from among its members.

   6.3.5   The TRAC shall prepare an annual report on the basis of a full review of all scientific and technical aspects of the program. This report, containing findings and recommendations, shall be submitted to the secretariat. The secretariat shall submit its comments (if any) to the standing committee, which shall then submit the report, comments of the secretariat (in any), and its own comments (if any) to the CARG.

   6.3.6   The chairman of the TRAC, or a member of the TRAC acting as deputy, shall attend all sessions of the CARG.

Part Five

THE FUTURE

32

Research Needs

DIXIE E. SNIDER, JR., and ROBERT C. GOOD

Centers for Disease Control and Prevention
Atlanta, Georgia

I. Introduction

Since the discovery of the tubercle bacillus by Robert Koch in 1882 (Koch, 1882), research in tuberculosis has resulted in many discoveries, some related directly to the disease and others with much broader application. These contributions have included the use of smear and culture techniques for presumptive diagnosis of tuberculosis and other mycobacterial infections; the discovery and use of tuberculin and other mycobacterial antigen preparations to identify persons infected with mycobacteria and to study cell-mediated immune responses; the development of bacille Calmette-Guérin (BCG) vaccine; the development of thoracic surgery techniques, antituberculosis drugs, and clinical trial methods; the elucidation of the principles of multidrug therapy; and the development and use of isoniazid preventive therapy.

In part because of the successes in tuberculosis research, the prevailing opinion, especially during the 1960s and 1970s, was that the tools for controlling tuberculosis were available and the methods for their application were well understood (World Health Organization [WHO], 1964). All that remained was establishing the commitment to use these tools and methods on a broad scale. As time has shown, this optimism was not justified. By the late 1970s, it was recognized that the global strategy for tuberculosis control was failing (Holm, 1984). Thereafter, a somewhat paradoxical opinion emerged; namely, that tuberculosis should not be accorded a high priority in health care programs because the control methods were so cumbersome and ineffective (Walsh and Warren, 1979).

In 1986, Dr. James O. Mason, then Director of the Centers for Disease Control (CDC) and, subsequently Assistant Secretary for Health, Department of Health and Human Services, challenged those involved in tuberculosis control activities to eliminate tuberculosis from the United States (Mason, 1986). In considering a response to that challenge, it was recognized that the goal of elimination could not be realized without the development of new technologies. Therefore, as one response to Dr. Mason's challenge, the Centers for Disease Control, the National Institutes of Health (NIH), the American Thoracic Society (ATS), and the Pittsfield [Massachusetts] Antituberculosis Association cosponsored a conference to identify priority areas for research that might lead to an accelerated decline in tuberculous morbidity and, ultimately, to elimination of tuberculosis from the United States. The report of that conference was published in the *American Review of Respiratory Disease* (American Thoracic Society et al., 1986) and was incorporated into the Department of Health and Human Services "Strategic Plan for the Elimination of Tuberculosis in the United States" (CDC, 1989).

Subsequent to the 1985 conference, some progress was made in carrying out the recommended research agenda. With the development of gene probes and the application of polymerase chain reaction amplification, more rapid methods for diagnosis began to emerge (Brisson-Noel et al., 1989; Pao et al., 1990). With the nationwide implementation of an individual tuberculosis case report system in 1985, the epidemiology of tuberculosis in the United States on a "macrolevel" was better understood (Rieder et al., 1989). The concomitant development of restriction fragment length polymorphism analysis has begun to enhance our understanding of the epidemiology of tuberculosis on the "microlevel" (Hermans et al., 1990). Significant progress was also made in understanding the antigens of *Mycobacterium tuberculosis* and the immune response to these antigens (American Thoracic Society, 1988). Strategies for the development of new tuberculosis vaccines were developed (Bloom, 1989).

Those attending the 1985 conference did not fully appreciate how the tuberculosis problem was changing in the United States in the mid-1980s. Since 1985, the steady downward trend in tuberculous cases, noted since nationwide reporting of the disease was instituted in 1953, was reversed. In 1985 through 1991, the United States experienced an 18% increase in reported cases. It is now apparent that the human immunodeficiency virus (HIV) epidemic is one cause of these increases and its effect on tuberculosis morbidity in the United States is likely to continue for the foreseeable future. Furthermore, tuberculosis has increasingly become a disease of the poor and the socioeconomically disenfranchised. It has become a disease of the young, minority adult and, alarmingly, cases have begun to increase among children. Tuberculosis among the foreign-born continues to increase. Outbreaks of drug-resistant tuberculosis have become more common, especially among persons with HIV infection. Patient noncompliance with screening programs and with therapy and preventive therapy recommendations continues to thwart control efforts. Cutbacks in health department resources for tuberculosis control, or level funding in the face of increasing morbidity, further complicate matters, as have shortages of antituberculosis drugs.

At the global level, the epidemic of HIV has exposed the weaknesses of tuberculosis control programs and health care systems in many developing countries (Slutkin et al., 1988; WHO/International Union Against Tuberculosis and Lung Disease, 1989). Inadequate control programs in the areas of high incidence of HIV infection have been unable to deal with the dual epidemic. The long period of research inactivity has left us with no new tools with which to confront this situation.

In view of the changing nature of the tuberculosis problem and the increasing need for new technologies, a workshop was held in December 1990, at the National Institutes of Health (NIH) to define a tuberculosis research agenda for the 1990s. Many of the ideas in this chapter are drawn from presentations and discussions at that workshop.

In retrospect, the nation's failure to continue an adequate investment in tuberculosis research was shortsighted, and we must now reinvigorate tuberculosis research to get tuberculosis back under control and eventually eliminate the disease. There are some who fear that funding tuberculosis research will divert precious health care resources away from funding control programs. Although it is clear that control programs also need more funding, it is equally clear that many of our current problems (e.g., delays and other difficulties in diagnosis, long waits for drug susceptibility test results, and the inability to cure some patients with drug-resistant disease) are not going to be solved by doing things the same old ways. Research is needed to solve new problems as well as to help us learn to use our old technologies more efficiently and effectively.

In this chapter, we will use the terms research and technology in their broadest sense. Our concept of *research* is any activity designed to obtain new information. This new information is new technology in its broadest sense. Perhaps *innovation* is a better word than *technology*. Innovations can consist of hardware, software, or both (Rogers, 1983). We make these points because some have argued that we do not need new technologies as much as we need to learn to change people's behavior so that they will appropriately use the technologies we now have. Although we strongly support continuing attempts to modify patient and provider behavior through educational activities, behavioral research is desperately needed to show us how to do this better. Furthermore, attempting behavioral change is a never-ending task with each new patient and provider. Research could lead to the development of new "hardware" that would make behavioral change less necessary. For example, patient noncompliance would be less of a problem if we could find drugs that would cure the disease with a few doses. An example from another discipline is the use of passive-restraint systems and air bags in automobiles, which is a much easier approach to passenger safety than attempting to change people's behavior in their use of seat belts.

II. Research on Diagnostic Methods

Rapid diagnosis of tuberculosis will contribute to overall case reduction by providing identification of infectious and noninfectious cases, so that they can be treated and removed from the chain of transmission. Currently, isolation and identification of *M. tuberculosis* from clinical specimens is required for confirmation of a case. Presumptive identification is provided by results of the acid-fast stain, which should be available within 24 hr of specimen collection. Development of fluorescent acid-fast-staining procedures have simplified the reading of smears and have speeded the availability of results. Because of slow growth of tubercle bacilli, i.e., a 12–18 hr generation time versus about 29 min for a bacterium such as *Escherichia coli*, extended incubation periods on specific media in controlled atmospheres are necessary. Isolation and identification of *M. tuberculosis* can take up to 8 weeks or longer. Development of a radiometric procedure has made it possible to reduce this time by approximately one-half. Once 10^5–10^7 cells are available, DNA probes or determination of the unique mycolic acid pattern by high-performance liquid chromatography (HPLC) can be used as a 4-hr identification test.

Progress in diagnostic methods still needs to be made to reduce the overall period required for definitive species identification. Antigen detection tests with monoclonal and polyclonal antibodies need to be investigated using newer techniques for increasing sensitivity. DNA amplification is promising. Further research may also lead to the recognition of unique antigenic materials such as complexes of protein, polysaccharide, and lipid, or more simple compounds that can be used for rapid diagnosis of disease. Investigators must be encouraged to explore the immunologic relations and chemical structures that will lead to development of better procedures. These procedures are discussed further below.

III. Epidemiological Research

In recent years, groups of persons at high risk for tuberculosis have been identified by national surveillance systems. The question naturally arises of why some groups have higher tuberculosis case rates than others. Is it because they contain a higher proportion of infected persons, or do infected persons in these groups have a higher risk of developing disease? Or is it some combination of these risks? Epidemiological research is needed to sort out the reasons for the group differences.

A major research question is the reason(s) for the recent reversal of the downward trend in tuberculosis incidence in the United States. Although much of the recent increase in tuberculosis morbidity is probably due to the HIV epidemic, this hypothesis has not been adequately studied.

The magnitude and trends in the influence of the HIV epidemic on the incidence of tuberculosis need to be determined by (1) collecting HIV serostatus information on all tuberculous cases reported in each state; or (2) collecting HIV status of tuberculous patients, using active surveillance in selected areas with known population base (countries, states, cities). Additional investigations of the epidemiology of tuberculosis in demographic groups that are not known to be at high risk for HIV is needed—as defined by age, sex, race–ethnicity, and location. Determining the cause(s) of the recent increases in tuberculosis among children is of particularly high priority.

There has been no national surveillance of the prevalence of tuberculous infection since the 1972 National Health and Nutrition Examination Survey (NHANES) I study. The development of efficient methods for periodically ascertaining the prevalence of infection in the United States is important for providing a complete picture of the tuberculosis problem. The level and trend of infection are, in many ways, the fundamental measurement of the effectiveness of tuberculosis control, and their quantitation is essential information for planning tuberculosis screening and prevention strategies.

Studies of the epidemiology of susceptibility to antituberculous drugs have recently assumed greater importance because of reported outbreaks of drug-resistant disease. Drug resistance decreases the effectiveness of standard treatment and preventive treatment regimens and increases the costs of therapy. Surveillance for drug resistance should be reinstituted in the United States. This could be either in the form of active surveillance, with a representative sample of *M. tuberculosis* isolates being tested in a central laboratory, or by passive surveillance in which data from state and local laboratories are collected. In addition to developing information concerning the magnitude and distribution of drug resistance, demographic and clinical information concerning patients from whom the organisms were isolated should be collected.

Studies of factors associated with seeking, or not seeking, care for tuberculosis should be investigated. If patients with disease do not seek or are unable to access medical care, then diagnosis and effective treatment of disease are delayed, and transmission of infection in the community will continue to occur. If infected persons who are at high risk of disease do not seek care, then there will continue to be reservoirs of infection—a portion of which will progress to develop infectious disease. Studies designed to identify perceived or existing barriers to care are needed.

Studies of the risk factors associated with transmission and acquisition of infection and disease should be conducted. Although there is considerable information available concerning factors associated with transmission and acquisition of infection, many unknowns remain. Questions have arisen concerning whether modes of transmission and rates of acquisition of infection are the same in new risk groups, such as HIV-infected persons, as in non–HIV-infected persons. Other questions include: Are all strains of *M. tuberculosis* equally transmissible and equally infections? What are the environmental circumstances that favor transmission? Are there periods of short, high-intensity exposure that might go unnoticed in standard epidemiological investigations? Can persons at increased risk of infection be identified? What are the demographic or clinical characteristics of persons at greatest risk of developing tuberculosis? Answers to these questions are of great relevance in developing appropriate infection control measures, in targeting preventive interventions, and in investigation of outbreaks.

Additional studies to determine why tuberculosis is not prevented are needed. Tuberculosis is preventable through preventive therapy for infected individuals. Each new case of tuberculosis represents a failure in prevention. Many opportunities to prevent tuberculosis are being missed (Glassroth, et al., 1990). Additional investigations to identify these missed opportunities could result in improved quality of care and perhaps identify new locations where screening and prevention programs could be introduced.

Studies of methods for reducing transmission of *M. tuberculosis* in settings of intense exposure are needed. Potential methods of reducing transmission include ventilation, ultraviolet lamps, high-efficiency filters, and disposable particulate respirators (CDC, 1990). None of these methods has been subjected to rigorous investigation for efficacy and cost-effectiveness.

IV. Therapy

There are multiple problems with current approaches to treatment of tuberculosis, including the length of treatment, development of resistance, lack of alternative agents, and toxicity of existing agents. In addition, there is a critical lack of knowledge about the growth, physiology–biochemistry, and molecular biology of *M. tuberculosis*, which is a serious impediment to the development of more effective chemotherapeutic agents.

The ideal antituberculosis agent would be bactericidal for both actively growing and quiescent bacilli and administered over a short period. Other important features would include a long half-life, minimal toxicity, and relatively complete absorption from the gastrointestinal tract. Resistance to the drug should not develop during the course of therapy.

It has been two decades since a new drug for the treatment of tuberculosis was introduced. Unfortunately, there is no comprehensive program to screen new compounds for antituberculosis activity; potentially effective agents are identified only serendipitously. Meager progress has been made in identifying potentially useful new compounds, but the development of new classes of antimicrobials (e.g., quinolones and macrolides) for the treatment of other bacterial infections has led to tests of their application to the treatment of *M. avium* complex disease.

To achieve progress in this area, a coordinated system of drug development, involving the public and private sectors, is required. Comprehensive in vitro screening of new compounds, testing of active agents in appropriate in vivo systems, and coordinated clinical trials are needed. A close working relationship involving the private sector (pharmaceutical and biologics companies), public funding agencies (NIH and CDC), and regulatory agencies (FDA) is essential.

To identify more effective agents, the mechanism of action of existing agents at the molecular level needs to be investigated. A better understanding of biosynthetic and catabolic pathways of *M. tuberculosis* would help identify chemotherapeutic targets within these pathways. Genetic approaches could be used to define steps in the synthesis of important cell wall components, such as arabinogalactan, lipoarabinomannan, or mycolic acids. In addition, mechanisms of resistance should be defined for existing agents and new agents. A molecular approach to this problem would be to clone and sequence drug-resistance genes or, alternatively, to develop probes to conserved regions of resistance markers defined in other systems.

An important obstacle to the development of effective new agents may be the impermeability of the mycobacterial cell wall and membrane to many existing classes of drugs. There is a need to elucidate, using both genetic and physiological methods, the role of permeability in drug resistance in *M. tuberculosis*. Basic studies directed at understanding the mechanisms of mycobacteriophage infection and replication may reveal other targets or chemotherapeutic strategies and should be included in long-range approaches to this problem.

Persistent tubercle bacilli, probably sequestered within macrophages, represent another therapeutic challenge. Efforts should be made to both define the metabolic state of persistence and to identify agents that are active against these organisms.

There is a need to develop rapid methods for measuring the quantitative susceptibility [minimum inhibitory concentrations (MICs) and minimum bactericidal concentrations (MBCs)] of *M. tuberculosis* to antimicrobial agents. Conventional growth-dependent methods are not amenable either to screening large numbers of compounds for activity or for systematic structure–activity relationship studies. Methods based on luciferase-reporter mycobacteriophage replication, enzyme activity assays, and measures of macromolecular synthesis offer the potential for the development of growth-independent assays.

There is an urgent need for methods to rapidly detect resistant tubercle bacilli in clinical specimens, perhaps by employing polymerase chain reaction (PCR) amplification and hybridization with probes directed against resistance-defining nucleotide sequences. The growing problem of multidrug-resistant tuberculosis and the need to provide treatment regimens that are conducive to patient compliance are major considerations.

Despite the availability of regimens that offer the potential for high-response rates and very low relapse rates, the results of the treatment of tuberculosis under field conditions are far less successful. The major factor in these disappointing results is *noncompliance* (failure to take medicine as prescribed). A wide variety of inducements and enforcements have been employed in the effort to combat noncompliance. However, they have met with limited success. Directly observed intermittent therapy has been used, but not without considerable expense, since it is labor-intensive. If methods could be found to lengthen the interval between doses, substantial progress in solving the problem of noncompliance could be anticipated. Alternative delivery systems that should be investigated include biodegradable polymer matrix sustained-release systems (already tested in animal models with encouraging results; Gangadharam, 1981) and liposome-encapsulated chemotherapeutic agents.

Immunotherapy of tuberculosis could reduce the duration of chemotherapy necessary to effect cure. Specific agents that should be investigated include recombinant molecules, such as interleukin-2 (IL-2) and interferon gamma; inducers of modifiers of lymphokines; such as indomethacin, muramyl dipeptides, vitamins A or D; and living bacterial vaccines.

V.   Preventive Therapy for Tuberculosis

Preventive therapy, the secondary prevention of tuberculosis in individuals infected with *M. tuberculosis*, is the only intervention that might dramatically change the epidemiology of tuberculosis in a relatively short period. In a country with a low annual risk of infection, such as the United States, the vast majority of incident cases of tuberculosis arise from a group of persons who have carried their infection for more than 2 years. However, the effectiveness of preventive therapy programs is limited by the risk of hepatotoxicity and long duration of therapy associated with isoniazid, the only drug evaluated in clinical trials of preventive therapy. Also, the increase in the number of cases of tuberculosis with bacilli resistant to both isoniazid and rifampin, and the proved transmission from these cases, creates a demand for new drugs or other approaches to preventive therapy.

Improvements in preventive therapy must focus on shortening the length of therapy and improving the safety of the intervention. Most of the studies outlined in the previous section have the potential for contributing to improvements in preventive therapy as well. In addition, studies should be done to identify and describe where the tubercle bacilli reside in infected persons and their metabolic state. It will also be important to better characterize the immunologic relations between the human host and the parasite, the tubercle bacillus.

An important undertaking will be the development of animal models of latent infection with *M. tuberculosis* so that new and existing drugs can be tested for their value in preventive therapy. Promising drugs, dosages, and rhythms of administration could then be identified for use in human clinical trials. Those drugs that are prime candidates for preventive therapy act directly on the earliest metabolic activities, reach high tissue and macrophage concentrations, and have minimal toxic effects. Promising candidates include the long-acting rifamycin derivatives, rifabutin and rifapentine, and several of the quinolones, such as ciprofloxacin, ofloxacin, and sparfloxacin (AT4140). One of the new macrolide antibiotics (e.g., azithromycin) may also be useful in preventive therapy.

Another important area of research is behavioral research on how different people perceive the risk of tuberculosis and the benefit of preventive strategies. Additionally, operational research will be needed to evaluate new preventive strategies as they are developed.

VI. Behavioral, Economic, and Operational Studies

The limited resources available for tuberculosis control activities mandate the efficient use of these resources. Both economic studies to determine the most cost-effective preventive and therapeutic interventions and operational studies to determine optimal methods of delivering these services are needed.

Behavioral studies of patient and provider compliance are needed. To generate hypotheses to be tested in more formal studies, focus group techniques might be used to identify individual, sociocultural, and external factors possibly facilitating and impeding adherence. The factors thought most important could then be evaluated in prospective studies. As a final step, intervention studies to determine the value of specific adherence-enhancing measures should be undertaken.

Similarly, studies of providers are needed to define the determinants of compliance with recommended treatment and preventive practices.

VII. Immunology

Interest in the immune response to mycobacterial antigens has increased remarkably in the past few years. Research has advanced the understanding of the microbial targets of T-cell reactivity, yet the immunodominant antigens remain undefined; the induction of gamma–delta T cells, yet the function of these cells is uncertain; and the mechanisms of immunosuppression, yet the relevant mediators are undefined. Therefore, enthusiasm concerning progress must be tempered by the knowledge that some of the information that is most critical to the application of these advances to the design of improved methods of diagnosis and prevention of tuberculosis is incomplete or missing. Continuing research in tuberculosis, combined with advances in cellular immunology and biomedical technology, should allow researchers to address many of the unanswered questions concerning the immune response to *M. tuberculosis* and, particularly, the microbial targets of T-cell reactivity. Once these issues are clarified, the approach to the development of improved reagents for the diagnosis and prevention of tuberculosis will be on sounder footing and, therefore, more likely to succeed.

A vaccine that prevents primary or reactivation tuberculosis would be of tremendous benefit. No experimental product yet tested has offered greater protection in animals than live BCG. It is unclear whether there is a single or multiple protective antigens. An array of antigens deficient in immunosuppressive mycobacterial constituents and enriched with protective antigens might prove to be a promising vaccine. Attempts to identify these antigens and engineer vaccines that express them should be made.

Currently, there is no reliable means of assessing protective immunity in humans, other than by longitudinal observation. Animal models in which protective efficacy can be evaluated are urgently needed. In vitro assays of T-cell function should be studied for correlation with these models. More knowledge of the mechanisms of in vivo mycobacterial killing or growth inhibition is needed.

The development of better diagnostic reagents is of critical importance. Present methods of recognizing latent infection based on tuberculin skin testing and in vitro correlates of cell-mediated immunity lack both sensitivity and specificity. Because the bacillary burden is small and the infectious process is largely confined to the primary focus and regional lymph nodes, priority should be placed on finding techniques that recognize the host response rather than on those that detect the parasite. Emphasis should be placed on defining and characterizing the specific epitopes of mycobacterial antigens. Assays of T-cell responses are needed that are inexpensive, rapid, and applicable in the field.

For the detection of active disease, attempts to develop simple and specific serodiagnostic tests should be undertaken. Antigen detection systems must also be explored, especially for use in HIV-infected persons. Studies of nonimmunologic pathogen and host factors (e.g., tuberculostearic acid detection; adenosine deaminase levels) should be continued.

Basic studies of the immunology of tuberculosis should be performed to determine the relative importance of defined T-cell populations (CD4, CD8, gamma–delta) in acquired immunity to tuberculosis and to better define T cells that mediate memory and immunity.

Systematic approaches should be undertaken to define key protective antigens in tuberculosis. Studies should be performed to evaluate the capacity of mycobacterial antigens to elicit antimycobacterial activity by human lymphocytes and macrophages in vitro, to evaluate mycobacterial antigens that stimulate protective immunity in animal models, and to assess the response to antigens in patients with differing manifestations of disease.

Investigations into the mechanisms and pathways of antigen processing and presentation are important; the roles of various cytokines in tuberculosis also deserve further investigation.

It is widely accepted that the monocyte–macrophage is the central host cell that influences the ultimate outcome of infection. The functions of the monocyte–macrophage in tuberculosis appear paradoxical. This cell is apparently responsible for providing a protective niche for the replicative microbe under some circumstances, while exerting bacteriostatic (perhaps bactericidal) effects given appropriate activation signals. To control tuberculosis, we must better understand the nature of the macrophage-pathogen interaction.

High priority should be given to research that addresses the following questions:

1. What are the molecules mediating complement fixation and uptake of mycobacteria? What is the intracellular compartment in which the mycobacteria are contained and what are the physiochemical features of this environment (e.g., pH, O_2 tension, enzyme content)?

2. How does the intracellular environment of the monocyte–macrophage alter the physiology of the mycobacteria? What is the relation between these alterations in bacterial physiology and virulence? Are mycobacteria growing intracellularly different from organisms grown on artificial media?

3. What is the influence of the maturational state of the monocyte–macrophage on its ability to support the growth of, or kill, mycobacteria? How does infection alter the physiology of host cells at different stages of development in terms of cellular metabolism, receptor expression, response to cytokines, or other?

4. What is the process by which macrophages become activated (e.g., external signals, gene activation, alterations in intracellular environment)? Which other cells (e.g. T lymphocytes) are involved, which cytokines are required, and how is their production triggered? Which of the many metabolic changes that accompany macrophage activation are actually responsible for bacteriostasis or killing?

5.   What is the role of the monocyte–macrophage in persistence or dormancy of mycobacteria in chronically infected hosts?

6.   What is the contribution of extracellular immunologic factors to the survival or destruction of mycobacteria? Where and how does this extracellular host–parasite interaction occur?

7.   How do antimycobacterial drugs penetrate infected macrophages, what regulates their intracellular compartmentalization, and how does the physiological state of the macrophage affect drug efficacy on mycobacteria growing (or dormant) intracellularly?

VIII. Molecular Biology

Recent developments in the field of molecular biology offer tremendous promise in providing novel tools for controlling tuberculosis. Tremendous progress has been made toward the development of both the methods and vectors that permit efficient transfer of recombinant DNA from mycobacteria to *E. coli* (Bloom, 1989). Recent developments in mycobacterial genetics have provided new opportunities to genetically manipulate this pathogen and to address, from a new perspective, old problems. Research should be directed at determining genomic sequence, developing methods for genetic manipulation, studying mechanisms of gene expression, and understanding the genetic basis of drug action and resistance. The end result of this research will be a fuller understanding of the mechanisms of pathogenesis of tuberculosis, the mechanisms of drug resistance, the construction of effective vaccines, and the development of improved diagnostic methods.

With the introduction of DNA fingerprinting, usually restriction fragment length polymorphism (RFLP) analysis, a very specific system for distinguishing strains is available. DNA fingerprinting offers great promise for the precise identification of sources of infection and for the identification of common source outbreaks. There is, however, a need for additional techniques for subdividing strains of *M. tuberculosis*. These techniques need to be rapid and simple to allow the screening of many strains. Possible techniques include nucleic acid fingerprinting, using probes for repetitive insertion elements or ribosomal RNA genes; mycolic acid pattern analysis; two-dimensional electrophoresis maps of proteins; nuclear magnetic resonance (NMR) profiles; and multilocus enzyme electrophoresis.

Molecular biology can help define the targets for existing antituberculosis drugs (isoniazid, ethambutol, rifampin, pyrazinamide, and others), analyze the mode of action of these drugs, and determine the mechanisms of drug resistance. The basic approaches involve molecular cloning of the specific genes that encode targets of drug action, DNA sequencing, and comparison of sequences from susceptible and resistant strains.

The complex cell wall of *M. tuberculosis* plays a role in permeability of drugs. Genetic approaches, using various mutants, may define the role of structures such as arabinogalactan, lipoarabinomannan (LAM), or mycolic acids in permeability. Genetic analysis may also elucidate specific transport systems of *M. tuberculosis*, such as those that are used to transport nutrients into tubercle bacilli in macrophages. This may allow the synthesis of antimicrobial agents linked to carriers that are specifically transported into the bacilli. Molecular biology may also be applied to rapid drug susceptibility testing as discussed earlier.

With the development of mycobacterial genetics and the new capabilities to genetically manipulate mycobacteria, a variety of fresh approaches can be applied to the development of a vaccine. However, the potential of these powerful methods will be realized only if a substantial effort is placed on additional basic genetic studies, including the identification of protective and suppressive antigens.

Several approaches to vaccine development need study. These include further development of the existing BCG vaccine strains, construction of genetically defined vaccine strains, and evaluation of nonmycobacterial vaccine delivery systems. It may also be possible to improve the effective processing of BCG by macrophages and, thereby, increase its immunogenicity.

References

American Thoracic Society, Centers for Disease Control, National Institutes of Health, Pittsfield Antituberculosis Association. (1986). *Am. Rev. Respir. Dis.* **134**:401–402.

American Thoracic Society Committee on Priorities for Tuberculosis Research (1988). Future research in tuberculosis: Research initiatives in the immunology of tuberculosis. *Am. Rev. Respir. Dis.* **138**:1327–1329.

Bloom, B.R. (1989). An ordinary mortal's guide to the molecular biology of mycobacteria. *Bull. Int. Union Tuberc. Lung Dis.* **64**:50–58.

Brisson-Noel, A., Lecossier, D., Nassif, X., Gicquel, B., Levy-Freba-ult, V., and Hance, A.J. (1989). Rapid diagnosis of tuberculosis by amplification of mycobacterial DNA in clinical samples. *Lancet* **2**:1069–1071.

Centers for Disease Control (1989). A strategic plan for the elimination of tuberculosis in the United States *MMWR* **38** (S-3):1–25.

Centers for Disease Control (1990). Guidelines for preventing the transmission of tuberculosis in health-care settings, with special focus on HIV-related issues. *MMWR* **39** (RR-7):1–29.

Centers for Disease Control—National Institute for Allergy and Infectious Disease—Pittsfield Antituberculosis Association (1986). Future research in tuberculosis. *Am. Rev. Respir. Dis.* **134**D:401–423.

Gangadharam, P.R.J., Ashtekar, D.R., Farhi, D.C., and Wise D.L., (1991). Sustained release of isoniazid in vivo from a single implant of a biodegradable polymer. *Tubercle* **72**:115–122.

Glassroth, J., Bailey, W.C., Hopewell, P.C., Schecter, G., and Harden, J.W. (1990). What tuberculosis is not prevented. *Am. Rev. Respir. Dis.* **141**:1236–1240.

Hermans, P.W.M., VanSoolingen, D., Dale, J.W., et al. (1990). Insertion element IS986 from *Mycobacterium tuberculosis*: A useful tool for diagnosis and epidemiology of tuberculosis. *J. Clin. Microbiol.* **28**:2051–2058.

Holm, J. (1984). Tuberculosis control in the developing world: It's time for a change. *World Health Forum* **5**:103–107.

Koch, R. (1932). Die Aethiologie der Tuberculose, a translation by Berna Pinner and Max Pinner with an introduction by Allen K. Krause. *Am. Rev. Tuberc.* **25**:285–323.

Mason, J.O. (1986). Opportunities for the elimination of tuberculosis. *Am. Rev. Respir. Dis.* **134**:201–203.

Pao, C.C., Yen, T.S.B., You, J.B., Maa, J.S., Fiss, E.H., and Chang, C.H. (1990). Detection and identification of *Mycobacterium tuberculosis* by DNA amplification. *J. Clin. Microbial.* **28**:1877–1880.

Rieder, H.L., Cauthen, G.M., Comstock, G.W., and Snider, D.E. (1989). Epidemiology of tuberculosis in the United States. *Epidemiol. Rev.* **11**:79–98.

Rogers, E.M. (1983). *Diffusions of Innovations*, 3rd ed. Free Press, New York.

Slutkin, G., Leoski, J., and Mann, J. (1988). Tuberculosis and AIDS. The effects of the AIDS epidemic on the tuberculosis problem and tuberculosis programmes. *Bull. Int. Union Tuberc. Lung Dis.* **63**:21–24.

Walsh, J.A., and Warren, K.S. (1979). Selective primary health care: An interim strategy for disease control in developing countries. *N. Engl. J. Med.* **301**:967–979.

World Health Organization Expert Committee on Tuberculosis (1964). Eighth report. WHO Technical Report, Ser. 290.

World Health Organization –International Union Against Tuberculosis and Lung Disease (1989). Tuberculosis and AIDS. *Bull. Int. Union Tuberc. Lung Dis.* **64**:8–11.

INDEX

Z